Lymphoid Organs: Advances in Immunology

Lymphoid Organs: Advances in Immunology

Editor: Quinn Houghton

FOSTER ACADEMICS
www.fosteracademics.com

www.fosteracademics.com

FOSTER ACADEMICS

Cataloging-in-Publication Data

Lymphoid organs : advances in immunology / edited by Quinn Houghton.
p. cm.
Includes bibliographical references and index.
ISBN 978-1-64646-604-7
1. Lymphatics. 2. Lymphatics--Immunology. 3. Lymphoid tissue. 4. Immune system. 5. Immunology.
I. Houghton, Quinn.
QP115 .L96 2023
612.42--dc23

Foster Academics,
118-35 Queens Blvd., Suite 400,
Forest Hills, NY 11375, USA

ISBN 978-1-64646-604-7 (Hardback)

Contents

Preface

The world is advancing at a fast pace like never before. Therefore, the need is to keep up with the latest developments. This book was an idea that came to fruition when the specialists in the area realized the need to coordinate together and document essential themes in the subject. That's when I was requested to be the editor. Editing this book has been an honour as it brings together diverse authors researching on different streams of the field. The book collates essential materials contributed by veterans in the area which can be utilized by students and researchers alike.

Lymphoid organs are comprised of lymphoid tissue and are the site of lymphocyte activation and lymphocyte production. The structure of lymphoid organs includes primary lymphoid organs, secondary lymphoid organs and tertiary lymphoid organs. Primary lymphoid organs produce lymphocytes, the spleen and lymph nodes, through immature progenitor cells. Secondary lymphoid organs maintain mature lymphocytes, while initiating adaptive immune response. Tertiary lymphoid organs (TLOs) develop in peripheral tissues in adult organisms as a response to non-resolving inflammation. TLOs related diseases include chronic infection, allograft rejection, cancer and autoimmune diseases. They contain an active germinal center which is surrounded by a network of follicular dendritic cells (FDCs). The lymphatic system as a whole provides accessory return route for the blood. Furthermore, immune defense is another significant function of the lymphatic system. This book is a compilation of chapters that discuss the most vital advances in the field of Immunology with respect to lymphoid organs. It will provide comprehensive knowledge to the readers.

Each chapter is a sole-standing publication that reflects each author's interpretation. Thus, the book displays a multi-facetted picture of our current understanding of application, resources and aspects of the field. I would like to thank the contributors of this book and my family for their endless support.

Editor

1

Lymphoid Neogenesis and Tertiary Lymphoid Organs in Transplanted Organs

*Alice Koenig[1,2,3] and Olivier Thaunat[1,2,3]**

[1] *Service de Transplantation, Néphrologie et Immunologie Clinique, Hôpital Edouard Herriot, Hospices Civils de Lyon, Lyon, France,* [2] *INSERM UMR1111, Lyon, France,* [3] *Université de Lyon, Lyon, France*

Correspondence:
Olivier Thaunat
olivier.thaunat@chu-lyon.fr

The progressive organization of immune effectors into functional ectopic lymphoid structures, named tertiary lymphoid organs (TLO), has been observed in many conditions in which target antigens fail to be eliminated by the immune system. Not surprisingly, TLO have been recurrently identified in chronically rejected allografts. Although significant progress has been made over the last decades in understanding the molecular mechanisms involved in TLO development (a process named lymphoid neogenesis), the role of intragraft TLO (if any) in chronic rejection remains elusive. The prevailing dogma is that TLO contribute to graft rejection by generating and propagating local humoral and cellular alloimmune responses. However, TLO have been recently observed in long-term accepting allografts, suggesting that they might also be able to regulate alloimmune responses. In this review, we discuss our current understanding of how TLO are induced and propose a unified model in which TLO can play deleterious or regulatory roles and therefore actively modulate the kinetics of chronic rejection.

Keywords: transplantation, lymphoid neogenesis, tertiary lymphoid organs, chronic rejection, tolerance

INTRODUCTION: THE CHALLENGE OF CHRONIC REJECTION IN TRANSPLANTATION

Vital organ failure is a life-threatening condition where a vital organ (i.e., kidney, heart, liver, or lung…) does not perform its expected function. Recent lifestyle changes in developed countries, and the increased incidence of chronic diseases such as hypertension, obesity, and diabetes, have set the stage for accelerated risk for, and the occurrence of, vital organ failure. As a result, vital organ failure is currently recognized as the leading cause of debility and premature death worldwide (www.who.int). In France alone, the personal, societal, and economic consequences of vital organ failure have a cost of more than €70 billion a year (25% of total health expenditures).

Transplantation consists in the restoration of vital physiologic functions through the surgical substitution of a defective organ by a functioning graft retrieved from a donor. Patients with end-stage vital organ failure depend on solid organ transplantation, which is their best (often their only) therapeutic option.

In clinical transplantation, the donor is from the same species but genetically different. Consequently, the immune system of the recipient inevitably recognizes the antigenic determinants (alloantigens) that differ between the recipient and the donor, particularly the highly polymorphic molecules from the major histocompatibility complex [i.e., human leukocyte antigen (HLA)] in humans. The alloimmune response that develops against the donor-specific HLA molecules is responsible for tissue damage, which leads to the failure of the transplanted organ, a process named "rejection."

In the absence of a clinically applicable protocol able to induce the specific tolerance of the allogenic transplant by the recipient's immune system (1, 2), the prevention of rejection is currently dependent upon immunosuppressive drugs (3). These drugs produce generalized immunosuppression, which means that any reduction in immune responsiveness to the allograft is accompanied by reduced immunity to infections and malignant diseases. Chronic immune injuries that result from the incomplete blockade of the recipient's alloimmune response (i.e., chronic rejection) are currently the main factor limiting graft function duration (4). No significant progress has been made on this issue over the last decades as highlighted by the stagnation of graft half-life (5). A better understanding of the pathophysiology of chronic rejection is therefore a mandatory step in identifying innovative approaches that would prolong graft function duration.

INTRAGRAFT TERTIARY LYMPHOID ORGANS (TLO)

Rejected grafts are characterized by interstitial infiltration of cellular effectors, mainly T cells and macrophages, but also dendritic cells, NK cells, B cells, and plasma cells.

In contrast with acute rejection, where infiltrates exhibit no particular spatial organization, during chronic rejection immune cells tend to organize themselves in structures that morphologically resemble the secondary lymphoid organs.

Analyzing all sorts of human kidney grafts removed for terminal chronic rejection, we and others showed that in the majority of chronically rejected grafts the immune cells were grouped, conferring a nodular organization to the infiltrate (6, 7). These nodules exhibited a highly organized microarchitecture with clear cell subset segregation: the core, made of the B cells intermingled with a network of follicular dendritic cells, was surrounded by T cells and mature dendritic cells. CD138-expressing plasma cells were found within or in close vicinity to TLO, suggesting that part of these cells differentiated locally. As in canonical secondary lymphoid organs the compartmentalization of the different cell subsets appeared to be mediated by gradients of homeostatic chemokines CCL21 (in the T cell area) and CXCL13 (in the B cell area). Furthermore, neolymphatic vessels and PNAd-expressing high endothelial venules (HEVs) were observed in the periphery of the nodules (8).

The structural organization of immune effectors observed in chronically rejected renal grafts (**Figure 1**) does not seem specific of this type of transplant since similar lymphoid structures have been observed in chronically rejected pancreas, livers, hearts (7, 9–11), lungs (12), and even composite transplants (13–15). This phenomenon is not specific of the alloimmune setting either, since the very same lymphoid structures have previously been observed in various inflammatory conditions, including chronic infections, autoimmune diseases, and cancers (16, 17). Structural organization of immune effectors therefore appears as a generic response of the chronically stimulated immune system that cannot eradicate targeted antigens.

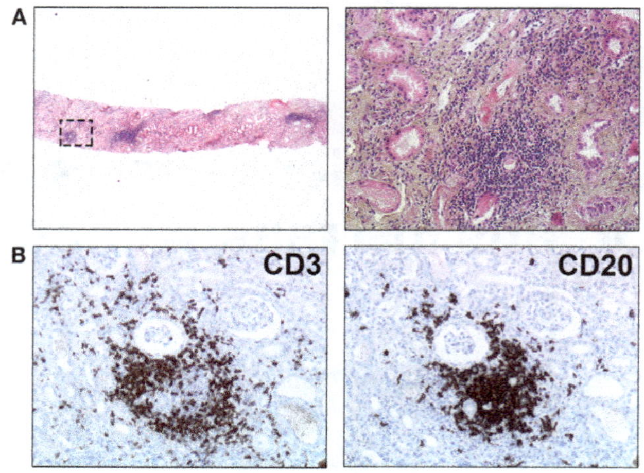

FIGURE 1 | Tertiary lymphoid organs in a chronically rejected renal transplant. Biopsy of a renal transplant was performed for progressive deterioration of graft function, suggestive of chronic rejection. **(A)** HES staining revealed nodular infiltrates of mononuclear cells within graft parenchyma (original magnification: left panel, ×20; right panel, ×200). **(B)** Immunostainings unraveled the organized distribution of T cells (CD3+, left panel) and B cells (CD20, right panel). Original magnification: ×200.

Because the microarchitecture of organized immune infiltrates is highly reminiscent of that of secondary lymphoid organs, these lymphoid structures have been named TLO.

MOLECULAR MECHANISMS INVOLVED IN THE DEVELOPMENT OF SECONDARY LYMPHOID ORGANS

Primary immune responses are initiated in secondary lymphoid organs, which are located at strategic sites where antigens are most likely to be encountered.

The development of secondary lymphoid organs, a process named lymphoid organogenesis, is initiated during embryogenesis independently of antigen recognition at predetermined sites as a result of complex interactions between hematopoietic, mesenchymal, and endothelial cells (18, 19). Lymphoid organogenesis can be schematically divided into two consecutive steps: first the induction, then the organization phase.

The induction phase depends on lymphoid-tissue inducer cells, which arise in the fetal liver. Under the influence of TRANCE (at sites of peripheral lymph node development) or IL-7 (at mucosal sites) lymphoid-tissue inducer cells express membrane-bound lymphotoxin: a heterotrimer containing lymphotoxin α and lymphotoxin β that allow lymphoid-tissue inducer cells to interact with the lymphotoxin β receptor (LTβR) of stromal cells. Signaling through the LTβR initiates NFκB signaling in stromal cells, which promotes the production of homeostatic chemokines (18, 19).

Homeostatic chemokines are crucial for the organization phase. CXCL13 recruits circulating B cells to what becomes the B cell area of lymphoid tissues, and the T zone chemokines (CCL19 and CCL21) attract T and dendritic cells to shape the T cell area

(18, 19). The lymphotoxin signaling pathway is also crucial in promoting the differentiation of HEVs, which are postcapillary venules expressing specific adhesion molecules (known as addressins) that have a crucial role in lymphocyte trafficking to secondary lymphoid organs (18, 19).

MOLECULAR MECHANISMS OF LYMPHOID NEOGENESIS IN TRANSPLANTATION

Chronic rejection provides optimal conditions for studying the molecular mechanisms involved in the development of TLO (**Figure 2**). Indeed, (i) TLO have systematically been detected in chronically rejected grafts; (ii) the antigens targeted by the immune system are known (recipient-mismatched HLA antigens of the transplanted tissues); and (iii) chronically rejected grafts are sometimes removed, providing a large amount of diseased tissue, which can be comprehensively analyzed.

In-depth analysis of a series of detransplanted human renal grafts revealed the heterogenous nature of the cellular composition of TLO (8). Two types of B cell nodules could be identified: nodules composed of a uniform CD20^{pos} B cell population expressing IgD and Bcl-2 were similar to primary follicles, while nodules with a core of CD20^{pos}IgD^{neg}Bcl-2^{neg} B cells, highly expressing Bcl-6 that had pushed aside the CD20^{pos}IgD^{pos}Bcl-2^{pos} B cells, resembled secondary follicles, i.e., germinal centers (8). The ratio between these two types of structures differed between samples, and the number of ectopic germinal centers did not increase with the quantity of primary nodules. The phenotypic heterogeneity of TLO correlated more with the expression profile of a set of genes (*CCL19, CCL21, CXCL12, CXCL13*, CCR7, *CXCR4*, and *CXCR5*)

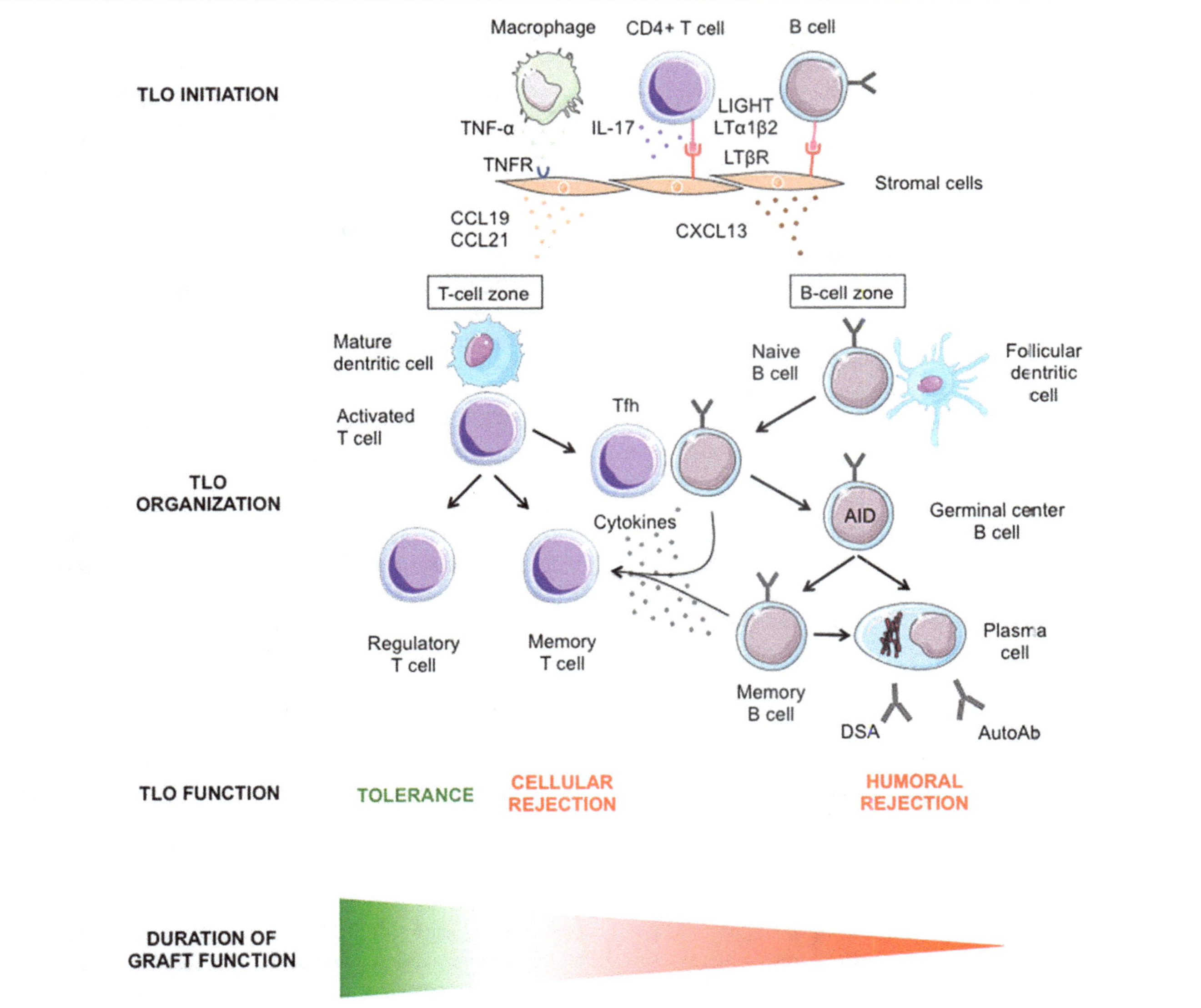

FIGURE 2 | Graphical summary of our current understanding of intragraft lymphoid neogenesis. The main molecular mechanisms involved in the initiation (upper row) and the subsequent organization (middle row) of tertiary lymphoid organs (TLO) within transplanted organs are showed. The diverse functions of intragraft TLO and their respective impact on graft survival are presented (lower row).

involved in the formation and the maintenance of canonical secondary lymphoid organs (i.e., the lymphoid organogenesis described in the previous section) (18, 19). The complete recapitulation of this genetic program in chronically rejected grafts resulted in the generation of fully functional ectopic germinal centers that allowed for the efficient maturation of B cells into memory B cells and plasma cells (**Figure 2**). In contrast, when this recapitulation was incomplete, local B cell maturation was impeded (8). These results highlighted the similarity between the molecular processes involved in the development of canonical secondary lymphoid organs and those involved in the organization of immune effectors during chronic inflammation, a process named lymphoid neogenesis.

If the molecular mechanisms responsible for the organization and maintenance of secondary lymphoid organs and TLO appear similar, the initiation of the cascade is likely to be different (**Figure 2**). The formation of secondary lymphoid organs in the embryo is developmentally programed and results from the interaction between lymphotoxin-$\alpha_1\beta_2$-expressing lymphoid-tissue inducer cells and lymphotoxin-β receptor-expressing stromal organizer cells (18, 19). In contrast, TLO development seems independent of lymphoid-tissue inducer cells (20, 21). Yet, several studies have documented the importance of the lymphotoxin pathway in lymphoid neogenesis (21, 22), including in a transplantation setting (23), by demonstrating that the development of TLO was abolished by treatment with inhibitory LTβR–Ig fusion protein. We must then ask who provides lymphotoxin signaling in the chronic rejection setting. Beyond lymphoid-tissue inducer cells, lymphotoxin-α and lymphotoxin-β are also expressed by activated lymphocytes (24). It is therefore conceivable that activated T and/or B cells replace lymphoid-tissue inducer cells to initiate lymphoid neogenesis in rejected grafts (**Figure 2**) as already demonstrated for the induction of TLO in the gut (21). Another possibility is that lymphotoxin is dispensable for the formation of TLO. Lymphotoxin-α and lymphotoxin-β are two related members of the large TNF ligand family (25). Since homologous genes and gene products often have redundant physiological functions, it seems reasonable to propose that other ligands and/or receptors of the TNF superfamily could act as alternative pathways for TLO induction (**Figure 2**). In line with this hypothesis, the provision of the alternative LTβR ligand LIGHT (aka tumor necrosis factor superfamily member 14) by activated T cells infiltrating inflamed pancreas have been shown to be crucial for the formation of TLO (26). Furthermore, TNF-α, which is produced within rejected grafts (27), has been shown to be critical for the development of TLO in a murine model of atherosclerosis (20). TNF-α does not bind to LTβR but to distinct TNF receptors (25). Using apolipoprotein E-deficient mice, which spontaneously develop atherosclerotic lesions in their aorta, the Antonino Nicoletti's group recently demonstrated that the blockade of LTβR signaling had no effect, whereas that of TNFR1/2 signaling reduced the expression of homeostatic chemokines and the subsequent development of TLO (20). Finally, it has recently been reported that IL-17 produced by CD4+ T cells (i.e., Th17 cells) was essential for the formation of both (i) TLO in the central nervous system of mice during experimental autoimmune encephalomyelitis (the animal model of multiple sclerosis) (28) and (ii) the development of inducible bronchus-associated lymphoid tissue, an ectopic lymphoid tissue that forms in the lungs after pulmonary inflammation (29, 30). In the latter setting, IL-17 acted by triggering the expression of homeostatic chemokines independently of lymphotoxin signaling (**Figure 2**). If this hypothesis was proven true in transplantation, initiation of lymphoid neogenesis in chronically rejected grafts could therefore be totally independent of both lymphoid-tissue inducer cells and the lymphotoxin/TNF pathway. Interestingly, we have recently reported that a Th17 polarization of CD4+ T cells infiltrating the graft was associated with increased TLO development during clinical chronic rejection (31).

It is conceivable that instead of conflicting with each other, these different works reveal the fact that several pathways can promote the initiation of TLO depending on the initiating events. This hypothesis was recently substantiated by the demonstration that the development of bronchus-associated lymphoid tissue was triggered by different pathways according to the pathogen responsible for lung inflammation (29).

While significant progress has been made in the identification of the molecular mechanisms that participate to the development of TLO, the endogenous signals capable of inhibiting the lymphoid neogenesis are far more elusive. Through evaluation of synovial tissues from rheumatoid arthritis patients it has been recently reported that low interleukin-27 (IL-27) expression corresponds with an increased incidence of TLO and gene signatures associated with their development and activity. The presence of synovial TLO was also noted in mice deficient in the IL-27 receptor after the onset of inflammatory arthritis (32). IL-27 might therefore represent a negative regulator of TLO development. Whether this is also true for chronic rejection remains to be demonstrated.

DO INTRAGRAFT TLO PROMOTE CHRONIC REJECTION?

Tertiary lymphoid organs differ from canonical secondary lymphoid organs inasmuch as they develop in an inflammatory milieu (31, 33), enriched in neoantigens released from injured tissue and trapped by defective lymphatic drainage (34). Comparing the cellular composition of TLO of chronically rejected grafts with one of the secondary lymphoid organs, we observed a drastic increase in the percentage of activated and memory CD4+ T cell in intragraft TLO and a symmetric decrease in T regulatory subsets (IL-10-producing Tr1 cells and Foxp3^{pos} Tregs) in both a murine experimental model and human samples (33, 35).

These peculiarities suggest that the local immune response that develops in intragraft TLO might be less tightly regulated than in secondary lymphoid organs and are therefore more aggressive. In line with this hypothesis, we (33) and others (23) have shown that intragraft TLO are a major site where B cell tolerance breakdown occurs during chronic rejection (**Figure 2**). Interestingly, the generation of autoantibodies following solid organ transplantation has long been reported to correlate with chronic rejection, and the deleterious impact of some autoantibodies on graft survival has been demonstrated (36, 37). Furthermore, comparing the alloimmune responses elicited in intragraft TLO, spleen, and draining lymph nodes in a rat model of chronic rejection, our group observed increased production of anti-HLA antibodies in TLO as compared with canonical secondary lymphoid organs (35). Not only were the humoral alloimmune responses elicited in TLO quantitatively enhanced but they also displayed a more diverse repertoire, a finding that we confirmed in the clinical setting by the analysis of chronically rejected human kidney allografts (8).

Tertiary lymphoid organs could also contribute to chronic destruction of the graft through antibody-independent functions of B cells. B cells are indeed unique antigen-presenting cells because (i) they have an antigen-specific receptor (B cell receptor), which when engaged by surface-tethered antigens leads to the formation of an immunological synapse that coordinates cell signaling events and promotes antigen uptake for presentation on MHC class II molecules (38), even when the antigen is membrane-tethered or is present in limiting quantities and (ii) B cells have the capacity to clonally expand, thereby becoming the numerically dominant antigen-presenting cells. Interestingly, it has been reported that the presence of B cell clusters within the graft during rejection was associated with reduced graft survival and resistance to steroid therapy, independently of C4d (a breakdown product generated during classical complement pathway activation) deposition or alloantibody detection (39). Some authors have proposed that this could be due to the local presentation of antigen to effector T cells by intragraft B cells (40). This hypothesis is supported by experimental data from the group of Fadi Lakkis, who showed that in a murine skin graft model, TLO perpetuate the rejection process by supporting naïve T cell activation within the graft (41). Strikingly, the same authors also demonstrated that TLO generate T cell memory immune responses (41).

In addition to presenting antigen, B cells can also enhance T cell-mediated immune responses through the secretion of cytokines and chemokines. Studies from the group of Frances Lund (42) have shown that B cells can be functionally subdivided based on their cytokine profile. B cells activated in the presence of TH1-type cytokines (referred to as Be-1 cells) secrete IFNγ and IL-12 but not IL-4, IL-13, or IL-2. By contrast, B cells activated in the presence of TH2-type cytokines (Be-2 cells) secrete IL-2, lymphotoxin, IL-4, and IL-13 but make minimal amounts of IFNγ and IL-12. Both Be-1 and Be-2 cells seem able to produce IL-10, TNFα, and IL-6. The importance of B cell cytokines in promoting T cell responses has been illustrated in several models. For example, *in vitro* generated effector B cells that produced either TH1- or TH2-type cytokines were shown to promote the activation and differentiation of naïve T cells into effector TH1 and TH2 cells, respectively (43). The importance of B cell cytokines in promoting T cell responses has been confirmed *in vivo*. In a murine model of *Toxoplasma gondii* infection, TNF production by B cells was shown to be required for the generation of an optimal TH1 cell protective response (44). In another set of experiments, the generation of a protective TH2 memory response to *H. polygyrus* was shown to depend on IL-2-producing B cells (45). The exact role of cytokine-producing B cells in enhancing intra-TLO T cell responses remains to be evaluated.

Since grafts in which TLO were harboring germinal center reactions had a shorter life expectancy (**Figure 2**), we have proposed that lymphoid neogenesis could play a detrimental role during chronic rejection (8). However, the validity of this conclusion is limited by the fact that only explanted grafts have been analyzed, i.e., organs displaying extreme rejection damage that are sometimes (notably in the case of renal grafts) removed after immunosuppressive therapy withdrawal. The definitive demonstration that TLO are involved in the pathophysiology of chronic rejection would require selectively impairing the development of intragraft TLO while leaving the rest of the recipient's immune system unaffected. Addressing this issue is not trivial because, as discussed above, TLO share many biological pathways with canonical lymphoid tissue, and hence an adequate experimental model is not currently available. Therefore, most of the attempts to validate the data obtained in murine experimental models and in human detransplanted grafts have relied on graft biopsies. The identification of TLO within the grafts before the development of the lesions indeed appears as a prerequisite for confirming the role of lymphoid neogenesis in chronic rejection. This implies a study of protocol biopsies, which has long been introduced as standard follow up in transplantation (46). Unfortunately, the numerous studies aiming at evaluating the correlation between the presence of TLO in protocol biopsies and the later development of chronic rejection have reached conflicting conclusions (**Table 1**).

The absence of an unequivocal deleterious role for B cell clusters has led to the conclusion that these structures could be like "fish in a sunken ship," i.e., although fish are frequently seen in a sunken boat, they play no role in the process responsible for the shipwreck.

INTRAGRAFT TLO: FRIENDS AND FOES?

An alternative explanation could reconcile these apparently conflicting results. As discussed above, the proportion of B cells that infiltrate chronically rejected kidney grafts does not correlate with the functionality of intragraft TLO (8). The attraction of B cells within inflamed tissue appears therefore to be a generic phenomenon with no intrinsic deleterious consequences on the graft. However, when intragraft B cells meet the appropriate microenvironment, and upon the complete recapitulation of the lymphoid organogenesis program, B cell nodules organize themselves into functional ectopic germinal centers, which harbor the development of a local aggressive immune response. Because graft biopsies provide only a very limited amount of tissue (which is already an important limitation for evaluation in a patchy process such as lymphoid neogenesis), they do not allow for functional analysis of the ectopic lymphoid organs and are therefore inappropriate for analyzing the role of B cell clusters in rejected grafts.

Another layer of complexity has recently been brought into the picture by experimental evidence that certain B cell subsets are endowed with an immune regulatory role (47). For instance, IL-10-producing B cells have been shown to efficiently prevent the induction of autoimmune disease in several mouse models (48–50). Tolerance in transplantation is defined as the maintenance of graft function in the absence of therapeutic immunosuppression for at least 12 months. About 100 tolerant patients have been identified among renal transplant recipients over the last decade (51). These patients, defined as "operationally tolerant,"

TABLE 1 | Summary of biopsy-based studies evaluating the role of graft-infiltrating B cells.

Reference	Population	Biopsy indication	Histologic criteria	Key findings
KIDNEY RECIPIENTS				
Sarwal et al. (39)	51 patients	Biopsy with acute graft rejection	CD20+ cell count >275/HPF	B cell clusters associated with glucocorticoid resistance and graft loss
Hippen et al. (58)	27 patients	Biopsy with Banff 1A or 1B acute rejection	CD20+ if "strong and diffuse staining"	CD20+ correlated with steroid-resistance rejection and reduced graft survival
Kayler et al. (59)	120 patients	Biopsy with first episode of acute cellular rejection	Cluster of ≥15 CD20+ cells in the tubulo-interstitial compartment	CD20+ clusters are not prognostic factors for glucocorticoid resistance and graft loss
Bagnasco et al. (60)	58 patients (74 biopsies)	Biopsy with type 1 and type 2 acute cellular rejection during the first year post-Tx	B cell-rich when ≥1 cluster containing 100 CD20+ cells/HPF	No correlation between B cell-rich biopsies and worst graft outcome
Scheepstra et al. (61)	50 patients (54 biopsies)	Biopsy with clinically suspect and histologically confirmed acute rejection	B cell (CD20+) count >275/HPF CD20+ cluster if >30 cells CD20+ without the interposition of tubules	Presence of B cells does not correlate with response to conventional therapy or graft outcome
Hwang et al. (62)	54 patients (67 biopsies)	Biopsy with acute cellular rejection	CD20+ count >275/HPF CD38+ if >30% infiltration	CD38+ B cells ± CD20+ B cells correlated with poor clinical outcomes
Martin et al. (63)	18 patients	Serial biopsies for 10 recipients with chronic dysfunction and 8 with long-term normal graft function	Plasma cells count Cd4 deposits DSA elution from biopsy	Patients developing chronic rejection present plasma cells, DSA, and C4d depositions more often than control group on their biopsy
Abbas et al. (64)	50 patients	Biopsy for cause	Plasma cell-rich acute rejection if >10% plasma cells	Plasma cell-rich acute rejection correlated with a poor graft outcome when associated with DSA
HEART RECIPIENTS				
Yamani et al. (65)	140 patients	Systematic biopsy	Nodular endocardial infiltrates (quilty lesions)	Quilty lesions are associated with increased development of coronary vasculopathy at 1 year
Chu et al. (66)	285 patients	Systematic biopsy	Quilty lesions	Patients with quilty lesions and no anti-HLA class II DSA are more likely to develop graft arteriosclerosis at 5 years
Hiemann et al. (67)	873 patients (9,713 biopsies)	Systematic biopsy	Quilty lesions	Quilty lesions are associated with an increased risk for stenotic microvasculopathy and a poor graft outcome
Zakliczynski et al. (68)	344 patients	Systematic biopsy	Quilty lesions	Positive correlation between quilty lesions and an increased risk of acute rejection but not with the occurrence of coronary artery vasculopathy
Frank et al. (69)	79 patients (37 with DSA)	Biopsy with or without graft dysfunction	Ratios of T:B cells and CD4:CD8 T cells	Patients with DSA have lower CD4:CD8 T cell ratio than controls T:B cell ratio was similar in patients with and without DSA
COMPOSITE TISSUE RECIPIENTS				
Hautz et al. (14)	6 human hand recipients (187 biopsies)	Systematic and for cause biopsies	CD3, CD4, CD8, CD20 PNAd stainings	PNAd expression in graft vessels correlated with rejection and T- and B-cell infiltration

DSA, donor-specific antibodies; HLA, human leukocyte antigen; HPF, high power field; PNAd, peripheral lymph node addressin; Tx, transplantation.

are healthy, do not exhibit more infections or malignancies than healthy volunteers, and do not display clinical evidence of immune incompetence (51). When compared with transplanted patients with stable graft function under pharmacologic immunosuppression, operationally tolerant patients exhibited an increase in both absolute number and frequency of total B cells (52). Furthermore, two independent microarray analyses of PBMC revealed a higher expression of B cell-related genes and their associated molecular pathways in tolerant recipients (53, 54). It is therefore conceivable that in certain conditions intragraft B cell infiltrate, instead of being neutral or deleterious, could actually promote graft survival (**Figure 2**). This theory has been nicely illustrated by murine experimental studies that recently reported the formation of TLO within tolerated allografts (55–57). If such a local protective response can prevent terminal failure of grafts, then not only would such samples having "tolerogenic" TLO be absent from the studies based on the analysis of detransplanted grafts but it could also explain the difficulty of biopsy-based studies to reach an unequivocal conclusion.

CONCLUSION

Transplanted organ expresses donor-specific alloantigens, which stimulate a recipient's immune system. Prevention of acute rejection of the graft is achieved using a combination of non-specific immunosuppressive drugs that can only partially block the alloimmune effectors. The residual enduring alloimmune response promotes immune injuries known as chronic rejection, the main cause of late allograft loss. As in other chronic immune diseases, immune effectors within chronically rejected allografts progressively organize into functional TLO that display the same micro-architecture as secondary lymphoid organs, a process known as lymphoid neogenesis. Because biopsy-based studies have reached conflicting conclusions regarding the pathological significance of these TLO, it has been proposed that the presence of TLO in rejected grafts is a non-specific response to local inflammation-induced production of chemokines. While that can indeed sometimes be the case, it should not be excluded that under appropriate conditions, lymphoid neogenesis turns non-functional TLO into ectopic germinal centers, in which a local aggressive humoral immune response can be elicited. Alternatively, functional TLO can also regulate immune responses and slow down the destruction process.

Therefore, we propose that TLO be considered as active players, able to modulate the kinetics of the natural history of chronic rejection. Future works will determine if the versatility of TLO can be manipulated to design innovative therapeutic interventions that would improve graft life expectancy.

AUTHOR CONTRIBUTIONS

All the authors listed have made substantial, direct, and intellectual contribution to the work and approved it for publication.

ACKNOWLEDGMENTS

The authors wish to thank the Drs. Maud Rabeyrin and Brigitte McGregor, from the Pathology Department of Edouard Herriot Hospital (Lyon University Hospital), for their help in collecting the pathological samples. The authors wish to thank Mathilde Koenig and Servier Medical Art (creativecommons.org/licenses/by/3.0/fr/) for their contribution to the design of the figure.

FUNDING

OT is supported by the Agence Nationale pour la Recherche (ANR-12-PDOC-0019), the Agence de la Biomédecine (AOR-2013), the Société Françophone de Transplantation, and the Etablissement Français du Sang.

REFERENCES

1. Leventhal J, Abecassis M, Miller J, Gallon L, Ravindra K, Tollerud DJ, et al. Chimerism and tolerance without GVHD or engraftment syndrome in HLA-mismatched combined kidney and hematopoietic stem cell transplantation. *Sci Transl Med* (2012) 4:124ra28. doi:10.1126/scitranslmed.3003509
2. Cetrulo CL, Drijkoningen T, Sachs DH. Tolerance induction via mixed chimerism in vascularized composite allotransplantation: is it time for clinical application? *Curr Opin Organ Transplant* (2015) 20:602–7. doi:10.1097/MOT.0000000000000248
3. Halloran PF. Immunosuppressive drugs for kidney transplantation. *N Engl J Med* (2004) 351:2715–29. doi:10.1056/NEJMra033540
4. Sellarés J, de Freitas DG, Mengel M, Reeve J, Einecke G, Sis B, et al. Understanding the causes of kidney transplant failure: the dominant role of antibody-mediated rejection and nonadherence. *Am J Transplant* (2012) 12:388–99. doi:10.1111/j.1600-6143.2011.03840.x
5. Lodhi SA, Lamb KE, Meier-Kriesche HU. Solid organ allograft survival improvement in the United States: the long-term does not mirror the dramatic short-term success. *Am J Transplant* (2011) 11:1226–35. doi:10.1111/j.1600-6143.2011.03539.x
6. Kerjaschki D, Regele HM, Moosberger I, Nagy-Bojarski K, Watschinger B, Soleiman A, et al. Lymphatic neoangiogenesis in human kidney transplants is associated with immunologically active lymphocytic infiltrates. *J Am Soc Nephrol* (2004) 15:603–12. doi:10.1097/01.ASN.0000113316.52371.2E
7. Thaunat O, Field A-C, Dai J, Louedec L, Patey N, Bloch M-F, et al. Lymphoid neogenesis in chronic rejection: evidence for a local humoral alloimmune response. *Proc Natl Acad Sci U S A* (2005) 102:14723–8. doi:10.1073/pnas.0507223102
8. Thaunat O, Patey N, Caligiuri G, Gautreau C, Mamani-Matsuda M, Mekki Y, et al. Chronic rejection triggers the development of an aggressive intragraft immune response through recapitulation of lymphoid organogenesis. *J Immunol* (2010) 185:717–28. doi:10.4049/jimmunol.0903589
9. Thaunat O, Patey N, Morelon E, Michel J-B, Nicoletti A. Lymphoid neogenesis in chronic rejection: the murderer is in the house. *Curr Opin Immunol* (2006) 18:576–9. doi:10.1016/j.coi.2006.07.006
10. Thaunat O, Nicoletti A. Lymphoid neogenesis in chronic rejection. *Curr Opin Organ Transplant* (2008) 13:16–9. doi:10.1097/MOT.0b013e3282f3df15
11. Wehner JR, Fox-Talbot K, Halushka MK, Ellis C, Zachary AA, Baldwin WM. B cells and plasma cells in coronaries of chronically rejected cardiac transplants. *Transplantation* (2010) 89:1141–8. doi:10.1097/TP.0b013e3181d3f271
12. Sato M, Hirayama S, Hwang DM, Lara-Guerra H, Wagnetz D, Waddell TK, et al. The role of intrapulmonary de novo lymphoid tissue in obliterative bronchiolitis after lung transplantation. *J Immunol* (2009) 182:7307–16. doi:10.4049/jimmunol.0803606
13. Kanitakis J, Karayannopoulou G, Lanzetta M, Petruzzo P. Graft vasculopathy in the skin of a human hand allograft: implications for diagnosis of rejection of vascularized composite allografts. *Transpl Int* (2014) 27:e118–23. doi:10.1111/tri.12399
14. Hautz T, Zelger BG, Nasr IW, Mundinger GS, Barth RN, Rodriguez ED, et al. Lymphoid neogenesis in skin of human hand, nonhuman primate, and rat vascularized composite allografts. *Transpl Int* (2014) 27:966–76. doi:10.1111/tri.12358
15. Thaunat O, Badet L, Dubois V, Kanitakis J, Petruzzo P, Morelon E. Immunopathology of rejection: do the rules of solid organ apply to vascularized composite allotransplantation? *Curr Opin Organ Transplant* (2015) 20:596–601. doi:10.1097/MOT.0000000000000242
16. Dieu-Nosjean M-C, Giraldo NA, Kaplon H, Germain C, Fridman WH, Sautès-Fridman C. Tertiary lymphoid structures, drivers of the anti-tumor responses in human cancers. *Immunol Rev* (2016) 271:260–75. doi:10.1111/imr.12405
17. Pitzalis C, Jones GW, Bombardieri M, Jones SA. Ectopic lymphoid-like structures in infection, cancer and autoimmunity. *Nat Rev Immunol* (2014) 14:447–62. doi:10.1038/nri3700

18. Randall TD, Carragher DM, Rangel-Moreno J. Development of secondary lymphoid organs. *Annu Rev Immunol* (2008) 26:627–50. doi:10.1146/annurev.immunol.26.021607.090257
19. Van de Pavert SA, Mebius RE. New insights into the development of lymphoid tissues. *Nat Rev Immunol* (2010) 10:664–74. doi:10.1038/nri2832
20. Guedj K, Khallou-Laschet J, Clement M, Morvan M, Gaston A-T, Fornasa G, et al. M1 macrophages act as LTβR-independent lymphoid tissue inducer cells during atherosclerosis-related lymphoid neogenesis. *Cardiovasc Res* (2014) 101:434–43. doi:10.1093/cvr/cvt263
21. Lochner M, Ohnmacht C, Presley L, Bruhns P, Si-Tahar M, Sawa S, et al. Microbiota-induced tertiary lymphoid tissues aggravate inflammatory disease in the absence of RORgamma t and LTi cells. *J Exp Med* (2011) 208:125–34. doi:10.1084/jem.20100052
22. Columba-Cabezas S, Griguoli M, Rosicarelli B, Magliozzi R, Ria F, Serafini B, et al. Suppression of established experimental autoimmune encephalomyelitis and formation of meningeal lymphoid follicles by lymphotoxin beta receptor-Ig fusion protein. *J Neuroimmunol* (2006) 179:76–86. doi:10.1016/j.jneuroim.2006.06.015
23. Motallebzadeh R, Rehakova S, Conlon TM, Win TS, Callaghan CJ, Goddard M, et al. Blocking lymphotoxin signaling abrogates the development of ectopic lymphoid tissue within cardiac allografts and inhibits effector antibody responses. *FASEB J* (2012) 26:51–62. doi:10.1096/fj.11-186973
24. Ware CF, Crowe PD, Grayson MH, Androlewicz MJ, Browning JL. Expression of surface lymphotoxin and tumor necrosis factor on activated T, B, and natural killer cells. *J Immunol* (1992) 149:3881–8.
25. Locksley RM, Killeen N, Lenardo MJ. The TNF and TNF receptor superfamilies: integrating mammalian biology. *Cell* (2001) 104:487–501. doi:10.1016/S0092-8674(01)00237-9
26. Lee Y, Chin RK, Christiansen P, Sun Y, Tumanov AV, Wang J, et al. Recruitment and activation of naive T cells in the islets by lymphotoxin beta receptor-dependent tertiary lymphoid structure. *Immunity* (2006) 25:499–509. doi:10.1016/j.immuni.2006.06.016
27. Krams SM, Falco DA, Villanueva JC, Rabkin J, Tomlanovich SJ, Vincenti F, et al. Cytokine and T cell receptor gene expression at the site of allograft rejection. *Transplantation* (1992) 53:151–6. doi:10.1097/00007890-199201000-00031
28. Peters A, Pitcher LA, Sullivan JM, Mitsdoerffer M, Acton SE, Franz B, et al. Th17 cells induce ectopic lymphoid follicles in central nervous system tissue inflammation. *Immunity* (2011) 35:986–96. doi:10.1016/j.immuni.2011.10.015
29. Fleige H, Ravens S, Moschovakis GL, Bölter J, Willenzon S, Sutter G, et al. IL-17-induced CXCL12 recruits B cells and induces follicle formation in BALT in the absence of differentiated FDCs. *J Exp Med* (2014) 211:643–51. doi:10.1084/jem.20131737
30. Rangel-Moreno J, Carragher DM, de la Luz Garcia-Hernandez M, Hwang JY, Kusser K, Hartson L, et al. The development of inducible bronchus-associated lymphoid tissue depends on IL-17. *Nat Immunol* (2011) 12:639–46. doi:10.1038/ni.2053
31. Deteix C, Attuil-Audenis V, Duthey A, Patey N, McGregor B, Dubois V, et al. Intragraft Th17 infiltrate promotes lymphoid neogenesis and hastens clinical chronic rejection. *J Immunol* (2010) 184:5344–51. doi:10.4049/jimmunol.0902999
32. Jones GW, Bombardieri M, Greenhill CJ, McLeod L, Nerviani A, Rocher-Ros V, et al. Interleukin-27 inhibits ectopic lymphoid-like structure development in early inflammatory arthritis. *J Exp Med* (2015) 212:1793–802. doi:10.1084/jem.20132307
33. Thaunat O, Graff-Dubois S, Fabien N, Duthey A, Attuil-Audenis V, Nicoletti A, et al. A stepwise breakdown of B-cell tolerance occurs within renal allografts during chronic rejection. *Kidney Int* (2012) 81:207–19. doi:10.1038/ki.2011.317
34. Thaunat O, Kerjaschki D, Nicoletti A. Is defective lymphatic drainage a trigger for lymphoid neogenesis? *Trends Immunol* (2006) 27:441–5. doi:10.1016/j.it.2006.08.003
35. Thaunat O, Graff-Dubois S, Brouard S, Gautreau C, Varthaman A, Fabien N, et al. Immune responses elicited in tertiary lymphoid tissues display distinctive features. *PLoS One* (2010) 5:e11398. doi:10.1371/journal.pone.0011398
36. Dragun D, Müller DN, Bräsen JH, Fritsche L, Nieminen-Kelhä M, Dechend R, et al. Angiotensin II type 1-receptor activating antibodies in renal-allograft rejection. *N Engl J Med* (2005) 352:558–69. doi:10.1056/NEJMoa035717
37. Sicard A, Chen C-C, Morelon E, Thaunat O. Alloimmune-induced intragraft lymphoid neogenesis promotes B-cell tolerance breakdown that accelerates chronic rejection. *Curr Opin Organ Transplant* (2016) 21:368–74. doi:10.1097/MOT.0000000000000329
38. Carrasco YR, Batista FD. B cell recognition of membrane-bound antigen: an exquisite way of sensing ligands. *Curr Opin Immunol* (2006) 18:286–91. doi:10.1016/j.coi.2006.03.013
39. Sarwal M, Chua M-S, Kambham N, Hsieh S-C, Satterwhite T, Masek M, et al. Molecular heterogeneity in acute renal allograft rejection identified by DNA microarray profiling. *N Engl J Med* (2003) 349:125–38. doi:10.1056/NEJMoa035588
40. Zarkhin V, Kambham N, Li L, Kwok S, Hsieh S-C, Salvatierra O, et al. Characterization of intra-graft B cells during renal allograft rejection. *Kidney Int* (2008) 74:664–73. doi:10.1038/ki.2008.249
41. Nasr IW, Reel M, Oberbarnscheidt MH, Mounzer RH, Baddoura FK, Ruddle NH, et al. Tertiary lymphoid tissues generate effector and memory T cells that lead to allograft rejection. *Am J Transplant* (2007) 7:1071–9. doi:10.1111/j.1600-6143.2007.01756.x
42. Lund FE, Randall TD. Effector and regulatory B cells: modulators of CD4+ T cell immunity. *Nat Rev Immunol* (2010) 10:236–47. doi:10.1038/nri2729
43. Harris DP, Haynes L, Sayles PC, Duso DK, Eaton SM, Lepak NM, et al. Reciprocal regulation of polarized cytokine production by effector B and T cells. *Nat Immunol* (2000) 1:475–82. doi:10.1038/82717
44. Menard LC, Minns LA, Darche S, Mielcarz DW, Foureau DM, Roos D, et al. B cells amplify IFN-gamma production by T cells via a TNF-alpha-mediated mechanism. *J Immunol* (2007) 179:4857–66. doi:10.4049/jimmunol.179.7.4857
45. Wojciechowski W, Harris DP, Sprague F, Mousseau B, Makris M, Kusser K, et al. Cytokine-producing effector B cells regulate type 2 immunity to *H. polygyrus*. *Immunity* (2009) 30:421–33. doi:10.1016/j.immuni.2009.01.006
46. Thaunat O, Legendre C, Morelon E, Kreis H, Mamzer-Bruneel M-F. To biopsy or not to biopsy? Should we screen the histology of stable renal grafts? *Transplantation* (2007) 84:671–6. doi:10.1097/01.tp.0000282870.71282.ed
47. Rosser EC, Mauri C. Regulatory B cells: origin, phenotype, and function. *Immunity* (2015) 42:607–12. doi:10.1016/j.immuni.2015.04.005
48. Fillatreau S, Gray D, Anderton SM. Not always the bad guys: B cells as regulators of autoimmune pathology. *Nat Rev Immunol* (2008) 8:391–7. doi:10.1038/nri2315
49. Bouaziz J-D, Yanaba K, Tedder TF. Regulatory B cells as inhibitors of immune responses and inflammation. *Immunol Rev* (2008) 224:201–14. doi:10.1111/j.1600-065X.2008.00661.x
50. Thaunat O, Morelon E, Defrance T. Am"B"valent: anti-CD20 antibodies unravel the dual role of B cells in immunopathogenesis. *Blood* (2010) 116:515–21. doi:10.1182/blood-2010-01-266668
51. Brouard S, Pallier A, Renaudin K, Foucher Y, Danger R, Devys A, et al. The natural history of clinical operational tolerance after kidney transplantation through twenty-seven cases. *Am J Transplant* (2012) 12:3296–307. doi:10.1111/j.1600-6143.2012.04249.x
52. Pallier A, Hillion S, Danger R, Giral M, Racapé M, Degauque N, et al. Patients with drug-free long-term graft function display increased numbers of peripheral B cells with a memory and inhibitory phenotype. *Kidney Int* (2010) 78:503–13. doi:10.1038/ki.2010.162
53. Newell KA, Asare A, Kirk AD, Gisler TD, Bourcier K, Suthanthiran M, et al. Identification of a B cell signature associated with renal transplant tolerance in humans. *J Clin Invest* (2010) 120:1836–47. doi:10.1172/JCI39933
54. Sagoo P, Perucha E, Sawitzki B, Tomiuk S, Stephens DA, Miqueu P, et al. Development of a cross-platform biomarker signature to detect renal transplant tolerance in humans. *J Clin Invest* (2010) 120:1848–61. doi:10.1172/JCI39922

55. Brown K, Sacks SH, Wong W. Tertiary lymphoid organs in renal allografts can be associated with donor-specific tolerance rather than rejection. *Eur J Immunol* (2011) 41:89–96. doi:10.1002/eji.201040759
56. Le Texier L, Thebault P, Lavault A, Usal C, Merieau E, Quillard T, et al. Long-term allograft tolerance is characterized by the accumulation of B cells exhibiting an inhibited profile. *Am J Transplant* (2011) 11:429–38. doi:10.1111/j.1600-6143.2010.03336.x
57. Li W, Bribriesco AC, Nava RG, Brescia AA, Ibricevic A, Spahn JH, et al. Lung transplant acceptance is facilitated by early events in the graft and is associated with lymphoid neogenesis. *Mucosal Immunol* (2012) 5:544–54. doi:10.1038/mi.2012.30
58. Hippen BE, DeMattos A, Cook WJ, Kew CE, Gaston RS. Association of CD20+ infiltrates with poorer clinical outcomes in acute cellular rejection of renal allografts. *Am J Transplant* (2005) 5:2248–52. doi:10.1111/j.1600-6143.2005.01009.x
59. Kayler LK, Lakkis FG, Morgan C, Basu A, Blisard D, Tan HP, et al. Acute cellular rejection with CD20-positive lymphoid clusters in kidney transplant patients following lymphocyte depletion. *Am J Transplant* (2007) 7:949–54. doi:10.1111/j.1600-6143.2007.01737.x
60. Bagnasco SM, Tsai W, Rahman MH, Kraus ES, Barisoni L, Vega R, et al. CD20-positive infiltrates in renal allograft biopsies with acute cellular rejection are not associated with worse graft survival. *Am J Transplant* (2007) 7:1968–73. doi:10.1111/j.1600-6143.2007.01885.x
61. Scheepstra C, Bemelman FJ, van der Loos C, Rowshani AT, van Donselaar-Van der Pant KAMI, Idu MM, et al. B cells in cluster or in a scattered pattern do not correlate with clinical outcome of renal allograft rejection. *Transplantation* (2008) 86:772–8. doi:10.1097/TP.0b013e3181860a74
62. Hwang HS, Song JH, Hyoung BJ, Lee SY, Jeon YJ, Kang SH, et al. Clinical impacts of CD38+ B cells on acute cellular rejection with CD20+ B cells in renal allograft. *Transplantation* (2010) 89:1489–95. doi:10.1097/TP.0b013e3181dd35b8
63. Martin L, Charon-Barra C, Bocrie O, Guignier F, D'Athis P, Dautin G, et al. Detection of plasma cells, C4d deposits and donor-specific antibodies on sequential graft biopsies of renal transplant recipients with chronic dysfunction. *Transpl Immunol* (2010) 22:110–4. doi:10.1016/j.trim.2009.11.001
64. Abbas K, Mubarak M, Zafar MN, Aziz T, Abbas H, Muzaffar R, et al. Plasma cell-rich acute rejections in living-related kidney transplantation: a clinicopathological study of 50 cases. *Clin Transplant* (2015) 29:835–41. doi:10.1111/ctr.12589
65. Yamani MH, Ratliff NB, Starling RC, Tuzcu EM, Yu Y, Cook DJ, et al. Quilty lesions are associated with increased expression of vitronectin receptor (alphavbeta3) and subsequent development of coronary vasculopathy. *J Heart Lung Transplant* (2003) 22:687–90. doi:10.1016/S1053-2498(02)01181-6
66. Chu KE, Ho EK, de la Torre L, Vasilescu ER, Marboe CC. The relationship of nodular endocardial infiltrates (Quilty lesions) to survival, patient age, anti-HLA antibodies, and coronary artery disease following heart transplantation. *Cardiovasc Pathol* (2005) 14:219–24. doi:10.1016/j.carpath.2005.03.009
67. Hiemann NE, Knosalla C, Wellnhofer E, Lehmkuhl HB, Hetzer R, Meyer R. Quilty indicates increased risk for microvasculopathy and poor survival after heart transplantation. *J Heart Lung Transplant* (2008) 27:289–96. doi:10.1016/j.healun.2007.11.573
68. Zakliczynski M, Nozynski J, Konecka-Mrowka D, Pyka L, Trybunia D, Swierad M, et al. Quilty effect correlates with biopsy-proven acute cellular rejection but does not predict transplanted heart coronary artery vasculopathy. *J Heart Lung Transplant* (2009) 28:255–9. doi:10.1016/j.healun.2008.12.011
69. Frank R, Dean SA, Molina MR, Kamoun M, Lal P. Correlations of lymphocyte subset infiltrates with donor-specific antibodies and acute antibody-mediated rejection in endomyocardial biopsies. *Cardiovasc Pathol* (2015) 24:168–72. doi:10.1016/j.carpath.2014.11.001

2

High Endothelial Venules and Other Blood Vessels: Critical Regulators of Lymphoid Organ Development and Function

*Ann Ager**

Division of Infection and Immunity, School of Medicine and Systems Immunity Research Institute, Cardiff University, Cardiff, UK

***Correspondence:**
Ann Ager
agera@cardiff.ac.uk

The blood vasculature regulates both the development and function of secondary lymphoid organs by providing a portal for entry of hemopoietic cells. During the development of lymphoid organs in the embryo, blood vessels deliver lymphoid tissue inducer cells that initiate and sustain the development of lymphoid tissues. In adults, the blood vessels are structurally distinct from those in other organs due to the requirement for high levels of lymphocyte recruitment under non-inflammatory conditions. In lymph nodes (LNs) and Peyer's patches, high endothelial venules (HEVs) especially adapted for lymphocyte trafficking form a spatially organized network of blood vessels, which controls both the type of lymphocyte and the site of entry into lymphoid tissues. Uniquely, HEVs express vascular addressins that regulate lymphocyte entry into lymphoid organs and are, therefore, critical to the function of lymphoid organs. Recent studies have demonstrated important roles for CD11c^{+} dendritic cells in the induction, as well as the maintenance, of vascular addressin expression and, therefore, the function of HEVs. Tertiary lymphoid organs (TLOs) are HEV containing LN-like structures that develop inside organized tissues undergoing chronic immune-mediated inflammation. In autoimmune lesions, the development of TLOs is thought to exacerbate disease. In cancerous tissues, the development of HEVs and TLOs is associated with improved patient outcomes in several cancers. Therefore, it is important to understand what drives the development of HEVs and TLOs and how these structures contribute to pathology. In several human diseases and experimental animal models of chronic inflammation, there are some similarities between the development and function of HEVs within LN and TLOs. This review will summarize current knowledge of how hemopoietic cells with lymphoid tissue-inducing, HEV-inducing, and HEV-maintaining properties are recruited from the bloodstream to induce the development and control the function of lymphoid organs.

Keywords: blood vessels, high endothelial venules, peripheral node addressin, mucosal addressin, lymph nodes, tertiary lymphoid organs, ectopic lymphoid structures

INTRODUCTION

Secondary lymphoid organs (SLOs) are sites in which immune responses are initiated and maintained in order to generate protective immunity against exogenous pathogens and tolerance to self-antigens and commensal organisms (1, 2). These specialized structures include lymph nodes (LNs), Peyer's patches (PPs), tonsils, appendix, bronchus-associated lymphoid tissue (BALT), nasal-associated lymphoid tissue (NALT), isolated lymphoid follicles, and the spleen. All SLOs develop in the embryo, apart from NALT and BALT, which develop neonatally and in adults, respectively. As well as supplying oxygen and nutrients, the vasculature regulates the development of SLOs by recruiting a distinct population of hemopoietic cells that is essential to initiate lymphoid organogenesis. In adults, the blood vasculature in lymphoid organs is different from that found in other organs due to the requirement for efficient recruitment of lymphocytes under non-inflammatory, homeostatic conditions. Specialized blood vessels called high endothelial venules (HEVs) perform this function in all lymphoid organs except the spleen (3).

Tertiary lymphoid organs (TLOs) are lymph node-like immune cell clusters that develop inside non-lymphoid organs in response to chronic immune-mediated inflammation stimulated by persistent infections, chronic graft rejection, autoimmunity, and cancer (4). Defining features of TLOs are those that define SLOs: HEVs, lymphoid stromal cells, separate T-lymphocyte, and B-lymphocyte-rich compartments, follicular dendritic cell (FDC)-containing germinal centers, and antigen-presenting cells, including dendritic cells (DCs). However, in contrast to SLOs, TLOs are not encapsulated organs and are also known as tertiary lymphoid structures or ectopic lymphoid structures (ELS). TLOs are sites of active immune responses in autoimmune patients and animal models of autoimmunity (5, 6). There is evidence implicating TLOs in generating destructive immunity to self-antigens (7) although the relative contributions of TLOs and SLOs to disease progression are difficult to dissect during ongoing disease. Retrospective studies have correlated the presence of TLOs in resected solid cancers with prolonged patient outcome following resection of the primary cancer in several cancers (8). In some cancers, the density of HEVs alone predicted patient outcome (9, 10), indicating the critical role that HEVs play in orchestrating anti-cancer immunity. Importantly however, the formation of TLOs does not correlate with improved cancer patient outcome for all cancers. In virus-induced hepatic cellular carcinoma, TLOs promote carcinogenesis (11). In *Helicobacter pylori*-infected humans and mice, TLO development precedes carcinogenesis but whether TLOs promote the development of gastric cancer is not clear (12, 13). Therefore, there is much interest in how HEVs and TLOs develop and their exact roles in different chronic inflammatory diseases.

The development of LNs and PPs is well characterized, but how TLOs form is less clear because they develop during ongoing diseases. The similarities in structure between SLOs and TLOs suggest that underlying mechanisms driving their development may be conserved. Much attention has focused on the role of hemopoietic lymphoid tissue inducer (LTi) cells in driving the differentiation of local mesenchyme into lymphoid tissue organizer (LTo) cells during the development of LNs and PPs in mice (14–16). LTo cells are gp38$^+$ fibroblasts and are precursors of lymphoid stromal cells such as fibroblast reticular cells (FRCs) and FDCs. Lymphotoxin (LT)-αβ on hemopoietic LTi cells engaging lymphotoxin β receptor (LTβR) on LTo cells plays a dominant role in differentiating LTo into chemokine-secreting, adhesion molecule expressing fibroblasts that are able to recruit and retain LTis in the developing lymphoid tissue. An equally important, but unanswered question, is how embryonic blood vessels deliver LTi cells from their site of generation in fetal liver to predetermined sites where LNs are to develop. A role for inflamed blood vessels in initiating TLO development is implied by the finding that myeloid cells recruited into inflamed tissues drive the differentiation of gp38$^+$ fibroblasts that share properties with lymphoid stromal cells and are likely precursors of LTo cells (17). However, the mechanisms underlying myeloid cell recruitment by inflamed blood vessels were not determined in this study.

In adults, HEVs continually recruit naive and memory lymphocytes from the bloodstream into lymphoid organs in an antigen-independent manner where they survey DCs for cognate antigen (3). In peripheral LN draining the skin, HEVs express the peripheral addressin, peripheral node addressin (PNAd), whereas in PPs, HEVs express the mucosal addressin, mucosal addressin cell adhesion molecule (MAdCAM)-1. HEVs in some LNs (mesenteric, sacral, cervical) express both PNAd and MAdCAM-1. It has long been known that PNAd expression by HEV is actively maintained since PNAd levels on HEVs are rapidly downregulated following disruption of, or isolation from, the lymphoid microenvironment (18–20). Interestingly, HEVs in peripheral LN of newborn mice express the mucosal addressin but not the peripheral addressin (21, 22). During the first 2–3 weeks of life, HEV maturation is completed by a switch in vascular addressin expression from MAdCAM-1 to PNAd. How the vascular addressin switch is regulated and PNAd expression maintained on HEV in adult SLOs have been unclear. Recent studies have identified critical roles for CD11c$^+$ DCs in the vascular addressin switch (23) as well as the maintenance of PNAd-expressing HEV in adult mice (24). Therefore, the blood vasculature plays a central role in recruiting distinct populations of hemopoietic cells at precise stages of lymphoid organ development that are essential to initiate lymphoid organogenesis, induce HEV maturation, and maintain fully differentiated HEV. These points will be addressed in greater detail in the following section.

A key step in the recruitment of lymphoid cells is their selection from the total pool of blood-borne leukocytes by binding to the inner blood vessel surface prior to transmigration across the vessel wall and entry into lymphoid organs. This involves a sequence of adhesive interactions between leukocytes and vascular endothelial (VE) cells, which can be divided into distinct stages of rolling and activation-induced arrest. In general, selectins mediate rolling and chemokines immobilized on the endothelial cell (EC) surface activate leukocyte integrins to arrest rolling cells. How hemopoietic cells with LT-inducing, HEV-inducing, and HEV-maintaining properties are recruited into lymphoid organs is central to understanding both the development of lymphoid tissues and the mechanisms regulating adaptive immune responses and disease pathologies.

BLOOD VESSELS AND THE DEVELOPMENT OF SLOs

The earliest event in LN development is the formation of lymphatic vasculature around embryonic day 10.5 (E10.5) by budding from larger veins and establishing a primordial lymph sac or anlagen (**Figure 1**) (25). CD45$^+$ CD4$^+$ CD3$^-$ IL7Rα$^+$

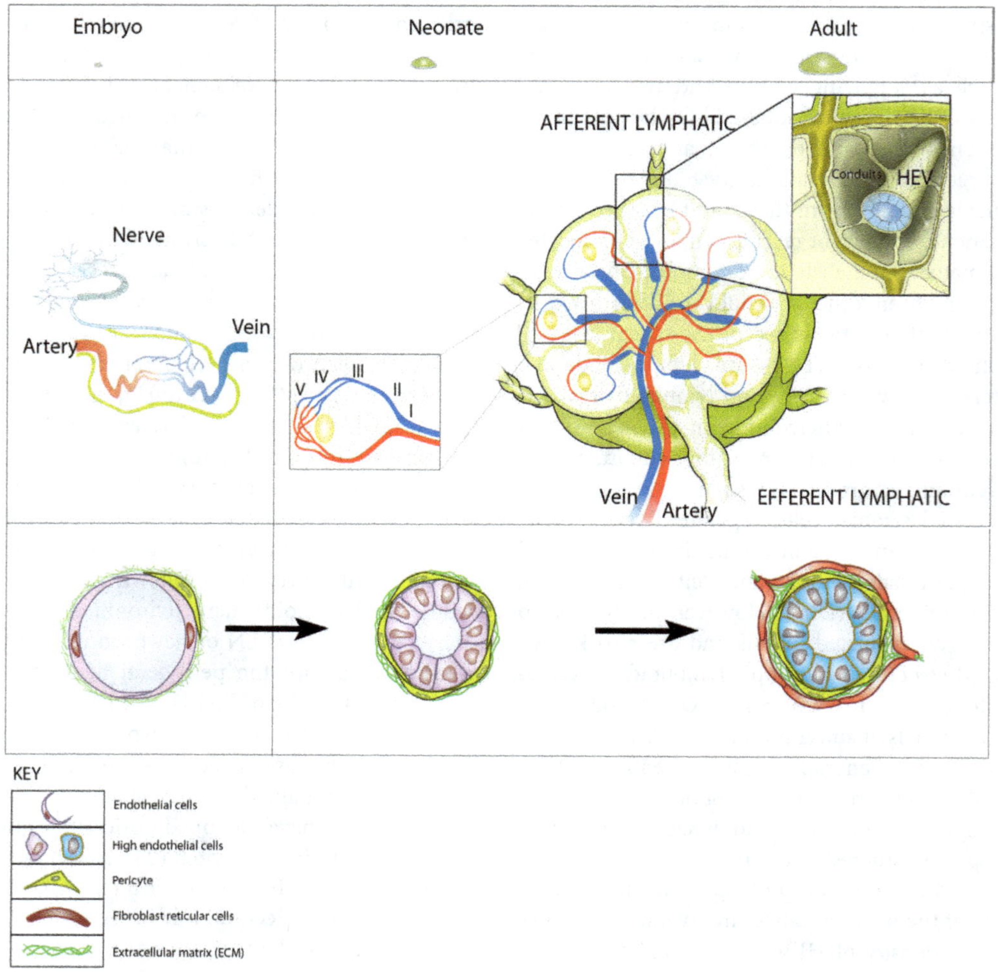

FIGURE 1 | Blood vessels and high endothelial venules (HEVs) in the development of lymph nodes (LNs). Top: LN development represented as relative sizes of (left) embryonic and (right) neonatal and adult LNs. Middle (left): in the embryo, neuronal stimulation induces retinoic acid-dependent expression of CXCL13 by mesenchymal cells that can be reverse transcytosed and presented on the inner surface of embryonic blood vessels. (Right) In LNs of adults, the HEV network extends from the cortical/paracortical junction adjacent to B cell follicles to large collecting veins in the hilar region gradually increasing in diameter from the smallest, order V venules to the largest order I venules (left hand inset). HEV connect directly to afferent lymphatics via fibroblast reticular cell-coated conduits that form the supporting internal scaffold on which lymphocytes and antigen presenting cells crawl during immunosurveillance (right hand insert). This enables the recruitment of fetal liver-derived CXCR5^{+} $\alpha 4\beta 7$ integrin-expressing lymphoid tissue inducer cells to the sites where LN develop. (Right) At birth, structurally distinct MAdCAM-1-expressing HEV lined with cuboidal endothelial cells and supported by a thickened fibronectin containing basal lamina are visible. During the first weeks of life, MAdCAM-1-expressing HEV recruit CD11c^{+} neonatal migratory dendritic cells mobilized from the intestinal lamina propria, undergo a switch from MAdCAM-1 to peripheral node addressin expression and become ensheathed by fibroblast reticular cells. The vascular addressin switch is followed by rapid growth and a concomitant increase in cellularity and expansion in LN.

RORγt^{+}, Id2^{+} lymphoid tissue-inducing (LTi) cells (members of the group 3 category of innate lymphoid cells) are recruited into the anlagen and drive the development of gp38^{+} LTo cells from local mesenchyme (26). CXCL13 and IL7, produced by local mesenchymal fibroblasts in response to retinoic acid (RA) generated by neuronal stimulation, recruit CXCR5 and IL7 receptor-expressing LTi cells at sites where LNs are to develop (14). In the embryonic intestine, myeloid cell expression of the tyrosine kinase receptor, RET, is important to localize LTi to sites where PPs develop (27). LT$\alpha\beta$ is upregulated on the surface of incoming LTis and stimulates LTβR-dependent upregulation of MAdCAM-1, vascular cell adhesion molecule (VCAM)-1, and intercellular adhesion molecule (ICAM)-1 and the secretion of homeostatic chemokines CXCL13, CCL19, and CCL21 by lymphoid stromal LTo cells. This enables LTo cells to retain recruited LTi cells in the developing anlagen. The continual recruitment and retention of LTi cells during embryogenesis is required to differentiate sufficient numbers of LTo cells to support the full development and organization of LNs and PPs (22).

During embryogenesis, LTi cells are generated in the fetal liver so how are they recruited to the sites at which LNs and PPs are to develop? A key finding is that all embryonic venous blood vessels express MAdCAM-1 (28). LTis express the integrin $\alpha 4\beta 7$, which binds to MAdCAM-1 and $\alpha 4\beta 7$-MAdCAM-1 binding is a dominant pathway for leukocyte recruitment from the bloodstream into developing LNs (21). In adults, homeostatic and inflammatory chemokines released by stromal cells are reverse transcytosed and presented on the inner blood vessel surface using Duffy antigen-related receptor-dependent and independent pathways (29–32). By analogy, CXCL13 released by activated fibroblasts presented on the inner surface of embryonic blood vessels together with cell surface MAdCAM-1, recruits CXCR5 expressing LTis from the bloodstream to initiate lymphoid organogenesis. Key questions, therefore, are what controls MAdCAM-1 expression on blood vessels in the embryo and is MAdCAM-1 essential for lymphoid organogenesis? MAdCAM-1 is expressed by all venous blood vessels as early as E9.5 in mice and expression is maintained throughout lymphoid organogenesis (28). In adults, MAdAM-1 expression by cultured EC is induced by classical Rel A/NF-κB signaling stimulated by factors such TNF-α, LT-α, IL-1-β, and LPS (33–35). Whether constitutive MAdCAM-1 expression on blood vessels in the LN anlagen is driven by NF-κB signaling or is ontologically determined, for example, by the transcription factor NKX2.3 (36), has not been determined. Interestingly, MAdCAM-1 expression by embryonic blood vessels is not essential for lymphoid organogenesis since LNs and PPs develop in MAdCAM-1 ko mice (37). LTis also express α4β1 integrin, which binds to VCAM-1 and could substitute for MAdCAM-1, however, mice globally deficient in VCAM-1 die in utero (38) and the role of VCAM-1 in lymphoid organogenesis is undetermined. ICAM-1 expression by LTo cells is not essential for lymphoid organogenesis since LNs develop in ICAM-1-deficient mice (39). However, MAdCAM-1, VCAM-1, and ICAM-1 are not redundant in adult mice because they regulate lymphocyte recirculation through SLOs and/or recruitment to inflamed tissues (1, 3).

Lymph nodes and PPs do not develop in LTα ko mice (40). Administration of an LTβR agonist to pregnant mice bypasses the requirement for LTi cells and induces LN development (41). The initiation of LN and PP organogenesis is time restricted; mesenteric LN starts around E9–10 and PPs around E16 with peripheral LN (axillary, brachial, inguinal, and popliteal) between E10 and E16. However, exogenous administration of LTβR agonists outside of these times will not initiate LN formation. Administration of antagonistic LTβR-Ig to pregnant wildtype mice also blocks the development of LN in a similar time-dependent manner (42). What controls the timing of LN development is not clear but one possibility is the ability of embryonic blood vessels to recruit LTi cells. For example, the expression of sufficient MAdCAM-1, immobilized chemokines, or other, as yet unidentified, homing-associated molecules that recruit LTi cells from the bloodstream into to the LN anlagen may be time dependent. The local generation of RA drives lymphoid organogenesis and RA is required to mature developing blood vessels in the embryo (43). It is possible that locally generated RA facilitates LTi recruitment by promoting the expression or activity of homing-associated molecules on growing vessels in the LN anlagen, but we know very little about when RA is produced and how this is regulated.

Although LTαβ–LTβR is a dominant NF-κB signaling pathway and CXCL13 a dominant chemokine in the development of peripheral LN and PP, other pathways can substitute during the development of mucosal and visceral draining LN. For example, mesenteric, cervical (submandibular), sacral, and lumbar LN (44) develop in LTβ-, LTβR-, or CXCL13-deficient mice (15, 22). LTβR engagement by membrane LTαβ stimulates both classical NF-κB signaling *via* Iκκβ and p50/RelA as well as non-classical signaling *via* Iκκα and p52/RelB, and there is considerable interplay between these two pathways (45). LN and PP do not develop in mice globally deficient in either RelA or Rel B, key components of classical and non-classical NF-κB signaling, respectively, although the impact of classical NF-κB signaling on LN development may be *via* upregulation of non-classical NF-κB signaling substrates such as NF-κB2 and RelB (46, 47). In mice deficient in NFkB2, the substrate for p52 in the non-classical pathway, mesenteric and some peripheral LN develop but lymphoid organs that form later in embryogenesis (inguinal, popliteal, and PPs) are small or do not develop at all (48). It is suggested that p50/RelB can substitute for p52/RelB in these mice but the signal strength is weaker and so, although LTi cells are recruited, the induction of CAMs is not enough to retain sufficient LTi cells to maintain development and organize the full structure of late developing lymphoid organs. Non-classical NF-κB signaling is important for the proper development of HEVs since the small LN that develop in LTβ- or NFkB2-deficient mice have poorly developed HEVs, as do peripheral LNs that develop in mice expressing a signaling-deficient mutant of the non-classical NK-κB pathway, Iκκα (48, 49). The widespread expression of LTβR on the developing vasculature as well as LTo cells makes it difficult to assess their relative contributions to the development of lymphoid organs or of HEVs in mice globally deficient in either LTαβ–LTβR or following administration of antagonistic LTβR-Ig. Recent studies have shown that the development of peripheral LNs in 25–40% of pups is completely blocked in mice selectively deficient in LTβR in blood and lymphatic ECs, but the underlying mechanism is not clear (50). Further work will be required to dissect the roles of NF-κB signaling in the blood vs the lymphatic vasculature during lymphoid organogenesis and how this integrates into the scheme of lymphoid organogenesis driven by gp38$^+$ lymphoid stromal LTo cells.

THE DEVELOPMENT AND FUNCTION OF HIGH ENDOTHELIAL VENULES IN SLOs

The Vascular Addressin Switch

The recruitment of naïve T and B cells into all lymphoid organs, apart from spleen, is dependent on the differentiation of a subset of blood vessels into HEVs. Structurally distinct HEVs are not apparent in LN of mice until birth when a branching network of HEV blood vessels starts to organize around B cell follicles during the first days after birth in PPs (28). A key event in neonatal maturation and expansion of LN is a switch in vascular addressin expression by HEV (21). In LNs of newborn mice, all HEVs express the mucosal addressin MAdCAM-1; during the first few weeks of life MAdCAM-1 is downregulated and expression of the PNAd is upregulated. PNAd comprises a mixture of ligands for L-selectin (CD34, podocalyxin, GlyCAM-1, MAdCAM-1, nepmucin, and endomucin) that are modified by 6-sulfo sialyl Lewis[x] on extended core 1 O-linked oligosaccharides and detected by monoclonal antibody MECA79 (51). PNAd expressed on the inner, apical surface of HEVs co-operates with the arrest chemokine CCL21 to select L-selectin/CD62L$^+$, CCR7$^+$ lymphocytes from the bloodstream for entry into LN allowing postnatal colonization of LN by naive T and B lymphocytes as they are released into the circulation from the thymus and fetal liver/bone marrow, respectively. Interestingly, PNAd is also expressed on the basolateral surfaces of ECs lining HEVs but it is not involved in recruiting lymphocytes directly from the bloodstream. Distinct sulfotransferases generate apical and basolateral PNAd and the expression of GlcNAc6ST-2 (HEC-6ST; CHST4), which is required to generate apically expessed PNAd, is restricted to HEV ECs, whereas GlcNAc6ST-1 (CHST2), which generates basolaterally expressed PNAd, is more widely expressed in stromal cells (51). The PNAd-expressing HEV network grows alongside the growth of other stromal components resulting in a rapid increase in the size and cellularity of LN during the first weeks of life (23). Although PNAd is a well-characterized ligand for L-selectin, it only accounts for 50% of L-selectin-dependent recruitment into peripheral LNs. Important non-PNAd ligands on HEV that regulate L-selectin-dependent recruitment into peripheral LN include 6-sulpho sialyl Lewis X modified N-linked glycans such as CD34, as well as a minor role for core 2-branched O-linked glycans (51, 52).

Vascular addressins expressed on the inner, luminal surface of ECs lining HEV bind to homing receptors on lymphocytes; therefore, addressins define the specialized property of HEV in driving lymphocyte recruitment into LNs and PPs. PNAd was originally described in HEVs of peripheral LNs draining the skin (inguinal, axillary, brachial, and popliteal) (53) and MAdCAM-1 in mucosal-associated lymphoid tissues such as PPs (54). However, analysis of other mucosal and viscera-draining SLOs in mice shows that PNAd expression is upregulated and MAdCAM-1 variably downregulated. For example, MAdCAM-1 expression is not completely downregulated in mesenteric and sacral LNs where individual high endothelial cells (HECs) co-express PNAd and MAdCAM-1. However, mucosal addressin is completely downregulated in lymphoid tissues draining other mucosal sites such as cervical (submandibular) LN or NALT (4). Similarly, LNs draining visceral organs, such as lumbar LN, express PNAd and not mucosal addressin (44); therefore PNAd expression is not restricted to subcutaneous LN and is widely expressed by mucosal and visceral LN in mice. PNAd expression was originally reported to be restricted to the basolateral surfaces of HEVs in PPs (54). However, in different mouse strains and other species, PNAd expression in PPs is comparable with that in peripheral LN, which may reflect increased antigenic stimulation (51). Why MAdCAM-1 expression is maintained by HEVs in PPs and some mucosal LN whereas other HEVs completely switch to PNAd expression is not clear, but MAdCAM-1 expression is regulated by the transcription factor NKX2.3 (55).

The Connection with Afferent Lymph

A unique feature of HEV is the connection with afferent lymph. HEVs are supported by a perivascular sheath composed of FRCs that are connected to the FRC coated conduit system within LN. The conduit system allows communication between afferent lymph and HEV whereby incoming lymph-borne soluble factors, such as chemokines and cytokines, are delivered directly to the basal lamina of HEV (**Figure 1**) (56). Early studies showed that ligation of afferent lymphatics, which drain fluid and immune cells into popliteal LN, resulted in a gradual flattening of HECs and although some PNAd expression was retained it was restricted to the basolateral surfaces of HECs (18, 19, 57). Other changes in HECs included a transient induction of MAdCAM-1 expression, which peaked 4 days following deafferentization suggesting reversion of mature HEVs to an immature state. Lymphocyte recruitment by HEV decreased and was no longer detectable 8 days after deafferentization. HEVs reverted to fully functional vessels expressing PNAd at the luminal surface following regrowth of afferent lymphatics demonstrating the complete reversibility of HEV differentiation. Early studies indicated a dominant role for LTβR signaling in maintaining PNAd expression since chronic administration of LTβR blocking reagents to adult mice recapitulates the effects of deafferentization in that HEVs downregulate PNAd and MAdCAM-1, and therefore lose the ability to support lymphocyte homing (58). The flattened appearance of PNAd-positive HEV in deafferentized LNs is seen in peripheral LNs that develop in mice in the absence of endothelial expression of LTβR (50) and in inguinal LNs developing in the absence of either NFKB2 or IKKα (48, 49), indicating a key role for LTβR stimulated non-canonical NFκB signaling in driving luminal expression of PNAd by HECs. Which cells engage LTβR on HECs to induce and maintain PNAd expression has been unclear, however, recent studies identify dominant roles for CD11c$^+$ DCs in the induction, as well as the maintenance, of PNAd expression by HEV.

Role of CD11c$^+$ Cells in the Vascular Addressin Switch

An important finding is that during the first weeks of life CD11c$^+$, CD11b$^+$, CD103$^+$ DCs mobilized from the gut lamina propria in response to microbial colonization induce the switch from mucosal to peripheral addressin expression by HEV in peripheral LN (23). RA-dependent signaling is critical for these so-called neonatal migratory DCs to induce the vascular switch; cells that do not express retinaldeyhde dehydrogenase (RALDH), which generates RA from retinaldehyde, a derivative of Vitamin A, are unable to induce the vascular addressin switch. This important finding came from studies of adult germ-free mice in which peripheral LN HEVs express MAdCAM-1, but not PNAd, and LN are small without clear compartmentalization into T and B-cell areas, similar to LN in newborn mice. When germ-free mice were co-housed with conventionally housed mice, HEVs underwent the vascular addressin switch with consequent increases in lymphocyte homing and LN cellularity. These effects could be reproduced by administration of RALDH$^+$ neonatal migratory DCs isolated from conventionally housed adult mice to young germ-free mice. Migration of neonatal migratory DCs to peripheral LN was dependent on MAdCAM-1 expression by HEVs in peripheral LN. Interestingly, the migration of these cells to peripheral LN was highest around 2 weeks after birth and subsided after 6 weeks, presumably because of the loss of MAdCAM-1 expression by peripheral LN HEVs.

In adult mice, CD11c$^+$ cells have been shown to maintain PNAd-expressing, fully functional HEVs by stimulating LTβR-dependent signaling in HECs (24, 50). Moussion and Girard used transgenic mice expressing the diphtheria toxin (DT) receptor under the CD11c promoter (CD11c-DTR mice) and DT to deplete CD11c$^+$ cells (24). They noted a gradual loss of PNAd expression, a transient expression of MAdCAM-1, and a reduction in lymphocyte entry *via* HEVs over 8 days, which was prevented by administration of exogenously generated LTαβ-expressing CD11c$^+$ DCs. Since ligands for LTβR are membrane bound, LTαβ DCs might be expected to make frequent contacts with HECs under homeostatic conditions in order to maintain PNAd expression. Migration of DCs into LN of adult mice has focused on entry from surrounding tissues *via* incoming, afferent lymphatics. DCs entering *via* this route do not come into cellular contact with HECs since they do not penetrate the surrounding pericytic sheath (59, 60). However, DCs entering from surrounding tissues *via* afferent lymphatics do locate around HEVs (61); it is therefore possible that protruding DC membranes or exosomes released by DC (62, 63) could cross the pericytic sheath and contact with HECs. Precursors of classical DCs that are recruited from the bloodstream into LN of adult mice spend up to 5 h in the walls of HEVs are a possible HEV-maintaining cell. In this scenario, the critical role of afferent lymph in maintaining fully differentiated HEVs is not as an entry point for DCs but to supply the chemoattractants necessary to recruit LT-expressing DCs from the bloodstream, enabling DC-HEC contact to sustain LTβR signaling.

Interestingly, CCR7$^+$ expression by CD11c$^+$ cells is required to control the homeostatic expansion of PNAd-expessing HEV but in the absence of CCR7 expession, CD11c$^+$ cells are still able to induce the switch in addressin expression to PNAd (64). The increase in size of the HEV network and associated increase in LN cellularity and volume is due, in part, to the release of angiogenic stimuli such as VEGF-A by FRC and DCs (65, 66). These findings suggest that the differentiation of fully functional, PNAd-expressing HEV and the expansion of the HEV network are controlled by different types of CD11c$^+$ cells in adult mice. It will be interesting to determine whether RA signaling is required for CD11c$^+$ DCs to maintain PNAd expression and expand HEV in adult mice as has been shown in neonates (23).

High Endothelial Venules in Homeostatic Lymphocyte Trafficking

Together, the SLOs are uniquely placed to survey the whole body for incoming pathogens and self-antigens derived from the skin, mucosal surfaces, or directly into the bloodstream, mount an appropriate immune response and clear invading pathogens from the body. To achieve this, rare lymphocytes with appropriate antigen receptor must be selected from the total pool of lymphocytes each with its own unique receptor; this occurs inside SLOs. Pathogens are first degraded and presented as MHC-binding peptides on DCs bound to gp38$^+$ FRCs. The total pool of lymphocytes in the body is then exposed to pathogen peptide-enriched DCs. Lymphocytes with antigen receptors able to respond to the level of peptide presented are removed from the circulating pool of cells and undergo proliferation and differentiation to effector, memory, or regulatory lymphocytes before returning to the circulation. Blood vessels are critical components of adaptive immunity since they recruit naïve and central memory lymphocyte irrespective of antigen receptor specificity and deliver them to DCs inside lymphoid organ under homeostatic conditions. Postcapillary venules (PCV) lined with continuous ECs are the preferred sites of lymphocyte extravasation in LNs and other organs such as the skin and GI tract. The increase in diameter as blood vessels transition from capillaries to PCV alters hemodynamics such that leukocytes move to the outer stream or margin of flowing blood adjacent to the inner surface of the vessel (67). Here lymphocytes tether, roll, and arrest on the inside surface without obstructing flow that would happen in smaller capillaries. In other organs where the microvessels are lined with sinusoidal endothelium, such as the spleen, liver, and bone marrow, shear stress at the vessel wall–blood interface may be significantly reduced that the requirement for selectins for capture from flowing blood is not necessary and other homing-associated molecules such as leukocyte integrins perform this role (67). In LNs and PPs, the trafficking of naïve lymphocytes is restricted to specialized postcapillary venules called HEVs. These vessels are structurally adapted to support large-scale lymphocyte trafficking without compromising vascular integrity. The spleen does not have HEV and, in mice, lymphocytes enter the spleen from capillaries in the marginal zone using incompletely defined molecular recognition pathways. The structure of human spleen differs from that in mice and the route of lymphocyte entry has not been identified (68).

Arteries feeding the LN enter at the hilar region and arborize into nutrient- and oxygen-transporting capillary beds surrounding B cell follicles in the outer cortex and in the T cell zone. The capillary beds lead directly (or indirectly *via* arteriovenous shunts) into the postcapillary venular network, which extends throughout the paracortex (T cell area) of the LN; HEVs form part of this postcapillary network (**Figure 1**). HEVs are readily distinguished from other blood vessels; the cuboidal (high) ECs, which line HEV and give these vessels their name, contrast with flat ECs lining other vessels. In addition, HEVs are supported by a thickened basal lamina comprising overlapping pericytes and a perivascular sheath of FRC that together generate a structural and functional unit exquisitely adapted to support high levels of lymphocyte recruitment and transendothelial migration to deliver lymphocytes to the LN parenchyma. The ECs lining HEVs express a number of pan-endothelial markers such as VE-cadherin and CD31 as well as the master venous regulator Nr2f2 (69), which suggests that they differentiate from local postcapillary venules. Invitavital imaging of lymphocyte recruitment allows HEVs to be ordered according to size and location. The smallest vessels (order V) are found at the junction between the B cell-enriched cortex and the T cell-enriched paracortex. HEVs gradually increase in size to larger vessels (order II) at the junction between the paracortex and medulla where they merge into order I collecting venules which drain into hilar vein (70) (**Figure 1**). The majority of lymphocytes recruited into LN and PPs are from the higher order vessels III–V. In peripheral LN, L-selectin dependent recruitment from lower order vessels does occur but the vascular ligand on HEC is distinct from PNAd (71). How this complex branching network of differentiated HEVs develops and is maintained in LN is not clear but it is likely to be connected with development of the highly organized secondary structures of FRC-coated conduits that connect the draining lymphatics with the HEVs (29). The dominant roles of LTβR signaling in maintaining fully differentiated PNAd-expressing HEVs as well as T/B compartmentalization in LNs are likely to cooperate in forming an organized HEV network.

The ability to image the behavior of leukocytes inside post-capillary venules using intravital microscopy has identified the molecular interactions between lymphocytes and HEVs in LN and PPs that control recruitment from flowing blood. The multi-step adhesion cascade describes the sequence of tethering, rolling and activation-induced arrest, which selects lymphocytes for transendothelial migration and entry into lymphoid organs. The cascade is best exemplified by the fact that neutrophils undergo L-selectin-depending rolling in HEVs but they are unable to undergo activation-induced arrest by CCL21 immobilized on the inner HEV surface because they do not express CCR7 and are, therefore, not recruited into LN under homeostatic conditions (70). The selectin, chemokines, and integrins that regulate rolling and activation-induced arrest of naive and central memory T and B cells and the non-random recruitment of T and B lymphocytes in HEV of LN and PP of mice have been described in detail elsewhere (1, 3, 72–74). The regulated expression of peripheral node and mucosal addressins by HEV and their roles in lymphocyte recruitment are conserved in LNs of larger animals as well as humans indicating that studies in mice have clinical relevance (75–79). This review will summarize recent advances in understanding the structure and function of HEV and its role in regulating adaptive immunity.

In LNs, L-selectin mediates tethering and rolling of lymphocytes. In comparison with T cells, B cells express lower L-selectin and are reduced in LNs but highly enriched in PPs. Although L-selectin supports lymphocyte rolling in HEVs of PPs, it is not a dominant homing molecule under homeostatic conditions since, in contrast to peripheral LN, the cellularity of PPs in L-selectin deficient mice is not reduced (80). The B-cell expressed lectin that supports preferential recruitment by HEVs of PPs was unknown until a detailed comparison of transcriptomes expressed by HECs isolated from PPs and peripheral LN of mice demonstrated preferential expression of the enzyme β-galactoside α-2,6-sialyltransferease I (ST6GaI 1) by PP HECs. ST6Gal 1 generates high affinity α-2,6-sialylated glycan ligands for the B cell lectin CD22 (Siglec-2) and was shown to function as a B cell selective mucosal addressin in PPs (69).

Apart from addressin expression and their location inside LN, a characteristic histological feature of HEV is lymphocytes embedded in the walls of HEV, which suggests that transmigration is a rate-determining step in lymphocyte recruitment from the bloodstream into the LN parenchyma. Transmigration is a rapid event taking 3 min to cross the endothelial lining and 10 min to complete migration across the underlying basal lamina (81–83). The molecules and signaling pathways that regulate transmigration are not completely understood. Whether lymphocytes move through the junctions between HECs (paracellular route) or penetrate the EC cytoplasm (transcellular route) has long been debated (84, 85). It is important to understand how lymphocytes transmigrate the walls of HEV since the potential for bi-directional signaling in lymphocytes and HECs may prime transmigrating lymphocytes for interstitial motility and immunosurveillance. Recent studies have demonstrated that lymphocytes are held in the so-called HEV pockets that are extracellular spaces between HECs and the surrounding pericyte-containing basal lamina (86). The accumulation of transmigrating lymphocytes, particularly T cells, contributes to the height of HECs (81, 87). Residence in HEV pockets provides an opportunity for cellular contacts with HECs or with other transmigrating cells, such as DCs, which may facilitate rapid transmigration in comparison with vessels lined with flat EC (81). It is also possible that antigen could be passed from the basolateral adjoining conduits to DCs inside HEV pockets for presentation to incoming lymphocytes. HEVs are contractile vessels responding to locally released vasoactive agents (88). Arterial pressure and vasoconstriction can regulate the height of HECs measured in histological sections of LN (89). Dynamic changes in shear stress at the vessel wall interface generated by HEV contractility may enhance the capture of lymphocytes from flowing blood.

Lymphocytes form very close, intercellular, gap-like junctions of 2–4 nm with HECs during transmigration (90), which may be the *in vivo* equivalent of the docking structures between lymphocytes and ECs reported *in vitro* (91, 92). ECs lining HEVs express a range of junctional proteins that are found in other vascular beds, including VE-cadherin, CD31, JAM-A, JAM-B, JAM-C, and ESAM-1 (93). Engagement of EC junctional proteins by complementary receptors on lymphocytes may regulate migration across the endothelial lining of HEVs, as shown for leukocytes transmigrating inflamed blood vessels (67). Unlike other types of endothelium, HEV ECs lack tight junctions and vascular specific claudin-5. These distinct structural features may facilitate paracellular transmigration of lymphocytes and/or lymphocyte accumulation inside HEV pockets.

Some progress has been made in dissecting the molecular events driving entry and exit of lymphocytes from HEV pockets and subsequent penetration of the underlying basal lamina to enter the LN parenchyma (94). Lymphocytes are retained in HEV pockets of FTY720 treated mice, and this was thought to be due to lack of space in the LN parenchyma (86). However, as well as blocking lymphocyte exit from LN *via* lymphatics, FTY720 inhibits T cell recruitment from the bloodstream across HEVs (95). An alternative explanation is that incoming T cells drive the exit from HEV pockets and, in the absence of incoming T cells in FTY720 treated mice, lymphocytes do not complete transmigration, as has been shown *in vitro* (96). There are other mechanisms controlling lymphocyte retention in HEV pockets. T cells accumulate in the endothelial lining of HEVs in mice treated with dual specificity MMP/ADAM inhibitors (87), suggesting that exit from HEV pockets may be metalloproteinase-dependent. L-selectin is proteolytically cleaved from T cells as they transmigrate HEVs (97) and lymphocytes expressing a metalloproteinase-resistant mutant of L-selectin take longer to transmigrate the endothelial lining of HEVs (98). Proteolytic shedding of L-selectin following cross-linking by basolaterally expressed ligands such as PNAd may polarize transmigrating T cells, as recently demonstrated in monocytes (99) and neutrophils (100) and allow directed migration into the LN parenchyma in response to HEC-derived lipids such as autoaxin and lymphoid stromal cell-derived chemokines such as CCL19 and CCL21 (101, 102).

The Impact of Immunization and Infection on High Endothelial Venules

There are marked changes to HEVs in LNs draining sites of immunization or infection. These include increased blood flow, expansion of the HEV network, and marked changes in expression of homing-associated molecules. Changes in HEV function cooperate to alter the size and composition of the leukocyte infiltrate. In particular, altered expression of homing molecules on HEV enables the recruitment of activated lymphocytes and innate immune cells that are normally excluded by HEVs because they lack expression of L-selectin or CCR7. The impact of altered immune cell recruitment *via* HEV on ongoing immunity is only just starting to be analyzed (94).

Innate immune cells remodel feeding arterioles to increase blood supply and, thereby, increase the delivery of naïve lymphocytes into draining LNs (103). This allows a major fraction of the full repertoire of lymphocytes to pass through antigen-activated LNs within a few days (104). The HEV network grows to accommodate the increase in blood supply and the accompanying increase in lymphocyte trafficking. For example, the total length of HEVs increases threefold from approximately 10–30 cm in antigen-reactive LN in parallel with a threefold size increase of LN volume (105). LT and VEGF family members regulate expansion of the HEV network. LTβR activation of FRCs by DCs induces release of VEGF-A, an angiogenic factor that stimulates HEV growth (65, 106). VEGF-A is also produced by activated DCs, which, following injection into the skin, stimulate the growth of HEV in LN draining the site of injection (66).

Other changes to HEV in antigen-challenged LN relate directly to links with afferent lymphatics. For example, the plasticity of HEV revealed by afferent lymphatic ligation (19) or isolation from the LN environment (20) is directly relevant to adaptive immune responses. Antigen administration is accompanied by a temporary shutdown of afferent lymphatics between days 2 and 5 and concomitant dedifferentiation of HEV (107). Interestingly, the loss of luminal PNAd by HEV following antigen administration is accompanied by transient induction of MAdCAM-1 as found following deafferentization or CD11c$^+$ cell depletion. By limiting the influx of lymphocytes, the loss of PNAd expression may serve to prevent the dilution of lymphocytes already in contact with antigen-laden DCs and promote the generation of memory cells. The reversion of PNAd-expressing HEV to MAdCAM-1-expressing HEV may allow entry of LTis or other α4β7 integrin-expressing innate lymphoid cells (108), for repair or remodeling of LN during the later stages of virus infection to restore preinfection architecture (109).

Vascular changes in antigen-stimulated LNs are accompanied by increased growth of afferent lymphatics and remodeling of the FRC network that alters the availability of chemokines for presentation by HEVs. For example, the dramatic reduction in CCL21 and CXCL13 expression by LN stroma following viral or bacterial infection (110) impacts on T and B lymphocyte recruitment since stromal cell-derived chemokines are presented by HEVs to blood-borne lymphocytes (32). The increased delivery of DCs and other immune cells mobilized from inflamed tissues *via* expanded afferent lymphatics may have, as yet unexplored, effects on HEV function. However, as the immune response subsides, CD11c$^+$ cells are required to remodel the perivascular FRC sheath surrounding HEVs and restore vascular permeability and HEV function (111). These observations suggest a regulatory loop based on HEV that controls the size of LN, preventing uncontrolled growth of inflamed lymphoid tissue. How the structure of LNs and other secondary lymphoid tissues is restored to the preactivated state is largely unknown. This is likely to be relevant to understanding TLOs that develop in chronically inflamed tissues.

BLOOD VESSELS, HIGH ENDOTHELIAL VENULES, AND THE DEVELOPMENT OF TLOs

Tertiary lymphoid organs or ELS develop inside non-lymphoid organs. TLOs form in response to chronic immune-mediated inflammation stimulated by persistent antigens such as infection, allograft rejection or ulcerative colitis but also in several autoimmune conditions such as rheumatoid arthritis and Hashimoto's thyroiditis (112). TLOs have been reported by histology in biopsied or surgically removed clinical tissues from the majority of organs in the body including the CNS and atherosclerotic aorta. TLOs are also found associated with cancerous tissues. TLOs are highly organized lymph node-like structures containing discrete T and B-cell rich areas supported by stromal cells that share markers with FRCs and FDCs in LNs. TLOs contain PNAd-expressing blood vessels that resemble structurally distinct HEV in LNs; they are the presumed sites of entry of blood-borne lymphocyte and, therefore, critical to the function of TLOs. PNAd-expressing blood vessels lined by flat ECs are found inside cancer-induced ectopic lymphoid aggregates that are not organized into distinct T/B cell areas. These could represent immature HEV-containing structures in the process of forming TLOs, or TLOs that are distintegrating during the resolution of chronic inflammation (113). Interestingly, PNAd-expressing blood vessels that form following depletion of Foxp3$^+$ regulatory T cells from cancer-bearing mice are not associated with histologically distinct, lymphoid cell aggregates (114) which indicates that HEV neogenesis can precede lymphoid neo-organogenesis. The development of HEV in the absence of full-blown TLOs correlates with cancer regression in this experimental model highlighting the important role of HEV in controlling immunity to cancers. Interestingly gp38$^+$ (podoplanin) stromal cells are induced locally by CD11b$^+$ myeloid cells recruited to inflamed skin of mice, recapitulating the earliest stages of lymphoid stromal cell development, but whether CD11b$^+$ myeloid cells drive the development HEV and/or TLOs in chronic inflammation is not known (17).

How HEVs form during ongoing chronic diseases is difficult to dissect but insights to the stimuli and signaling pathways that control HEV neogenesis and function have come from experimental studies in mice. In experimental animals, organized lymphocytic infiltrates containing PNAd-expressing blood vessels develop in exocrine tissue of the pancreas and thyroid in response to ectopic expression of homeostatic chemokines and cytokines that control LN development (115–118) and virus-induced autoantibody production in the salivary gland (119). However, as found in chronic diseases, the size, location, and composition of lymphoid infiltrates that develop at ectopic sites vary depending on the stimulus. For example, when LTα is expressed in pancreatic β cells PNAd expressing blood vessels are found inside the small lymphoid infiltrates that form around some islets (120). Development is independent of endogenous LTβ and dependent on signaling *via* the type I TNFR. However, the infiltrates comprise mainly memory T cells that express low levels of L-selectin, which may be due to the predominantly abluminal expression of PNAd, which is unable to recruit L-selectin expressing lymphocytes (118). Co-expression of both LTα and LTβ and consequent LTβR signaling in the exocrine pancreas is required to develop large, organized lymphoid aggregates that contain HEV expressing PNAd at the luminal surface and, as in LNs, these ectopic TLOs are highly enriched in L-selectin-expressing T and B lymphocytes. LTαβ expressing cells other than LTis drive TLO formation, such as T and B cells which upregulate LTαβ in response to ectopic expression of CCL21 and CXCL13, respectively (116). PNAd expressing, structurally distinct HEV develop within 5 days of transferring T cells to RAG-deficient mice expressing CCL21 under the thyroglubulin promoter and, as found in LN, HEV development is dependent on LTαβ–LTβR signaling and DCs (117, 121). As in LN, the development of PNAd expressing HEV in cytokine or chemokine-induced TLOs is stunted in mice deficient in either LTα or LTβ. PNAd-expressing blood vessels lack the HEV-restricted sulfotransferase and, therefore, luminal expression of PNAd, and are lined with flat ECs typical of immature HEVs in LN unable to support high levels of lymphocyte traffic. The lack of HEV maturation in the absence of LTα or LTβ correlates with and, most likely, contributes to the reduced size and cellularity of lymphoid infiltrates in these mice (118).

The development of PNAd-expressing HEV in mouse models of cytokine- or inflammation-induced cancer correlates with increased T cell infiltration and priming and reduced tumor growth (114, 122, 123). In tumor cell transplant models, PNAd expression is induced on tumor blood vessels by infiltrating tumor-specific effector CD8$^+$ T cells as well as NK cells (124). In marked contrast to HEV development in LN and TLO, PNAd expression is not dependent on LTβR signaling but is stimulated by CD8$^+$ T and NK cell-derived LTα3 activation of TNFR. Interestingly, expression of the arrest chemokine CCL21 is not induced by the same stimuli that induce PNAd expression, but instead by IFN-γ released by activated T and NK cells. However, the tumor-associated HEVs are distinct from conventional mature HEVs in LN since PNAd expression is exceptionally low and the endothelial lining is flat, rather than the characteristic, LTβR-dependent cuboidal morphology found in LNs (50). Although comprising <10% of the tumor vascular network and lined by flat EC, these PNAd-expressing tumor blood vessels are functional in that they recruit naïve, L-selectin-expressing T cells from the bloodstream into the tumor where they are activated to kill tumor tissue (124). These findings suggest that TNFR signaling in ECs stimulates the development of PNAd-expressing blood vessels resembling immature HEVs in LNs and that these vessels promote anti-tumour immunity by recruiting naïve T cells into cancerous tissues. This allows T cell priming and reactivation inside solid cancers, thus avoiding the dilution of tumoricidal T cells during redistribution from their LN site of priming *via* the efferent lymphatics and bloodstream (123).

The presence of HEV-containing TLO is highly correlated with active disease and for persistent infections such as *H. pylori*, TLOs in the gastric mucosa disappear when the infection is cleared (125). In the case of solid, vascularized cancers, the presence of TLO in resected solid cancers has been correlated with prolonged patient outcome following resection of the primary cancer in breast cancer (126, 127), melanoma (128, 129), lung (130), and colorectal cancer, although in the latter case the correlation depends on the stage of the disease (131, 132). In separate studies of lung cancer, mature DC containing TLO enriched in CD8$^+$ effector memory T cells or expressing a LN-associated chemokine and adhesion molecule gene signature have both been correlated with improved patient outcome (133, 134). Importantly however, the formation of TLO does not always indicate improved cancer patient outcome. In virus-induced hepatic cellular carcinoma, TLOs provide a cytokine-rich niche, which promotes the development and survival of malignant hepatocyte progenitors (11). The density of HEV alone was sufficient to predict patient outcome in breast cancer and melanoma (9, 10), indicating the critical role that HEVs play in orchestrating anticancer immunity. It will be interesting to determine the expression of other markers of HEV differentiation such as MAdCAM-1, GlyCAM-1, GlcNAc6ST-2, and GlcNAc6ST-1 to further understand the precise roles of HEV development and maturation in protective immunity to clinical cancers.

Evidence of ongoing immune responses are seen inside TLOs; activation-induced cytidine deaminase is active in ectopic germinal centers in salivary glands of Sjorgren's syndrome patients (5) and T cell priming and epitope spreading occur in mouse models of multiple sclerosis and cancer (122, 135). In mice lacking all SLOs, Moyron-Quiroz and colleagues demonstrated that humoral and cellular immune responses develop in TLOs following influenza infection (136). The formation of TLO in clinical conditions may, therefore, reflect a lack of function in draining secondary LNs, which are no longer able to accept incoming antigen or antigen-presenting cells or that SLOs are operating at maximal capacity. The formation of TLOs is thought to exacerbate autoimmune diseases, at least in part, because effector lymphocytes generated within the target organ will not be diluted out during transit from the normal LN site of priming. However, the impact of TLO will depend on the nature of the ongoing immune response to the autoantigen, pathogen, or cancer antigen, which may be protective (CD8$^+$ T cells in cancer), inflammatory (Th17 cells in autoimmunity), or tolerance inducing (Foxp3$^+$ regulatory T cells), and this may be regulated by the activation status of PNAd-expressing HEVs and additional factors such as chemokines. Further studies are required to understand exactly how ectopic HEVs are formed and their impact on different types of chronic diseases. Such studies may reveal therapeutic targets for intervention in autoimmune diseases and cancers.

A Unifying Hypothesis of HEV Neogenesis

Extensive studies of SLOs and TLOs have shown that HEVs present as peripheral and/or mucosal addressin expressing blood vessels in which the endothelium is either characteristically cuboidal and filled with transmigrating lymphocytes or flat and, although PNAd-positive, lymphocyte-filled pockets are absent. Can we reconcile these divergent reports of HEV into a single, unifying model of HEV neogenesis in lymphoid and non-lymphoid tissues? Clues for this have come from studies in which cytokines ectopically expressed in pancreatic islets of mice stimulate the development of vascular addressin expressing blood vessels. Expression of LTα-induced PNAd and MAdCAM-1 on pancreatic blood vessels dependent on signaling through TNFR1 but the ECs are flat, do not express the HEV-restricted sulfotransferase (HEC-6ST/GlcNAc6ST-2) and PNAd expression was located to the basolateral EC surface where, in LN, it does not support high levels of lymphocyte recruitment. Structurally distinct, PNAd-expressing blood vessels, similar to HEVs in LN, were only formed when LTα and LTβ were co-expressed in pancreatic islets (137). Interestingly, LT-α drives the development of flat, PNAd-expressing blood vessels in mouse models of cancer which, although structurally similar to immature HEVs in LN, are able to recruit L-selectin-expressing T cells from the bloodstream *via* $PNAd^+$ ligands indicating they are not completely immature (124).

LTα and LTαβ activate the classical NF-κB pathway characterized by nuclear translocation of p50–RelA complexes. LTαβ also activates the alternative, non-canonical NF-κB pathway of NF-κB-inducing kinase (NIK)-dependent activation of IκB kinase (IKK)-α and nuclear translocation of p52–RelB complexes (138). Non-canonical NF-κB signaling plays a dominant role in the formation of HEVs in LNs since blockade of LTβR, but not TNFR, leads to loss of several HEV-specific markers such as GlyCAM-1, MAdCAM-1, CCL21, and the HEV-restricted sulfotransferase, HEC-6ST/GlcNAc6ST-2 (58). In addition, PNAd-expressing blood vessels that develop in IKKα(AA) mutant mice where non-canonical NF-κB signaling is defective lack GlyCAM-1 and HEC-6ST (49). Conversely, mice lacking full-length p100 protein, resulting in constitutively active p52, develop PNAd-positive HEVs in the spleen (139). The key event in non-canonical NF-κB activation is signal-induced protein stabilization of NIK that is normally degraded by a ubiquitin ligase complex comprising TRAF2, TRAF3, and cIAP1/2 (140, 141). LTβR ligation sequesters this NIK-targeting destruction complex leading to NIK accumulation. Importantly, signal-induced NIK stability is transient (142), suggesting that continual activation of the LTβR is required to maintain functional NIK expression levels and hence, sustain the activity of the non-canonical NF-κB pathway.

It is proposed that the development of HEVs is dissected into at least two distinct stages based on NF-κB signaling in blood vessel ECs (**Figure 2**). The first stage is driven by LTα-TNFR classical NF-κB signaling and generates MAdCAM-1-expressing HEV lined with flat, PNAd-expressing ECs. The second stage is driven by sustained LTβR non-canonical NF-κB signaling and induces the development of fully mature, PNAd-expressing HEVs lined by HECs and containing lymphocyte-filled pockets. However, these two stages may be not always be clearly delineated because there is overlap between classical and non-canonical NFκB signaling in blood ECs. For example, classical RelA/NF-κB signaling by TNFα, LTα, or LTαβ in EC cultured from human and mouse tissues induces expression of MAdCAM-1 protein and expression of the gene encoding HEC-6ST, which generates the PNAd epitope in LN HEVs (33–35, 143). However, LTβR signaling in isolated human EC has not been reported to induce the expression of PNAd modified glycoproteins (143). It is known that classical NF-κB-dependent signaling in human EC inhibits non-canonical NF-κB signaling (144). The outcome of LTβR signaling in ECs will, therefore, depend on the balance between classical and non-canonical NF-κB signaling. Recent studies have demonstrated that endothelial differentiation is regulated by components of the basal lamina (145). As in other types of postcapillary venule, structural support to the endothelial lining of HEV is provided by the basal lamina, which is known to regulate NF-κB signaling (146). Further studies on isolated blood ECs may identify the stimuli and signaling pathways that stimulate the synthesis of HEV-restricted PNAd-modified glycoproteins thereby controlling HEV neogenesis.

THERAPEUTIC STRATEGIES TO CONTROL HEV NEOGENESIS AND FUNCTION

If HEVs in TLO are critical to exacerbation of autoimmune diseases by allowing activation of tissue destroying lymphocytes within target tissues, can the development of HEVs be prevented? Since HEVs in SLOs are important for generating protective immunity to infection any such therapy would need to be targeted to TLO. Intuitively, this will require the identification of markers or signaling pathways in ectopic HEVs that are not shared by HEVs in LN. One candidate is TNFR signaling that is not required for the development or maintenance of HEVs in LN (58) but has been shown to induce PNAd-expressing ectopic HEVs able to recruit naïve T lymphocytes, at least in cancer (124). It is possible that the success of anti-TNF-α or TNFRII-Ig (Etanercept) therapies in rheumatoid arthritis patients may depend, in part, on reversing or blocking blood vessel differentiation toward an HEV-like phenotype. The formation of HEVs in cancerous tissues in the absence of TLO correlates with reduced tumor progression in experimental animals; HEV neogenesis may, therefore, be a possible therapy to control cancer growth but it is not clear how this would be achieved. Clinical and experimental data indicate that tumor blood vessels are poor at recruiting cytotoxic, effector T lymphocytes and present an immune checkpoint that limits effective immunotherapy (147). Several different strategies are being considered to achieve this including targeted delivery of TNF-α to tumor blood vessels, which may induce the development of PNAd-expressing blood vessels although this was not determined (148). Approaches to induce HEV-containing TLO formation in cancers are also being considered but it is worth bearing in mind that TLOs, like SLOs, could be sites of tolerance induction and, therefore, may limit effective antitumor immunity. The full impact of HEVs and/or TLO may only be revealed when

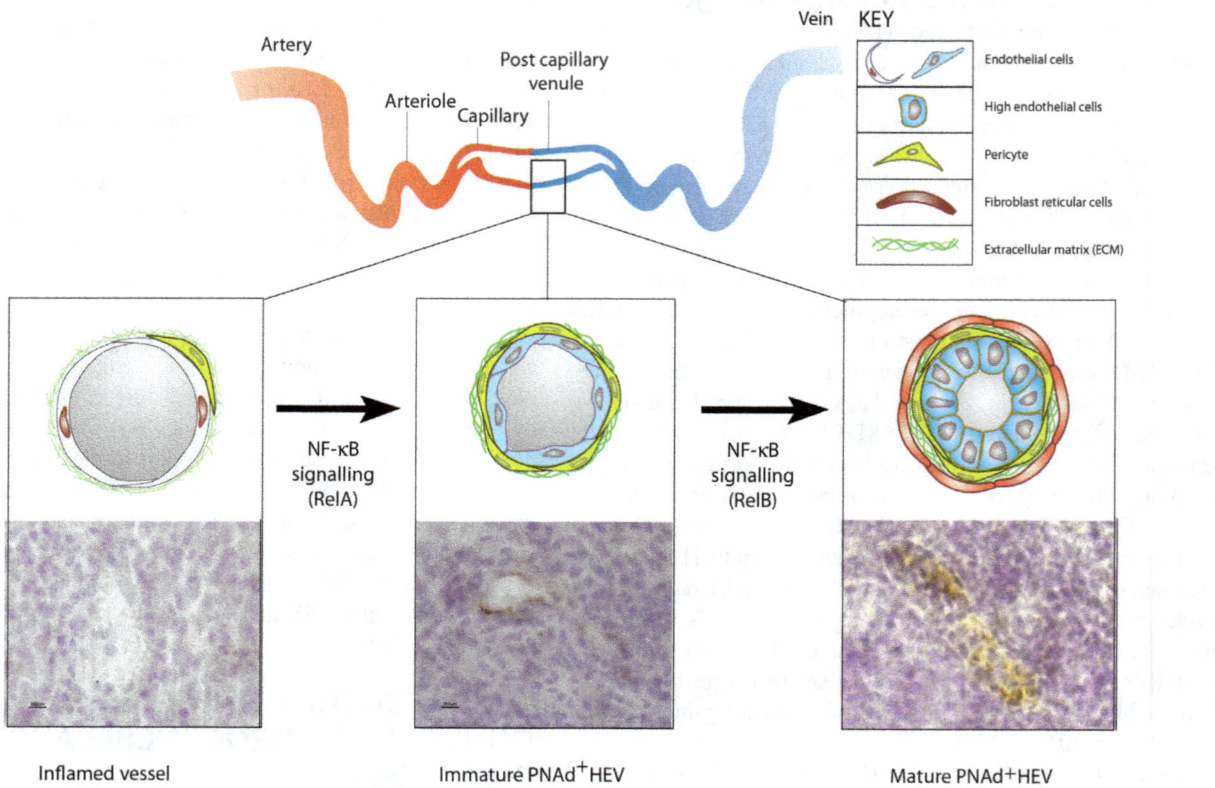

FIGURE 2 | The development of ectopic high endothelial venules (HEVs). Top: diagrammatic representation of blood vasculature in non-lymphoid organs and the location of postcapillary venules. Bottom (left): blood vessels in acutely inflamed tissues do not express vascular addressins but are able to recruit activated lymphoid cells. (Middle) TNFα, LTα, or LTαβ expressing T or NK cells recruited by inflamed blood vessels induce the expression of peripheral node addressin (PNAd) (and/or MAdCAM-1) in blood vessels lined with flat endothelial cells (ECs) by stimulating classical NF-κB (RelA) signaling in ECs. (Right) Sustained contact between LTαβ expressing activated lymphoid cells and PNAd expressing flat EC induces LTβR-dependent non-canonical NF-κB (RelB) signaling in ECs, which allows the full maturation of PNAd-expressing HEV lined with cuboidal ECs filled with transmigrating lymphocytes. It is not known if the recruitment of fibroblast reticular cells into the perivascular sheath surrounding HEV is driven by LTβR signaling in ECs or perivascular cells or both.

highly immunosuppressive cells such as Foxp3+ Tregs or myeloid-derived suppressor cells are depleted allowing effector T cells to exit TLO, infiltrate, and kill cancerous tissues (114, 149, 150). It will be important to determine which immune cells are recruited by cancer-associated HEVs to dissect their impact on cancer immunity. Further studies are required to determine the extent and role of HEV development in clinical cancers.

AUTHOR CONTRIBUTIONS

The author confirms being the sole contributor of this work and approved it for publication.

ACKNOWLEDGMENTS

I thank Mike May, Mark Coles, Jens Stein, Diana Costa Bento, and Emily Colbeck for stimulating discussions about HEV; Julia Ohme for images of vascular addressin expression; and Janice Sharp for the figures.

FUNDING

AA is supported by project grants from the Wellcome Trust (094511/Z/10/Z) and the Medical Research Council UK (MR/L008742/1).

REFERENCES

1. Masopust D, Schenkel JM. The integration of T cell migration, differentiation and function. *Nat Rev Immunol* (2013) 13(5):309–20. doi:10.1038/nri3442
2. Fletcher AL, Malhotra D, Turley SJ. Lymph node stroma broaden the peripheral tolerance paradigm. *Trends Immunol* (2011) 32(1):12–8. doi:10.1016/j.it.2010.11.002
3. Girard JP, Moussion C, Forster R. HEVs, lymphatics and homeostatic immune cell trafficking in lymph nodes. *Nat Rev Immunol* (2012) 12(11):762–73. doi:10.1038/nri3298
4. Drayton DL, Liao S, Mounzer RH, Ruddle NH. Lymphoid organ development: from ontogeny to neogenesis. *Nat Immunol* (2006) 7(4):344–53. doi:10.1038/ni1330
5. Bombardieri M, Barone F, Humby F, Kelly S, McGurk M, Morgan P, et al. Activation-induced cytidine deaminase expression in follicular dendritic cell

networks and interfollicular large B cells supports functionality of ectopic lymphoid neogenesis in autoimmune sialoadenitis and MALT lymphoma in Sjogren's syndrome. *J Immunol* (2007) 179(7):4929–38. doi:10.4049/jimmunol.179.7.4929

6. Astorri E, Bombardieri M, Gabba S, Peakman M, Pozzilli P, Pitzalis C. Evolution of ectopic lymphoid neogenesis and in situ autoantibody production in autoimmune nonobese diabetic mice: cellular and molecular characterization of tertiary lymphoid structures in pancreatic islets. *J Immunol* (2010) 185(6):3359–68. doi:10.4049/jimmunol.1001836
7. Lee Y, Chin RK, Christiansen P, Sun Y, Tumanov AV, Wang J, et al. Recruitment and activation of naive T cells in the islets by lymphotoxin beta receptor-dependent tertiary lymphoid structure. *Immunity* (2006) 25(3):499–509. doi:10.1016/j.immuni.2006.06.016
8. Sautes-Fridman C, Lawand M, Giraldo NA, Kaplon H, Germain C, Fridman WH, et al. Tertiary lymphoid structures in cancers: prognostic value, regulation, and manipulation for therapeutic intervention. *Front Immunol* (2016) 7:407. doi:10.3389/fimmu.2016.00407
9. Martinet L, Garrido I, Filleron T, Le Guellec S, Bellard E, Fournie JJ, et al. Human solid tumors contain high endothelial venules: association with T- and B-lymphocyte infiltration and favorable prognosis in breast cancer. *Cancer Res* (2011) 71(17):5678–87. doi:10.1158/0008-5472.CAN-11-0431
10. Martinet L, Le Guellec S, Filleron T, Lamant L, Meyer N, Rochaix P, et al. High endothelial venules (HEVs) in human melanoma lesions: major gateways for tumor-infiltrating lymphocytes. *Oncoimmunology* (2012) 1(6):829–39. doi:10.4161/onci.20492
11. Finkin S, Yuan D, Stein I, Taniguchi K, Weber A, Unger K, et al. Ectopic lymphoid structures function as microniches for tumor progenitor cells in hepatocellular carcinoma. *Nat Immunol* (2015) 16(12):1235–44. doi:10.1038/ni.3290
12. Wotherspoon AC, Doglioni C, Diss TC, Pan L, Moschini A, de Boni M, et al. Regression of primary low-grade B-cell gastric lymphoma of mucosa-associated lymphoid tissue type after eradication of *Helicobacter pylori*. *Lancet* (1993) 342(8871):575–7. doi:10.1016/0140-6736(93)91409-F
13. Kobayashi M, Lee H, Schaffer L, Gilmartin TJ, Head SR, Takaishi S, et al. A distinctive set of genes is upregulated during the inflammation-carcinoma sequence in mouse stomach infected by *Helicobacter felis*. *J Histochem Cytochem* (2007) 55(3):263–74. doi:10.1369/jhc.6A7097.2006
14. van de Pavert SA, Mebius RE. New insights into the development of lymphoid tissues. *Nat Rev Immunol* (2010) 10(9):664–74. doi:10.1038/nri2832
15. Randall TD, Carragher DM, Rangel-Moreno J. Development of secondary lymphoid organs. *Annu Rev Immunol* (2008) 26:627–50. doi:10.1146/annurev.immunol.26.021607.090257
16. Blum KS, Pabst R. Keystones in lymph node development. *J Anat* (2006) 209(5):585–95. doi:10.1111/j.1469-7580.2006.00650.x
17. Peduto L, Dulauroy S, Lochner M, Spath GF, Morales MA, Cumano A, et al. Inflammation recapitulates the ontogeny of lymphoid stromal cells. *J Immunol* (2009) 182(9):5789–99. doi:10.4049/jimmunol.0803974
18. Hendricks HR, Eestermans IL. Disappearance and reappearance of high endothelial venules and immigrating lymphocytes in lymph nodes deprived of afferent lymphatic vessels: a possible regulatory role of macrophages in lymphocyte migration. *Eur J Immunol* (1983) 13:663–9. doi:10.1002/eji.1830130811
19. Mebius RE, Streeter PR, Breve J, Duijvestijn AM, Kraal G. The influence of afferent lymphatic vessel interruption on vascular addressin expression. *J Cell Biol* (1991) 115(1):85–95. doi:10.1083/jcb.115.1.85
20. Lacorre DA, Baekkevold ES, Garrido I, Brandtzaeg P, Haraldsen G, Amalric F, et al. Plasticity of endothelial cells: rapid dedifferentiation of freshly isolated high endothelial venule endothelial cells outside the lymphoid tissue microenvironment. *Blood* (2004) 103(11):4164–72. doi:10.1182/blood-2003-10-3537
21. Mebius RE, Streeter PR, Michie S, Butcher EC, Weissman IL. A developmental switch in lymphocyte homing receptor and endothelial vascular addressin expression regulates lymphocyte homing and permits CD4+ CD3- cells to colonize lymph nodes. *Proc Natl Acad Sci U S A* (1996) 93(20):11019–24. doi:10.1073/pnas.93.20.11019
22. Mebius RE. Organogenesis of lymphoid tissues. *Nat Rev Immunol* (2003) 3(4):292–303. doi:10.1038/nri1054
23. Zhang Z, Li J, Zheng W, Zhao G, Zhang H, Wang X, et al. Peripheral lymphoid volume expansion and maintenance are controlled by gut microbiota via RALDH+ dendritic cells. *Immunity* (2016) 44(2):330–42. doi:10.1016/j.immuni.2016.01.004
24. Moussion C, Girard JP. Dendritic cells control lymphocyte entry to lymph nodes through high endothelial venules. *Nature* (2011) 479(7374):542–6. doi:10.1038/nature10540
25. Wigle JT, Oliver G. Prox1 function is required for the development of the murine lymphatic system. *Cell* (1999) 98(6):769–78. doi:10.1016/S0092-8674(00)81511-1
26. Mebius RE, Rennert P, Weissman IL. Developing lymph nodes collect CD4+CD3- LTbeta+ cells that can differentiate to APC, NK cells, and follicular cells but not T or B cells. *Immunity* (1997) 7(4):493–504. doi:10.1016/S1074-7613(00)80371-4
27. Veiga-Fernandes H, Coles MC, Foster KE, Patel A, Williams A, Natarajan D, et al. Tyrosine kinase receptor RET is a key regulator of Peyer's patch organogenesis. *Nature* (2007) 446(7135):547–51. doi:10.1038/nature05597
28. Hashi H, Yoshida H, Honda K, Fraser S, Kubo H, Awane M, et al. Compartmentalization of Peyer's patch anlagen before lymphocyte entry. *J Immunol* (2001) 166(6):3702–9. doi:10.4049/jimmunol.166.6.3702
29. Gretz JE, Norbury CC, Anderson AO, Proudfoot AE, Shaw S. Lymph-borne chemokines and other low molecular weight molecules reach high endothelial venules via specialized conduits while a functional barrier limits access to the lymphocyte microenvironments in lymph node cortex. *J Exp Med* (2000) 192(10):1425–40. doi:10.1084/jem.192.10.1425
30. Pruenster M, Mudde L, Bombosi P, Dimitrova S, Zsak M, Middleton J, et al. The Duffy antigen receptor for chemokines transports chemokines and supports their promigratory activity. *Nat Immunol* (2009) 10(1):101–8. doi:10.1038/ni.1675
31. Palframan RT, Jung S, Cheng CY, Weninger W, Luo Y, Dorf M, et al. Inflammatory chemokine transport and presentation in HEV: a remote control mechanism for monocyte recruitment to lymph nodes in inflamed tissues. *J Exp Med* (2001) 194(9):1361–73. doi:10.1084/jem.194.9.1361
32. Baekkevold ES, Yamanaka T, Palframan RT, Carlsen HS, Reinholt FP, von Andrian UH, et al. The CCR7 ligand ELC (CCL19) is transcytosed in high endothelial venules and mediates T cell recruitment. *J Exp Med* (2001) 193(9):1105–12. doi:10.1084/jem.193.9.1105
33. Sikorski EE, Hallmann R, Berg EL, Butcher EC. The Peyer's patch high endothelial receptor for lymphocytes, the mucosal vascular addressin, is induced on a murine endothelial cell line by tumor necrosis factor-alpha and IL-1. *J Immunol* (1993) 151(10):5239–50.
34. Takeuchi M, Baichwal VR. Induction of the gene encoding mucosal vascular addressin cell adhesion molecule 1 by tumor necrosis factor alpha is mediated by NF-kappa B proteins. *Proc Natl Acad Sci U S A* (1995) 92(8):3561–5. doi:10.1073/pnas.92.8.3561
35. Cuff CA, Schwartz J, Bergman CM, Russell KS, Bender JR, Ruddle NH. Lymphotoxin alpha3 induces chemokines and adhesion molecules: insight into the role of LT alpha in inflammation and lymphoid organ development. *J Immunol* (1998) 161(12):6853–60.
36. Pabst O, Forster R, Lipp M, Engel H, Arnold HH. NKX2.3 is required for MAdCAM-1 expression and homing of lymphocytes in spleen and mucosa-associated lymphoid tissue. *EMBO J* (2000) 19(9):2015–23. doi:10.1093/emboj/19.9.2015
37. Schippers A, Leuker C, Pabst O, Kochut A, Prochnow B, Gruber AD, et al. Mucosal addressin cell-adhesion molecule-1 controls plasma-cell migration and function in the small intestine of mice. *Gastroenterology* (2009) 137(3):924–33. doi:10.1053/j.gastro.2009.05.039
38. Gurtner GC, Davis V, Li H, McCoy MJ, Sharpe A, Cybulsky MI. Targeted disruption of the murine VCAM1 gene: essential role of VCAM-1 in chorioallantoic fusion and placentation. *Genes Dev* (1995) 9(1):1–14. doi:10.1101/gad.9.1.1
39. Xu H, Gonzalo JA, St Pierre Y, Williams IR, Kupper TS, Cotran RS, et al. Leukocytosis and resistance to septic shock in intercellular adhesion molecule 1-deficient mice. *J Exp Med* (1994) 180(1):95–109. doi:10.1084/jem.180.1.95
40. De Togni P, Goellner J, Ruddle NH, Streeter PR, Fick A, Mariathasan S, et al. Abnormal development of peripheral lymphoid organs in mice deficient in lymphotoxin. *Science* (1994) 264(5159):703–7. doi:10.1126/science.8171322

41. Rennert PD, James D, Mackay F, Browning JL, Hochman PS. Lymph node genesis is induced by signaling through the lymphotoxin beta receptor. *Immunity* (1998) 9(1):71–9. doi:10.1016/S1074-7613(00)80589-0
42. Rennert PD, Browning JL, Mebius R, Mackay F, Hochman PS. Surface lymphotoxin alpha/beta complex is required for the development of peripheral lymphoid organs. *J Exp Med* (1996) 184(5):1999–2006. doi:10.1084/jem.184.5.1999
43. Lai L, Bohnsack BL, Niederreither K, Hirschi KK. Retinoic acid regulates endothelial cell proliferation during vasculogenesis. *Development* (2003) 130(26):6465–74. doi:10.1242/dev.00887
44. Rennert PD, Browning JL, Hochman PS. Selective disruption of lymphotoxin ligands reveals a novel set of mucosal lymph nodes and unique effects on lymph node cellular organization. *Int Immunol* (1997) 9(11):1627–39. doi:10.1093/intimm/9.11.1627
45. May MJ, Ghosh S. Signal transduction through NF-kappa B. *Immunol Today* (1998) 19(2):80–8. doi:10.1016/S0167-5699(97)01197-3
46. Alcamo E, Hacohen N, Schulte LC, Rennert PD, Hynes RO, Baltimore D. Requirement for the NF-kappaB family member RelA in the development of secondary lymphoid organs. *J Exp Med* (2002) 195(2):233–44. doi:10.1084/jem.20011885
47. Weih F, Carrasco D, Durham SK, Barton DS, Rizzo CA, Ryseck RP, et al. Multiorgan inflammation and hematopoietic abnormalities in mice with a targeted disruption of RelB, a member of the NF-kappa B/Rel family. *Cell* (1995) 80(2):331–40. doi:10.1016/0092-8674(95)90416-6
48. Carragher D, Johal R, Button A, White A, Eliopoulos A, Jenkinson E, et al. A stroma-derived defect in NF-kappaB2-/- mice causes impaired lymph node development and lymphocyte recruitment. *J Immunol* (2004) 173(4):2271–9. doi:10.4049/jimmunol.173.4.2271
49. Drayton DL, Bonizzi G, Ying X, Liao S, Karin M, Ruddle NH. I kappa B kinase complex alpha kinase activity controls chemokine and high endothelial venule gene expression in lymph nodes and nasal-associated lymphoid tissue. *J Immunol* (2004) 173(10):6161–8. doi:10.4049/jimmunol.173.10.6161
50. Onder L, Danuser R, Scandella E, Firner S, Chai Q, Hehlgans T, et al. Endothelial cell-specific lymphotoxin-beta receptor signaling is critical for lymph node and high endothelial venule formation. *J Exp Med* (2013) 210(3):465–73. doi:10.1084/jem.20121462
51. Rosen SD. Ligands for L-selectin: homing, inflammation, and beyond. *Annu Rev Immunol* (2004) 22:129–56. doi:10.1146/annurev.immunol.21.090501.080131
52. Mitoma J, Bao X, Petryanik B, Schaerli P, Gauguet JM, Yu SY, et al. Critical functions of N-glycans in L-selectin-mediated lymphocyte homing and recruitment. *Nat Immunol* (2007) 8(4):409–18. doi:10.1038/ni1442
53. Streeter PR, Rouse BT, Butcher EC. Immunohistologic and functional characterization of a vascular addressin involved in lymphocyte homing into peripheral lymph nodes. *J Cell Biol* (1988) 107(5):1853–62. doi:10.1083/jcb.107.5.1853
54. Streeter PR, Berg EL, Rouse BT, Bargatze RF, Butcher EC. A tissue-specific endothelial cell molecule involved in lymphocyte homing. *Nature* (1988) 331(6151):41–6. doi:10.1038/331041a0
55. Kellermayer Z, Labadi A, Czompoly T, Arnold HH, Balogh P. Absence of Nkx2-3 homeodomain transcription factor induces the formation of LYVE-1-positive endothelial cysts without lymphatic commitment in the spleen. *J Histochem Cytochem* (2011) 59(7):690–700. doi:10.1369/0022155411410061
56. Anderson AO, Shaw S. T cell adhesion to endothelium: the FRC conduit system and other anatomic and molecular features which facilitate the adhesion cascade in lymph node. *Semin Immunol* (1993) 5(4):271–82. doi:10.1006/smim.1993.1031
57. Swarte VV, Joziasse DH, Van den Eijnden DH, Petryniak B, Lowe JB, Kraal G, et al. Regulation of fucosyltransferase-VII expression in peripheral lymph node high endothelial venules. *Eur J Immunol* (1998) 28(10):3040–7. doi:10.1002/(SICI)1521-4141(199810)28:10<3040::AID-IMMU3040>3.0.CO;2-5
58. Browning JL, Allaire N, Ngam-Ek A, Notidis E, Hunt J, Perrin S, et al. Lymphotoxin-beta receptor signaling is required for the homeostatic control of HEV differentiation and function. *Immunity* (2005) 23(5):539–50. doi:10.1016/j.immuni.2005.10.002
59. Lindquist RL, Shakhar G, Dudziak D, Wardemann H, Eisenreich T, Dustin ML, et al. Visualizing dendritic cell networks in vivo. *Nat Immunol* (2004) 5(12):1243–50. doi:10.1038/ni1139
60. Kissenpfennig A, Henri S, Dubois B, Laplace-Builhe C, Perrin P, Romani N, et al. Dynamics and function of Langerhans cells in vivo: dermal dendritic cells colonize lymph node areas distinct from slower migrating Langerhans cells. *Immunity* (2005) 22(5):643–54. doi:10.1016/j.immuni.2005.04.004
61. Bajenoff M, Granjeaud S, Guerder S. The strategy of T cell antigen-presenting cell encounter in antigen-draining lymph nodes revealed by imaging of initial T cell activation. *J Exp Med* (2003) 198(5):715–24. doi:10.1084/jem.20030167
62. Randolph GJ, Ochando J, Partida-Sanchez S. Migration of dendritic cell subsets and their precursors. *Annu Rev Immunol* (2008) 26:293–316. doi:10.1146/annurev.immunol.26.021607.090254
63. Choi JH, Do Y, Cheong C, Koh H, Boscardin SB, Oh YS, et al. Identification of antigen-presenting dendritic cells in mouse aorta and cardiac valves. *J Exp Med* (2009) 206(3):497–505. doi:10.1084/jem.20082129
64. Wendland M, Willenzon S, Kocks J, Davalos-Misslitz AC, Hammerschmidt SI, Schumann K, et al. Lymph node T cell homeostasis relies on steady state homing of dendritic cells. *Immunity* (2011) 35(6):945–57. doi:10.1016/j.immuni.2011.10.017
65. Chyou S, Ekland EH, Carpenter AC, Tzeng TC, Tian S, Michaud M, et al. Fibroblast-type reticular stromal cells regulate the lymph node vasculature. *J Immunol* (2008) 181(6):3887–96. doi:10.4049/jimmunol.181.6.3887
66. Webster B, Ekland EH, Agle LM, Chyou S, Ruggieri R, Lu TT. Regulation of lymph node vascular growth by dendritic cells. *J Exp Med* (2006) 203(8):1903–13. doi:10.1084/jem.20052272
67. Ley K, Laudanna C, Cybulsky MI, Nourshargh S. Getting to the site of inflammation: the leukocyte adhesion cascade updated. *Nat Rev Immunol* (2007) 7(9):678–89. doi:10.1038/nri2156
68. Steiniger B, Timphus EM, Barth PJ. The splenic marginal zone in humans and rodents: an enigmatic compartment and its inhabitants. *Histochem Cell Biol* (2006) 126(6):641–8. doi:10.1007/s00418-006-0210-5
69. Lee M, Kiefel H, LaJevic MD, Macauley MS, Kawashima H, O'Hara E, et al. Transcriptional programs of lymphoid tissue capillary and high endothelium reveal control mechanisms for lymphocyte homing. *Nat Immunol* (2014) 15(10):982–95. doi:10.1038/ni.2983
70. Warnock RA, Askari S, Butcher EC, von Andrian UH. Molecular mechanisms of lymphocyte homing to peripheral lymph nodes. *J Exp Med* (1998) 187(2):205–16. doi:10.1084/jem.187.2.205
71. M'Rini C, Cheng G, Schweitzer C, Cavanagh LL, Palframan RT, Mempel TR, et al. A novel endothelial L-selectin ligand activity in lymph node medulla that is regulated by alpha(1,3)-fucosyltransferase-IV.[see comment]. *J Exp Med* (2003) 198(9):1301–12. doi:10.1084/jem.20030182
72. Picker LJ, Butcher EC. Physiological and molecular mechanisms of lymphocyte homing. *Annu Rev Immunol* (1992) 10:561–91. doi:10.1146/annurev.iy.10.040192.003021
73. Gauguet JM, Bonaiso R, von Andrian UH. High endothelial venules. In: Aird WC, editor. *Endothelial BioMedcine*. New York, NY: Cambridge University Press (2007). p. 1568–88.
74. Ager A, Coles MC, Stein JV. Development of lymph node circulation and homing mechanisms. In: Balogh P, editor. *Developmental Biology of Lymphoid Organs*. Berlin: Springer-Verlag (2010). p. 75–94.
75. Michie SA, Streeter PR, Bolt PA, Butcher EC, Picker LJ. The human peripheral lymph node vascular addressin. An inducible endothelial antigen involved in lymphocyte homing. *Am J Pathol* (1993) 143(6):1688–98.
76. Abitorabi MA, Mackay CR, Jerome EH, Osorio O, Butcher EC, Erle DJ. Differential expression of homing molecules on recirculating lymphocytes from sheep gut, peripheral, and lung lymph. *J Immunol* (1996) 156(9):3111–7.
77. Briskin M, Winsor-Hines D, Shyjan A, Cochran N, Bloom S, Wilson J, et al. Human mucosal addressin cell adhesion molecule-1 is preferentially expressed in intestinal tract and associated lymphoid tissue. *Am J Pathol* (1997) 151(1):97–110.
78. Pullen N, Molloy E, Carter D, Syntin P, Clemo F, Finco-Kent D, et al. Pharmacological characterization of PF-00547659, an anti-human MAdCAM monoclonal antibody. *Br J Pharmacol* (2009) 157(2):281–93. doi:10.1111/j.1476-5381.2009.00137.x

79. Salmi M, Alanen K, Grenman S, Briskin M, Butcher EC, Jalkanen S. Immune cell trafficking in uterus and early life is dominated by the mucosal addressin MAdCAM-1 in humans. *Gastroenterology* (2001) 121(4):853–64. doi:10.1053/gast.2001.27968
80. Arbones ML, Ord DC, Ley K, Ratech H, Maynard-Curry C, Otten G, et al. Lymphocyte homing and leukocyte rolling and migration are impaired in L-selectin-deficient mice. *Immunity* (1994) 1(4):247–60. doi:10.1016/1074-7613(94)90076-0
81. Fossum S, Smith ME, Ford WL. The migration of lymphocytes across specialized vascular endothelium VII. The migration of T and B lymphocytes from the blood of the athymic, nude rat. *Scand J Immunol* (1983) 17(6):539–50. doi:10.1111/j.1365-3083.1983.tb00822.x
82. Bajenoff M, Egen JG, Koo LY, Laugier JP, Brau F, Glaichenhaus N, et al. Stromal cell networks regulate lymphocyte entry, migration, and territoriality in lymph nodes. *Immunity* (2006) 25(6):989–1001. doi:10.1016/j.immuni.2006.10.011
83. Boscacci RT, Pfeiffer F, Gollmer K, Sevilla AI, Martin AM, Soriano SF, et al. Comprehensive analysis of lymph node stroma-expressed Ig superfamily members reveals redundant and nonredundant roles for ICAM-1, ICAM-2, and VCAM-1 in lymphocyte homing. *Blood* (2010) 116(6):915–25. doi:10.1182/blood-2009-11-254334
84. Schoefl GI. The migration of lymphocytes across the vascular endothelium in lymphoid tissue. A reexamination. *J Exp Med* (1972) 136(3):568–88. doi:10.1084/jem.136.3.568
85. Engelhardt B, Wolburg H. Mini-review: transendothelial migration of leukocytes: through the front door or around the side of the house? *Eur J Immunol* (2004) 34(11):2955–63. doi:10.1002/eji.200425327
86. Mionnet C, Sanos SL, Mondor I, Jorquera A, Laugier JP, Germain RN, et al. High endothelial venules as traffic control points maintaining lymphocyte population homeostasis in lymph nodes. *Blood* (2011) 118(23):6115–22. doi:10.1182/blood-2011-07-367409
87. Faveeuw C, Preece G, Ager A. Transendothelial migration of lymphocytes across high endothelial venules into lymph nodes is affected by metalloproteinases. *Blood* (2001) 98(3):688–95. doi:10.1182/blood.V98.3.688
88. Sainte-Marie G, Peng FS. Dilatation of high endothelial venules in compartments of rat lymph nodes with abundant cortical mast cells. *J Anat* (1991) 174:163–70.
89. Belisle C, Sainte-Marie G. The narrowing of high endothelial venules of the rat lymph node. *Anat Rec* (1985) 211(2):184–91. doi:10.1002/ar.1092110210
90. Campbell FR. Intercellular contacts of lymphocytes during migration across high-endothelial venules of lymph nodes. An electron microscopic study. *Anat Rec* (1983) 207(4):643–52. doi:10.1002/ar.1092070413
91. Barreiro O, Yanez-Mo M, Serrador JM, Montoya MC, Vicente-Manzanares M, Tejedor R, et al. Dynamic interaction of VCAM-1 and ICAM-1 with moesin and ezrin in a novel endothelial docking structure for adherent leukocytes. *J Cell Biol* (2002) 157(7):1233–45. doi:10.1083/jcb.200112126
92. Carman CV, Springer TA. A transmigratory cup in leukocyte diapedesis both through individual vascular endothelial cells and between them. *J Cell Biol* (2004) 167(2):377–88. doi:10.1083/jcb.200404129
93. Pfeiffer F, Kumar V, Butz S, Vestweber D, Imhof BA, Stein JV, et al. Distinct molecular composition of blood and lymphatic vascular endothelial cell junctions establishes specific functional barriers within the peripheral lymph node. *Eur J Immunol* (2008) 38(8):2142–55. doi:10.1002/eji.200838140
94. Ager A, May MJ. Understanding high endothelial venules: lessons for cancer immunology. *Oncoimmunology* (2015) 4(6):e1008791. doi:10.1080/2162402X.2015.1008791
95. Halin C, Scimone ML, Bonasio R, Gauguet JM, Mempel TR, Quackenbush E, et al. The S1P-analog FTY720 differentially modulates T-cell homing via HEV: T-cell-expressed S1P1 amplifies integrin activation in peripheral lymph nodes but not in Peyer patches. *Blood* (2005) 106(4):1314–22. doi:10.1182/blood-2004-09-3687
96. Hourihan H, Allen TD, Ager A. Lymphocyte migration across high endothelium is associated with increases in alpha 4 beta 1 integrin (VLA-4) affinity. *J Cell Sci* (1993) 104(Pt 4):1049–59.
97. Klinger A, Gebert A, Bieber K, Kalies K, Ager A, Bell EB, et al. Cyclical expression of L-selectin (CD62L) by recirculating T cells. *Int Immunol* (2009) 21(4):443–55. doi:10.1093/intimm/dxp012
98. Galkina E, Tanousis K, Preece G, Tolaini M, Kioussis D, Florey O, et al. L-selectin shedding does not regulate constitutive T cell trafficking but controls the migration pathways of antigen-activated T lymphocytes. *J Exp Med* (2003) 198(9):1323–35. doi:10.1084/jem.20030485
99. Rzeniewicz K, Newe A, Rey Gallardo A, Davies J, Holt MR, Patel A, et al. L-selectin shedding is activated specifically within transmigrating pseudopods of monocytes to regulate cell polarity in vitro. *Proc Natl Acad Sci U S A* (2015) 112(12):E1461–70. doi:10.1073/pnas.1417100112
100. Hickey MJ, Forster M, Mitchell D, Kaur J, De Caigny C, Kubes P. L-selectin facilitates emigration and extravascular locomotion of leukocytes during acute inflammatory responses in vivo. *J Immunol* (2000) 165(12):7164–70. doi:10.4049/jimmunol.165.12.7164
101. Bai Z, Cai L, Umemoto E, Takeda A, Tohya K, Komai Y, et al. Constitutive lymphocyte transmigration across the basal lamina of high endothelial venules is regulated by the autotaxin/lysophosphatidic acid axis. *J Immunol* (2013) 190(5):2036–48. doi:10.4049/jimmunol.1202025
102. Kanda H, Newton R, Klein R, Morita Y, Gunn MD, Rosen SD. Autotaxin, an ectoenzyme that produces lysophosphatidic acid, promotes the entry of lymphocytes into secondary lymphoid organs. *Nat Immunol* (2008) 9(4):415–23. doi:10.1038/ni1573
103. Soderberg KA, Payne GW, Sato A, Medzhitov R, Segal SS, Iwasaki A. Innate control of adaptive immunity via remodeling of lymph node feed arteriole. *Proc Natl Acad Sci U S A* (2005) 102(45):16315–20. doi:10.1073/pnas.0506190102
104. Hay JB, Hobbs BB. The flow of blood to lymph nodes and its relation to lymphocyte traffic and the immune response. *J Exp Med* (1977) 145(1):31–44. doi:10.1084/jem.145.1.31
105. Kumar V, Scandella E, Danuser R, Onder L, Nitschke M, Fukui Y, et al. Global lymphoid tissue remodeling during a viral infection is orchestrated by a B cell-lymphotoxin-dependent pathway. *Blood* (2010) 115(23):4725–33. doi:10.1182/blood-2009-10-250118
106. Chyou S, Benahmed F, Chen J, Kumar V, Tian S, Lipp M, et al. Coordinated regulation of lymph node vascular-stromal growth first by CD11c+ cells and then by T and B cells. *J Immunol* (2011) 187(11):5558–67. doi:10.4049/jimmunol.1101724
107. Liao S, Ruddle NH. Synchrony of high endothelial venules and lymphatic vessels revealed by immunization. *J Immunol* (2006) 177(5):3369–79. doi:10.4049/jimmunol.177.5.3369
108. Sawa S, Cherrier M, Lochner M, Satoh-Takayama N, Fehling HJ, Langa F, et al. Lineage relationship analysis of RORgammat+ innate lymphoid cells. *Science* (2010) 330(6004):665–9. doi:10.1126/science.1194597
109. Scandella E, Bolinger B, Lattmann E, Miller S, Favre S, Littman DR, et al. Restoration of lymphoid organ integrity through the interaction of lymphoid tissue-inducer cells with stroma of the T cell zone. *Nat Immunol* (2008) 9(6):667–75. doi:10.1038/ni.1605
110. Mueller SN, Hosiawa-Meagher KA, Konieczny BT, Sullivan BM, Bachmann MF, Locksley RM, et al. Regulation of homeostatic chemokine expression and cell trafficking during immune responses. *Science* (2007) 317(5838):670–4. doi:10.1126/science.1144830
111. Tzeng TC, Chyou S, Tian S, Webster B, Carpenter AC, Guaiquil VH, et al. CD11c(hi) dendritic cells regulate the re-establishment of vascular quiescence and stabilization after immune stimulation of lymph nodes. *J Immunol* (2010) 184(8):4247–57. doi:10.4049/jimmunol.0902914
112. Pitzalis C, Jones GW, Bombardieri M, Jones SA. Ectopic lymphoid-like structures in infection, cancer and autoimmunity. *Nat Rev Immunol* (2014) 14(7):447–62. doi:10.1038/nri3700
113. Cipponi A, Mercier M, Seremet T, Baurain JF, Theate I, van den Oord J, et al. Neogenesis of lymphoid structures and antibody responses occur in human melanoma metastases. *Cancer Res* (2012) 72(16):3997–4007. doi:10.1158/0008-5472.CAN-12-1377
114. Hindley JP, Jones E, Smart K, Bridgeman H, Lauder SN, Ondondo B, et al. T-cell trafficking facilitated by high endothelial venules is required for tumor control after regulatory T-cell depletion. *Cancer Res* (2012) 72(21):5473–82. doi:10.1158/0008-5472.CAN-12-1912
115. Luther SA, Lopez T, Bai W, Hanahan D, Cyster JG. BLC expression in pancreatic islets causes B cell recruitment and lymphotoxin-dependent lymphoid neogenesis. *Immunity* (2000) 12(5):471–81. doi:10.1016/S1074-7613(00)80199-5

116. Luther SA, Bidgol A, Hargreaves DC, Schmidt A, Xu Y, Paniyadi J, et al. Differing activities of homeostatic chemokines CCL19, CCL21, and CXCL12 in lymphocyte and dendritic cell recruitment and lymphoid neogenesis. *J Immunol* (2002) 169(1):424–33. doi:10.4049/jimmunol.169.1.424
117. Martin AP, Coronel EC, Sano G, Chen SC, Vassileva G, Canasto-Chibuque C, et al. A novel model for lymphocytic infiltration of the thyroid gland generated by transgenic expression of the CC chemokine CCL21. *J Immunol* (2004) 173(8):4791–8. doi:10.4049/jimmunol.173.8.4791
118. Drayton DL, Ying X, Lee J, Lesslauer W, Ruddle NH. Ectopic LT alpha beta directs lymphoid organ neogenesis with concomitant expression of peripheral node addressin and a HEV-restricted sulfotransferase. *J Exp Med* (2003) 197(9):1153–63. doi:10.1084/jem.20021761
119. Barone F, Nayar S, Campos J, Cloake T, Withers DR, Toellner KM, et al. IL-22 regulates lymphoid chemokine production and assembly of tertiary lymphoid organs. *Proc Natl Acad Sci U S A* (2015) 112(35):11024–9. doi:10.1073/pnas.1503315112
120. Sacca R, Cuff CA, Lesslauer W, Ruddle NH. Differential activities of secreted lymphotoxin-alpha3 and membrane lymphotoxin-alpha1beta2 in lymphotoxin-induced inflammation: critical role of TNF receptor 1 signaling. *J Immunol* (1998) 160(1):485–91.
121. Marinkovic T, Garin A, Yokota Y, Fu YX, Ruddle NH, Furtado GC, et al. Interaction of mature CD3+CD4+ T cells with dendritic cells triggers the development of tertiary lymphoid structures in the thyroid. *J Clin Invest* (2006) 116(10):2622–32. doi:10.1172/JCI28993
122. Schrama D, thor Straten P, Fischer WH, McLellan AD, Brocker EB, Reisfeld RA, et al. Targeting of lymphotoxin-alpha to the tumor elicits an efficient immune response associated with induction of peripheral lymphoid-like tissue. *Immunity* (2001) 14(2):111–21. doi:10.1016/S1074-7613(01)00094-2
123. Yu P, Lee Y, Liu W, Chin RK, Wang J, Wang Y, et al. Priming of naive T cells inside tumors leads to eradication of established tumors. *Nat Immunol* (2004) 5(2):141–9. doi:10.1038/ni1029
124. Peske JD, Thompson ED, Gemta L, Baylis RA, Fu YX, Engelhard VH. Effector lymphocyte-induced lymph node-like vasculature enables naive T-cell entry into tumours and enhanced anti-tumour immunity. *Nat Commun* (2015) 6:7114. doi:10.1038/ncomms8114
125. Genta RM, Hamner HW. The significance of lymphoid follicles in the interpretation of gastric biopsy specimens. *Arch Pathol Lab Med* (1994) 118(7):740–3.
126. Gu-Trantien C, Loi S, Garaud S, Equeter C, Libin M, de Wind A, et al. CD4(+) follicular helper T cell infiltration predicts breast cancer survival. *J Clin Invest* (2013) 123(7):2873–92. doi:10.1172/JCI67428
127. Lee HJ, Park IA, Song IH, Shin SJ, Kim JY, Yu JH, et al. Tertiary lymphoid structures: prognostic significance and relationship with tumour-infiltrating lymphocytes in triple-negative breast cancer. *J Clin Pathol* (2016) 69(5):422–30. doi:10.1136/jclinpath-2015-203089
128. Ladanyi A, Kiss J, Somlai B, Gilde K, Fejos Z, Mohos A, et al. Density of DC-LAMP(+) mature dendritic cells in combination with activated T lymphocytes infiltrating primary cutaneous melanoma is a strong independent prognostic factor. *Cancer Immunol Immunother* (2007) 56(9):1459–69. doi:10.1007/s00262-007-0286-3
129. Messina JL, Fenstermacher DA, Eschrich S, Qu X, Berglund AE, Lloyd MC, et al. 12-Chemokine gene signature identifies lymph node-like structures in melanoma: potential for patient selection for immunotherapy? *Sci Rep* (2012) 2:765. doi:10.1038/srep00765
130. Dieu-Nosjean MC, Antoine M, Danel C, Heudes D, Wislez M, Poulot V, et al. Long-term survival for patients with non-small-cell lung cancer with intratumoral lymphoid structures. *J Clin Oncol* (2008) 26(27):4410–7. doi:10.1200/JCO.2007.15.0284
131. Di Caro G, Bergomas F, Grizzi F, Doni A, Bianchi P, Malesci A, et al. Occurrence of tertiary lymphoid tissue is associated with T-cell infiltration and predicts better prognosis in early-stage colorectal cancers. *Clin Cancer Res* (2014) 20(8):2147–58. doi:10.1158/1078-0432.CCR-13-2590
132. Bento DC, Jones E, Junaid S, Tull J, Williams GT, Godkin A, et al. High endothelial venules are rare in colorectal cancers but accumulate in extra-tumoral areas with disease progression. *Oncoimmunology* (2015) 4(3):e974374. doi:10.4161/2162402X.2014.974374
133. Goc J, Germain C, Vo-Bourgais TK, Lupo A, Klein C, Knockaert S, et al. Dendritic cells in tumor-associated tertiary lymphoid structures signal a Th1 cytotoxic immune contexture and license the positive prognostic value of infiltrating CD8+ T cells. *Cancer Res* (2014) 74(3):705–15. doi:10.1158/0008-5472.CAN-13-1342
134. de Chaisemartin L, Goc J, Damotte D, Validire P, Magdeleinat P, Alifano M, et al. Characterization of chemokines and adhesion molecules associated with T cell presence in tertiary lymphoid structures in human lung cancer. *Cancer Res* (2011) 71(20):6391–9. doi:10.1158/0008-5472.CAN-11-0952
135. McMahon EJ, Bailey SL, Castenada CV, Waldner H, Miller SD. Epitope spreading initiates in the CNS in two mouse models of multiple sclerosis. *Nat Med* (2005) 11(3):335–9. doi:10.1038/nm1202
136. Moyron-Quiroz JE, Rangel-Moreno J, Kusser K, Hartson L, Sprague F, Goodrich S, et al. Role of inducible bronchus associated lymphoid tissue (iBALT) in respiratory immunity. *Nat Med* (2004) 10(9):927–34. doi:10.1038/nm1091
137. Cuff CA, Sacca R, Ruddle NH. Differential induction of adhesion molecule and chemokine expression by LTalpha3 and LTalphabeta in inflammation elucidates potential mechanisms of mesenteric and peripheral lymph node development. *J Immunol* (1999) 162(10):5965–72.
138. Sun SC. The noncanonical NF-kappaB pathway. *Immunol Rev* (2012) 246(1):125–40. doi:10.1111/j.1600-065X.2011.01088.x
139. Guo F, Weih D, Meier E, Weih F. Constitutive alternative NF-kappaB signaling promotes marginal zone B-cell development but disrupts the marginal sinus and induces HEV-like structures in the spleen. *Blood* (2007) 110(7):2381–9. doi:10.1182/blood-2007-02-075143
140. Zarnegar BJ, Wang Y, Mahoney DJ, Dempsey PW, Cheung HH, He J, et al. Noncanonical NF-kappaB activation requires coordinated assembly of a regulatory complex of the adaptors cIAP1, cIAP2, TRAF2 and TRAF3 and the kinase NIK. *Nat Immunol* (2008) 9(12):1371–8. doi:10.1038/ni.1676
141. Vallabhapurapu S, Matsuzawa A, Zhang W, Tseng PH, Keats JJ, Wang H, et al. Nonredundant and complementary functions of TRAF2 and TRAF3 in a ubiquitination cascade that activates NIK-dependent alternative NF-kappaB signaling. *Nat Immunol* (2008) 9(12):1364–70. doi:10.1038/ni.1678
142. Razani B, Zarnegar B, Ytterberg AJ, Shiba T, Dempsey PW, Ware CF, et al. Negative feedback in noncanonical NF-kappaB signaling modulates NIK stability through IKKalpha-mediated phosphorylation. *Sci Signal* (2010) 3(123):ra41. doi:10.1126/scisignal.2000778
143. Pablos JL, Santiago B, Tsay D, Singer MS, Palao G, Galindo M, et al. A HEV-restricted sulfotransferase is expressed in rheumatoid arthritis synovium and is induced by lymphotoxin-alpha/beta and TNF-alpha in cultured endothelial cells. *BMC Immunol* (2005) 6:6. doi:10.1186/1471-2172-6-6
144. Madge LA, May MJ. Classical NF-kappaB activation negatively regulates noncanonical NF-kappaB-dependent CXCL12 expression. *J Biol Chem* (2010) 285(49):38069–77. doi:10.1074/jbc.M110.147207
145. Cooley LS, Handsley MM, Zhou Z, Lafleur MA, Pennington CJ, Thompson EW, et al. Reversible transdifferentiation of blood vascular endothelial cells to a lymphatic-like phenotype in vitro. *J Cell Sci* (2010) 123(Pt 21):3808–16. doi:10.1242/jcs.064279
146. Klein S, de Fougerolles AR, Blaikie P, Khan L, Pepe A, Green CD, et al. Alpha 5 beta 1 integrin activates an NF-kappa B-dependent program of gene expression important for angiogenesis and inflammation. *Mol Cell Biol* (2002) 22(16):5912–22. doi:10.1128/MCB.22.16.5912-5922.2002
147. Ager A, Watson HA, Wehenkel SC, Mohammed RN. Homing to solid cancers: a vascular checkpoint in adoptive cell therapy using CAR T-cells. *Biochem Soc Trans* (2016) 44(2):377–85. doi:10.1042/BST20150254
148. Calcinotto A, Grioni M, Jachetti E, Curnis F, Mondino A, Parmiani G, et al. Targeting TNF-alpha to neoangiogenic vessels enhances lymphocyte infiltration in tumors and increases the therapeutic potential of immunotherapy. *J Immunol* (2012) 188(6):2687–94. doi:10.4049/jimmunol.1101877
149. Joshi NS, Akama-Garren EH, Lu Y, Lee DY, Chang GP, Li A, et al. Regulatory T cells in tumor-associated tertiary lymphoid structures suppress

anti-tumor T cell responses. *Immunity* (2015) 43(3):579–90. doi:10.1016/j.immuni.2015.08.006

150. Lanca T, Silva-Santos B. The split nature of tumor-infiltrating leukocytes: implications for cancer surveillance and immunotherapy. *Oncoimmunology* (2012) 1(5):717–25. doi:10.4161/onci.20068

3

How Follicular Dendritic Cells Shape the B-Cell Antigenome

Jan Kranich[1]* and Nike Julia Krautler[2]*

[1] *Institute for Immunology, Ludwig Maximilian University Munich, Munich, Germany,* [2] *Institute of Microbiology, ETH Zurich, Zurich, Switzerland*

Correspondence:
Jan Kranich
jan.kranich@med.uni-muenchen.de;
Nike Julia Krautler
knike@ethz.ch

Follicular dendritic cells (FDCs) are stromal cells residing in primary follicles and in germinal centers of secondary and tertiary lymphoid organs (SLOs and TLOs). There, they play a crucial role in B-cell activation and affinity maturation of antibodies. FDCs have the unique capacity to bind and retain native antigen in B-cell follicles for long periods of time. Therefore, FDCs shape the B-cell antigenome (the sum of all B-cell antigens) in SLOs and TLOs. In this review, we discuss recent findings that explain how this stromal cell type can arise in almost any tissue during TLO formation and, furthermore, focus on the mechanisms of antigen capture and retention involved in the generation of long-lasting antigen depots displayed on FDCs.

Keywords: follicular dendritic cells, tertiary lymphoid organs, antigen, B-cell responses, antigenome, germinal centers, antigen trapping

Follicular dendritic cells (FDCs) are cells of stromal origin that are indispensable for secondary lymphoid organ (SLO) and tertiary lymphoid organ (TLO) development and maintenance. They are located in the central region of primary follicles and in the light zone of germinal centers [GCs; (1, 2)]. Their most striking feature is the ability to capture and retain native antigen. This was first observed in 1965, when Mitchell and Abbott analyzed the location of iodine-125 labeled flagella of *Salmonella Adelaide* in draining lymph nodes of mice using high-resolution electron microscopic autoradiographs (3). Since then, the role of FDCs as crucial players in antibody responses has been widely accepted. Their main function being the presentation of native antigen, in the form of immune complexes (ICs), to B cells, thereby driving their affinity maturation during the GC reaction.

In this review, we focus first on recent findings that help to explain, how FDCs can arise in almost any tissue undergoing TLO formation and, second, on their ability to retain antigen in B-cell follicles. For a more detailed description of FDC biology, we refer the reader to other recent reviews (4, 5).

REQUIREMENTS FOR FDC DEVELOPMENT

After the first mentioning of FDCs little more than half a decade ago, initial experiments, mainly using bone marrow chimeras (6, 7), indicated that FDCs are of stromal, radioresistant, and likely sessile character. In the meantime, extensive data were brought forward attributing important functions to FDCs in B-cell responses, such as the provision of the chemokine CXCL13, essential to allure B cells into the follicles in a CXCR5-dependent manner (8). Interestingly, the dependence of B cells and FDCs was found to be mutual; in the absence of B cells, FDCs did not form (9). B cells were shown to be the main source for lymphotoxins (LT) and tumor necrosis factors (TNF), which upon binding to their respective receptors, LTβR and TNFR1, present on the surface of FDCs and their precursors, acted as potent drivers of FDC maturation (9–16). Furthermore, after the initial generation of FDCs sustained LT signaling was shown to be required for keeping them in a differentiated and functional state (17).

While it was soon recognized that FDCs are a central component of B-cell follicles in spleen and in lymph nodes, their appearance was not limited to SLOs. FDCs were also shown to contribute to non-encapsulated lymphoid structures, such as the isolated lymphoid follicles of the intestine (18). In addition to this, FDCs were frequently observed during certain chronic inflammations in non-lymphoid tissues. As a result of an unresolved inflammation during autoimmunity (e.g., rheumatoid arthritis) or during chronic infections (e.g., hepatitis C infection), such tissues can undergo remodeling into TLOs (19–21), containing FDCs and microanatomically segregated T and B cell areas. Autoimmune diseases and chronic inflammations with FDC involvement are summarized in **Table 1**. The notion that FDCs can possibly be generated everywhere in the body suggests that their precursors sport either considerable motility or that they are derived from a non-migratory ancestor. Bone marrow chimera experiments, where FDCs in spleen and LN were generated from host cells, added evidence to the latter hypothesis (6, 7). The idea that FDCs could have differentiated from a local precursor, was further supported by the finding that FDCs shared markers with other stromal cells of SLOs and TLOs and showed similarities with fibroblasts and mesenchymal cells (1, 22, 23). In parabiont experiments, where the blood circulation of two mice was surgically connected for 3 months, no FDCs had been generated from the surgically attached counterpart (24). This also corroborated a model of a non-migratory and rather local precursor, giving rise to FDCs.

In a murine model of chronic inflammation, transgenic overexpression of LTα under the rat insulin promoter (RIP-*Lta*) leads to the formation of TLOs in kidneys, including fully matured FDCs (25–27). When these mice were treated with LTβR-Ig decoy receptors (17) to remove mature (renal) FDCs followed by transplantation of their kidneys into recipient mice, this led to the reformation of FDCs exclusively derived from cells of the transplanted donor kidneys. This finding proved that, even during the generation of TLOs, FDC precursors are tissue-intrinsic (25). Detailed analysis of the expression of the FDC-expressed molecule Mfge8 [FDC-M1; (28)] during splenic organogenesis as well as in mice lacking FDCs, further suggested that the earliest FDC precursor was located in the splenic perivascular space. These putative precursors expressed PDGFRβ and SMA. Since mature FDCs do not express PDGFRβ, lineage-tracing experiments (using Pdgfrb-Cre mice) were performed and confirmed that FDCs had derived from such PDGFRβ-positive precursors. The expression of PDGFRβ and SMA as well as their localization indicated that these cells were in fact mural vascular cells. Depending on the localization (surrounding small capillaries or larger vessel) and their appearance, mural cells are divided into single-layered pericytes or several layers of vascular smooth muscle cells. Mural cells can be isolated from the stromal-vascular fraction of white adipose tissue (29). The transplantation of PDGFRβ-positive cells, sort-purified from the stromal-vascular fraction, into the kidney capsule of mice lacking endogenous FDCs gave rise to artificial lymph nodes containing fully differentiated FDCs. This showed that FDCs are generated from perivascular cells. The ubiquity of such perivascular cells and, therefore, likely FDC precursors also explains why it is possible for FDCs to arise in any tissue or organ (25). It remains to be shown, whether any mural cell can give rise to FDCs or whether it needs to be derived from specific tissues, such as the adipose tissue. This is of particular interest as LN anlagen usually are inserted within fat pads. Indeed stimulation of LTβR signaling inhibits adipocyte differentiation and promotes a fibroblast-like phenotype (30).

Follicular dendritic cells are not the sole stromal cell of SLOs. Fibroblast reticular cells (FRCs) contribute to the structure and function of the T-cell zone, while marginal reticular cells (MRCs) are important for the function and the structure of the splenic marginal zone (MZ) (31). Recently, novel stromal subpopulations were identified, such as the versatile stromal cells at the T cell–B cell border of inflamed B-cell follicles [VSCs; (32)] and the CXCL12-expressing reticular cells of the GC dark zone [CRCs; (2)]. FDCs, MRCs, and FRCs share the expression of many markers, such as LTβR, BP-3, VCAM-1, and ICAM-1 (25, 33–35), which could also suggest a common precursor. To identify this potential precursor, labeling experiments were performed with fetal mesenchymal progenitors of spleen and lymph nodes. Splenic mesenchymal precursors were followed using either Nkx2-5-Cre or Islet1-Cre reporter mice and found to contribute to FDCs, FRCs, MRCs, and mural cells (36). A reporter mouse for neural crest cells (Wnt-1-Cre), embryonic progenitor cells that give rise to mesenchymal structures of the head and the neck region, was used to test if FDCs in auricular and cervical lymph nodes were derived from such cells. Indeed, Jarjour et al. could show that FDCs as well as MRCs and other stromal cells can be labeled with this technique (24). While the authors did not confirm if the Wnt-1-Cre reporter also labeled PDGRβ^{+}SMA^{+} perivascular precursors in lymph nodes, FRCs, and precursors thereof, have been attributed a pericyte-like character and reside as CCL21^{+}CCL19^{+}PDGFRβ^{-}SMA^{+} cells in perivascular locations of inguinal and popliteal lymph nodes (35, 37). The transplantation of fetal splenic Nkx2-5-reporter positive cells or adult adipose PDGFRβ stromal vascular cells generated artificial lymph nodes, further supporting the idea that these early precursors can contribute to all stromal compartments and

TABLE 1 | Human diseases with lymphoid neogenesis.

Autoimmune diseases	Chronic allograft rejection
Rheumatoid arthritis (88–91)	Organ transplantation (118, 119)
Hashimoto's thyroiditis and Graves' disease (92–95)	
Myasthenia gravis (96–98)	**Other chronic inflammations**
Sjogren's syndrome (99–101)	Ulcerative colitis (120, 121)
Multiple sclerosis (102–104)	Atherosclerosis (122, 123)
Cryptogenic fibrosing alveolitis (105, 106)	
Systemic lupus erythematosus (107, 108)	**Cancer**
	Non-small cell lung cancer (124, 125)
Infectious diseases	Colorectal carcinoma (126)
Chronic hepatitis C (109, 110)	Ductal breast carcinoma (127, 128)
Helicobacter pylori-induced gastritis (111–115)	Melanoma (metastasis) (129)
Chronic Lyme disease (116, 117)	Mucosal-associated lymphoid tissue lymphoma (115)

even includes stromal organizer cells able to initiate lymph node anlagen (25, 36). A model for FDC development is illustrated in **Figure 1**.

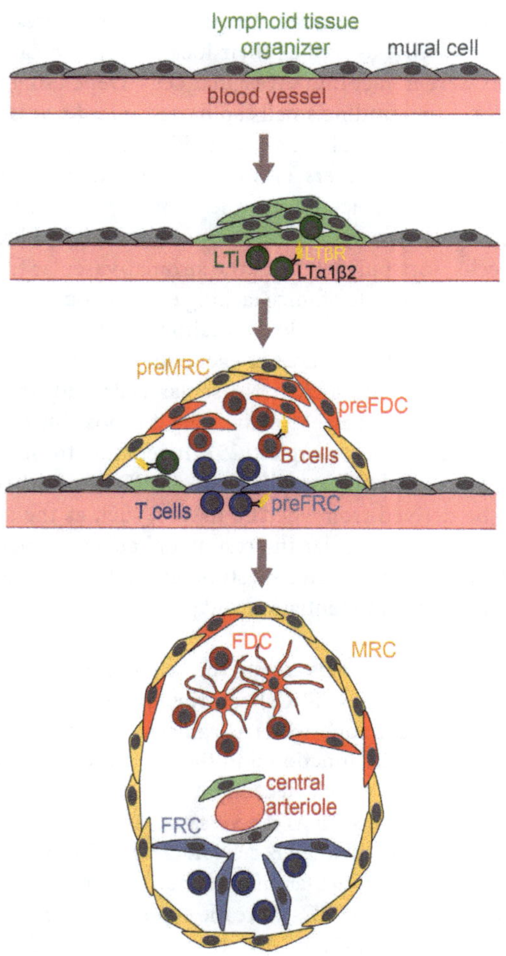

stromal cells of lympohid tissues

mural cell: PDGFRβ$^+$SMA$^{+/-}$NG2$^{+/-}$

lymphoid tissue organizer: ICAM1$^+$VCAM1$^+$CXCL13$^+$PDGFRβ$^+$SMA$^?$

MRC: MadCAM1$^+$CXCL13$^+$Mfge8$^+$ICAM1$^+$VCAM1$^+$PDGFRβ$^+$SMA$^+$

FDC: Mfge8$^+$CR1$^+$CXCL13$^+$ICAM1$^+$VCAM1$^+$PDGFRβ$^+$SMA$^-$

FRC: GP38$^+$ERTR7$^+$CCL19$^+$PDGFRβ$^+$SMA$^+$

FIGURE 1 | Model of FDC development. Mural cells and lymphoid tissue organizer cells line blood vessels (top panel) at places where future lymphoid tissues develop. The arriving lymphoid tissue inducer cells (LTi) express membrane bound LTα1β2 and trigger expansion of lymphoid tissue organizer cells and upregulation of the chemokine CXCL13 (second panel). Further recruitment of T and B lymphocytes provisioning LTα1β2 leads to the induction of marginal reticular cells (MRC), follicular dendritic cell (FDC), and fibroblast reticular cell (FRC) precursors, all likely to be generated from lymphoid tissue organizer cells (third panel). Shared expression of markers of MRC and FDC suggest a close lineage relationship, further supported by appearance of mature FDC next to MRC. The influx of T and B cells further leads to a zonal segregation and differentiation of blood vessel into marginal sinus and central arteriole as shown in case of the spleen (bottom panel). Markers used to identify specific stromal populations are highlighted in bold.

THE DISCOVERY OF FDCs

As mentioned above, the deposition of antigen within SLOs was studied extensively in the 1960s, using radioactively labeled microbial antigens, such as isolated flagellin derived from *Salmonella*. Immunofluorescent detection of antigens, which was a very new technique at that time, was also used in some of the studies (38, 39). A common observation was that even though most of the antigen was endocytosed by phagocytic cells, some remained extracellularly on the surface of cells, whose identity was obscure at that time. Miller and Nossal described that within the follicle cell surface-bound antigen was trapped on fine processes of cells, which at that point they believed to be a phagocytic cell subset (39). However, later electron-microscopy studies clarified that antigen was rather associated with the dendritic processes of non-phagocytic reticular cells and that these cells formed large web-like structures (3, 40, 41).

While further studies in the following years dealt with the exact distribution of antigen within the lymph node and GCs, the precise nature of these antigen-retaining reticular cells remained unclear for several more years. Various different names were used for these cells by the different laboratories that studied them. So they were also sometimes referred to as dendritic macrophages or dendritic reticular cells (40, 42). However, the common feature recognized by all these studies (43) was the extraordinary ability of these cells to retain antigen on their cell surface. Hence, these cells clearly differed from the typical phagocytic cells. In 1978, Chen et al. published a detailed anatomical and functional study of these cells. They introduced the name "FDCs" owing to their long cytoplasmic processes, and not because of relations to classical dendritic cells (DCs) (44). The authors realized that the name may not be ideal and suggested that at a later time point, when more would become known about these cells the name might need to be reconsidered (44). However, even when it became evident that FDCs lacked MHC class II expression, a molecule expressed at high levels by conventional, hematopoietic DCs, the name FDCs persisted (45) with the consequence that FDCs are still often confused with conventional DCs.

Using electron-dense tracers, Chen et al. showed that FDCs, unlike macrophages, do not actively endocytose (43, 44), a view that has recently been challenged by a study that showed that FDCs endocytose ICs, which they acquire from non-cognate B cells. In contrast to macrophages, ICs endocytosed by FDCs retain their native form and recycle to the cell surface (46), a feature essential for long-term antigen display. Electron microscopy further revealed that FDCs have unique cellular structures, including large, irregular nuclei, containing little heterochromatin, and only few organelles. One striking feature was that FDCs only had small cell bodies, while their cytoplasm extended into many filiform dendrites, forming an extensive net-like structure, which seemed to act like a cap covering the secondary follicle (43, 44).

IMMUNE-COMPLEX TRAPPING – THE CARDINAL FUNCTION OF FDCs

In the 1960s, researchers tried to address the molecular requirements for antigen retention in B-cell follicles. Nossal et al.

compared antigen distribution in non-immunized rats with those that either had received a passive or an active immunization against *Salmonella* prior to administration of radiolabeled *Salmonella* flagellin. Strikingly, they observed that immunization greatly influenced the distribution of antigen within the lymph node. Rats that were actively or passively immunized before they received radiolabeled antigen had a faster and more intense accumulation of antigen in their follicles than non-immunized animals. The increase in follicular antigen deposition seen in immunized rats led the authors to conclude that an opsonin was responsible for the efficient targeting of antigen to the follicle, and that this opsonin was likely to be an antibody (47). This observation was also confirmed to hold true in other species: Humphrey et al. immunized rabbits with non-microbial antigens (radiolabeled hemocyanin or human serum albumin). Prior to injection of radiolabeled antigen, the rabbits were either immunized with a single injection of unlabeled antigen, received repeated injections of antigen shortly after birth (inducing antigenic tolerance) or had remained untreated (naive). While uptake of radiolabeled antigen by medullary sinus macrophages did not differ between the three treatments, no antigen was retained by FDCs in the follicles of naive rabbits. Furthermore, tolerized rabbits had no detectable levels of antibody and showed no follicular antigen retention by FDCs. Thus, it was established that for the follicular retention of antigen the presence of antigen-specific antibodies was crucial (48).

Still, some studies had shown that low-level retention of antigen also occurred in non-primed animals (47). Hence, some doubts remained, whether the "follicular opsonin" was the antibody itself or if another, antibody-induced substance, was involved.

Experiments by Williams then showed that a substance produced by lymphocytes was important: he had previously seen a diminished uptake of *Salmonella* flagellin in lymphoid follicles after depletion of peripheral lymphocytes by partial irradiation with shielded bone marrow (49). This observation had led him to assume that lymphocytes produced substances with opsonizing activity. To test this hypothesis, he monitored the accumulation of flagellin in follicles in the absence of peripheral lymphocytes and assessed how the application of normal rat serum or antibody influenced follicular antigen deposition. A decline in the retention of radiolabeled antigen was observed from day 5 after irradiation onward. Jaroslow and Nossal had previously shown that FDCs are highly resistant to irradiation, so an impairment of FDC function could be excluded as the reason for reduced antigen accumulation following irradiation (50). To restore the antigen retention, normal rat serum or anti-flagellar immune serum was injected. Immune serum significantly improved antigen trapping, as did normal rat serum, but for the latter 25-times more volume was required. By contrast, fetal calf serum did not improve the antigen uptake in follicles, showing that serum-dependent antigen trapping was species specific. Furthermore, neither injection of lymphocytes nor supernatant from cultured lymphocytes showed an effect. While this study had pitfalls mainly due to the irradiation, still an important conclusion could be drawn from this study; immune serum contained large-amounts of the "follicular opsonin," also supporting the idea, that antibodies might be the crucial opsonin. However, the finding that non-immune serum also was able to restore antigen retention in the follicle even though at a much lower efficiency, suggested the presence of additional opsonins (49).

While it became generally accepted that antigen–antibody complexes were crucial for efficient targeting of native antigen to FDCs, years had to pass until other factors essential for IC-trapping, namely complement, were identified. Only in 1974 Pepys found that depletion of the complement component C3 by cobra venom factor, strongly reduced T-cell-dependent B-cell responses to sheep red blood cells (SRBC), illustrating the central role of C3 in the induction of antibody production (51). One year later evidence that complement was required to retain antigen in the GC came from Papamichail et al., who reported that complement inhibition with cobra venom factor blocked trapping of aggregated IgG in the splenic follicle (52). In line with this, Klaus and Humphrey observed that chronic depletion of C3 inhibited memory B-cell formation and concluded that the assembly of an antigen–antibody–C3 complex on FDCs is crucial for B-cell memory (53). More than 20 years later, the complement receptors 1 and 2 (CR1, CR2) were found to be responsible for capturing of C3-containing ICs (54). In humans, two separate genes encode for CR1 and CR2; in mice, however, the Cr2 locus encodes for both CR1 (CD35) and CR2 (CD21) and expression of either CR1 or CR2 is determined by alternative splicing. CR2 binds degradation products of C3, such as iC3bm C3d,g, C3d, while CR1 binds C3b and C4b (55). All mature B cells express CR2, but particularly high levels are found on MZ B cells. FDCs predominantly express CR1 (56). On B cells, CR2 acts as a B-cell receptor (BCR) co-receptor. Fusing antigen with one or more copies of C3d lowered the amount of antigen needed to induce B-cell responses up to 10,000 fold in a CR2-dependent manner (57). Several studies have shown that FDCs utilize CR1/2 to retain antigen on their surface (54, 56, 58, 59).

In addition to complement receptors, FDCs use other receptors to bind ICs. *Ex vivo* IC-trapping experiments on splenic cryosections of immunized mice were tested in presence or absence of serum for the retention of ICs. In presence of serum, most trapping depended on CR1/2, since CR1/2 blocking antibodies dramatically reduced IC-capturing. However, in absence of complement (without serum), some trapping on a subset of FDCs still occurred. This residual trapping could be blocked with anti-FcγRIIβ antibodies (59). The importance of Fc-receptors for IC-trapping by FDCs was also confirmed *in vivo*, since *Fcgr2b*$^{-/-}$ mice showed significantly reduced IC-trapping, and although primary antibody responses are unaltered in mice with FcγRIIβ-deficient FDCs, recall responses are diminished (60).

In summary, the crucial components to deliver antigen to FDCs are antigen-specific antibodies and complement factors. But how exactly antigen reaches FDCs has remained unclear for a long time.

MECHANISMS OF ANTIGEN DELIVERY TO FDCs

Already in 1983, Szakal et al. described antigen transport cells (ATCs) that supposedly transported antigen from the subcapsular

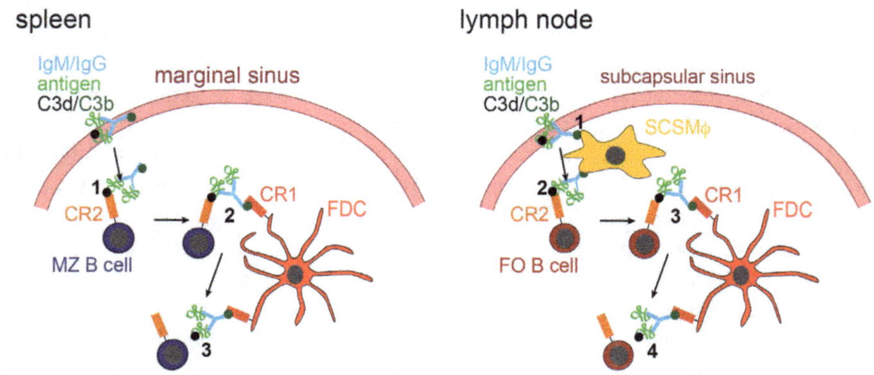

FIGURE 2 | IC acquisition. In the spleen (left panel), non-cognate marginal zone (MZ) B cells capture ICs, consisting of antigen, IgM or IgG, and C3 degradation products (C3d and C3b), from the blood stream (1). MZ B cells, which have captured ICs in a C3d/CR2-dependent fashion, then migrate into the follicle, where they transfer the ICs onto FDCs, which bind them via C3b and CR1 (2). The ICs are then released from the MZ B cell (3). In the lymph node (right panel), subcapsulary sinus macrophages (SCSMϕ) capture ICs consisting of antigen, IgM or IgG, and C3d and C3b degradation products from the lymph (1). SCSMϕ migrate into the follicle and transfer ICs to follicular (FO) B cells in a CR2-dependent manner (2). Subsequently, FO B cells transfer the ICs onto FDCs (3, 4).

sinus to the FDCs. These cells were non-phagocytic and had morphological similarities with FDCs, leading to the assumption that these cells might be pre-FDCs, an observation which remained unconfirmed (61, 62).

It was shown that in the spleen MZ B cells capture IgM-containing immune complexes (IgM-ICs) and transport and deposit them onto FDCs within the B-cell follicle (63, 64). This transfer was dependent on complement and CR1/CR2, and mice deficient for those factors, showed no accumulation of IgM-ICs on FDCs. Still, how would antigen be brought to FDCs in lymph nodes that lack MZ B cells? This was revealed by two-photon microscopy studies (65, 66). Phan et al. showed that in lymph nodes subcapsulary sinus (SCS) macrophages capture immunofluorescently labeled ICs [Phycoerythrin:ICs; (65)]. These macrophages monitor the lymph fluid that arrives in the subcapsular sinus, bind large amount of ICs and have little endocytic activity. ICs travel along the processes of these macrophages and transfer antigen onto non-cognate follicular B cells in a complement receptor-dependent manner. Subsequently, ICs are shuttled from the B cells onto FDCs (66). Mechanisms of IC delivery to FDCs are depicted in **Figure 2**.

THE ROLE OF FDC-BOUND ICs IN B-CELL RESPONSES

Immune complexes bound by FDCs are organized in a bead-like formation, as the so-called iccosomes. These IC-coated bodies can be endocytosed by tingible body macrophages (TBMϕs) and B cells (67). The effect on B-cell activation, GC development, affinity maturation, and memory B-cell maintenance of FDC-bound ICs has been studied in great detail (1). It is generally accepted that FDC function as storage of native antigen. During the GC reaction, high-affinity B cells access antigen, internalize, process, and display it to T helper cells, thereby receiving BCR stimulation as well as additional T helper cell-derived survival signals (68, 69). Early studies assessing the influence of FDCs on B-cell activation were performed *in vitro* using FDC-enriched clusters. They showed that only in the presence of FDCs, ICs (in the form of isolated iccosomes) were able to strongly activate B cells, evidenced by substantially increased antibody production against the cognate antigen. Hence, FDCs stimulate B cells via FDC-bound antigen, but also via antigen-independent FDC products (70). In addition to this, Boes et al. found that in the absence of secreted IgM antigen trapping by FDCs was reduced and GC formation as well as antibody affinity maturation impaired (71).

Based on these and other studies, the view that FDCs can take part in B-cell activation and play an important role during affinity maturation by displaying native antigen and by presenting survival signals to B cells and that they are involved in memory B-cell development has become generally accepted.

However, this view has been challenged by results obtained from mice that produce only membrane bound IgM, hence, unable to make ICs. These mice showed normal GC formation, despite absent IC-trapping by FDCs (72). Furthermore, CR1/2-deficient mice are also able to form GCs and B cells of such mice even undergo affinity maturation, although numbers and size of the GCs were reduced and antibody levels much lower than those in their wild-type counterparts (73, 74). The role of FDCs and ICs trapped by them has then been critically discussed (75, 76). Haberman and Shlomchik concluded that the role of FDCs in providing non-specific support for the GC reaction is undisputed, but ICs on FDCs might only be important under certain conditions. By contrast, Kosco-Vilbois stresses that immune responses are still most efficient in the presence of ICs on FDCs. Thus, an efficient vaccine should maximize the deposition of ICs on FDCs.

SPECULATIONS ON ADDITIONAL FUNCTIONS OF FDCs

While the consequences of IC-trapping by FDCs are still not fully understood, other functions of FDCs have been identified. The expression of cytokines directs B cells to primary and secondary follicles (1, 77), they supply B cells with trophic factors, such as B-cell activating factor [BAFF; (78)] or instruct TBMϕs to remove apoptotic GC B cells through the secretion of the phosphatidylserine-binding bridging molecule Mfge8 (28). The main functions of FDCs are shown in **Figure 3**.

However, we still think that apart from the role of FDCs in establishing the correct follicular microarchitecture and enabling the formation of GCs (79), one of the most important functions of FDCs lies in the trapping of antigen and activation of B cells. FDCs are the only known cell type that extensively trap ICs for long periods of time in a way that protects native antigen from degradation (46). Therefore, FDCs shape the antigenome – the sum of all native antigens that can be detected by B cells, in primary and secondary follicles. However, although evidence is lacking, we postulate that FDCs might not only trap antigen in the form of ICs, but also in a way that does not require the presence of antigen-specific antibodies, hence, would allow antigen trapping also in individuals that have not previously been exposed to the antigen.

The reasons why we think a trapping mechanism independent of antibodies might exist are the following. It is still widely unknown how naive B cells are activated in a non-immune host, where ICs are absent. While in immune hosts not only the capturing of antigen by FDCs is dependent on ICs but also the antigen transport into the follicle requires ICs. It has been shown that native antigen is captured by subcapsulary sinus macrophages (SCSMϕ) in lymph nodes (66) and by MZ B cells in the spleen (63) in an IC-dependent manner. These cells then transport the antigen inside the follicle and deposit it onto FDCs, where it then can activate naive B cells.

While natural IgM is certainly of importance to control infections before high-affinity antibodies are generated (80), natural IgM does not seem to be sufficient to deposit easily detectable amounts of antigen onto FDCs (47–49). Furthermore, it is known that some viral glycoproteins (such as HIV gp120) quite successfully evade recognition by antibodies, e.g., by shielding their epitopes with glycans (81). This makes it very hard for the infected host to develop antibodies against such antigens. In such a case, it seems counterintuitive that antibody-containing ICs are required to mount a B-cell response, especially since such an IC would potentially mask the rare epitope needed for the initial BCR engagement in order to activate the cognate B cell.

Another study showed that soluble antigen readily diffuses through the follicle and is capable of activating B cells (82). However, this study used adoptively transferred BCR transgenic B cells, with the consequence that an unphysiological high number of antigen-specific B cells are located in the follicles. If soluble antigen is efficient enough to trigger B-cell responses, in a more natural setting, where antigen, as well as antigen-specific B cells are limiting, remains an open question.

Using BCR transgenic B cells specific for HEL and DCs that were pulsed with HEL, Qi et al. showed in a two-photon

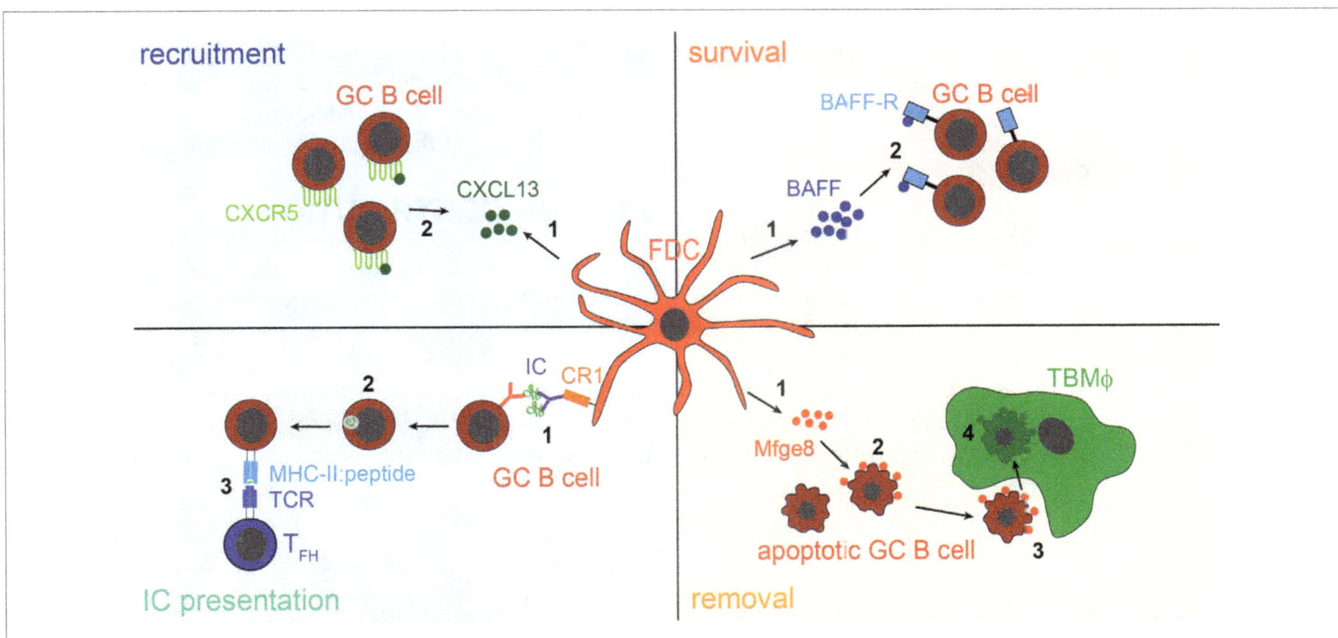

FIGURE 3 | FDC influence on B cells. *Recruitment:* FDCs secret the B cell attracting chemokine CXCL13 (1). GC B cells express the CXCL13-binding chemokine receptor CXCR5 and are thereby attracted towards the B cell follicle (2). *Survival:* FDCs produce B-cell activating factor [BAFF (1)], which is involved in regulating GC B cell survival (2). *IC presentation:* Via their CR1s FDCs present naive antigen to GC B cells (1). Antigen-specific GC B cells, recognizing the antigen via their BCR, endocytose, and process it into peptides (2), and subsequently present it to T follicular helper cells (T_{FH} cells) in form of peptide-MHCII (3). T_{FH} cells then supply cognate B cells with survival signals. It is assumed that after each round of somatic hypermutation, B cells with high-affinity BCRs are able to access antigen presented by FDCs and, thus are able to interact with T_{FH} cells. This leads to the positive selection of such B cells, while others bearing lower affinity receptors are unable to compete for binding to limiting amounts of antigen and undergo apoptosis. *Removal:* the large number of GC B cells that fail to bind antigen presented by FDCs and do not receive T_{FH} help die by apoptosis. To prevent autoimmunity, these cells have to be cleared efficiently. FDCs secrete the apoptotic cell binding protein Mfge8 (1). Mfge8-opsonized apoptotic cells (2) are then recognized and removed by tingible body macrophages (TBMϕs, 3, 4).

microscopy approach that DCs can carry unprocessed antigen into the lymph node and activate cognate B cells in extrafollicular regions (83). If this is a general mechanism of antigen transport into the lymph node and how efficiently this activates B cells under more physiological conditions remains to be addressed.

While all these possibilities are certainly able to trigger B-cell responses, the presentation of antigen via FDCs (46) seems to be the most intuitive and effective way to bring antigen in contact with antigen-specific B cells.

Secondary lymphoid organs are considered to be specialized structures to ensure that a DC, presenting pathogen-derived peptides via MHC class II molecules, finds and activates the rare cognate T cell that recognizes these peptides. Accordingly, we think that the network-like structure of FDCs within B-cell follicles ensures that a rare cognate B cell meets its specific antigen. To do so FDCs retain native antigen sufficiently long, protected from degradation and at the same time concentrating it at the location where many B cells reside. This strongly increases the likelihood of antigen-encounter by the rare cognate B cell. Such a mechanism is especially important when antigen and cognate B cells are limited. In artificial systems where large quantities of antigen are combined with a high frequency of antigen-specific B cells (like in models that use BCR transgenic B cells), naive B cells might readily get in contact with their antigen even without the need of FDCs. Thus, although, it is often assumed that FDCs play no or only a minor role in the initial priming of naive B cells (84), we, therefore, postulate that efficient mechanisms exist, which allow FDCs to capture, retain, and present antigen in non-immune hosts in an antibody-independent manner and, thus, can play an important role in the initial activation of B cells.

CONCLUDING REMARKS

The biology of FDCs has been extensively studied, nevertheless, many questions regarding these cells remain unanswered.

Although there have been some controversies about their importance in the past (75, 76), FDCs are now generally accepted as indispensable for efficient, high-affinity antibody responses. Importantly, FDCs are the only known cell type that functions as a long-term antigen depot. We think it is important to understand what the consequences of such antigen storage are for the activation of B cells, especially during chronic inflammations, where FDC-containing TLOs arise in non-lymphoid tissues, e.g., during rheumatoid arthritis (85). There, FDCs might function as a tissue-specific depot of antigen. Although, little is known, how antigen is acquired by FDCs in TLOs, it might differ from antigen acquisition in lymph nodes or spleen. Also the nature of the antigen might be different from antigen that circulates in the blood stream and is then captured by FDCs in the spleen or from antigen that is transported by the lymph flow to the draining lymph node. It is possible that FDCs in TLOs might preferentially capture antigens that are released in the affected tissue by local tissue damage and that this drives GC formation and chronic inflammation or autoimmunity in affected tissues. Hence, FDCs have long been considered an attractive target for therapeutic intervention, e.g., by administering LTβR-Ig fusion proteins, which lead to FDC ablation (86). However, clinical trials assessing efficacy of LTβR-Ig fusion proteins (Baminercept) in RA patients did not show a measurable effect in treated patients (87). Other studies, assessing, for example, the efficacy of Baminercept to treat Sjögren's syndrome are still ongoing (study ID NCT01552681).

Being "dynamic antigen libraries" (5), FDCs hold valuable information about antigens and antigen epitopes that trigger antibody responses. This information would be of relevance in autoimmunity, chronic inflammation, and cancers with intratumoral TLOs to identify antigenic triggers of disease or cancer antigens that can be used to fight tumors. However, there are currently no techniques available to screen and define the antigenome of FDCs. It would be important to develop techniques that allow the isolation of the FDC antigenome. Subsequent proteomic analysis of the FDC-trapped antigens would provide valuable information that could be exploited for development of novel vaccines or for therapeutics against chronic inflammation.

AUTHOR CONTRIBUTIONS

JK wrote the abstract, introduction, and following chapters: The discovery of FDCs, Immune complex trapping – the cardinal function of FDCs, Mechanisms of antigen delivery to FDCs, The role of FDC-bound ICs in B-cell responses, Speculations on additional functions of FDCs, and Concluding remarks. He also prepared Figures 1, 2, and 3. NK wrote the chapter "Requirements for FDC development," and prepared Table 1 and Figures 1, 2, and 3.

REFERENCES

1. Allen CD, Cyster JG. Follicular dendritic cell networks of primary follicles and germinal centers: phenotype and function. *Semin Immunol* (2008) 20(1):14–25. doi:10.1016/j.smim.2007.12.001
2. Rodda LB, Bannard O, Ludewig B, Nagasawa T, Cyster JG. Phenotypic and morphological properties of germinal center dark zone Cxcl12-expressing reticular cells. *J Immunol* (2015) 195(10):4781–91. doi:10.4049/jimmunol.1501191
3. Mitchell J, Abbot A. Ultrastructure of the antigen-retaining reticulum of lymph node follicles as shown by high-resolution autoradiography. *Nature* (1965) 208(5009):500–2. doi:10.1038/208500b0
4. Aguzzi A, Kranich J, Krautler NJ. Follicular dendritic cells: origin, phenotype, and function in health and disease. *Trends Immunol* (2014) 35(3):105–13 doi:10.1016/j.it.2013.11.001
5. Heesters BA, Myers RC, Carroll MC. Follicular dendritic cells: dynamic antigen libraries. *Nat Rev Immunol* (2014) 14(7):495–504. doi:10.1038/nri3689
6. Humphrey JH, Grennan D, Sundaram V. The origin of follicular dendritic cells in the mouse and the mechanism of trapping of immune complexes on them. *Eur J Immunol* (1984) 14(9):859–64. doi:10.1002/eji.1830140916
7. Yoshida K, Kaji M, Takahashi T, van den Berg TK, Dijkstra CD. Host origin of follicular dendritic cells induced in the spleen of SCID mice after transfer of allogeneic lymphocytes. *Immunology* (1995) 84(1):117–26.

8. Cyster JG, Ansel KM, Reif K, Ekland EH, Hyman PL, Tang HL, et al. Follicular stromal cells and lymphocyte homing to follicles. *Immunol Rev* (2000) 176:181–93. doi:10.1034/j.1600-065X.2000.00618.x
9. Futterer A, Mink K, Luz A, Kosco-Vilbois MH, Pfeffer K. The lymphotoxin beta receptor controls organogenesis and affinity maturation in peripheral lymphoid tissues. *Immunity* (1998) 9(1):59–70. doi:10.1016/S1074-7613(00)80588-9
10. Fu YX, Chaplin DD. Development and maturation of secondary lymphoid tissues. *Annu Rev Immunol* (1999) 17:399–433. doi:10.1146/annurev.immunol.17.1.399
11. Koni PA, Sacca R, Lawton P, Browning JL, Ruddle NH, Flavell RA. Distinct roles in lymphoid organogenesis for lymphotoxins alpha and beta revealed in lymphotoxin beta-deficient mice. *Immunity* (1997) 6(4):491–500. doi:10.1016/S1074-7613(00)80292-7
12. De Togni P, Goellner J, Ruddle NH, Streeter PR, Fick A, Mariathasan S, et al. Abnormal development of peripheral lymphoid organs in mice deficient in lymphotoxin. *Science* (1994) 264(5159):703–7. doi:10.1126/science.8171322
13. Fu YX, Molina H, Matsumoto M, Huang G, Min J, Chaplin DD. Lymphotoxin-alpha (LTalpha) supports development of splenic follicular structure that is required for IgG responses. *J Exp Med* (1997) 185(12):2111–20. doi:10.1084/jem.185.12.2111
14. Pasparakis M, Alexopoulou L, Episkopou V, Kollias G. Immune and inflammatory responses in TNF alpha-deficient mice: a critical requirement for TNF alpha in the formation of primary B cell follicles, follicular dendritic cell networks and germinal centers, and in the maturation of the humoral immune response. *J Exp Med* (1996) 184(4):1397–411. doi:10.1084/jem.184.4.1397
15. Le Hir M, Bluethmann H, Kosco-Vilbois MH, Muller M, di Padova F, Moore M, et al. Differentiation of follicular dendritic cells and full antibody responses require tumor necrosis factor receptor-1 signaling. *J Exp Med* (1996) 183(5):2367–72. doi:10.1084/jem.183.5.2367
16. Marino MW, Dunn A, Grail D, Inglese M, Noguchi Y, Richards E, et al. Characterization of tumor necrosis factor-deficient mice. *Proc Natl Acad Sci U S A* (1997) 94(15):8093–8. doi:10.1073/pnas.94.15.8093
17. Mackay F, Majeau GR, Lawton P, Hochman PS, Browning JL. Lymphotoxin but not tumor necrosis factor functions to maintain splenic architecture and humoral responsiveness in adult mice. *Eur J Immunol* (1997) 27(8):2033–42. doi:10.1002/eji.1830270830
18. Glaysher BR, Mabbott NA. Isolated lymphoid follicle maturation induces the development of follicular dendritic cells. *Immunology* (2007) 120(3):336–44. doi:10.1111/j.1365-2567.2006.02508.x
19. Aloisi F, Pujol-Borrell R. Lymphoid neogenesis in chronic inflammatory diseases. *Nat Rev Immunol* (2006) 6(3):205–17. doi:10.1038/nri1786
20. Dieu-Nosjean MC, Goc J, Giraldo NA, Sautes-Fridman C, Fridman WH. Tertiary lymphoid structures in cancer and beyond. *Trends Immunol* (2014) 35(11):571–80. doi:10.1016/j.it.2014.09.006
21. Neyt K, Perros F, GeurtsvanKessel CH, Hammad H, Lambrecht BN. Tertiary lymphoid organs in infection and autoimmunity. *Trends Immunol* (2012) 33(6):297–305. doi:10.1016/j.it.2012.04.006
22. Bofill M, Akbar AN, Amlot PL. Follicular dendritic cells share a membrane-bound protein with fibroblasts. *J Pathol* (2000) 191(2):217–26. doi:10.1002/(SICI)1096-9896(200006)191:2<217::AID-PATH586>3.3.CO;2-Y
23. Lee IY, Choe J. Human follicular dendritic cells and fibroblasts share the 3C8 antigen. *Biochem Biophys Res Commun* (2003) 304(4):701–7. doi:10.1016/S0006-291X(03)00649-1
24. Jarjour M, Jorquera A, Mondor I, Wienert S, Narang P, Coles MC, et al. Fate mapping reveals origin and dynamics of lymph node follicular dendritic cells. *J Exp Med* (2014) 211(6):1109–22. doi:10.1084/jem.20132409
25. Krautler NJ, Kana V, Kranich J, Tian Y, Perera D, Lemm D, et al. Follicular dendritic cells emerge from ubiquitous perivascular precursors. *Cell* (2012) 150(1):194–206. doi:10.1016/j.cell.2012.05.032
26. Seeger H, Heikenwalder M, Zeller N, Kranich J, Schwarz P, Gaspert A, et al. Coincident scrapie infection and nephritis lead to urinary prion excretion. *Science* (2005) 310(5746):324–6. doi:10.1126/science.1118829
27. Picarella DE, Kratz A, Li CB, Ruddle NH, Flavell RA. Insulitis in transgenic mice expressing tumor necrosis factor beta (lymphotoxin) in the pancreas. *Proc Natl Acad Sci U S A* (1992) 89(21):10036–40. doi:10.1073/pnas.89.21.10036
28. Kranich J, Krautler NJ, Heinen E, Polymenidou M, Bridel C, Schildknecht A, et al. Follicular dendritic cells control engulfment of apoptotic bodies by secreting Mfge8. *J Exp Med* (2008) 205(6):1293–302. doi:10.1084/jem.20071019
29. Tang W, Zeve D, Suh JM, Bosnakovski D, Kyba M, Hammer RE, et al. White fat progenitor cells reside in the adipose vasculature. *Science* (2008) 322(5901):583–6. doi:10.1126/science.1156232
30. Benezech C, Mader E, Desanti G, Khan M, Nakamura K, White A, et al. Lymphotoxin-beta receptor signaling through NF-kappaB2-RelB pathway reprograms adipocyte precursors as lymph node stromal cells. *Immunity* (2012) 37(4):721–34. doi:10.1016/j.immuni.2012.06.010
31. den Haan JM, Mebius RE, Kraal G. Stromal cells of the mouse spleen. *Front Immunol* (2012) 3:201. doi:10.3389/fimmu.2012.00201
32. Mionnet C, Mondor I, Jorquera A, Loosveld M, Maurizio J, Arcangeli ML, et al. Identification of a new stromal cell type involved in the regulation of inflamed B cell follicles. *PLoS Biol* (2013) 11(10):e1001672. doi:10.1371/journal.pbio.1001672
33. Mueller SN, Germain RN. Stromal cell contributions to the homeostasis and functionality of the immune system. *Nat Rev Immunol* (2009) 9(9):618–29. doi:10.1038/nri2588
34. Katakai T, Suto H, Sugai M, Gonda H, Togawa A, Suematsu S, et al. Organizer-like reticular stromal cell layer common to adult secondary lymphoid organs. *J Immunol* (2008) 181(9):6189–200. doi:10.4049/jimmunol.181.9.6189
35. Link A, Vogt TK, Favre S, Britschgi MR, Acha-Orbea H, Hinz B, et al. Fibroblastic reticular cells in lymph nodes regulate the homeostasis of naive T cells. *Nat Immunol* (2007) 8(11):1255–65. doi:10.1038/ni1513
36. Castagnaro L, Lenti E, Maruzzelli S, Spinardi L, Migliori E, Farinello D, et al. Nkx2-5(+)islet1(+) mesenchymal precursors generate distinct spleen stromal cell subsets and participate in restoring stromal network integrity. *Immunity* (2013) 38(4):782–91. doi:10.1016/j.immuni.2012.12.005
37. Chai Q, Onder L, Scandella E, Gil-Cruz C, Perez-Shibayama C, Cupovic J, et al. Maturation of lymph node fibroblastic reticular cells from myofibroblastic precursors is critical for antiviral immunity. *Immunity* (2013) 38(5):1013–24. doi:10.1016/j.immuni.2013.03.012
38. Nossal GJ, Ada GL, Austin CM. Antigens in immunity. IV. Cellular localization of 125-I- and 131-I-labelled flagella in lymph nodes. *Aust J Exp Biol Med Sci* (1964) 42:311–30. doi:10.1038/icb.1964.32
39. Miller JJ III, Nossal GJ. Antigens in immunity. VI. The phagocytic reticulum of lymph node follicles. *J Exp Med* (1964) 120:1075–86. doi:10.1084/jem.120.6.1075
40. Nossal GJ, Abbot A, Mitchell J, Lummus Z. Antigens in immunity. XV. Ultrastructural features of antigen capture in primary and secondary lymphoid follicles. *J Exp Med* (1968) 127(2):277–90. doi:10.1084/jem.127.2.277
41. Szakal AK, Hanna MG Jr. The ultrastructure of antigen localization and viruslike particles in mouse spleen germinal centers. *Exp Mol Pathol* (1968) 8(1):75–89. doi:10.1016/0014-4800(68)90007-5
42. White RG, French VI, Stark JM. A study of the localisation of a protein antigen in the chicken spleen and its relation to the formation of germinal centres. *J Med Microbiol* (1970) 3(1):65–83. doi:10.1099/00222615-3-1-65
43. Chen LL, Frank AM, Adams JC, Steinman RM. Distribution of horseradish peroxidase (HRP)-anti-HRP immune complexes in mouse spleen with special reference to follicular dendritic cells. *J Cell Biol* (1978) 79(1):184–99. doi:10.1083/jcb.79.1.184
44. Chen LL, Adams JC, Steinman RM. Anatomy of germinal centers in mouse spleen, with special reference to "follicular dendritic cells". *J Cell Biol* (1978) 77(1):148–64. doi:10.1083/jcb.77.1.148
45. Tew JG, Thorbecke GJ, Steinman RM Dendritic cells in the immune response: characteristics and recommended nomenclature (A report from the Reticuloendothelial Society Committee on Nomenclature). *J Reticuloendothel Soc* (1982) 31(5):371–80.
46. Heesters BA, Chatterjee P, Kim YA, Gonzalez SF, Kuligowski MP, Kirchhausen T, et al. Endocytosis and recycling of immune complexes by follicular dendritic cells enhances B cell antigen binding and activation. *Immunity* (2013) 38(6):1164–75. doi:10.1016/j.immuni.2013.02.023

47. Nossal GJ, Ada GL, Austin CM, Pye J. Antigens in immunity. 8. Localization of 125-I-labelled antigens in the secondary response. *Immunology* (1965) 9(4):349–57.
48. Humphrey JH, Frank MM. The localization of non-microbial antigens in the draining lymph nodes of tolerant, normal and primed rabbits. *Immunology* (1967) 13(1):87–100.
49. Williams GM. Antigen localization in lymphopenic states. II. Further studies on whole body x-irradiation. *Immunology* (1966) 11(5):475–88.
50. Jaroslow BN, Nossal GJ. Effect of x-irradiation on antigen localization in lymphoid follicles. *Aust J Exp Biol Med Sci* (1966) 44(6):609–27. doi:10.1038/icb.1966.60
51. Pepys MB. Role of complement in induction of antibody production in vivo. Effect of cobra factor and other C3-reactive agents on thymus-dependent and thymus-independent antibody responses. *J Exp Med* (1974) 140(1):126–45. doi:10.1084/jem.140.1.126
52. Papamichail M, Gutierrez C, Embling P, Johnson P, Holborow EJ, Pepys MB. Complement dependence of localisation of aggregated IgG in germinal centres. *Scand J Immunol* (1975) 4(4):343–7. doi:10.1111/j.1365-3083.1975.tb02635.x
53. Klaus GG, Humphrey JH. The generation of memory cells. I. The role of C3 in the generation of B memory cells. *Immunology* (1977) 33(1):31–40.
54. Fang Y, Xu C, Fu YX, Holers VM, Molina H. Expression of complement receptors 1 and 2 on follicular dendritic cells is necessary for the generation of a strong antigen-specific IgG response. *J Immunol* (1998) 160(11):5273–9.
55. Roozendaal R, Carroll MC. Complement receptors CD21 and CD35 in humoral immunity. *Immunol Rev* (2007) 219:157–66. doi:10.1111/j.1600-065X.2007.00556.x
56. Donius LR, Handy JM, Weis JJ, Weis JH. Optimal germinal center B cell activation and T-dependent antibody responses require expression of the mouse complement receptor Cr1. *J Immunol* (2013) 191(1):434–47. doi:10.4049/jimmunol.1203176
57. Dempsey PW, Allison ME, Akkaraju S, Goodnow CC, Fearon DT. C3d of complement as a molecular adjuvant: bridging innate and acquired immunity. *Science* (1996) 271(5247):348–50. doi:10.1126/science.271.5247.348
58. Qin D, Wu J, Carroll MC, Burton GF, Szakal AK, Tew JG. Evidence for an important interaction between a complement-derived CD21 ligand on follicular dendritic cells and CD21 on B cells in the initiation of IgG responses. *J Immunol* (1998) 161(9):4549–54.
59. Yoshida K, van den Berg TK, Dijkstra CD. Two functionally different follicular dendritic cells in secondary lymphoid follicles of mouse spleen, as revealed by CR1/2 and FcR gamma II-mediated immune-complex trapping. *Immunology* (1993) 80(1):34–9.
60. Qin D, Wu J, Vora KA, Ravetch JV, Szakal AK, Manser T, et al. Fc gamma receptor IIB on follicular dendritic cells regulates the B cell recall response. *J Immunol* (2000) 164(12):6268–75. doi:10.4049/jimmunol.164.12.6268
61. Szakal AK, Holmes KL, Tew JG. Transport of immune complexes from the subcapsular sinus to lymph node follicles on the surface of nonphagocytic cells, including cells with dendritic morphology. *J Immunol* (1983) 131(4):1714–27.
62. Tew JG, Mandel TE, Phipps RP, Szakal AK. Tissue localization and retention of antigen in relation to the immune response. *Am J Anat* (1984) 170(3):407–20. doi:10.1002/aja.1001700314
63. Ferguson AR, Youd ME, Corley RB. Marginal zone B cells transport and deposit IgM-containing immune complexes onto follicular dendritic cells. *Int Immunol* (2004) 16(10):1411–22. doi:10.1093/intimm/dxh142
64. Cinamon G, Zachariah MA, Lam OM, Foss FW Jr, Cyster JG. Follicular shuttling of marginal zone B cells facilitates antigen transport. *Nat Immunol* (2008) 9(1):54–62. doi:10.1038/ni1542
65. Phan TG, Green JA, Gray EE, Xu Y, Cyster JG. Immune complex relay by subcapsular sinus macrophages and noncognate B cells drives antibody affinity maturation. *Nat Immunol* (2009) 10(7):786–93. doi:10.1038/ni.1745
66. Phan TG, Grigorova I, Okada T, Cyster JG. Subcapsular encounter and complement-dependent transport of immune complexes by lymph node B cells. *Nat Immunol* (2007) 8(9):992–1000. doi:10.1038/ni1494
67. Szakal AK, Kosco MH, Tew JG. A novel in vivo follicular dendritic cell-dependent iccosome-mediated mechanism for delivery of antigen to antigen-processing cells. *J Immunol* (1988) 140(2):341–53.
68. MacLennan IC. Germinal centers. *Annu Rev Immunol* (1994) 12:117–39. doi:10.1146/annurev.iy.12.040194.001001
69. Victora GD, Nussenzweig MC. Germinal centers. *Annu Rev Immunol* (2012) 30:429–57. doi:10.1146/annurev-immunol-020711-075032
70. Wu J, Qin D, Burton GF, Szakal AK, Tew JG. Follicular dendritic cell-derived antigen and accessory activity in initiation of memory IgG responses in vitro. *J Immunol* (1996) 157(8):3404–11.
71. Boes M, Esau C, Fischer MB, Schmidt T, Carroll M, Chen J. Enhanced B-1 cell development, but impaired IgG antibody responses in mice deficient in secreted IgM. *J Immunol* (1998) 160(10):4776–87.
72. Hannum LG, Haberman AM, Anderson SM, Shlomchik MJ. Germinal center initiation, variable gene region hypermutation, and mutant B cell selection without detectable immune complexes on follicular dendritic cells. *J Exp Med* (2000) 192(7):931–42. doi:10.1084/jem.192.7.931
73. Ahearn JM, Fischer MB, Croix D, Goerg S, Ma M, Xia J, et al. Disruption of the Cr2 locus results in a reduction in B-1a cells and in an impaired B cell response to T-dependent antigen. *Immunity* (1996) 4(3):251–62. doi:10.1016/S1074-7613(00)80433-1
74. Chen Z, Koralov SB, Gendelman M, Carroll MC, Kelsoe G. Humoral immune responses in Cr2-/- mice: enhanced affinity maturation but impaired antibody persistence. *J Immunol* (2000) 164(9):4522–32. doi:10.4049/jimmunol.164.9.4522
75. Haberman AM, Shlomchik MJ. Reassessing the function of immune-complex retention by follicular dendritic cells. *Nat Rev Immunol* (2003) 3(9):757–64. doi:10.1038/nri1178
76. Kosco-Vilbois MH. Are follicular dendritic cells really good for nothing? *Nat Rev Immunol* (2003) 3(9):764–9. doi:10.1038/nri1179
77. Muppidi JR, Lu E, Cyster JG. The G protein-coupled receptor P2RY8 and follicular dendritic cells promote germinal center confinement of B cells, whereas S1PR3 can contribute to their dissemination. *J Exp Med* (2015) 212(13):2213–22. doi:10.1084/jem.20151250
78. Lesley R, Xu Y, Kalled SL, Hess DM, Schwab SR, Shu HB, et al. Reduced competitiveness of autoantigen-engaged B cells due to increased dependence on BAFF. *Immunity* (2004) 20(4):441–53. doi:10.1016/S1074-7613(04)00079-2
79. Wang X, Cho B, Suzuki K, Xu Y, Green JA, An J, et al. Follicular dendritic cells help establish follicle identity and promote B cell retention in germinal centers. *J Exp Med* (2011) 208(12):2497–510. doi:10.1084/jem.20111449
80. Jayasekera JP, Moseman EA, Carroll MC. Natural antibody and complement mediate neutralization of influenza virus in the absence of prior immunity. *J Virol* (2007) 81(7):3487–94. doi:10.1128/JVI.02128-06
81. West AP Jr, Scharf L, Scheid JF, Klein F, Bjorkman PJ, Nussenzweig MC. Structural insights on the role of antibodies in HIV-1 vaccine and therapy. *Cell* (2014) 156(4):633–48. doi:10.1016/j.cell.2014.01.052
82. Pape KA, Catron DM, Itano AA, Jenkins MK. The humoral immune response is initiated in lymph nodes by B cells that acquire soluble antigen directly in the follicles. *Immunity* (2007) 26(4):491–502. doi:10.1016/j.immuni.2007.02.011
83. Qi H, Egen JG, Huang AY, Germain RN. Extrafollicular activation of lymph node B cells by antigen-bearing dendritic cells. *Science* (2006) 312(5780):1672–6. doi:10.1126/science.1125703
84. Tew JG, Wu J, Fakher M, Szakal AK, Qin D. Follicular dendritic cells: beyond the necessity of T-cell help. *Trends Immunol* (2001) 22(7):361–7. doi:10.1016/S1471-4906(01)01942-1
85. Ruddle NH. Lymphatic vessels and tertiary lymphoid organs. *J Clin Invest* (2014) 124(3):953–9. doi:10.1172/JCI71611
86. Fava RA, Notidis E, Hunt J, Szanya V, Ratcliffe N, Ngam-Ek A, et al. A role for the lymphotoxin/LIGHT axis in the pathogenesis of murine collagen-induced arthritis. *J Immunol* (2003) 171(1):115–26. doi:10.4049/jimmunol.171.1.115
87. Genovese MC, Greenwald MW, Alloway JA, Baldassare AR, Chase W, Newman C, et al. Efficacy and safety of baminercept in the treatment of rheumatoid arthritis (RA) results of the phase 2B study in the TNF-IR population. *Arthritis Rheum* (2009) 60(Suppl 10): 417. doi:10.1002/art.25500

88. Randen I, Mellbye OJ, Forre O, Natvig JB. The identification of germinal centres and follicular dendritic cell networks in rheumatoid synovial tissue. *Scand J Immunol* (1995) 41(5):481–6. doi:10.1111/j.1365-3083.1995.tb03596.x
89. Takemura S, Braun A, Crowson C, Kurtin PJ, Cofield RH, O'Fallon WM, et al. Lymphoid neogenesis in rheumatoid synovitis. *J Immunol* (2001) 167(2):1072–80. doi:10.4049/jimmunol.167.2.1072
90. Young CL, Adamson TC III, Vaughan JH, Fox RI. Immunohistologic characterization of synovial membrane lymphocytes in rheumatoid arthritis. *Arthritis Rheum* (1984) 27(1):32–9. doi:10.1002/art.1780270106
91. Manzo A, Paoletti S, Carulli M, Blades MC, Barone F, Yanni G, et al. Systematic microanatomical analysis of CXCL13 and CCL21 in situ production and progressive lymphoid organization in rheumatoid synovitis. *Eur J Immunol* (2005) 35(5):1347–59. doi:10.1002/eji.200425830
92. Aust G, Sittig D, Becherer L, Anderegg U, Schutz A, Lamesch P, et al. The role of CXCR5 and its ligand CXCL13 in the compartmentalization of lymphocytes in thyroids affected by autoimmune thyroid diseases. *Eur J Endocrinol* (2004) 150(2):225–34. doi:10.1530/eje.0.1500225
93. Armengol MP, Cardoso-Schmidt CB, Fernandez M, Ferrer X, Pujol-Borrell R, Juan M. Chemokines determine local lymphoneogenesis and a reduction of circulating CXCR4+ T and CCR7 B and T lymphocytes in thyroid autoimmune diseases. *J Immunol* (2003) 170(12):6320–8. doi:10.4049/jimmunol.170.12.6320
94. Armengol MP, Juan M, Lucas-Martin A, Fernandez-Figueras MT, Jaraquemada D, Gallart T, et al. Thyroid autoimmune disease: demonstration of thyroid antigen-specific B cells and recombination-activating gene expression in chemokine-containing active intrathyroidal germinal centers. *Am J Pathol* (2001) 159(3):861–73. doi:10.1016/S0002-9440(10)61762-2
95. Knecht H, Saremaslani P, Hedinger C. Immunohistological findings in Hashimoto's thyroiditis, focal lymphocytic thyroiditis and thyroiditis de Quervain. Comparative study. *Virchows Arch A Pathol Anat Histol* (1981) 393(2):215–31. doi:10.1007/BF00431078
96. Bofill M, Janossy G, Willcox N, Chilosi M, Trejdosiewicz LK, Newsom-Davis J. Microenvironments in the normal thymus and the thymus in myasthenia gravis. *Am J Pathol* (1985) 119(3):462–73.
97. Roxanis I, Micklem K, McConville J, Newsom-Davis J, Willcox N. Thymic myoid cells and germinal center formation in myasthenia gravis; possible roles in pathogenesis. *J Neuroimmunol* (2002) 125(1–2):185–97. doi:10.1016/S0165-5728(02)00038-3
98. Thomas JA, Willcox HN, Newsom-Davis J. Immunohistological studies of the thymus in myasthenia gravis. Correlation with clinical state and thymocyte culture responses. *J Neuroimmunol* (1982) 3(4):319–35. doi:10.1016/0165-5728(82)90035-2
99. Salomonsson S, Jonsson MV, Skarstein K, Brokstad KA, Hjelmstrom P, Wahren-Herlenius M, et al. Cellular basis of ectopic germinal center formation and autoantibody production in the target organ of patients with Sjogren's syndrome. *Arthritis Rheum* (2003) 48(11):3187–201. doi:10.1002/art.11311
100. Salomonsson S, Larsson P, Tengner P, Mellquist E, Hjelmstrom P, Wahren-Herlenius M. Expression of the B cell-attracting chemokine CXCL13 in the target organ and autoantibody production in ectopic lymphoid tissue in the chronic inflammatory disease Sjogren's syndrome. *Scand J Immunol* (2002) 55(4):336–42. doi:10.1046/j.1365-3083.2002.01058.x
101. Barone F, Bombardieri M, Manzo A, Blades MC, Morgan PR, Challacombe SJ, et al. Association of CXCL13 and CCL21 expression with the progressive organization of lymphoid-like structures in Sjogren's syndrome. *Arthritis Rheum* (2005) 52(6):1773–84. doi:10.1002/art.21062
102. Prineas JW. Multiple sclerosis: presence of lymphatic capillaries and lymphoid tissue in the brain and spinal cord. *Science* (1979) 203(4385):1123–5. doi:10.1126/science.424741
103. Serafini B, Rosicarelli B, Magliozzi R, Stigliano E, Aloisi F. Detection of ectopic B-cell follicles with germinal centers in the meninges of patients with secondary progressive multiple sclerosis. *Brain Pathol* (2004) 14(2):164–74. doi:10.1111/j.1750-3639.2004.tb00049.x
104. Magliozzi R, Howell O, Vora A, Serafini B, Nicholas R, Puopolo M, et al. Meningeal B-cell follicles in secondary progressive multiple sclerosis associate with early onset of disease and severe cortical pathology. *Brain* (2007) 130(Pt 4):1089–104. doi:10.1093/brain/awm038
105. Campbell DA, Poulter LW, Janossy G, du Bois RM. Immunohistological analysis of lung tissue from patients with cryptogenic fibrosing alveolitis suggesting local expression of immune hypersensitivity. *Thorax* (1985) 40(6):405–11. doi:10.1136/thx.40.6.405
106. Wallace WA, Howie SE, Krajewski AS, Lamb D. The immunological architecture of B-lymphocyte aggregates in cryptogenic fibrosing alveolitis. *J Pathol* (1996) 178(3):323–9. doi:10.1002/(SICI)1096-9896(199603)178:3<323:AID-PATH467>3.0.CO;2-7
107. Chang A, Henderson SG, Brandt D, Liu N, Guttikonda R, Hsieh C, et al. In situ B cell-mediated immune responses and tubulointerstitial inflammation in human lupus nephritis. *J Immunol* (2011) 186(3):1849–60. doi:10.4049/jimmunol.1001983
108. Clark MR, Trotter K, Chang A. The pathogenesis and therapeutic implications of tubulointerstitial inflammation in human lupus nephritis. *Semin Nephrol* (2015) 35(5):455–64. doi:10.1016/j.semnephrol.2015.08.007
109. Mosnier JF, Degott C, Marcellin P, Henin D, Erlinger S, Benhamou JP. The intraportal lymphoid nodule and its environment in chronic active hepatitis C: an immunohistochemical study. *Hepatology* (1993) 17(3):366–71. doi:10.1002/hep.1840170304
110. Murakami J, Shimizu Y, Kashii Y, Kato T, Minemura M, Okada K, et al. Functional B-cell response in intrahepatic lymphoid follicles in chronic hepatitis C. *Hepatology* (1999) 30(1):143–50. doi:10.1002/hep.510300107
111. Genta RM, Hamner HW, Graham DY. Gastric lymphoid follicles in *Helicobacter pylori* infection: frequency, distribution, and response to triple therapy. *Hum Pathol* (1993) 24(6):577–83. doi:10.1016/0046-8177(93)90235-9
112. Genta RM, Hamner HW. The significance of lymphoid follicles in the interpretation of gastric biopsy specimens. *Arch Pathol Lab Med* (1994) 118(7):740–3.
113. Stolte M, Eidt S. Lymphoid follicles in antral mucosa: immune response to *Campylobacter pylori*? *J Clin Pathol* (1989) 42(12):1269–71. doi:10.1136/jcp.42.12.1269
114. Eidt S, Stolte M. Prevalence of lymphoid follicles and aggregates in *Helicobacter pylori* gastritis in antral and body mucosa. *J Clin Pathol* (1993) 46(9):832–5. doi:10.1136/jcp.46.9.832
115. Mazzucchelli L, Blaser A, Kappeler A, Scharli P, Laissue JA, Baggiolini M, et al. BCA-1 is highly expressed in *Helicobacter pylori*-induced mucosa-associated lymphoid tissue and gastric lymphoma. *J Clin Invest* (1999) 104(10):R49–54. doi:10.1172/JCI7830
116. Steere AC, Duray PH, Butcher EC. Spirochetal antigens and lymphoid cell surface markers in Lyme synovitis. Comparison with rheumatoid synovium and tonsillar lymphoid tissue. *Arthritis Rheum* (1988) 31(4):487–95. doi:10.1002/art.1780310405
117. Ghosh S, Steere AC, Stollar BD, Huber BT. In situ diversification of the antibody repertoire in chronic Lyme arthritis synovium. *J Immunol* (2005) 174(5):2860–9. doi:10.4049/jimmunol.174.5.2860
118. Thaunat O, Patey N, Caligiuri G, Gautreau C, Mamani-Matsuda M, Mekki Y, et al. Chronic rejection triggers the development of an aggressive intragraft immune response through recapitulation of lymphoid organogenesis. *J Immunol* (2010) 185(1):717–28. doi:10.4049/jimmunol.0903589
119. Sato M, Hirayama S, Matsuda Y, Wagnetz D, Hwang DM, Guan Z, et al. Stromal activation and formation of lymphoid-like stroma in chronic lung allograft dysfunction. *Transplantation* (2011) 91(12):1398–405. doi:10.1097/TP.0b013e31821b2f7a
120. Carlsen HS, Baekkevold ES, Johansen FE, Haraldsen G, Brandtzaeg P. B cell attracting chemokine 1 (CXCL13) and its receptor CXCR5 are expressed in normal and aberrant gut associated lymphoid tissue. *Gut* (2002) 51(3):364–71. doi:10.1136/gut.51.3.364
121. Kaiserling E. Newly-formed lymph nodes in the submucosa in chronic inflammatory bowel disease. *Lymphology* (2001) 34(1):22–9.
122. Guedj K, Khallou-Laschet J, Clement M, Morvan M, Delbosc S, Gaston AT, et al. Inflammatory micro-environmental cues of human atherothrombotic arteries confer to vascular smooth muscle cells the capacity to trigger lymphoid neogenesis. *PLoS One* (2014) 9(12):e116295. doi:10.1371/journal.pone.0116295

123. Houtkamp MA, de Boer OJ, van der Loos CM, van der Wal AC, Becker AE. Adventitial infiltrates associated with advanced atherosclerotic plaques: structural organization suggests generation of local humoral immune responses. *J Pathol* (2001) 193(2):263–9. doi:10.1002/1096-9896(2000)9999:9999<:AID-PATH774>3.0.CO;2-N
124. Dieu-Nosjean MC, Antoine M, Danel C, Heudes D, Wislez M, Poulot V, et al. Long-term survival for patients with non-small-cell lung cancer with intratumoral lymphoid structures. *J Clin Oncol* (2008) 26(27):4410–7. doi:10.1200/JCO.2007.15.0284
125. Germain C, Gnjatic S, Tamzalit F, Knockaert S, Remark R, Goc J, et al. Presence of B cells in tertiary lymphoid structures is associated with a protective immunity in patients with lung cancer. *Am J Respir Crit Care Med* (2014) 189(7):832–44. doi:10.1164/rccm.201309-1611OC
126. Vayrynen JP, Sajanti SA, Klintrup K, Makela J, Herzig KH, Karttunen TJ, et al. Characteristics and significance of colorectal cancer associated lymphoid reaction. *Int J Cancer* (2014) 134(9):2126–35. doi:10.1002/ijc.28533
127. Coronella JA, Spier C, Welch M, Trevor KT, Stopeck AT, Villar H, et al. Antigen-driven oligoclonal expansion of tumor-infiltrating B cells in infiltrating ductal carcinoma of the breast. *J Immunol* (2002) 169(4):1829–36. doi:10.4049/jimmunol.169.4.1829
128. Nzula S, Going JJ, Stott DI. Antigen-driven clonal proliferation, somatic hypermutation, and selection of B lymphocytes infiltrating human ductal breast carcinomas. *Cancer Res* (2003) 63(12):3275–80.
129. Cipponi A, Mercier M, Seremet T, Baurain JF, Theate I, van den Oord J, et al. Neogenesis of lymphoid structures and antibody responses occur in human melanoma metastases. *Cancer Res* (2012) 72(16):3997–4007. doi:10.1158/0008-5472.CAN-12-1377

4

Model-Driven Experimentation: A New Approach to Understand Mechanisms of Tertiary Lymphoid Tissue Formation, Function and Therapeutic Resolution

*James A. Butler[1,2,3†], Jason Cosgrove[1,2,3†], Kieran Alden[2,3], Jon Timmis[2,3] and Mark Christopher Coles[1,3]**

[1] Centre for Immunology and Infection, Department of Biology, Hull York Medical School, York, UK, [2] Department of Electronics, University of York, York, UK, [3] York Computational Immunology Laboratory, University of York, York, UK

***Correspondence:**
Mark Christopher Coles
mark.coles@york.ac.uk

†Co-first authors.

The molecular and cellular processes driving the formation of secondary lymphoid tissues have been extensively studied using a combination of mouse knockouts, lineage-specific reporter mice, gene expression analysis, immunohistochemistry, and flow cytometry. However, the mechanisms driving the formation and function of tertiary lymphoid tissue (TLT) experimental techniques have proven to be more enigmatic and controversial due to differences between experimental models and human disease pathology. Systems-based approaches including data-driven biological network analysis (gene interaction network, metabolic pathway network, cell–cell signaling, and cascade networks) and mechanistic modeling afford a novel perspective from which to understand TLT formation and identify mechanisms that may lead to the resolution of tissue pathology. In this perspective, we make the case for applying model-driven experimentation using two case studies, which combined simulations with experiments to identify mechanisms driving lymphoid tissue formation and function, and then discuss potential applications of this experimental paradigm to identify novel therapeutic targets for TLT pathology.

Keywords: multi-scale modeling, tertiary lymphoid tissue, systems immunology, mechanistic modelling, model-driven experimentation

FORMATION AND FUNCTION OF SECONDARY AND TERTIARY IMMUNE MICROENVIRONMENTS

Lymphoid tissues are responsible for the orchestration of functional immune responses. This is achieved through the development and maintenance of niches that support the retention, activation, and proliferation of adaptive immune cells in response to antigenic stimulation. Adult lymphoid tissue architecture is organized by an underlying network of stromal cells that produce extracellular matrix (e.g., collagens) and provide survival (e.g., BAFF, IL-7), migratory (CCL19/21, CXCL13), and immune activation [the storage and presentation of immune complexes by follicular dendritic cell (FDC)] signals (1). Distinct stromal subsets with unique secretion profiles (chemokines, other cytokines, and survival factors) develop in response to signaling from lymphocytes with a key role for TNF superfamily receptors; this stromal–lymphocyte cross talk ensures the correct cell type is stimulated (or regulated) at the right time and place. Sustained cross talk between mesenchymal stroma and lymphocyte subsets is a core feature of lymphoid tissue formation and maintenance and occurs irrespective of the tissue type or anatomical location.

Formation of lymphoid tissues can occur by different cellular and molecular mechanisms. During fetal development, secondary lymphoid tissues form in a process dependent on the RAR-related orphan receptor gamma transcription factor expressing lymphoid tissue inducer cells (LTi) responding to localized chemotactic gradients leading to the formation of lymph nodes (LN) and Peyer's patches (PPs) in a lymphotoxin β (LTβ)-dependent process (2). Localized mesenchyme, lymphoid tissue organizer (LTo) cells differentiate into adult marginal reticular cells, fibroblastic reticular cells, and FDCs (3). Likewise, in the adult, innate lymphoid cells type 3, the adult equivalent of LTi cells, have a key role in regulating cryptopatches that can mature into isolated lymphoid follicles (4). These specialized lymphoid structures contain predominantly B cells and often contain germinal center (GC) reactions.

In humans, tertiary lymphoid tissues (TLTs) are found in inflammatory immune responses associated with chronic pathology from hip joint replacements, keloids, tissues in autoimmune disease (e.g., the salivary gland in Sjogren's syndrome, multiple sclerosis, and rheumatoid arthritis) to solid tumors and follicular lymphomas in the bone marrow (5–9). Although the role of specific cell types has been controversial, there is an emerging paradigm of a multistep process where localized inflammation induces stromal cell activation in a lymphocyte independent process, leading to localized microenvironments permissive for T and B cells entry (10). These lymphocytes have the potential to drive the formation of organized tertiary tissue in an autocrine-dependent process. This process closely resembles the capacity of naive B cells to drive B cell follicle formation in secondary lymphoid tissues in a TNFα- and LTβ-dependent process and the capacity of activated B cells to generate the GC, a transient microenvironment that drives high-affinity immune responses in a self-regulating autocrine-dependent process. In both secondary immune tissues (LN, PPs, and spleen) and TLTs including ILFs and TLT, activated B cells prime the formation of the GC reaction. This specialized microenvironment contains both activated and proliferating B cells and different stromal compartments of CXCL12-secreting stroma (dark zone) and CXCL13-secreting FDCs (light zone). This facilitates the cyclic selection and expansion of antigen-specific B cells (11).

Non-lymphoid inflammatory immune structures, granulomas, can form in the liver, intestine, adipose tissue (crown-like structures), and lung induced by chronic infection/inflammation associated with tuberculosis, sarcoidosis leishmaniasis, schistosomiasis, cell death, and Crohn's disease (12–14). The formation of these highly dynamic microenvironments superficially resembles TLT; however, their formation and organization is driven by activated macrophages rather than by the mesenchymal–lymphocyte cross talk observed in lymphoid tissues thus do not exhibit lymphocyte compartmentalization. Granuloma structures are very heterogeneous in presentation within individual patients in a continuum between early macrophage centric granulomas, self-resolving granulomas, and fibroblastic structures, these often being fibrotic rather than taking on a supportive stromal network phenotype. The triggers that drive granuloma formation instead of TLT formation appear not to be due to differences in the different chemotactic cues delivered by activated macrophages compared to those delivered by activated stromal fibroblasts, leading to a very different cellular make up to the inflammatory foci of leukocytes [primarily myelomonocytic (granuloma) vs. lymphocytic (TLT)].

CURRENT APPROACHES TO STUDYING LYMPHOID TISSUE FORMATION: LIMITS, CHALLENGES, AND NEW APPROACHES

Experimental studies, principally performed in gene knockout, lineage-specific fluorescent protein, and Cre reporter mouse lines have contributed significant insights into the roles of multiple different cell types and molecules in lymphoid tissue formation and function. This has been further validated using histology and flow cytometry analysis on human secondary lymphoid tissues. However, in contrast to secondary lymphoid tissues, there are some distinct differences in human tissue pathologies to those found in mice including the cellular composition of TLTs, granulomas, and other inflammatory tissues. This arises in part from genetic and physiological differences between human and mice including the timing and duration of the immune response (chronic vs. acute inflammation), the inflammatory triggers (infection, autoimmunity, and cancer), and transcriptional differences in immune cells in the different species. In general, mouse models of immune-mediated inflammatory disease are acute and fail to replicate the chronic human disease characterized by disease flairs followed by remission, limiting their translational capacity to human disease. Infection and tumor models in mice either rapidly resolve (too quickly for chronic pathology to establish) or lead to the mouse having to by euthanized for health and welfare prior to tertiary lymphoid pathology occurring. In comparison, humans may live the rest of their life with the disease pathology, particularly in the context of treatment with biologics and small molecules; thus, pathology has the opportunity to evolve from localized inflammation to fibrotic tissue failure, systemic inflammation, and autoimmunity working together to prevent disease resolution. Increasingly, human 3-dimensional tissue culture models containing both stroma and lymphocytes have become increasingly common and useful in understanding underlying molecule mechanisms of TLT formation. However, it is not currently possible to represent the full complexity of chronic human pathology *in vitro*.

Experimental systems (*in vivo* and *in vitro*) to date have proven limited in their ability to explain chronic clinical pathology and resolve established Sjogren's pathology, although TNF has an important role in FDC differentiation and B cell organization, anti-TNF fails to induce resolution disease (15). To better understand the form and function of TLTs, current knowledge of stromal regulation through molecular signals and immune cell behavior within lymphoid tissue must be consolidated and considered in a quantitative, systems-based approach. The development of systems-level stochastic computational models can bring together a broad understanding across spatiotemporal scales of how genetic and molecular factors relate to cellular and tissue level form and function and give rise to the complex, functional architectures observed in secondary lymphoid organs and disease-specific TLTs. These models permit *in silico* experimentation providing a unique platform driving further experimentation and assessing novel mechanistic targets and intervention strategies where *in vivo* observed heterogeneity can be replicated.

Alan Turing (of code breaking fame) in seminal early work in mathematical biology (16) noted that gastrulation arose from symmetry breaking, and this leads to fundamental insights and principles that drive modern mathematical and computational biology: the notion that chaotic, non-linear behavior of individual biological processes, including the self-organization of complex biological structures (e.g., TLT), can result in emergent properties that cannot be understood from consideration of each individual component in isolation. The development of models that capture the essential, emergent behavior of specific biological processes, with extraneous components excluded, enables understanding of how complex molecular and cellular interactions govern complex, emergent biological processes and can therefore lead to new insights and quantitative predictions (17). Emergent properties in a TLT model would include stromal networks, lymphocyte organization, migration and interactions with antigen-presenting cells, and localized cytokine/chemokine production.

APPLICATION OF MODEL-DRIVEN EXPERIMENTATION (MDE) TO UNDERSTAND MECHANISMS OF LYMPHOID TISSUE DEVELOPMENT AND FUNCTION

Advances in computing resources and computational modeling technology have provided the capacity to generate complex *in silico* models of lymphoid tissues that incorporate space, time, and cellular heterogeneity found in immune tissues including TLT. Applying *in silico* approaches to understand secondary lymphoid tissue formation and function requires the integration of experimental data across cellular, molecular, and tissue levels of organization. Ensuring that the biological processes are appropriately described requires a fine balance between model abstraction and interpretation (quantitative and qualitative) of experimental data. A number of different modeling approaches may be utilized (summarized in **Table 1**), increasingly, integration of different mathematical/computational techniques into a hybrid model is a common strategy to address the limitations of using each technique in isolation This approach also facilitates the consolidation of data across different levels of organization (molecular, cellular, tissue, and patient) into a single multi-scale model. For example, an agent-based model can capture an individual cell, which in turn incorporates a differential equation-based model capturing a "lower-level" aspect of that individual's behavior, such as surface expression of a receptor (42). Adopting an *in silico* approach provides a platform that can

TABLE 1 | Mathematical and computational techniques for modeling immune processes.

Technique	Description	Comments
ODE	Ordinary differential equations: describe the rate of change with respect to one other variable (e.g., population change over time, *t*)	Commonly used technique that can be used to quantify changes in population size over time
PDE	Partial differential equations: describe rate of change of a function of more than one variable with respect to one of those variables (e.g., motion through space *x*, *y*, and *z* as a function of time *t*)	Often used to describe changes occurring over both time and multiple spatial dimensions
Monte Carlo	Statistical random sampling method where outcomes are determined at random from input probability distribution functions	Stochastic technique to model deterministic processes, very frequently integrated within ABM, CPM, and other stochastic modeling approaches
Petri nets	Graph-based model describing network of events or "transitions" that occur depending on given conditions or "places," a stochastic methodology	Computationally efficient can be effectively defined using SBML2. Capturing explicit spatial representation can be difficult
ABMs	Agent-based models are composed of individual entities specified as agents, which exist independently in a well-defined state: a set of attributes at a specific point in, e.g., time and space, with state transitions governed by a rule-set, often described in terms of finite state machines and other diagrammatic constructs using the Unified Modeling Language	There are a number of methodologies to generate ABMs. There are tools with user interfaces for constructing simpler lattice-based ABMS or "unconstrained" models manually coded as software in languages such as Java and C++
(Extended) cellular Potts modeling	A lattice-based modeling technique for simulating the collective behavior of cells. A cell is defined as a set of pixels within a lattice (sharing a "spin state") and is updated pixel-by-pixel according to a mathematical function, which incorporates cell volume and surface/adhesion energies	Similar to an ABM but relies on effective energy functions (the Hamiltonian) to describe cellular adhesion, signaling, motility, and other physical phenomena
Hybridized models	Bringing together a range of different techniques generally within the context of an ABM or CPM, incorporating differential equations and a variety of other mathematical and computational techniques to effectively capture phenomena occurring over different spatiotemporal scales (e.g., intracellular activity)	Can take advantage of different modeling techniques, particularly applicable where there are multiple processes occurring in different scales of time and space

provide insights and generate predictions that can be verified *in vivo*: verification that can lead to increased biological understanding and incrementally improved *in silico* models for further experimentation. This iterative approach of combining *in vivo*, *in vitro*, and *in silico* approaches has been termed "model-driven experimentation" (18).

CASE STUDY 1: INSIGHTS FROM MDE TO SECONDARY LYMPHOID TISSUE FORMATION

Peyer's patches are specialized secondary lymphoid tissues of the intestine that develop during a fixed window in fetal development and have an essential role in maintaining intestinal immunity. PPs form stochastically along the midgut, with mice developing 8–12 patches; however, as the absence of or reduction in the number of PPs is observed in several different gene knockouts, the molecular process that triggers patch formation was unclear (19). Using an MDE-based approach had the potential to provide new insight into how different signaling pathways (RET, chemokine receptors, cytokine receptors, TNF superfamily, and adhesion molecules) might integrate to induce PP development *in silico* and to subsequently design key experiments to test hypotheses *in vivo*. PPSim is an agent-based PP simulator that captures key processes during the 72-h period of tissue development in prenatal mice and replicates (statistically similar) emergent cell behaviors found *in vivo*, specifically populations of hematopoietic cells, known as lymphoid tissue initiator (LTin) and lymphoid tissue inducer (LTi) cells, migrates into the developing gut, with data from laboratory observations suggesting these cells follow a random motion. Both cell populations express receptors for the adhesion molecule VCAM-1, expressed by stromal LTo cells residing in the gut wall (20, 21). In this computational model, LTi and LTin are captured as individual entities that migrate into the developing midgut serosa and undergo a random walk, interacting with their localized simulated environment through signaling pathways including GDRFs/Ret signaling pathways, adhesion molecules, and chemokine receptors, as is observed *in vivo*. On ensuring PPsim adequately represented individual cell responses, statistical analysis techniques, specifically sensitivity analyses, were used to explore mechanisms driving prenatal lymphoid organ formation (22, 23). This exploration of the simulated biological pathways revealed which pathways had significant impacts on simulated cell behavior at different time points during PP development. By examining correlations in the level of activity of simulated pathways and cell behavior, the hypothesis was derived that contact between LTin and LTo cells that leads to the localized upregulation of VCAM-1 on stromal cells was the key triggering event that determined the site of PP formation on the midgut (21). Utilizing this prediction, an *in vitro* assay imaging fetal midgut explants incubated in the presence or absence of anti-VCAM-1 antibodies was developed. Using this assay, it was verified that early upregulation of VCAM-1 was the triggering event that was essential for the initiation of LTi and LTin cell clustering. The model simulation results, supported by replicated experimentation and safety-critical systems-based fitness-for-purpose argumentation that details the knowledge integration in model composition, provide evidence that the simulation was fit for the purpose of aiding exploration of this specific research question: understanding the triggering of lymphoid tissue development, which was not possible by conventional genetic approaches (24, 25).

CASE STUDY 2: APPLYING MDE TO UNDERSTAND GC DYNAMICS AND FUNCTION

The GC reaction is a transient microenvironment in which affinity maturation occurs in response to immunization and infection, bearing key similarities to TLT in its evolution in the role of lymphocytes in inducing highly organized stromal networks, the essential role of TNF superfamily members in regulating its induction and the induction of chemokine gradients (10, 26). However, in comparison to TLT, the GC is a self-resolving tertiary lymphoid microenvironment. Recent technological advances, particularly the advent of intravital multiphoton imaging including photo-activated fluorescent proteins has led to the unprecedented availability of data on the dynamics B-cell migration and selection (27–30). However, imaging datasets provide a narrow window of insight into a process that occurs over a timescale of days and weeks. Furthermore, as imaging techniques are optimized for a given time and length scale, they are limited in their ability to link molecular, cellular, and tissue level processes. This has made the interpretation of imaging datasets in the context of the wider literature challenging. To address this issue, modeling approaches have been used to test the validity of different hypotheses of mechanisms controlling B-cell migration and selection within the GC (31–34).

In the GC reaction, model-derived insights have proved useful not only in the analysis of existing datasets but also as a driver for further experimentation. Specifically, an MDE approach has been used to examine the effects of antibody feedback on the process of affinity maturation (35). Analysis of an *in silico* GC reaction yielded the prediction that GC B-cells, which require antigen on FDCs for positive selection, were competing for antigen by early low-affinity antibodies. Only higher affinity B-cells were able to outcompete for antigen to receive the necessary survival signals. To experimentally validate this prediction, the authors manipulated the GC response with monoclonal antibodies of defined affinities and were able to confirm that antibody feedback provides a dynamic selection threshold to maximize Ig affinities (35). A similar approach was employed to investigate the role of toll-like receptor 4 (TLR4) on the GC where an iterative cycle of *in silico* and *in vivo* experimentation dissected the importance of TLR4 signaling on the maturation of FDCs, key regulators of B-cell selection in the light zone of the GC (36). Both of these MDE examples highlight the use of *in silico* experimentation as a means of refining experimental design through the identification of key time points and conditions to test *in vivo*. These case studies together provide example of how theoretical models can consolidate data from different

TABLE 2 | Key questions on tertiary lymphoid tissue (TLT) formation and maintenance that can be address in hybridized TLT models.

Formation
What are the minimum cellular requirements to initiate TLT formation? Is this driven by different types of stroma, lymphocytes, dendritic cells, or tissue-resident macrophage?
What is the relative importance of inflammation and antigen in TLT induction? Is autoantigen required for induction or just an outcome of the pathology?
What is the role of different cytokines and chemotactic signals on TLT formation?
Maintenance
What is the relative role of inflammatory cytokines, lymphocyte—stromal cross talk, immune cell entry, cell death, antigenic stimulation on TLT maintenance?
What are the key signaling pathways required to maintain TLT once it has formed? Can these pathways be targeted to induce TLT resolution?
Can TLT self-resolve in humans? If so, what is the balance between new TLT induction and resolution of existing structures?

sources as a platform for the development novel hypotheses and a driver for further experimentation.

PERSPECTIVE ON MDE AS APPLIED TO TLT FORMATION, FUNCTION, AND THERAPEUTIC RESOLUTION

When computational modeling is combined with knowledge derived from imaging, multi-dimensional cytometry, and gene expression analysis of human TLT pathology, MDE has the potential to provide novel insights to key questions on molecular and cellular mechanisms involved in TLT formation, maintenance, and function similar to its capacity to impact on our understanding of lymphoid stromal network and granuloma dynamics (**Table 2**) (37–40). One of the key advantages of applying multi-scale modeling is it permits capture of a wide range of different phenomena that occur on different orders of magnitude in terms of time and length scales that are critical in the stochastic processes involved in TLT induction. These include different cell types, states and interactions, inflammatory molecules, extracellular matrix, adhesion molecules, and chemotactic signals all in the context of an evolving tissue microenvironment. Developing *in silico* models permits temporal inhibition of different signaling pathways and cellular depletions during different stages of TLT pathology using statistical tools (**Figure 1**). This permits identification of key pathways that could be targeted to induce resolution of pre-existing TLT rather than inhibiting its formation as has been used to make *in silico* predictions for the treatment of tuberculosis (41). A large number of novel antibody therapies, biologics, and small molecular inhibitors have been developed to target immune function for the treatment of immune-mediated inflammatory diseases. These therapies are unlikely to show maximal efficacy against existing tissue pathology when used as monotherapies, rather it is more likely that use of therapeutic combinations that is most likely to show clinical efficacy. The clinical challenge is that there are already over 20,000 possible different combinations using existing therapeutics that would need to be trialed to find optimal targeting strategy to resolve TLT pathology. Thus, MDE-based approaches provide a rational approach to identify novel combination therapeutic regimes that have a best potential in clinical trials (42).

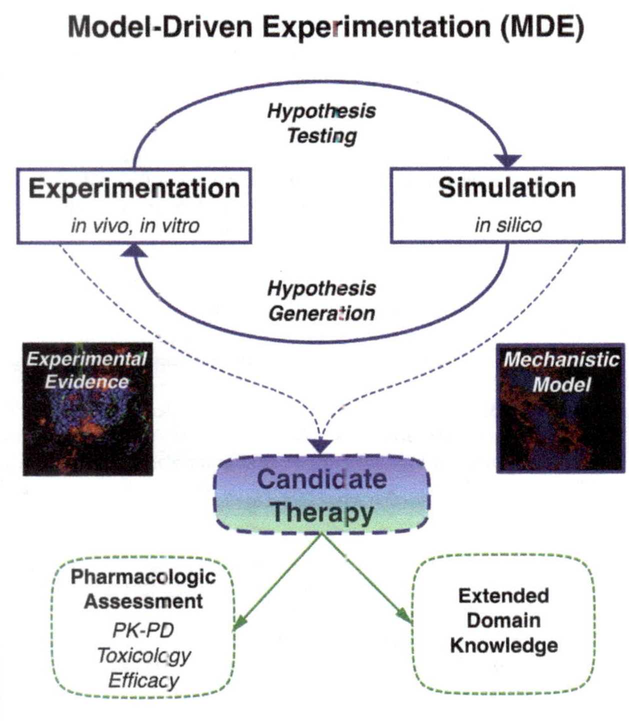

FIGURE 1 | **Application of model-driven experimentation to develop new mechanistic understanding of tertiary lymphoid tissue (TLT) formation and maintenance permitting identification of novel therapeutic approaches to resolve localized TLT pathology.**

Although the adoption of MDE has only recently started to impact on immunology research, it is starting to have a very significant impact on other areas of biology. We propose that the increased accessibility of computational models, the high-performance computing resources, the increased familiarity and understanding of simulations as tools to understand immune function, and the capacity to apply *in silico* approaches to identify potential therapeutic approaches and disease biomarkers will accelerate the application of MDE as a methodology understand and target disease resolution.

AUTHOR CONTRIBUTIONS

MC wrote this paper and is the corresponding author. JB, JC, KA and JT contributed to the writing of this perspective.

FUNDING

JC is supported by Wellcome Trust (Computational Approaches in Translational Science) WT095024MA. Research in MC providing a basis for this perspective is supported by MRC MR/K021125/1.

REFERENCES

1. Junt T, Scandella E, Ludewig B. Form follows function: lymphoid tissue microarchitecture in antimicrobial immune defence. *Nat Rev Immunol* (2008) 8:764–75. doi:10.1038/nri2414
2. van de Pavert SA, Mebius R. New insights into the development of lymphoid tissues. *Nat Rev Immunol* (2010) 10:664–74. doi:10.1038/nri2832
3. Jarjour M, Jorquera A, Mondor I, Wienert S, Narang P, Coles M, et al. Fate mapping reveals origin and dynamics of lymph node follicular dendritic cells. *J Exp Med* (2014) 211(6):1109–22. doi:10.1084/jem.20132409
4. Mowat A, Agace W. Regional specialization within the intestinal immune system. *Nat Rev Immunol* (2014) 14:667–85. doi:10.1038/nri3738
5. Mittal S, Revell M, Barone F, Hardie DL, Matharu GS, Davenport AJ, et al. Lymphoid aggregates that resemble tertiary lymphoid organs define a specific pathological subset in metal-on-metal hip replacements. *PLoS One* (2013) 8(5):e63470. doi:10.1371/journal.pone.0063470
6. Bombardieri M, Barone F, Lucchesi D, Nayar S, van den Berg WB, Proctor G, et al. Inducible tertiary lymphoid structures, autoimmunity, and exocrine dysfunction in a novel model of salivary gland inflammation in C57BL/6 mice. *J Immunol* (2012) 189(7):3767–76. doi:10.4049/jimmunol.1201216
7. Bagabir R, Byers RJ, Chaudhry IH, Müller W, Paus R, Bayat A. Site-specific immunophenotyping of keloid disease demonstrates immune upregulation and the presence of lymphoid aggregates. *Br J Dermatol* (2012) 167(5):1053–66. doi:10.1111/j.1365-2133.2012.11190.x
8. Dieu-Nosjean MC, Giraldo NA, Kaplon H, Germain C, Fridman WH, Sautès-Fridman C. Tertiary lymphoid structures, drivers of the anti-tumor responses in human cancers. *Immunol Rev* (2016) 271(1):260–75. doi:10.1111/imr.12405
9. Guilloton F, Caron G, Ménard C, Pangault C, Amé-Thomas P, Dulong J, et al. Mesenchymal stromal cells orchestrate follicular lymphoma cell niche through the CCL2-dependent recruitment and polarization of monocytes. *Blood* (2012) 119(11):2556–67. doi:10.1182/blood-2011-08-370908
10. De Silva NS, Klein U. Dynamics of B cells in germinal centres. *Nat Rev Immunol* (2015) 15:137–48. doi:10.1038/nri3804
11. Zhang Y, Garcia-Ibanez L, Toellner KM. Regulation of germinal center B-cell differentiation. *Immunol Rev* (2016) 270(1):8–19. doi:10.1111/imr.12396
12. Sandor M, Weinstock JV, Wynn TA. Granulomas in schistosome and mycobacterial infections: a model of local immune responses. *Trends Immunol* (2003) 24(1):44–52. doi:10.1016/S1471-4906(02)00006-6
13. Kaye PM, Beattie L. Lessons from other diseases: granulomatous inflammation in leishmaniasis. *Semin Immunopathol* (2016) 38(2):249–60. doi:10.1007/s00281-015-0548-7
14. Bolus WR, Gutierrez DA, Kennedy AJ, Anderson-Baucum EK, Hasty AH. CCR2 deficiency leads to increased eosinophils, alternative macrophage activation, and type 2 cytokine expression in adipose tissue. *J Leukoc Biol* (2015) 98(4):467–77. doi:10.1189/jlb.3HI0115-018R
15. Sankar V, Brennan MT, Kok MR, Leakan RA, Smith JA, Manny J, et al. Etanercept in Sjogren's syndrome: a twelve-week randomized, doubleblind, placebo-controlled pilot clinical trial. *Arthritis Rheum* (2004) 50:2240–5. doi:10.1002/art.20299
16. Turing AM. The chemical basis of morphogenesis. *Philos Trans R Soc Lond B Biol Sci* (1952) 237(641):37–72. doi:10.1098/rstb.1952.0012
17. Callard RE, Yates AJ. Immunology and mathematics: crossing the divide. *Immunology* (2005) 115(1):21–33. doi:10.1111/j.1365-2567.2005.02142.x
18. Ganesan A, Levchenko A. Principles of model building: an experimentation-aided approach to development of models for signaling networks. *Methods Cell Biol* (2012) 110:1–17. doi:10.1016/B978-0-12-388403-9.00001-1
19. Veiga-Fernandes H, Coles MC, Foster KE, Patel A, Williams A, Natarajan D, et al. Tyrosine kinase receptor RET is a key regulator in Peyer's patch organogenesis. *Nature* (2007) 446(7135):547–51. doi:10.1038/nature05597
20. Alden K, Timmis J, Andrews PS, Veiga-Fernandes H, Coles M. Pairing experimentation and computational modelling to understand the role of tissue inducer cells in the development of lymphoid organs. *Front Immunol* (2012) 3:172. doi:10.3389/fimmu.2012.00172
21. Patel N, Harker L, Moreira-Santos M, Ferreira K, Alden J, Timmis K, et al. Differential RET signaling pathways drive development of the enteric lymphoid and nervous systems. *Sci Signal* (2012) 5:235. doi:10.1126/scisignal.2002734
22. Alden K, Read M, Timmis J, Andrews P, Veiga-Fernades H, Coles M. Spartan: a comprehensive tool for understanding uncertainty in simulations of biological systems. *PLoS Comput Biol* (2013) 9(2):e1002916. doi:10.1371/journal.pcbi.1002916
23. Butler JA, Alden K, Veiga Fernandex H, Timmis J, Coles M. Novel approaches to the visualization and quantification of biological simulations by emulating experimental techniques. *ALIFE 14: Proceedings of the Fourteenth International Conference on the Synthesis and Simulation of Living Systems* (Vol. 14), New York: MIT Press (2014). p. 614–21.
24. Alden K, Andrews PS, Veiga-Fernandes H, Timmis J, Coles M. Utilising a simulation platform to understand the effect of domain model assumptions. *Nat Comput* (2015) 14(1):99–107. doi:10.1007/s11047-014-9428-7
25. Alden K, Andrews PS, Polack FA, Veiga-Fernandes H, Coles MC, Timmis J. Using argument notation to engineer biological simulations with increased confidence. *J R Soc Interface* (2015) 12(104):20141059. doi:10.1098/rsif.2014.1059
26. Victora GD, Mesin L. Clonal and cellular dynamics in germinal centers. *Curr Opin Immunol* (2014) 28:90–6. doi:10.1016/j.coi.2014.02.010
27. Allen CDC, Okada T, Tang HL, Cyster JG. Imaging of germinal center selection events during affinity maturation. *Science* (2007) 315:528–31. doi:10.1126/science.1136736
28. Schwickert TA, Lindquist RL, Shakhar G, Livshits G, Skokos D, Kosco-Vilbois MH, et al. In vivo imaging of germinal centres reveals a dynamic open structure. *Nature* (2007) 446:83–7. doi:10.1038/nature05573
29. Shulman Z, Gitlin AD, Targ S, Jankovic M, Pasqual G, Nussenzweig MC, et al. T follicular helper cell dynamics in germinal centers. *Science* (2013) 341:673–7. doi:10.1126/science.1241680
30. Shulman Z, Gitlin AD, Weinstein JS, Lainez B, Esplugues E, Flavell RA, et al. Dynamic signaling by T follicular helper cells during germinal center B cell selection. *Science* (2014) 345:1058–62. doi:10.1126/science.1257861
31. Chan C, Billard M, Ramirez SA, Schmidl H, Monson E, Kepler TB. A model for migratory B cell oscillations from receptor down-regulation induced by external chemokine fields. *Bull Math Biol* (2013) 75:185–205. doi:10.1007/s11538-012-9799-9
32. Figge MT, Garin A, Gunzer M, Kosco-Vilbois M, Toellner K-M, Meyer-Hermann M. Deriving a germinal center lymphocyte migration model from two-photon data. *J Exp Med* (2008) 205:3019–29. doi:10.1084/jem.20081160
33. Meyer-Hermann ME, Maini PK, Iber D. An analysis of B cell selection mechanisms in germinal centers. *Math Med Biol* (2006) 23:255–77. doi:10.1093/imammb/dql012
34. Meyer-Hermann M, Mohr E, Pelletier N, Zhang Y, Victora GD, Toellner K-M. A theory of germinal center B cell selection, division, and exit. *Cell Rep* (2012) 2:162–74. doi:10.1016/j.celrep.2012.05.010
35. Zhang Y, Meyer-Hermann M, George LA, Figge MT, Khan M, Goodall M, et al. Germinal center B cells govern their own fate via antibody feedback. *J Exp Med* (2013) 210:457–64. doi:10.1084/jem.20120150
36. Garin A, Meyer-Hermann M, Contie M, Figge MT, Buatois V, Gunzer M, et al. Toll-like receptor 4 signaling by follicular dendritic cells is pivotal for germinal center onset and affinity maturation. *Immunity* (2010) 33:84–95. doi:10.1016/j.immuni.2010.07.005
37. Kislitsyn A, Savinkov R, Novkovic M, Onder L, Bocharov G. Computational approach to 3D modeling of the lymph node geometry. *Computation* (2015) 3(2):222–34. doi:10.3390/computation3020222
38. Novkovic M, Onder L, Cupovic J, Abe J, Bomze D, Cremasco V, et al. Topological small-world organization of the fibroblastic reticular cell network determines lymph node functionality. *PLoS Biol* (2016) 14(7):e1002515. doi:10.1371/journal.pbio.1002515
39. Warsinske HC, Wheaton AK, Kim KK, Linderman JJ, Moore BB, Kirschner DE. Computational modeling predicts simultaneous targeting of fibroblasts and epithelial cells is necessary for treatment of pulmonary fibrosis. *Front Pharmacol* (2016) 23(7):183. doi:10.3389/fphar.2016.00183
40. Marino S, Gideon HP, Gong C, Mankad S, McCrone JT, Lin PL, et al. Computational and empirical studies predict *Mycobacterium tuberculosis*-specific T cells as a biomarker for infection outcome. *PLoS Comput Biol* (2016) 12(4):e1004804. doi:10.1371/journal.pcbi.1004804

41. Pienaar E, Dartois V, Linderman JJ, Kirschner DE. In silico evaluation and exploration of antibiotic tuberculosis treatment regimens. *BMC Syst Biol* (2015) 9:79. doi:10.1186/s12918-015-0221-8
42. Cosgrove J, Butler J, Alden K, Read M, Kumar V, Cucurull-Sanchez L, et al. Agent-based modeling in systems pharmacology. *CPT Pharmacometrics Syst Pharmacol* (2015) 4(11):615–29. doi:10.1002/psp4.12018

5

High Endothelial Venules and Lymphatic Vessels in Tertiary Lymphoid Organs: Characteristics, Functions and Regulation

*Nancy H. Ruddle**

Department of Epidemiology of Microbial Diseases, School of Public Health, Yale University School of Medicine, New Haven, CT, USA

***Correspondence:**
Nancy H. Ruddle
nancy.ruddle@yale.edu

High endothelial venules (HEVs) and lymphatic vessels (LVs) are essential for the function of the immune system, by providing communication between the body and lymph nodes (LNs), specialized sites of antigen presentation and recognition. HEVs bring in naïve and central memory cells and LVs transport antigen, antigen-presenting cells, and lymphocytes in and out of LNs. Tertiary lymphoid organs (TLOs) are accumulations of lymphoid and stromal cells that arise and organize at ectopic sites in response to chronic inflammation in autoimmunity, microbial infection, graft rejection, and cancer. TLOs are distinguished from primary lymphoid organs – the thymus and bone marrow, and secondary lymphoid organs (SLOs) – the LNs, spleen, and Peyer's patches, in that they arise in response to inflammatory signals, rather than in ontogeny. TLOs usually do not have a capsule but are rather contained within the confines of another organ. Their structure, cellular composition, chemokine expression, and vascular and stromal support resemble SLOs and are the defining aspects of TLOs. T and B cells, antigen-presenting cells, fibroblast reticular cells, and other stromal cells and vascular elements including HEVs and LVs are all typical components of TLOs. A key question is whether the HEVs and LVs play comparable roles and are regulated similarly to those in LNs. Data are presented that support this concept, especially with regard to TLO HEVs. Emerging data suggest that the functions and regulation of TLO LVs are also similar to those in LNs. These observations support the concept that TLOs are not merely cellular accumulations but are functional entities that provide sites to generate effector cells, and that their HEVs and LVs are crucial elements in those activities.

Keywords: lymph node, lymphatic vessel, high endothelial venule, tertiary lymphoid organ, autoimmunity, inflammation, cancer, lymphotoxin

INTRODUCTION

Goals

Lymphoid and stromal cells accumulate and organize into tertiary lymphoid organs (TLOs) at ectopic sites in response to chronic inflammation in autoimmunity, microbial infection, graft rejection, and cancer where they assume structural and cellular characteristics of lymph nodes (LNs). High endothelial venules (HEVs) and lymphatic vessels (LVs) play key roles in LNs in transporting cells

---

Abbreviations: HEV, high endothelial venule; LEC, lymphatic endothelial cell; LN, lymph node; LT, lymphotoxin; LV, lymphatic vessel; SLO, secondary lymphoid organ; TLO, tertiary lymphoid organ.

and antigens from and to the body. The questions to be addressed here are whether the HEVs and LVs in TLOs function and are regulated in a manner similar to those in LNs.

Background

My research group became intrigued by the concept of TLOs in the course of two apparently unrelated series of investigations. The first was the characterization of mice that were transgenic for a construct of the rat insulin promoter driving expression of lymphotoxin alpha (LTα) (1) (in those days known as TNFβ, despite having been described as LT previous to the discovery of TNF). We made the rat insulin promoter lymphotoxin (RIPLT) mouse in order to develop a model of type 1 diabetes, since we knew that LT could induce inflammation. The transgene was not only expressed in the β cells in the islets of Langerhans in the pancreas as expected but also in the kidney and skin, most likely because the entire promoter with its negative regulatory elements was not included in the construct. At all sites of transgene expression, lymphoid cells accumulated, which were organized into distinct T and B cell areas ("compartmentalization"). Despite several attempts to drive the animals to β cell destruction and diabetes, the mice were healthy (2) unless a costimulator molecule such as B7-1 was also expressed in the β cells. Thus, the model resembled the early peri insulitis and non-destructive insulitis of diabetes. At the same time, we were collaborating with David Chaplin on the LTα knock out mouse that has no LNs (3). We realized that the consequence of ectopic expression of LT in the RIPLT mouse was the production of organized infiltrates that resembled LNs. We called them TLOs (4), a term that had been previously used to designate any lymphoid infiltrate (5). The process by which TLOs arise and organize was designated as lymphoid neogenesis (4).

In later years, I became especially interested in the vasculature of TLOs as I realized that understanding how cells enter into TLOs would provide insight into this accumulation and would indicate whether or not the apparent organization reflected function. That is, the presence of HEVs might indicate that naïve cells could enter the TLO, and the presence of LVs could indicate a method of entrance of antigen-presenting cells, thus providing in a single location, the elements to generate an immune response. This manuscript addresses these questions.

TERTIARY LYMPHOID ORGANS

Characteristics

Tertiary lymphoid organs, which have been described in almost every organ of the body, are also known as tertiary lymphoid structures, ectopic lymphoid tissues, or tertiary lymphoid tissues. They are distinguished from primary lymphoid organs – the thymus and bone marrow, and secondary lymphoid organs (SLOs) – the LNs, spleen, and Peyer's patches, in that they arise in response to inflammation or inflammatory cues, rather than in ontogeny and are ectopic to canonical lymphoid organs. They usually do not have a capsule but are rather contained within the confines of another organ.

Tertiary lymphoid organs are similar to LNs (6) with regard to their cellular content, stromal components, lymphoid chemokines (7), vasculature, and organization. Cells include compartmentalized T and B cells and antigen-presenting cells, including follicular dendritic cells and dendritic cells. CD8 and CD4 subsets include naïve, Treg, and T follicular helper cells (8, 9). B cells may be organized into germinal centers with plasma cells. HEVs (10), LVs (11, 12) (**Figure 1**), and conduits with fibroblastic reticular cells (13), all components of LNs, have also been described. In LNs, CCL19 and CCL21 direct T cells and DCs to the paracortical region, and CXCL13 directs B cells to the B cell follicles. These chemokines and cells that express their receptors are also expressed in TLOs (7). TLOs can be distinguished from acute inflammation; they generally include few granulocytes, and they are not necessarily destructive, although they may transform into tissue damaging entities. The plasticity of TLOs is seen in the case of the infiltrates in the pancreas in type 1 diabetes in the NOD mouse. Initially, the cellular infiltrates are disorganized and lack HEVs; then the infiltrates assume the characteristics of TLOs, with T and B compartmentalization and HEVs and LVs (14, 15); later, the lymphoid cells become activated, β cells are destroyed, and eventually the inflammation and thus, the TLO, is resolved as antigen is eliminated.

Tertiary lymphoid organs differ from LNs in that they generally do not have a capsule, they are not confined to a fixed location in the body, they develop postnatally, and as noted above, they exhibit plasticity. This is not to say that LNs do not respond to their environment; they most certainly do with proliferation and changes in vasculature and cell and antigen accessibility in the course of inflammation [see, e.g., Ref. (16)].

Functions

Tertiary lymphoid organ functions vary depending on the location, stimulus and kinetics of inflammation, and cellular

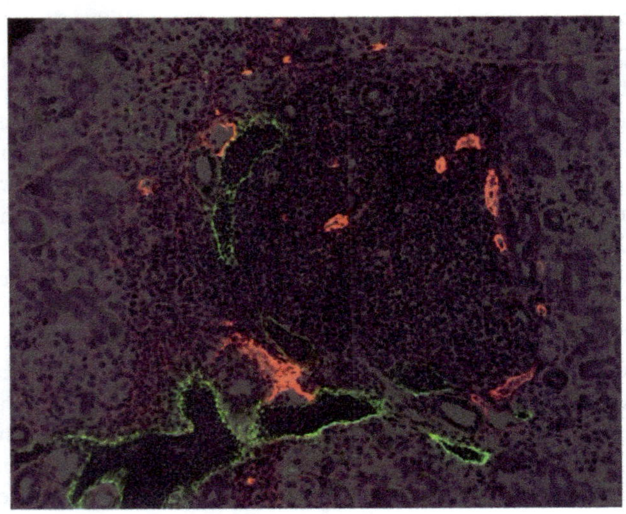

FIGURE 1 | High endothelial venules and lymphatic vessels in a TLO. A mouse salivary gland TLO. HEVs are stained red with an antibody to MECA-79. LVs are stained green with an antibody to LYVE-1. From "Transgenic LacZ under control of Hec-6ST regulatory sequences recapitulates endogenous gene expression on high endothelial venules" by Liao et al. (11).

activation. The strongest evidence that TLOs are harmful in exacerbating autoimmune disease derives from studies in rheumatoid arthritis. In some patients, evidence that somatic mutation and affinity maturation occur in the locus of the TLO in the joint provides support for a harmful role leading to determinant spreading. On the other hand, the presence of Tregs in some TLOs (17) suggests that they can play a beneficial role by limiting inflammation. Additional evidence for a beneficial role is provided from several clinical studies of cancer, which indicate that the presence of TLOs in tumors in breast, colon, or lung predicts a favorable outcome, suggesting that the TLO site provides a locus for antigen activation and destruction of tumor, reducing dissemination of the malignant cells through the body (18). Nevertheless, Tregs in tumor TLOs can act as brakes on their defensive role (19, 20).

HEVs: CHARACTERISTICS, FUNCTIONS, AND REGULATION IN TLOs

Characteristics

The presence of HEVs could be considered an essential trait distinguishing TLOs from acute inflammation. The endothelial cells in postcapillary venules in TLOs, as in LNs, tonsils, and Peyer's patches, exhibit a typical cuboidal appearance. LN HEVs express a particular set of genes that facilitate their interactions with blood stream naïve and central memory cells that result in rolling, firm adhesion, and transmigration from the vessel into the parenchyma. HEVs in TLOs express the same molecules: CCL21 (7), ICAM-1 (4), and peripheral and/or mucosal addressins, PNAd (10) and MAdCAM-1 (4). Expression of these proteins allows the egress from the blood stream into the parenchyma of LNs of cells of the naïve and central memory phenotype that express CCR7, LFA-1, L-selectin (CD62L), and $\alpha4\beta7$.

Functions

The evidence is quite strong that HEVs in TLOs function similarly to those in LNs, allowing naïve and central memory cells to leave the blood stream and enter into the parenchyma of the tissue where they can interact with their cognate antigen. First, as noted above, they express the molecules that allow naïve and central memory cells to interact. Second, cells expressing CCR7, LFA-1, L-selectin (CD62L), and $\alpha4\beta7$, the ligands for the receptors on HEVs, are found in TLOs. Third, several instances of T cell activation and memory generation occurring directly in the TLO have been described. These include generation of memory cells for graft rejection in skin TLOs (21) and presentation and activation of Teffector or Treg cells (19, 22). *In vivo* imaging of the transit of naïve cells into TLOs and their interaction with antigen-presenting cells will solidify the conclusion that HEVs function similarly in LNs and TLOs, and that HEVs in TLOs are the sites of entrance of naïve cells to undergo activation and differentiation and generation of memory cells.

Regulation

High endothelial venules are regulated similarly in TLOs and SLOs. LTα alone induces MAdCAM-1 in endothelial cells *in vitro* (23, 24), *in vivo* in mesenteric LN HEVs (16), and in HEVs in TLOs (23) through TNFR1 (25). Abluminal PNAd in LN HEVs is generated through modification of a variety of glycoproteins. These modifications include sulfation, which is essential for PNAd (also called L-selectin ligand) interaction with its receptor, L-selectin (CD62L) that is expressed on the surface of naïve and central memory lymphocytes. Sulfation is induced in peripheral LN HEVs by sulfotransferases (26, 27). LT$\alpha\beta$ regulates the HEV sulfotransferase in both LNs (16, 28) and TLOs (10) through the alternative NFκB pathway (29).

LVs: CHARACTERISTICS, FUNCTIONS, AND REGULATION IN TLOs

Characteristics

Lymphatic vessels play key roles in the body in fluid and lipid balance. They are crucial in the immune system in providing communication of the lymphoid organs with the rest of the body. Lymphatic capillaries are thin-walled, blind-ended vessels that express CCL21, LYVE-1, PROX-1, podoplanin, VEGFR-2, and VEGFR-3 and are the initial entry point into LNs from the tissues for antigen and antigen-presenting cells. The endothelial cells on the tips of lymphatic capillaries are most frequently in a zipper-like arrangement (30). They connect to collecting vessels whose cells exhibit a button-like arrangement that are usually low or negative for LYVE-1, but do express PROX-1. The latter is especially highly expressed in valves that are characteristic of collecting vessels. A layer of smooth muscle cells surrounding collecting vessels contributes to their pumping action. Afferent collecting vessels carry substances to LNs, whereas efferent vessels allow egress of activated cells from the LN into the next LN in the chain and eventually into the blood stream *via* the right or left subclavian veins. In addition to serving as routes of fluid, lipid, cell, and cytokine transport, recent publications attest to the ability of LN LVs to present self or foreign antigens, either directly or by transfer to antigen-presenting cells (31–34).

Thin-walled vessels that are positive for lymphatic markers, including LYVE-1, PROX-1, podoplanin in mouse and human or D2-40 in human have been noted in many TLOs [summarized in Ref. (12)]. These include chronic kidney rejection (35, 36), cardiac allografts (37), transgenic mouse models (38), age-related Sjögren's-like disease in the mouse (11), and a transgenic model of primary Sjögren's in the mouse (Truman et al., in preparation). Confusingly, a *reduced* number of LVs in kidneys of mouse strains with a higher preponderance of spontaneous kidney TLOs have been noted (39). However, the latter report did not indicate the actual location of the LVs (i.e., in the vicinity or not of the TLO). CCL21-expressing TLO-associated vessels have been described in rheumatoid arthritis, Crohn's disease, Sjögren's syndrome, chronic allograft rejection (40), and pancreatic infiltrates in NOD (15) and RIPLTα mice (7). Nevertheless, much still needs to be learned. Collecting vessels with valves and smooth muscle cells neither have been specifically identified entering or leaving TLOs nor have the vessel walls been characterized with regard to their zipper or button-like morphology.

Functions

Do the LVs in TLOs carry out the same functions as those in LNs? It is likely that they contribute to fluid drainage, although this has not been carefully analyzed. Do LVs carry antigen and cells to TLOs and cells away from TLOs, as do afferent and efferent vessels in LNs? TLO LVs frequently contain cells (11, 39), supporting the concept that they act as transporters as does their expression of CCL21 indicating they interact with CCR7-expressing cells. However, the fact that LVs in some TLOs appear to be packed with cells suggests that there could be a defect in cellular drainage and that their efferent function is compromised. Sphingosine-1 phosphate (S1P) is expressed in lymph and downregulates its receptor (S1P1) on lymphocytes. Lymphocytes in LNs reexpress the receptor and migrate toward the S1P in lymph and egress from the LN. FTY720 (fingolimod) is an agent that is used in transplantation and multiple sclerosis treatment that acts as an agonist for the receptor, causing its internalization resulting in lymphocyte accumulation in LNs (41), thus acting as an immunosuppressant. When NOD mice with pancreatic TLOs are treated with this agent, they are protected from islet destruction and diabetes, consistent with the concept that their LVs carry out an efferent function (42). In our hands, this treatment inhibits disease only at the time that the mice exhibit TLOs (15), although others have determined that FTY720 treatment is partially effective even after the development of elevated blood sugar (43). The pancreatic TLOs exhibit an increased insulitis score after FTY720 treatment, indicating that cells are trapped in these structures. Within days of cessation of drug treatment, islet destruction and diabetes occurs (15, 42). These data are consistent with the concept that the S1P gradient affects lymphocyte trafficking in TLO LVs. Further supporting the concept that the FTY720 effects are at least partially due to an effect on the TLOs is the observation that FTY720 treatment inhibits cellular migration from inflamed tissues into afferent LVs (44, 45). It must be noted that FTY720 treatment is also most likely affecting trafficking from LNs in this context, complicating interpretation of the data. This needs to be evaluated in situations where the events in TLOs can be isolated from LNs, as was done in a previous transplantation model (21). A straightforward test of these conclusions would be to determine if LVs in TLOs produce S1P as they do in LNs (46). If so, systemic inhibitors of lymphocyte trafficking may function directly at the TLO site by preventing traffic to the LNs from the TLO, a potential site of self antigen presentation.

Lymphatic vessels transport soluble or cell-associated antigens into LNs. Recently, it has become apparent that plasmalemma vesicle-associated protein (PLVAP), visualized by reactivity with the MECA-32 antibody, heretofore considered limited to blood vessels, is also expressed on the lymphatic endothelial cells in the lymphatic sinus in the LN. PLVAP positive lymphatic endothelial cells contribute to sieving of lymphocytes and high molecular weight antigens entering the LN *via* the conduits (47). Since TLOs include conduits (13), it seems reasonable to ask whether LVs in TLOs perform antigen and cell transport and sieving functions similar to those in LNs. Antigen transport may be less important than in SLOs because the antigen is an actual component of the TLO. As long as antigen-presenting cells are in the TLO (as they usually are), the issue is moot. Proteins such as insulin in the pancreatic islet are in immediate proximity or, as constituents of β cells, even contribute to the structure of the TLO in type 1 diabetes. With regard to the sieving function, an analysis of expression of PLVAP in TLOs by co-staining with MECA-32 and LYVE-1 or PROX-1 should be fairly straightforward. Functional analysis by crossing PLVAP-deficient mice to mice with TLOs or MECA-32 inhibition of migration of cells or labeled antigen to TLOs could address the function of LVs in TLOs. As noted above, LVs in LNs present self antigens (31–34), either directly through their expression of MHC molecules or by passing antigen on to "classical" antigen-presenting cells. Such presentation of self antigen by LVs (31) could be a way to induce either tolerance or T cell activation in LNs or in TLOs. The ability of TLO LVs to present antigen to induce either of these outcomes has not been investigated. Tregs are found in tumor TLOs and can inhibit cytotoxic T cells from attacking the tumor (19), indicating that understanding the mechanisms of self and tumor presentation to both potential effector T cells and Tregs is crucial to our ability to harness TLOs for both prophylaxis and therapy of cancer and autoimmune diseases.

Regulation

The most commonly accepted scenario for the development of LVs in ontogeny is that they sprout from veins (48) under the influence of SOX18, PROX-1, growth factors and their receptors (VEGF-C and VEGF-D and VEGFR-2 and VEGFR-3), and platelets (49) [reviewed in Ref. (50)]. Although the evidence is quite strong for this mechanism in the case of the LVs sprouting from the cardinal vein, it has become apparent that the situation is somewhat more complex. The first indication that additional mechanisms of lymphangiogenesis existed was the discovery of lymphangioblasts that could be distinguished from blood endothelial cells, in developing animals as distinct as tadpoles (51), chickens (52), and mice (53–55). Several recent studies have revealed that the origin of LVs is quite heterogeneous. Mahadevan et al. reported that LVs in the intestine are derived from arteries, rather than veins (56); Stanczuk et al. described hemangiogenic precursors that contribute to mesenteric LVs (57); Martinez-Corral et al. described the non-venous origin of dermal LVs in a process these authors termed lymphvasculogenesis (58); Klotz et al. also described a non-venous origin of cardiac LVs (59); and Nicenboim et al. reported that LVs derive from angioblasts in zebra fish (60).

Given the rapidly emerging data regarding the heterogeneity and the likelihood of organ-specific regulation of lymphangiogenesis in ontogeny (61), it becomes more important, and perhaps even more daunting, to understand the regulation of lymphangiogenesis in inflammation, particularly in chronic inflammation in TLOs. Do LVs in TLOs arise from veins? The presence of angiogenesis and platelets in inflammation supports such a scenario, as does the existence of vessels that express both HEV and LV markers in the inflamed LN (16). On the other hand, host-derived bone marrow precursors have been noted in association with LVs in the TLOs of chronically rejecting kidneys (36) suggesting a non-venous origin. Lymphangiogenesis in inflammation could occur by sprouting from existing LVs. But what cells orchestrate these events? DCs, macrophages, T and B cells have been implicated in the regulation of LVs in acute inflammation (16, 62–64), but different cells may be important at different times in different tissues. For example, B cells appear to be important in stimulating lymphangiogenesis that occurs in LNs during inflammation, but only at the early stages after immunization (16, 62) suggesting that they may be of lesser importance in chronic inflammation in TLOs. The participation of macrophages in lymphangiogenesis in acute inflammation has been documented, although the precise nature of their role is controversial. Various possibilities include integration into LVs, trans differentiation into lymphatic endothelial cells (65), and provision of growth factors [summarized in Ref. (66)] and cytokines. The expression of LYVE-1 by macrophages is supportive evidence for the former possibility; on the other hand, the expression of this marker on both macrophages and LECs may be serendipitous.

Several studies have evaluated the negative and positive roles of cytokines in lymphangiogenesis, although the bulk of these studies have evaluated acute inflammation rather than TLOs. There have been reports of negative regulation of lymphangiogenesis by IFNγ (67) and TH2 cytokines IL-4 and IL-13 (68) and positive regulation by IL-17 (69), LTα, and TNF (38, 70). LT is crucial for both lymphoid organ development and TLOs, and $LT\alpha_3$ contributes to lymphangiogenesis in development (38). LVs are apparent in RIPLT TLOs even in the absence of LTβ and before extensive cellular infiltration, suggesting a direct activity of the cytokine (38). On the other hand, LVs are inhibited by treatment with a LTβR-Ig in a CXCL13-induced model of a thyroid TLO (71). Further analysis of lymphangiogenesis in spontaneous TLOs, such as Sjögren's syndrome, rheumatoid arthritis, and type 1 diabetes, may reveal which cytokines regulate this process. Additional studies *in vivo* and *in vitro* should reveal the mechanism of cytokines' regulation as direct effects on lymphatic endothelial cells and/or as indirect effects through the facilitation of lymphatic growth factor producing cells.

Recent research reveals LV plasticity in gene function and regulation. It is obvious that their different environments (mesentery, skin, etc.) influence their gene expression. Inflammation in these diverse locales also contributes to changes in cytokine and growth factor expression. TNF and oxazolone treatment induce higher levels of CCL21 on dermal LVs, and presumably enhance cellular migration (72). Immunofluorescence and microarray studies revealed an increase in several additional inflammatory genes (73), although some genes, including *VEGFR-3 and PROX-1,* are downregulated. As yet, no such comparisons have included TLO LECs, which would be of particular interest because of the chronic nature of stimulation. Recently described methods to isolate LVs by virtue of their transgenically induced expression of a tomato red fluorescent protein should allow direct comparison of gene expression and function of LVs from different sites and acute and chronic inflammation (74, 75) and provide precise characterization of TLO LVs.

CONCLUDING REMARKS

In this communication, I have provided background from a personal perspective of the development of the TLO field, and more particularly the role of the vasculature present and employed in TLOs. Although questions remain concerning the precise functions of HEVs and LVs in TLOs, the evidence is quite strong that they do behave as they do in LNs. The appropriate experimental tools (*in vivo* imaging, mice with fluorescent HEVs and LVs) are available to address these issues. The answers to these questions will provide insight, not only into TLOs but also into processes of antigen presentation in LNs and tissue destruction in acute inflammation. This is turn will provide understanding and methods to induce or inhibit TLOs in autoimmunity, microbial infection, organ rejection, and cancer.

AUTHOR CONTRIBUTIONS

The author confirms being the sole contributor of this work and approved it for publication.

ACKNOWLEDGMENTS

The author gratefully acknowledges the contributions of her many colleagues, collaborators, and trainees who have provided data and insight that gave rise to the concept of TLOs.

FUNDING

This work was supported by 13-SCD-YALE-27, a grant from the Connecticut Regenerative Medicine Research Fund of Connecticut Innovations.

REFERENCES

1. Picarella DE, Kratz A, Li CB, Ruddle NH, Flavell RA. Insulitis in transgenic mice expressing tumor necrosis factor beta (lymphotoxin) in the pancreas. *Proc Natl Acad Sci U S A* (1992) 89(21):10036–40. doi:10.1073/pnas.89.21.10036
2. Picarella DE, Kratz A, Li CB, Ruddle NH, Flavell RA. Transgenic tumor necrosis factor (TNF)-alpha production in pancreatic islets leads to insulitis, not diabetes. Distinct patterns of inflammation in TNF-alpha and TNF-beta transgenic mice. *J Immunol* (1993) 150(9):4136–50.
3. De Togni P, Goellner J, Ruddle NH, Streeter PR, Andrea F, Mariathasan S, et al. Abnormal development of peripheral lymphoid organs in mice deficient in lymphotoxin. Science. 1994. 264: 703-707. *J Immunol* (2014) 192(5):2010–4. doi:10.1126/science.8171322
4. Kratz A, Campos-Neto A, Hanson MS, Ruddle NH. Chronic inflammation caused by lymphotoxin is lymphoid neogenesis. *J Exp Med* (1996) 183(4):1461–72. doi:10.1084/jem.183.4.1461
5. Picker LJ, Butcher EC. Physiological and molecular mechanisms of lymphocyte homing. *Annu Rev Immunol* (1992) 10:561–91. doi:10.1146/annurev.iy.10.040192.003021
6. Drayton DL, Liao S, Mounzer RH, Ruddle NH. Lymphoid organ development: from ontogeny to neogenesis. *Nat Immunol* (2006) 7(4):344–53. doi:10.1038/ni1330
7. Hjelmstrom P, Fjell J, Nakagawa T, Sacca R, Cuff CA, Ruddle NH. Lymphoid tissue homing chemokines are expressed in chronic inflammation. *Am J Pathol* (2000) 156(4):1133–8. doi:10.1016/S0002-9440(10)64981-4
8. Kielczewski JL, Horai R, Jittayasothorn Y, Chan CC, Caspi RR. Tertiary lymphoid tissue forms in retinas of mice with spontaneous autoimmune uveitis

and has consequences on visual function. *J Immunol* (2016) 196(3):1013–25. doi:10.4049/jimmunol.1501570

9. Gu-Trantien C, Willard-Gallo K. Tumor-infiltrating follicular helper T cells: the new kids on the block. *Oncoimmunology* (2013) 2(10):e26066. doi:10.4161/onci.26066
10. Drayton DL, Ying X, Lee J, Lesslauer W, Ruddle NH. Ectopic LT alpha beta directs lymphoid organ neogenesis with concomitant expression of peripheral node addressin and a HEV-restricted sulfotransferase. *J Exp Med* (2003) 197(9):1153–63. doi:10.1084/jem.20021761
11. Liao S, Bentley K, Lebrun M, Lesslauer W, Ruddle FH, Ruddle NH. Transgenic LacZ under control of Hec-6st regulatory sequences recapitulates endogenous gene expression on high endothelial venules. *Proc Natl Acad Sci U S A* (2007) 104(11):4577–82. doi:10.1073/pnas.0700334104
12. Ruddle NH. Lymphatic vessels and tertiary lymphoid organs. *J Clin Invest* (2014) 124(3):953–9. doi:10.1172/JCI71611
13. Stranford S, Ruddle NH. Follicular dendritic cells, conduits, lymphatic vessels, and high endothelial venules in tertiary lymphoid organs: parallels with lymph node stroma. *Front Immunol* (2012) 3:350. doi:10.3389/fimmu.2012.00350
14. Astorri E, Bombardieri M, Gabba S, Peakman M, Pozzilli P, Pitzalis C. Evolution of ectopic lymphoid neogenesis and in situ autoantibody production in autoimmune nonobese diabetic mice: cellular and molecular characterization of tertiary lymphoid structures in pancreatic islets. *J Immunol* (2010) 185(6):3359–68. doi:10.4049/jimmunol.1001836
15. Penaranda C, Tang Q, Ruddle NH, Bluestone JA. Prevention of diabetes by FTY720-mediated stabilization of peri-islet tertiary lymphoid organs. *Diabetes* (2010) 59(6):1461–8. doi:10.2337/db09-1129
16. Liao S, Ruddle NH. Synchrony of high endothelial venules and lymphatic vessels revealed by immunization. *J Immunol* (2006) 177(5):3369–79. doi:10.4049/jimmunol.177.5.3369
17. Grabner R, Lotzer K, Dopping S, Hildner M, Radke D, Beer M, et al. Lymphotoxin beta receptor signaling promotes tertiary lymphoid organogenesis in the aorta adventitia of aged ApoE-/- mice. *J Exp Med* (2009) 206(1):233–48. doi:10.1084/jem.20080752
18. Martinet L, Garrido I, Filleron T, Le Guellec S, Bellard E, Fournie JJ, et al. Human solid tumors contain high endothelial venules: association with T- and B-lymphocyte infiltration and favorable prognosis in breast cancer. *Cancer Res* (2011) 71(17):5678–87. doi:10.1158/0008-5472.CAN-11-0431
19. Joshi NS, Akama-Garren EH, Lu Y, Lee DY, Chang GP, Li A, et al. Regulatory T cells in tumor-associated tertiary lymphoid structures suppress anti-tumor T cell responses. *Immunity* (2015) 43(3):579–90. doi:10.1016/j.immuni.2015.08.006
20. Martinet L, Filleron T, Le Guellec S, Rochaix P, Garrido I, Girard JP. High endothelial venule blood vessels for tumor-infiltrating lymphocytes are associated with lymphotoxin beta-producing dendritic cells in human breast cancer. *J Immunol* (2013) 191(4):2001–8. doi:10.4049/jimmunol.1300872
21. Nasr IW, Reel M, Oberbarnscheidt MH, Mounzer RH, Baddoura FK, Ruddle NH, et al. Tertiary lymphoid tissues generate effector and memory T cells that lead to allograft rejection. *Am J Transplant* (2007) 7(5):1071–9. doi:10.1111/j.1600-6143.2007.01756.x
22. Hu D, Mohanta SK, Yin C, Peng L, Ma Z, Srikakulapu P, et al. Artery tertiary lymphoid organs control aorta immunity and protect against atherosclerosis via vascular smooth muscle cell lymphotoxin beta receptors. *Immunity* (2015) 42(6):1100–15. doi:10.1016/j.immuni.2015.05.015
23. Cuff CA, Sacca R, Ruddle NH. Differential induction of adhesion molecule and chemokine expression by LTalpha3 and LTalphabeta in inflammation elucidates potential mechanisms of mesenteric and peripheral lymph node development. *J Immunol* (1999) 162(10):5965–72.
24. Cuff CA, Schwartz J, Bergman CM, Russell KS, Bender JR, Ruddle NH. Lymphotoxin alpha3 induces chemokines and adhesion molecules: insight into the role of LT alpha in inflammation and lymphoid organ development. *J Immunol* (1998) 161(12):6853–60.
25. Sacca R, Cuff CA, Lesslauer W, Ruddle NH. Differential activities of secreted lymphotoxin-alpha3 and membrane lymphotoxin-alpha1beta2 in lymphotoxin-induced inflammation: critical role of TNF receptor 1 signaling. *J Immunol* (1998) 160(1):485–91.
26. Bistrup A, Bhakta S, Lee JK, Belov YY, Gunn MD, Zuo FR, et al. Sulfotransferases of two specificities function in the reconstitution of high endothelial cell ligands for L-selectin. *J Cell Biol* (1999) 145(4):899–910. doi:10.1083/jcb.145.4.899
27. Hemmerich S, Bistrup A, Singer MS, van Zante A, Lee JK, Tsay D, et al. Sulfation of L-selectin ligands by an HEV-restricted sulfotransferase regulates lymphocyte homing to lymph nodes. *Immunity* (2001) 15(2):237–47. doi:10.1016/S1074-7613(01)00188-1
28. Browning JL, Allaire N, Ngam-Ek A, Notidis E, Hunt J, Perrin S, et al. Lymphotoxin-beta receptor signaling is required for the homeostatic control of HEV differentiation and function. *Immunity* (2005) 23(5):539–50. doi:10.1016/j.immuni.2005.10.002
29. Drayton DL, Bonizzi G, Ying X, Liao S, Karin M, Ruddle NH. Ikappa B kinase complex alpha kinase activity controls chemokine and high endothelial venule gene expression in lymph nodes and nasal-associated lymphoid tissue. *J Immunol* (2004) 173(10):6161–8. doi:10.4049/jimmunol.173.10.6161
30. Baluk P, Fuxe J, Hashizume H, Romano T, Lashnits E, Butz S, et al. Functionally specialized junctions between endothelial cells of lymphatic vessels. *J Exp Med* (2007) 204(10):2349–62. doi:10.1084/jem.20062596
31. Cohen JN, Guidi CJ, Tewalt EF, Qiao H, Rouhani SJ, Ruddell A, et al. Lymph node-resident lymphatic endothelial cells mediate peripheral tolerance via Aire-independent direct antigen presentation. *J Exp Med* (2010) 207(4):681–8. doi:10.1084/jem.20092465
32. Rouhani SJ, Eccles JD, Riccardi P, Peske JD, Tewalt EF, Cohen JN, et al. Roles of lymphatic endothelial cells expressing peripheral tissue antigens in CD4 T-cell tolerance induction. *Nat Commun* (2015) 6:6771. doi:10.1038/ncomms7771
33. Tewalt EF, Cohen JN, Rouhani SJ, Guidi CJ, Qiao H, Fahl SP, et al. Lymphatic endothelial cells induce tolerance via PD-L1 and lack of costimulation leading to high-level PD-1 expression on CD8 T cells. *Blood* (2012) 120(24):4772–82. doi:10.1182/blood-2012-04-427013
34. Tamburini BA, Burchill MA, Kedl RM. Antigen capture and archiving by lymphatic endothelial cells following vaccination or viral infection. *Nat Commun* (2014) 5:3989. doi:10.1038/ncomms4989
35. Kerjaschki D, Huttary N, Raab I, Regele H, Bojarski-Nagy K, Bartel G, et al. Lymphatic endothelial progenitor cells contribute to de novo lymphangiogenesis in human renal transplants. *Nat Med* (2006) 12(2):230–4. doi:10.1038/nm1340
36. Kerjaschki D, Regele HM, Moosberger I, Nagy-Bojarski K, Watschinger B, Soleiman A, et al. Lymphatic neoangiogenesis in human kidney transplants is associated with immunologically active lymphocytic infiltrates. *J Am Soc Nephrol* (2004) 15(3):603–12. doi:10.1097/01.ASN.0000113316.52371.2E
37. Motallebzadeh R, Rehakova S, Conlon TM, Win TS, Callaghan CJ, Goddard M, et al. Blocking lymphotoxin signaling abrogates the development of ectopic lymphoid tissue within cardiac allografts and inhibits effector antibody responses. *FASEB J* (2012) 26(1):51–62. doi:10.1096/fj.11-186973
38. Mounzer RH, Svendsen OS, Baluk P, Bergman CM, Padera TP, Wiig H, et al. Lymphotoxin-alpha contributes to lymphangiogenesis. *Blood* (2010) 116(12):2173–82. doi:10.1182/blood-2009-12-256065
39. Huang Y, Caputo CR, Noordmans GA, Yazdani S, Monteiro LH, van den Born J, et al. Identification of novel genes associated with renal tertiary lymphoid organ formation in aging mice. *PLoS One* (2014) 9(3):e91850. doi:10.1371/journal.pone.0091850
40. Nykanen AI, Sandelin H, Krebs R, Keranen MA, Tuuminen R, Karpanen T, et al. Targeting lymphatic vessel activation and CCL21 production by vascular endothelial growth factor receptor-3 inhibition has novel immunomodulatory and antiarteriosclerotic effects in cardiac allografts. *Circulation* (2010) 121(12):1413–22. doi:10.1161/CIRCULATIONAHA.109.910703
41. Mandala S, Hajdu R, Bergstrom J, Quackenbush E, Xie J, Milligan J, et al. Alteration of lymphocyte trafficking by sphingosine-1-phosphate receptor agonists. *Science* (2002) 296(5566):346–9. doi:10.1126/science.1070238
42. Maki T, Gottschalk R, Ogawa N, Monaco AP. Prevention and cure of autoimmune diabetes in nonobese diabetic mice by continuous administration of FTY720. *Transplantation* (2005) 79(9):1051–5. doi:10.1097/01.TP.0000161220.87548.EE
43. Tsuji T, Inoue M, Yoshida Y, Fujita T, Kaino Y, Kohno T. Therapeutic approach for type 1 diabetes mellitus using the novel immunomodulator FTY720 (fingolimod) in combination with once-daily injection of insulin glargine in non-obese diabetic mice. *J Diabetes Investig* (2012) 3(2):132–7. doi:10.1111/j.2040-1124.2011.00160.x

44. Brown MN, Fintushel SR, Lee MH, Jennrich S, Geherin SA, Hay JB, et al. Chemoattractant receptors and lymphocyte egress from extralymphoid tissue: changing requirements during the course of inflammation. *J Immunol* (2010) 185(8):4873–82. doi:10.4049/jimmunol.1000676
45. Ledgerwood LG, Lal G, Zhang N, Garin A, Esses SJ, Ginhoux F, et al. The sphingosine 1-phosphate receptor 1 causes tissue retention by inhibiting the entry of peripheral tissue T lymphocytes into afferent lymphatics. *Nat Immunol* (2008) 9(1):42–53. doi:10.1038/ni1534
46. Pham TH, Baluk P, Xu Y, Grigorova I, Bankovich AJ, Pappu R, et al. Lymphatic endothelial cell sphingosine kinase activity is required for lymphocyte egress and lymphatic patterning. *J Exp Med* (2010) 207(1):17–27. doi:10.1084/jem.20091619
47. Rantakari P, Auvinen K, Jappinen N, Kapraali M, Valtonen J, Karikoski M, et al. The endothelial protein PLVAP in lymphatics controls the entry of lymphocytes and antigens into lymph nodes. *Nat Immunol* (2015) 16(4):386–96. doi:10.1038/ni.3101
48. Srinivasan RS, Dillard ME, Lagutin OV, Lin FJ, Tsai S, Tsai MJ, et al. Lineage tracing demonstrates the venous origin of the mammalian lymphatic vasculature. *Genes Dev* (2007) 21(19):2422–32. doi:10.1101/gad.1588407
49. Abtahian F, Guerriero A, Sebzda E, Lu MM, Zhou R, Mocsai A, et al. Regulation of blood and lymphatic vascular separation by signaling proteins SLP-76 and Syk. *Science* (2003) 299(5604):247–51. doi:10.1126/science.1079477
50. Tammela T, Alitalo K. Lymphangiogenesis: molecular mechanisms and future promise. *Cell* (2010) 140(4):460–76. doi:10.1016/j.cell.2010.01.045
51. Ny A, Koch M, Schneider M, Neven E, Tong RT, Maity S, et al. A genetic *Xenopus laevis* tadpole model to study lymphangiogenesis. *Nat Med* (2005) 11(9):998–1004. doi:10.1038/nm1285
52. Wilting J, Aref Y, Huang R, Tomarev SI, Schweigerer L, Christ B, et al. Dual origin of avian lymphatics. *Dev Biol* (2006) 292(1):165–73. doi:10.1016/j.ydbio.2005.12.043
53. Buttler K, Badar M, Seiffart V, Laggies S, Gross G, Wilting J, et al. De novo hem- and lymphangiogenesis by endothelial progenitor and mesenchymal stem cells in immunocompetent mice. *Cell Mol Life Sci* (2013) 71(8):1513–27. doi:10.1007/s00018-013-1460-8
54. Buttler K, Ezaki T, Wilting J. Proliferating mesodermal cells in murine embryos exhibiting macrophage and lymphendothelial characteristics. *BMC Dev Biol* (2008) 8:43. doi:10.1186/1471-213X-8-43
55. Buttler K, Kreysing A, von Kaisenberg CS, Schweigerer L, Gale N, Papoutsi M, et al. Mesenchymal cells with leukocyte and lymphendothelial characteristics in murine embryos. *Dev Dyn* (2006) 235(6):1554–62. doi:10.1002/dvdy.20737
56. Mahadevan A, Welsh IC, Sivakumar A, Gludish DW, Shilvock AR, Noden DM, et al. The left-right Pitx2 pathway drives organ-specific arterial and lymphatic development in the intestine. *Dev Cell* (2014) 31(6):690–706. doi:10.1016/j.devcel.2014.11.002
57. Stanczuk L, Martinez-Corral I, Ulvmar MH, Zhang Y, Lavina B, Fruttiger M, et al. cKit Lineage hemogenic endothelium-derived cells contribute to mesenteric lymphatic vessels. *Cell Rep* (2015) 10(10)1708–21. doi:10.1016/j.celrep.2015.02.026
58. Martinez-Corral I, Ulvmar MH, Stanczuk L, Tatin F, Kizhatil K, John SW, et al. Nonvenous origin of dermal lymphatic vasculature. *Circ Res* (2015) 116(10):1649–54. doi:10.1161/CIRCRESAHA.116.306170
59. Klotz L, Norman S, Vieira JM, Masters M, Rohling M, Dube KN, et al. Cardiac lymphatics are heterogeneous in origin and respond to injury. *Nature* (2015) 522(7554):62–7. doi:10.1038/nature14483
60. Nicenboim J, Malkinson G, Lupo T, Asaf L, Sela Y, Mayseless O, et al. Lymphatic vessels arise from specialized angioblasts within a venous niche. *Nature* (2015) 522(7554):56–61. doi:10.1038/nature14425
61. Ulvmar MH, Makinen T. Heterogeneity in the lymphatic vascular system and its origin. *Cardiovasc Res* (2016) 111(4):310–21. doi:10.1093/cvr/cvw175
62. Angeli V, Ginhoux F, Llodra J, Quemeneur L, Frenette PS, Skobe M, et al. B cell-driven lymphangiogenesis in inflamed lymph nodes enhances dendritic cell mobilization. *Immunity* (2006) 24(2):203–15. doi:10.1016/j.immuni.2006.01.003
63. Chyou S, Benahmed F, Chen J, Kumar V, Tian S, Lipp M, et al. Coordinated regulation of lymph node vascular-stromal growth first by CD11c+ cells and then by T and B cells. *J Immunol* (2011) 187(11):5558–67. doi:10.4049/jimmunol.1101724
64. Muniz LR, Pacer ME, Lira SA, Furtado GC. A critical role for dendritic cells in the formation of lymphatic vessels within tertiary lymphoid structures. *J Immunol* (2011) 187(2):828–34. doi:10.4049/jimmunol.1004233
65. Maruyama K, Ii M, Cursiefen C, Jackson DG, Keino H, Tomita M, et al. Inflammation-induced lymphangiogenesis in the cornea arises from CD11b-positive macrophages. *J Clin Invest* (2005) 115(9):2363–72. doi:10.1172/JCI23874
66. Ran S, Montgomery KE. Macrophage-mediated lymphangiogenesis: the emerging role of macrophages as lymphatic endothelial progenitors. *Cancers (Basel)* (2012) 4(3):618–57. doi:10.3390/cancers4030618
67. Kataru RP, Kim H, Jang C, Choi DK, Koh BI, Kim M, et al. T lymphocytes negatively regulate lymph node lymphatic vessel formation. *Immunity* (2011) 34(1):96–107. doi:10.1016/j.immuni.2010.12.016
68. Shin K, Kataru RP, Park HJ, Kwon BI, Kim TW, Hong YK, et al. TH2 cells and their cytokines regulate formation and function of lymphatic vessels. *Nat Commun* (2015) 6:6196. doi:10.1038/ncomms7196
69. Chauhan SK, Jin Y, Goyal S, Lee HS, Fuchsluger TA, Lee HK, et al. A novel pro-lymphangiogenic function for Th17/IL-17. *Blood* (2011) 118(17):4630–4. doi:10.1182/blood-2011-01-332049
70. Seeger H, Bonani M, Segerer S. The role of lymphatics in renal inflammation. *Nephrol Dial Transplant* (2012) 27(7):2634–41. doi:10.1093/ndt/gfs140
71. Furtado GC, Marinkovic T, Martin AP, Garin A, Hoch B, Hubner W, et al. Lymphotoxin beta receptor signaling is required for inflammatory lymphangiogenesis in the thyroid. *Proc Natl Acad Sci U S A* (2007) 104(12):5026–31. doi:10.1073/pnas.0606697104
72. Johnson LA, Jackson DG. Inflammation-induced secretion of CCL21 in lymphatic endothelium is a key regulator of integrin-mediated dendritic cell transmigration. *Int Immunol* (2010) 22(10):839–49. doi:10.1093/intimm/dxq435
73. Vigl B, Aebischer D, Nitschke M, Iolyeva M, Rothlin T, Antsiferova O, et al. Tissue inflammation modulates gene expression of lymphatic endothelial cells and dendritic cell migration in a stimulus-dependent manner. *Blood* (2011) 118(1):205–15. doi:10.1182/blood-2010-12-326447
74. Truman LA, Bentley KL, Smith EC, Massaro SA, Gonzalez DG, Haberman AM, et al. ProxTom lymphatic vessel reporter mice reveal Prox1 expression in the adrenal medulla, megakaryocytes, and platelets. *Am J Pathol* (2012) 180(4):1715–25. doi:10.1016/j.ajpath.2011.12.026
75. Truman LA, A-Gonzalez N, Bentley KL, Ruddle NH. Lymphatic vessel function in head and neck inflammation. *Lymphat Res Biol* (2013) 11(3):187–92. doi:10.1089/lrb.2013.0013

6

Early IL-1 Signaling Promotes iBALT Induction after Influenza Virus Infection

*Katrijn Neyt[1,2], Corine H. GeurtsvanKessel[3], Kim Deswarte[1,2], Hamida Hammad[1,2] and Bart N. Lambrecht[1,2,4]**

[1] Laboratory of Immunoregulation, VIB Inflammation Research Center, Ghent, Belgium, [2] Department of Respiratory Medicine, Ghent University, Ghent, Belgium, [3] Department of Viroscience, Erasmus MC, Rotterdam, Netherlands, [4] Department of Pulmonary Medicine, Erasmus MC, Rotterdam, Netherlands

***Correspondence:**
Bart N. Lambrecht
bart.lambrecht@ugent.be

Inducible bronchus-associated lymphoid tissue (iBALT) is a long lasting tertiary lymphoid tissue that can be induced following influenza A virus (IAV) infection. Previous studies have shown that iBALT structures containing germinal center (GC) B cells protect against repeated infection by contributing locally to the cellular and humoral immune response. If we are to exploit this in vaccination strategies, we need a better understanding on how iBALT structures are induced. One hypothesis is that the strength of the initial innate response dictates induction of iBALT. In the present study, we investigated the role of interleukin (IL)-1 and IL-1R signaling on iBALT formation. Mice lacking the IL-1R had a delayed viral clearance and, thus, a prolonged exposure to viral replication, leading to increased disease severity, compared to wild-type mice. Contradictorily, iBALT formation following clearance of the virus was heavily compromised in *Il1r1*$^{-/-}$ mice. Quantification of gene induction after IAV infection demonstrated induction of IL-1α and to a much lesser extent of IL-1β. Administration of recombinant IL-1α to the lungs of wild-type mice, early but not late, after IAV infection led to more pronounced iBALT formation and an increased amount of GC B cells in the lungs. Bone marrow chimeric mice identified the stromal compartment as the crucial IL-1 responsive cell for iBALT induction. Mechanistically, Q-PCR analysis of lung homogenates revealed a strongly diminished production of CXCL13, a B cell-attracting chemokine, in *Il1r*$^{-/-}$ mice during the early innate phase of IAV infection. These experiments demonstrate that appropriate innate IL-1α–IL-1R signaling is necessary for IAV clearance and at the same time instructs the formation of organized tertiary lymphoid tissues through induction of CXCL13 early after infection. These findings are discussed in the light of recent insights on the pathogenesis of tertiary lymphoid organ formation in the lung in various diseases where the IL-1 axis is hyperactive, such as rheumatoid arthritis and COPD.

Keywords: influenza, innate immunity, TLO, IL-1, iBALT, CXCL13

INTRODUCTION

Influenza A virus (IAV) is a respiratory pathogen that causes seasonal or pandemic outbreaks with severe outcome in elderly and immune compromised patients. Epithelial cells are the first target cells for IAV infection (1, 2) and also coordinate the innate immune defense to prevent spreading of the virus, *via* production of type I interferons (IFNs). Interleukin (IL)-1α and IL-1β are among the first cytokines that are secreted by epithelial cells and macrophages at sites of IAV replication (3). Secretion of IL-1β requires activation of the Nlrp3 inflammasome that leads to activation of caspase-1 and cleavage of pro-IL-1β into IL-1β. Infection with IAV leads to activation of the Nlrp3 inflammasome in a process requiring the type I IFN-induced RNAse L/OAS system, while the virus actively suppresses IL-1β production and Nlrp3 activation *via* the NS1 protein (4–6). IL-1 induces the expression of endothelial adhesion molecules that promote the entry of innate inflammatory cells like neutrophils, NK cells, dendritic cells (DCs), and monocytes resulting in a double effect on the host. On the one hand, it promotes survival by killing virus-infected cells, clearing debris, and alarming the adaptive immune response. On the other hand, overzealous neutrophil recruitment can also cause inflammatory pathology that can ultimately lead to diffuse alveolar damage and death (6–10). Not surprisingly, the outcome of genetic deficiency of key components in IL-1 generation or signaling has been very different depending on the severity of the IAV infection (2, 9, 11).

Simultaneously with the activation of the innate immune response, adaptive immune responses are initiated in the draining lymph nodes by antigen-presenting migratory DCs. The architecture of lymph nodes promotes contact between antigen-presenting DCs and rare antigen-specific T cells and B cells of the adaptive immune system to maximize the immune response against a certain antigen. Antigen-specific T lymphocytes undergo clonal proliferation upon encounter with antigen presented by antigen-presenting cells and migrate back to the site of inflammation as T effector memory (T_{EM}) cells or become central memory T cells (T_{CM}) or T resident memory (T_{RM}) cells (12). Antibody production is initiated from B lymphocytes that differentiate into plasmablasts, immediately, or become plasma cells after going through a germinal center (GC) reaction that promotes somatic hypermutation and affinity maturation of B cells (13).

The coordinated events of T and B cell activation induced by virus-laden DCs mainly occur in secondary lymphoid organs (SLOs) like lymph nodes and spleen that develop during embryogenesis at predefined areas, often at the crossroads of lymphatic vessels (14). However, highly organized structures of T and B cells can also be formed in the lung after birth as an adaptation to the increased demand for a localized immune response. Various names, such as lymphoid tissue neogenesis, ectopic lymphoid tissue, and tertiary lymphoid structures have been used to describe these structures. Furthermore, they are often named after the anatomical region in which they occur. In the lungs, for example, lymphoid aggregations can often be found in close proximity to bronchi, and hence, these are called inducible bronchus-associated lymphoid tissues (iBALT). As they resemble SLOs anatomically and functionally, yet, only develop after birth as a result of chronic immune stimulation, they can also be called tertiary lymphoid organs (TLOs), even when found within the boundaries of another organ.

Tertiary lymphoid organs have been implicated in protection against IAV. Mice that lack SLOs can mount a rapid CD8 T cell response during IAV infection due to the induction iBALT (15), induced after clearance of IAV infection. Such TLO structures are generally formed in close proximity to bronchi after IAV infection, but can also be observed in the lung interstitium and are fully formed 17 dpi. iBALT structures that are induced in mice with functional lymph nodes can serve as an additional priming site for T cells (16) and can also contribute to the humoral immune responses (17). Once formed, iBALT structures can mount high affinity immune responses to other antigenic stimuli than the initiating stimulus due to the presence of GCs that allow somatic hypermutation and affinity maturation, complementing the immune response in the draining lymph nodes (16, 18). Furthermore, iBALT structures could be the perfect environment for depots of viral antigen that were described long after viral clearance and recovery from viral infection and possibly related to the induction or maintenance of virus-specific T_{RM} cells (19, 20).

Despite morphological and functional similarities between SLOs and TLOs, the pathways that control formation and maintenance of TLOs are less clear. Generally, the molecular pathway that organizes T and B cells in discrete areas resembles the highly regulated inductive pathway for SLO development. Production of CCL19, CCL21, CXCL12, and CXCL13 by stromal cells and B cells helps to organize and retain T and B cells in discrete areas (21–26). Also IL-7 seems required for TLO formation, e.g., in joints of rheumatoid arthritis patients and mouse models (27–30) and lungs of idiopathic pulmonary hypertension (IPAH) patients (31). It is more controversial which cells give the initial instruction for stromal cells to produce these chemokines. During SLO development in the fetal period, this is the distinct task of lymphoid tissue inducer (LT_i) cells, a cell type that develops from $Flt3^+$ and $Flt3^-$ $\alpha_4\beta_7$ integrin-positive common progenitors that also forms innate lymphoid cells (ILC), and get expanded in response to Flt3L injections (32, 33). During formation of the lymph nodes and spleen, LT_i cells provide signals for lymphoid organogenesis like lymphotoxin-beta (LTβ) acting on the LTβR on stromal cells, but the precise signals might differ from organ to organ. *Flt3l*$^{-/-}$ mice for example have reduced LT_i cells and lack Peyer's patches, but still have lymph nodes (33). However, research in *Id2*$^{-/-}$ and *Rorc*$^{-/-}$ mice, which lack LT_i cells, showed that LT_i cells were dispensable for the initial TLO induction after IAV infection or other forms of TLO induction (15, 34–38). Although LT_i cells seem not strictly necessary for TLO induction, an instructive LTβ–LTβR signal remains essential for proper TLO development (25, 39). B cells, T cells, and DCs are heavily induced during inflammatory processes and all express $LT\alpha1\beta2$ on their cell surface (17, 35, 40, 41); therefore, they are perfect candidates to function as a substitute for LT_i cells.

Whatever the precise molecular mechanisms of TLO induction might be, these TLO structures are virtually always seen at sites of inflammation. Yet, which inflammatory cytokines contribute to TLO induction is currently unknown. After many insults to the lung, including viral or bacterial infection, IL-1α and IL-1β are among the first cytokines to be secreted (3). IL-1 secretion induces the expression of endothelial adhesion molecules that promote the entry of innate and adaptive immune cells and could, thus, promote TLO formation. On the other hand, it is also known that IL-1R$^{-/-}$ mice have a delayed viral clearance and, thus, a longer exposure to viral particles (7). Chronic immune stimulation is often assumed to lead to TLO formation (42). If IL-1 limits viral replication, it could reduce the trigger for TLO induction.

In this paper, we addressed the role of IL-1 and IL-1R in TLO formation in the lung. We show that the iBALT-inducing events are initiated early after infection, long before the virus is cleared. More specifically, we show that early IL-1R signaling is necessary for proper IAV-associated iBALT and GC induction and that prolonged viral presence does not automatically lead to iBALT induction.

MATERIALS AND METHODS

Ethics Statement

All experiments were approved by the independent animal ethics committee "Ethische Commissie Proefdieren – faculteit Wetenschappen Universiteit Gent en VIB-site Ardoyen" (identification number: EC 2013_070). Animal care and used protocols adhere to the Belgian Royal Degree of 29th May, 2013 for protection of experimental animals. European guideline 2010/63/EU is incorporated in this Belgian legislation.

Mice

C57Bl/6 mice (8–10 weeks) were purchased from Harlan Laboratories. IL-1R$^{-/-}$ mice were bred in-house and housed in specific pathogen-free housing.

To create chimeric mice, IL-1R$^{-/-}$ or wild-type acceptor mice were irradiated sublethally (9 Gy) and reconstituted with 2×10^6 bone marrow cells i.v. from wild-type or IL-1R$^{-/-}$ donor mice respectively 4 h after irradiation. Mice were used for experiment at least 10 weeks after reconstitution.

Influenza Virus Infection

Mice were infected intranasally with 10^5 TCID50 H3N2 influenza virus X-31 (Medical Research Council) or mock (allantoic fluid of uninfected eggs); diluted in 50 µl PBS. Weight loss was monitored daily. For suppletion assays, mice were treated intratracheally with 80 µg carrier-free recombinant IL-1α (R&D) at 2 or 10 dpi.

TCID50 Assay Viral Titers

Lungs were homogenized with a tissue homogenizer in 1 ml PBS and centrifuged (5 min, 400 *g*) to remove cellular debris before storage at −80°C. Titers of infectious virus were determined in triplicate by titration on MDCK cells in serum-free TPCK-treated trypsin-containing medium. Viral titers were determined by measuring chicken red blood cell agglutination activity in the cell supernatant after 7 days of infection of MDCK cells by using the calculation method of Reed and Muench.

Isolation of Lung Cells

Mice were sacrificed and the lungs were removed. Single-cell suspensions were prepared by digestion in collagenase/DNase solution for 30 min at 37°C. After digestion, the suspension was filtered over a 100 µm filter and red blood cells were lysed with osmotic lysis buffer (10 mM $KHCO_3$, 155 mM NH_4Cl, 0.1 mM EDTA in ddH_2O).

Flow Cytometry

Lung cells were stained extracelullarly with anti-CD3 (17A2, conjugated to AF700, eBioscience), anti-CD19 (1D3, conjugated to APC, BD Bioscience), anti-IgM (R6-60.2, conjugated to PerCp-Cy5.5, BD Bioscience), anti-IgD (11-26c.2a, conjugated to PE, BD Bioscience), anti-CD95 (Jo2, conjugated to PE-Cy7, BD Bioscience), anti-GL7 (GL7, conjugated to Fitc, BD Bioscience), and a fixable live-dead marker (conjugated to eFl506, eBioscience).

Acquisition of samples was performed on a LSR II or Fortessa cytometer equipped with FACSDiva software (BD biosciences). GC B cells were defined as CD3$^-$CD19$^+$IgM$^-$IgD$^-$CD95$^+$GL7$^+$. Final analysis and graphical output were performed using FlowJo software v9 (Tree Star, Inc.).

Real-time Quantitative RT-PCR

Quantitative RT-PCR for IL-1α, IL-1β, LTβ, CCL19, CCL21, CXCL12, and CXCL13 were performed on RNA obtained from whole lung homogenates. Total RNA was extracted using Tripure reagent (Roche) according to the manufacturer's protocol. RNA was resuspended in diethyl-polycarbonate (DEPC, Sigma)-treated water. A total of 1 µg RNA was used for reverse transcription using the Transcriptor High Fidelity Reverse Transcriptase kit (Roche) according to the manufacturer's protocol. The subsequent target amplification on triplicates of each cDNA sample was performed using the Universal Probe Library system from Roche, which contains fluorescent hydrolysis probes of eight locked nucleic acids (LNA). Primers were designed with the help of the web-based application Probefinder (https://qpcr.probefinder.com), and a minimum of two primer pairs per target were analyzed. Primers were validated first using the LC480 SybrGreenI Master (Roche) with melting curve analysis (TM calling) in the LC480 Software and then using the LC480 Probes Master. Aspecific primer pairs were discarded. **Table 1** shows a comprehensive view of the primer/probe combinations chosen. PCR conditions were: 5′ pre-incubation at 95°C followed by 45 amplification cycles of 10″ at 95°C, 10″ at 60°C, and 20″ at 72°C using a Lightcycler 480 (Roche). PCR amplifications for the housekeeping genes encoding *Hprt* or *L27* were performed during each run for each sample to allow normalization between samples.

Histology

Lungs were inflated with 1 ml 1:1 PBS-OCT (Tissue Tec), snap frozen in liquid nitrogen and stored at −80°C. Frozen 8 µm sections were fixed in 4% PFA and blocked in a 1% blocking buffer (Roche).

Immunofluorescence staining was performed by staining for B220 (RA3-6B2, Rat-a-mB220 conjugated to PE, BD Bioscience + Goat-a-Rat conjugated to AF555, Invitrogen), CD4 (RM4-5, Rat-a-CD4 conjugated to Fitc, eBioscience + Rab-a-Fitc conjugated to AF488, Invitrogen), CD8 (53-6.7, Rat-a-CD8 conjugated to Fitc, BD bioscience + Rab-a-Fitc conjugated to AF488, Invitrogen), CD11c (N418, Hamster-a-mCD11c conjugated to AF647, eBioscience), and GL7 (GL7, Rat-a-mGL7 Fitc, BD bioscience + a-Fitc conjugated to HRP, Jackson + a-HRP conjugated to Fitc, Jackson). Where necessary, slides were incubated with 10% normal rat serum to prevent aspecific binding of antibodies.

TABLE 1 | Q-PCR primers.

Target	Ensemble transcript	Fwd primer	Rvs primer	Probe #
CXCL12	ENSMUSG00000061353	GGTTCTTCGAGAGCCACATC	TTCTTCAGCCGTGCAACA	21
CXCL13	ENSMUSG00000023078	CAGAATGAGGCTCAGCACAG	ATGGGCTTCCAGAATACCG	80
CCL19	ENSMUSG00000071005	GGTGCCTGCTGTTGTGTTC	CTGGTGCTGTTGCCTTTGT	29
CCL21	ENSMUSG00000094121	ACCCAAGGCAGTGATGGA	GCTTCCGGGGTAAGAACAG	74
IL-1α	ENSMUSG00000027399	TTGGTTAAATGACCTGCAACA	GAGCGCTCACGAACAGTTG	52
IL-1β	ENSMUSG00000027398	AAAGCTTGGTGATGTCTGGTC	AAAGGACATGGAGAACACCACT	10

Slides were counterstained with Dapi and digitized on a LSM710 microscope (Zeiss). All depicted pictures are representative of at least five mice per group. Images were analyzed using Imaris software (Bitplane).

Statistical Analysis

All experiments were performed using three to six animals per group. All experiments were performed at least two times. The difference between groups was calculated using the Student's *t* test for unpaired data (Prism version 6; GraphPad Software, Inc.). Data are depicted as mean ± SEM. Differences were considered significant when $p < 0.05$.

Analysis of the repeated relative body weight data was performed using the residual maximum likelihood (REML) as implemented in Genstat v17 (43). The following linear mixed model (random terms underlined) was fitted to the data: $Y_{ijkt} = \mu + \text{genotype}_j + \text{treatment}_k + \text{time}_t + (\text{genotype}\cdot\text{treatment})_{jk} + (\text{genotype}\cdot\text{time})_{jt} + (\text{treatment}\cdot\text{time})_{kt} + (\text{genotype}\cdot\text{treatment}\cdot\text{time})_{jkt} + (\text{mouse}\cdot\text{time})_{it} + \textit{residual}_{ijkt}$, where Y_{ijkt} is the relative body weight of i-th mouse having genotype j, k-treated, and measured at time point t ($t = 3$–17 days; unequally spaced) and μ is the overall mean calculated for all mice considered across all time points. A first order antedependence covariance structure was used to model the within-subject correlation. The significance of the comparison between WT-X31 and KO-X31 across time was assessed by an *F*-test.

A log-linear model (Poisson distribution and log link) was fitted to the amount of viral particles measured by hemagglutination inhibiton assay. The dispersion parameter was set as free. Significance of main effects GENOTYPE and TIME and the GENOTYPE·TIME interaction effect was assessed by an *F*-test.

RESULTS

Il1r1$^{-/-}$ Mice Have Prolonged Viral Load but Are Unable to Induce iBALT

To assess the immune response to IAV infection in mice lacking signaling *via* IL-1R, we infected *Il1r1*$^{-/-}$ mice and monitored weight loss and viral load in the lungs. Wild-type mice showed maximum weight loss around 6 dpi, and bodyweight was fully restored around 10 dpi. *Il1r1*$^{-/-}$ mice lost weight with slower and prolonged kinetics, and reaching a nadir at 8 dpi. Like wild-type mice they did manage to gain weight again, but did not recover to their starting bodyweight before 17 dpi (**Figure 1A**). This difference in the weight loss curve was also reflected in the viral load in the lungs (**Figure 1B**). Viral load in wild-type mice peaked around 6 dpi, yet was cleared at 8 dpi. *Il1r1*$^{-/-}$ mice had systematically higher viral loads during the entire course of infection and did not clear the infection completely at 8 dpi as an estimated remaining titer of 100,000 viral particles is detected at this time point.

Viral clearance depends on induction of adaptive immunity by DCs that activate CD8 and CD4 T cells and a humoral immune response by B cells. Total numbers and kinetics of increase of T and B cells and conventional DCs were not altered in *Il1r1*$^{-/-}$ mice in response to IAV infection. Lung conventional DCs consist of various subsets that have different functions and can be discriminated based on cell surface markers CD11b and CD103 (44, 45). As soon as there is inflammation in the lung, monocytes can also be recruited and these can rapidly differentiate into a MHCII$^+$CD11c$^+$ cell type (so called monocyte-derived DC, MoDC) that also expresses the macrophage marker CD64 (46). In contrast to the conventional CD103$^+$ and CD11b$^+$ DCs, the accumulation of CD11c$^+$CD64$^+$ MoDCs was reduced in the lungs of *Il1r1*$^{-/-}$ mice (**Figure 1C**).

To evaluate the effect of the higher and prolonged viral exposure on IAV-associated iBALT formation, we visualized iBALT structures in the lungs by hematoxilin staining. Generally, clusters of cells near the bronchi were more readily detected in wild-type mice than in *Il1r1*$^{-/-}$ mice (**Figure 1D**). Because a hematoxilin stain did not allow us to evaluate if the inflammatory clusters of cells were organized and immunologically active iBALT structures, we stained frozen lung sections for B cells, T cells, DCs, and GC B cells and analyzed them by confocal microscopy. In wild-type mice, we could easily detect organized structures composed of B cells, T cells, and DCs and B cell aggregates that contain GC B cells, but we were unable to detect similar infiltrates in *Il1r1*$^{-/-}$ mice (**Figure 1E**). To quantify the presence or absence of iBALT structures we measured the proportion of GC B cells in the lungs at 17 dpi by flow cytometry as a measure for biologically active iBALT. As GL7$^+$ GC B cells are not found in the lungs of mice in the absence of iBALT, we believe this is a good approximation of the amount of iBALT formed (17). Wild-type mice showed an induction of GC B cells upon IAV infection, but this induction was absent in *Il1r1*$^{-/-}$ mice (**Figure 1F**). Taken together, these data suggest that although *Il1r1*$^{-/-}$ mice had a higher and prolonged exposure to viral particles in the lung, they were unable to form organized iBALT structures in the lung, pointing to an essential role for IL-1 cytokines in TLO induction following influenza virus infection.

IL-1α Administration Promotes Induction of iBALT Structures in the Lung

As the mere presence of viral particles was not enough to trigger the iBALT initiation and IL-1R signaling was necessary, we

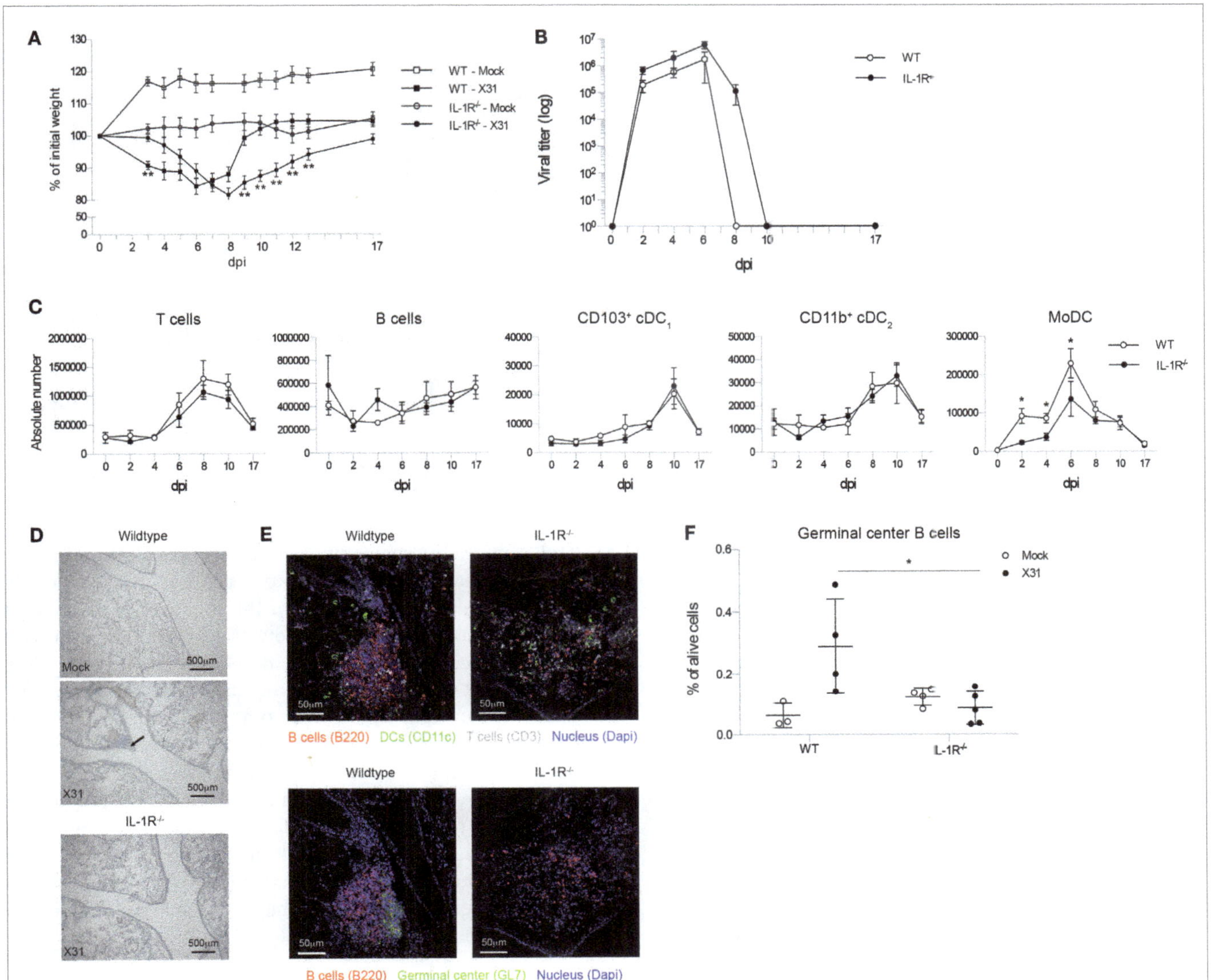

FIGURE 1 | *Il1r1*$^{-/-}$ mice have a prolonged viral load in the lungs, but do not develop iBALT structures. (A) Weight loss curve as percentage of the initial bodyweight for wild-type (squares) and *Il1r1*$^{-/-}$ mice (circles) that have been infected with mock (white) or X31 (black) virus. The significance of the comparison between WT-X31 and KO-X31 across time was assessed by an *F*-test ($F < 0.001$), differences between individual time points were assessed by a *t* test. **(B)** Viral titers in the lung of wild-type (white) or *Il1r1*$^{-/-}$ (black) mice determined by hemagglutination-inhibition assay after culture with MDCK cells. Significance of main effects GENOTYPE and TIME and the GENOTYPE·TIME interaction effect was assessed by an *F*-test ($F = 0.022$; $F < 0.01$; $F = 0.984$, respectively). **(C)** Numbers of T and B cells, CD103+ cDC_1 and CD11b+ cDC_2 DCs, and monocyte-derived cells (MoDC) in the lungs of wild-type (white) and *Il1r1*$^{-/-}$ mice (black).
(D) Hematoxylin-stained lung sections 17 dpi of wild-type and *Il1r1*$^{-/-}$ mice. Images are representative for at least three mice per group. **(E)** Confocal images of lung sections of wild-type and *Il1r1*$^{-/-}$ mice at 17 dpi. Sections were stained with either B220 (red), CD11c (Green), CD3 (Gray) and dapi (blue) or B220 (red), GL7 (Green), and dapi (Blue). Shown images are representative for five mice per group. **(F)** Proportion of germinal center B cells (GL7+) in the lungs of wild-type and *Il1r1*$^{-/-}$ mice infected with mock (white) or X31 (black) virus at 17 dpi determined by flow cytometry. All experiments were performed at least twice with 4–6 mice per group. $^{*}p < 0.05$; $^{**}p < 0.01$.

quantified expression of IL-1α and IL-1β, which signal both *via* IL-1R, in the lungs after IAV infection. Both cytokines were induced after infection in a bimodal curve with a first peak around 4 dpi and a second, but smaller, peak around 10 dpi (**Figure 2A**). In general, the induction of mRNA for IL-1α was more pronounced compared with IL-1β.

We, next, addressed if administration of IL-1 cytokine would be enough to further boost iBALT induction in IAV-infected mice. Since IL-1α and IL-1β have similar effects on the IL-1R, and as induction of IL-1α was more pronounced after IAV infection, we chose to only administer IL-1α. When recombinant IL-1α was administered i.t. 2 days post IAV infection in wild-type mice, clustering of inflammatory cells could be detected more readily on lung sections compared to PBS-treated IAV-infected mice (**Figure 2B**). To quantify biologically active iBALT, we again quantified the proportion of GC B cells by flow cytometry. Administration of recombinant IL-1α at 2 dpi resulted in a higher proportion of GC B cells in the lungs 17 dpi compared to PBS

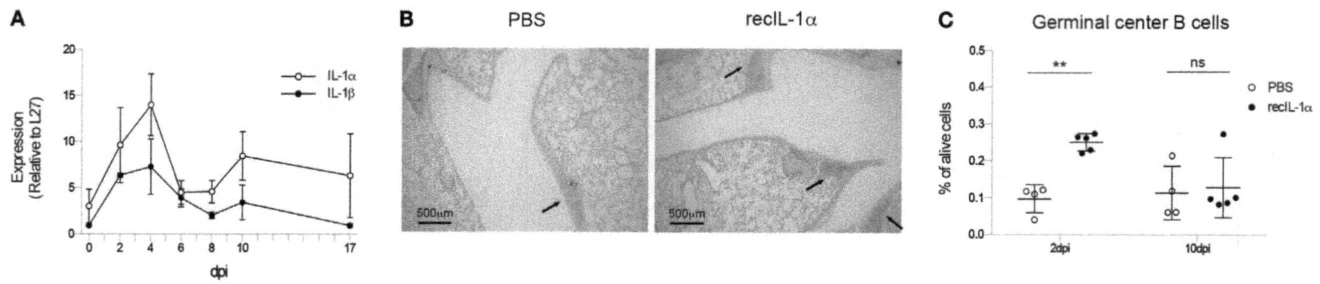

FIGURE 2 | Early IL-1α signaling is sufficient and necessary for iBALT induction. (A) mRNA expression of IL-1α (white) and IL-1β (black) relative to the housekeeping gene L27 in the lungs of wild-type mice. **(B)** Hematoxylin-stained lung sections 17 dpi of mice treated with PBS or recIL-1α 2dpi. Images are representative for at least three mice per group. **(C)** Proportion of germinal center B cells 17 dpi in the lungs of wild-type mice treated with PBS (white) or recombinant IL-1α (black) i.t. 2 or 10 dpi. All experiments were performed at least twice with 3–5 mice per group. ns, not significant. $^{**}p < 0.01$.

administration (**Figure 2C**). However, when the administration of recombinant IL-1α was only initiated at 10 dpi, no differences in the proportion of GC B cells could be observed between IL-1α and PBS-treated groups (**Figure 2C**). This suggests that early, but not late, IL-1R signaling is necessary and sufficient to promote GC B cell positive iBALT structures.

IL-1R Signaling on Stromal Cells Is Necessary to Induce GC B Cells

As early IL-1R signaling is necessary to induce iBALT structures in the lung, we sought to identify the cell type that is responsive to IL-1 signals. Therefore, we constructed bone marrow chimeric mice in which either the radiosensitive hematopoietic or the radioresistant stromal compartment was deficient for *Il1r1*. As a control, we also reconstituted *Il1r1*$^{-/-}$ mice with *Il1r1*$^{-/-}$ bone marrow as a substitute for intact *Il1r1*$^{-/-}$ mice and control for irradiation effects. *Il1r1*$^{-/-}$ mice that received wild-type bone marrow followed a weight loss curve characterized by a longer weight loss and slower recovery, as observed in *Il1r1*$^{-/-}$ mice. In contrast, wild-type mice that were reconstituted with *Il1r1*$^{-/-}$ bone marrow cells followed a weight loss curve that resembled the one observed in wild-type mice with a maximum of approximately 15% weight loss. Surprisingly, *Il1r1*$^{-/-}$ mice that were reconstituted with IL-1R sufficient bone marrow had a tendency to lose more weight than the *Il1r1*$^{-/-}$ mice that were reconstituted with IL-1R-deficient bone marrow (**Figure 3A**). We also counted the proportion of GC B cells in the lung. Wild-type mice with IL-1R-deficient hematopoietic cells were able to induce a higher proportion of GC B cells than *Il1r1*$^{-/-}$ mice with normal hematopoietic cells (**Figure 3B**), suggesting that IL-1 boosts the formation of iBALT structures by signaling to radioresistant stromal cells.

CXCL13 Expression Is Reduced in *Il1r1*$^{-/-}$ Mice

To define which downstream iBALT-instructive signals are induced by IL-1R signaling in radioresistant cells, we measured the expression level of the chemokines CXCL12, CXCL13, CCL19, and CCL21, which all have been implicated in iBALT formation. The chemokines CCL19 and CCL21 instruct the organization of T cell zones in iBALT structures, but were not impaired in *Il1r1*$^{-/-}$ mice (**Figure 4**). The chemokine CXCL12 is important for B cell lymphopoiesis, but expression of this chemokine was only slightly reduced early after infection in *Il1r1*$^{-/-}$ mice. The chemokine CXCL13 functions as an LT_i and B cell chemoattractant, and its expression was reduced 4 dpi in *Il1r1*$^{-/-}$ mice (**Figure 4**). None of the chemokines involved in iBALT formation and organization was differentially expressed at 17 dpi, when iBALT had fully developed in wild-type mice, showing that the instructive chemokine signals are given early after infection when the virus is not yet cleared from the lungs. Although CXCL13 expression was impaired early after infection, the total amount of B cells in the lungs was not significantly altered at the time iBALT was present (**Figure 1C**), suggesting that it is not recruitment of B cells to the lungs that is impaired in *Il1r1*$^{-/-}$ mice but that the B cells in the lung fail to cluster into organized iBALT structures. Whether this is a direct or indirect effect of defective IL-1R signaling on stromal cells remains a subject for future experiments.

DISCUSSION AND REVIEW OF THE LITERATURE

The IL-1 axis has been described previously to be responsible for inflammatory pathology in the lung, resulting in increased mortality, increased viral titers, and neutrophil recruitment following IAV infection (7). *Il1r1*$^{-/-}$ mice indeed suffered more from the mild X31 IAV infection and displayed a tendency to higher viral titers in the lung, but did manage to clear infection with delayed kinetics, leading to a presumably higher viral exposure over time. Despite this increased viral exposure, they hardly formed iBALT structures in the lung. Conversely, when recombinant IL-1 was administered early after IAV infection to wild-type mice, the formation of iBALT structures was facilitated. Mechanistically, we found impaired CXCL13 chemokine induction early after infection in *Il1r1*$^{-/-}$ mice. Later, at the time when iBALT was fully formed in wild-type mice, we could not detect any differences in CXCL13 levels, suggesting that the instructive signals that condition the lung for clustering adaptive immune cells are given very early (2–4 dpi) after infection. By studying iBALT formation in chimeric mice, we found that

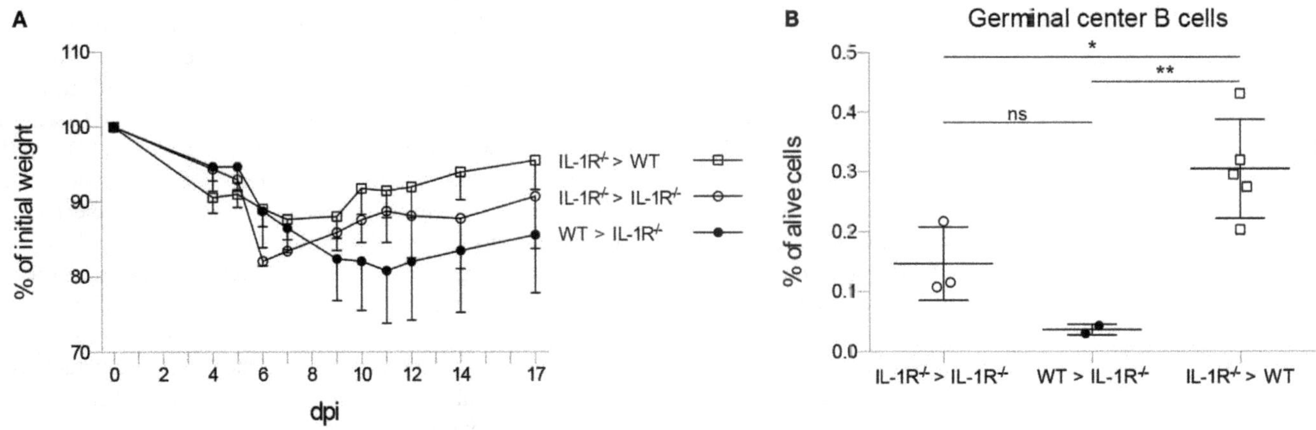

FIGURE 3 | IL-1R signaling on stromal cells is necessary to induce germinal center B cells in the lung. (A) Weight loss curve after infection with X31 virus as percentage of the initial bodyweight for wild-type (squares) and IL-1R$^{-/-}$ (circles) mice reconstituted with wild-type (black) or IL-1R$^{-/-}$ bone marrow (white). **(B)** Proportion of germinal center B cells 17 dpi in the lungs of wild-type (squares) and IL-1R$^{-/-}$ (circles) mice reconstituted with wild-type (black) or IL-1R$^{-/-}$ bone marrow (white). ns, not significant. *$p < 0.05$. **$p < 0.01$.

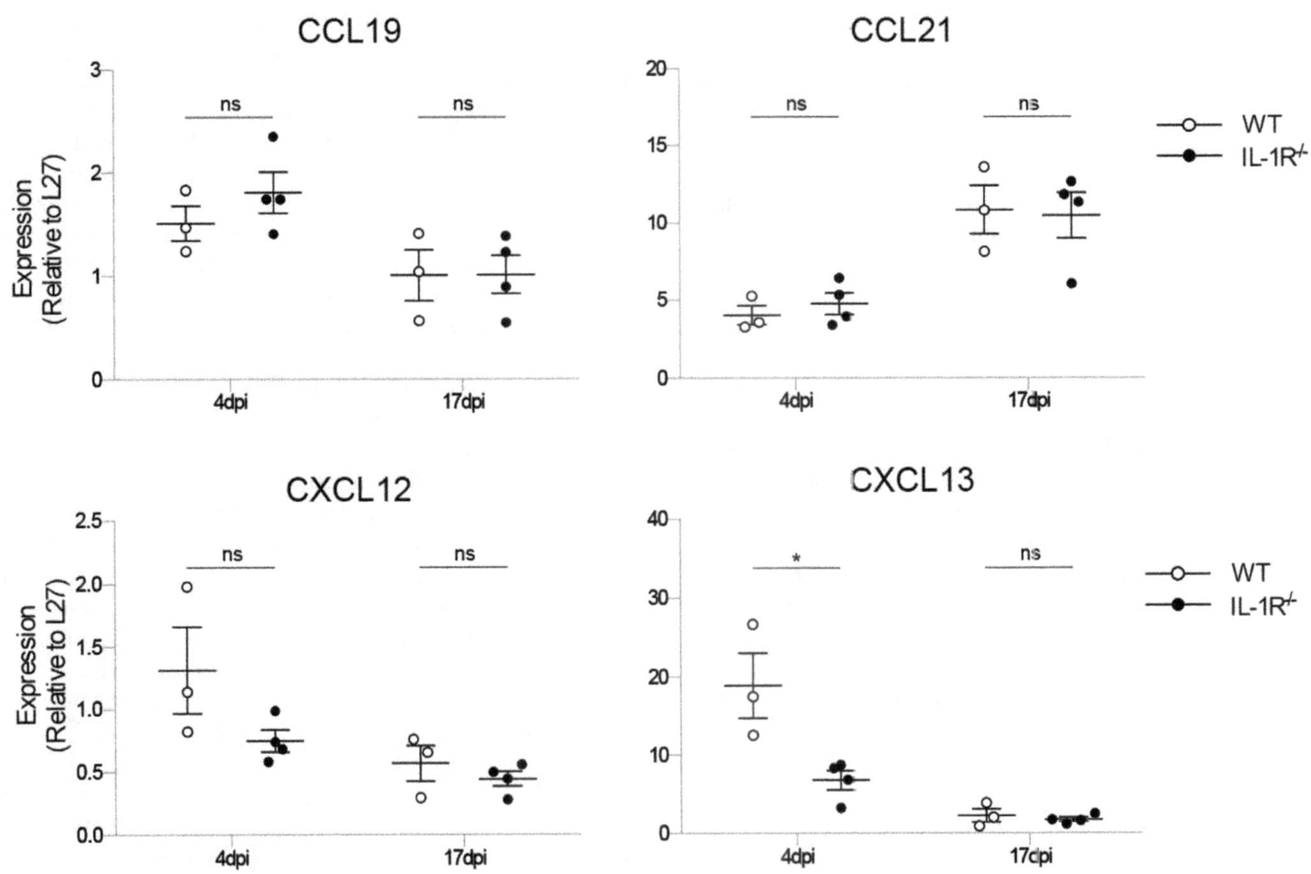

FIGURE 4 | *Il1r1*$^{-/-}$ mice have a defect in the production of the iBALT-inducing chemokine CXCL13. mRNA expression levels of the chemokines involved in iBALT induction: CXCL12, CXCL13, CCL19, CCL21 relative to the expression of housekeeping gene L27. The experiment was performed twice with three to five mice per group. ns, not significant. *$p < 0.05$.

IL-1R expression on stromal cells is necessary for proper iBALT formation. The exact cell type of stromal cells that is needed to induce GC B cells, however, still needs to be defined. Whether this stromal cell type is directly responsible for the CXCL13 production needed to initiate iBALT formation or an intermediate cell type is involved remains a matter of debate.

As we observed a decreased induction in MoDCs and these cells are previously described as being major cytokine and chemokine producers (46), it is a possibility that these cells are involved in the CXCL13 induction. Alternatively, LTβ-sufficient B cells can support the progression toward mature, fully structured TLOs (35, 47) most likely *via* a positive feedback loop of CXCL13 production and LTβ expression (24). According to this hypothesis B cells are activated *via* TLR signaling, induce expression of LTβ on their surface, and interact on its turn with LTβR bearing B cells. This LTβ signaling will induce CXCL13 production and release, which attracts more B cells and upregulates LTβ expression. It is an attractive hypothesis that IL-1 might also induce LTβ expression on B cells, although this is hard to reconcile with our observation that a radioresistant cell type responds to IL-1 in our model.

We can only speculate about the source of IL-1α. Previous research has shown that IL-1α can be released by dying cells (48). In this respect, virus-infected lung epithelial cells might be a possible source of IL-1α as it has been observed that IL-1α exerts feedback on epithelial cells and induces a second cytokine and chemokine wave during innate immune responses in the lung (3, 49). We have only measured the mRNA for IL-1β. Secretion of bioactive IL-1β requires activation of the Nlrp3 inflammasome that leads to activation of caspase-1 and cleavage of pro-IL-1β into IL-1β. Infection with IAV leads to activation of the Nlrp3 inflammasome in a process requiring the type I IFN-induced RNAse L/OAS system, while the virus actively suppresses IL-1β production and Nlrp3 activation *via* the NS1 protein (4, 5). Although others have shown that the NLRP3 inflammasome controls severity of infection (9, 11, 50, 51), future studies will have to address if lack of key components of this inflammasome also leads to reduced iBALT formation.

Generally, TLOs are absent in the lungs of healthy adults (52), but bronchus-associated lymphoid tissue can be observed in the lungs of children who are frequently infected by respiratory viruses (53) and in the lungs of adults who suffer from rheumatoid arthritis (28, 54), transplant rejection (55), COPD (56), and IPAH (31). We can only speculate that IL-1 might also be involved in the formation of these TLO structures. IL-1 is certainly a cytokine that has been implicated in the pathogenesis of rheumatoid arthritis, and targeting the IL-1 pathway *via* IL1RA (anakinra) has been used as an alternative biological treatment in patients failing therapy on TNFα blockade. A very common risk factor for rheumatoid arthritis development is smoking, which also leads to COPD. End-stage COPD is also accompanied by TLO formation in the lungs, and these can be sites of production of antibodies to citrullinated antigens, typical of RA patients. In a preclinical model of smoking-induced TLO formation, the production of autoantibodies and TLO structures was reduced in *Il1r1*$^{-/-}$ mice, accompanied by a reduced CXCL13-production in the lungs (57).

During development, neuronal cells give an LTα1β2-independent instructive signal to local fibroblasts to produce CXCL13 and, hereby, attract CD3$^-$CD4$^+$CD45$^+$ LT$_i$ cells (58, 59). The crucial step for SLO development is the interaction of LT$_i$ cells with stromal lymphoid tissue organizer (LT$_o$) cells. This process happens *via* interaction of LTβ expressed on LT$_i$ cells and the LTβR expressed on LT$_o$ cells. Upon this interaction, LT$_o$ cells produce homeostatic chemokines that drive the recruitment of lymphocytes. T cells and DCs are attracted by chemokine CC ligand (CCL)19 and CCL21; B cells are attracted by chemokine CXC ligand (CXCL)13. Expression of vascular cell adhesion molecule (VCAM)1, intercellular adhesion molecule (ICAM)1, and mucosal addressin cell adhesion molecule (MADCAM)1 allow the attracted cells to cluster together. IL-1 has been very well known for its effects of stimulating adhesion molecules on endothelial cells (60). It is tempting to speculate that the effects of IL-1 on radioresistant cells is *via* induction of the crucial adhesion molecules that initially tether a LT$_i$-like cell to the circulation and subsequently to initiate a communication between stromal cells and lymphoid cells, that initiates the CXCL13 production.

The LT$_i$-potential of T cells was first addressed in a model of thyroid overexpression of CCL21, where it was shown that CD3$^+$CD4$^+$-activated T cells interacted with DCs at sites of chronic inflammation and subsequently acted as LT$_i$ cells in the absence of Id2 activity (37). It has also been suggested that IL-17 signaling is involved during the initiation phase of iBALT formation by inducing CXCL13, but this role for IL-17 remains controversial (34). In two studies on neonatal mice exposed to endotoxin inhalation and on mice with experimental autoimmune encephalomyelitis, respectively, an activated Th17 CD4 T cell population was found to be involved in inducing TLO structures (34, 61). RORC$^+$ IL-17-producing cells were also found inside lung TLOs of patients with IPAH. In humans, Th17 cells express the CCR6 receptor, and in the bloodstream of IPAH patients circulating CCR6$^+$ cells were fewer, while the ligand CCL20 was produced in the perivascular TLOs (31). However, TLOs seem to develop normally in *Ccr6*$^{-/-}$ mice (34). The induction of TLOs by Th17 cells was dependent on expression of podoplanin, but why this is the case remains unknown. One possibility is that podoplanin is required for retention of Th17 cells at sites of TLO formation (34, 61). The role of Th17 as LT$_i$-like cells is still under debate, and it remains to be seen whether all forms of TLO depend on IL-17 production and whether IL-17A and/or IL-17F is involved. In this regard, iBALT induced by infection with modified vaccinia virus Ankara or influenza virus is not affected by deficiency of IL-17A, while *Pseudomonas aeruginosa*-induced iBALT is dependent on IL-17 signaling (35, 62). As IL-17 production by γδ T cells and Th17 cells can be induced by IL-1 (63–66), we also considered the possibility that IL-17 is part of the cascade leading to IL-1α driven iBALT formation. In our hands, IAV infection indeed gave rise to a higher amount of IL-17$^+$ CD4 T cells, but treatment with IL-1α 2 dpi could not increase the amount of IL-17$^+$ CD4 T cells in the lung, and experiments in which we administered IL-1 to IAV-infected *Il17ra*$^{-/-}$ mice were inconclusive (data not shown). This suggests that, in contrast to SLO formation, the instructive signals can differ depending on the source of initiating antigen or the inflammatory stimulus that is elicited by the used model.

In almost all TLO structures that have been described, the T cell area contained antigen-presenting DCs (17, 31). As DCs activate T cells, it has been suggested that DCs are sufficient for TLO induction (67). This hypothesis is supported by the observation that repeated injection of DCs into the lungs of mice is sufficient for induction of iBALT structures accompanied by induction of myofibroblast differentiation (17, 68). During formation of Peyer's patches, a CD11c⁺ cell type expressing LTαβ accumulates at the LN anlagen and is necessary for instruction of stromal cells (59). DCs might also directly instruct stromal cells irrespectively of their effects on T cells. In TLO structures induced in the thymus, DCs were specifically necessary for induction of lymph angiogenesis from stromal cells (69), but how DCs induce TLOs is less clear. In virus-induced iBALT, mainly $CD11b^+$ DCs or monocyte-derived cells accumulate; these cells express instructive $LT\alpha_1\beta_2$ while also producing the homeostatic chemokines CXCL13 and CCL19/CCL21 (17). However, in some models, mostly pDCs accumulate, suggesting a functional role for type I IFN. As is the case in TLOs found in end-stage COPD patients and in a murine SLE model (56, 70). Three studies have shown that depletion of DCs leads to disappearance of existing TLO structures, suggesting that DCs are necessary for structural organization and maintenance of TLOs, most likely through trans-presentation of chemokines, or by providing a continuous source of antigen presentation to T cells (16, 17, 69). We did observe reduced numbers of monocyte-derived DCs in *Il1r1*$^{-/-}$ mice, but have not performed experiments in which only DCs lacked IL-1R to study if the effects of IL-1 were cell-intrinsic or resulting from effects of IL-1 on epithelial cells. Indeed, IL-1R triggering on lung epithelial cells is a very well-known trigger for the production of GM-CSF, one of the major cytokines driving activation of monocytes to adopt a DC-like phenotype (49).

In conclusion, we have described a novel role for early IL-1 production in IAV infection to control the formation of iBALT structures *via* induction of CXCL13 in a stromal cell compartment. Future studies will have to address if this effect of one of the best-known proinflammatory and innate cytokines is a general feature of TLO formation at sites of acute and chronic immune stimulation such as infectious disease and autoimmune pathologies and if this can be exploited to induce iBALT formation as part of a mucosal vaccination strategy (71).

AUTHOR CONTRIBUTIONS

KN was responsible for conceptualization of mouse experiments, experimentation, data analysis, and preparation of the manuscript. HH and KD provided experimental support for confocal imaging. CG, HH, and BL assisted in conceptualization of experiments and discussion of data and provided feedback for the manuscript. All authors read and approved the final manuscript.

ACKNOWLEDGMENTS

We thank the technical and logistic support of Sofie De Prijck, Manon Vanheerswynghels, Gert Van Isterdael, Justine Van Moorleghem, and Karl Vergote and the statistical support of Marnik Vuylsteke.

FUNDING

KN is supported by a grant from FWO Flanders. CG is supported by an ESMCID grant. BL is supported by Project grants of FWO Flanders, by an ERC Consolidator grant, by an Interuniversity Attraction Pole grant, and by a Ghent University MRP Grant (Group-ID consortium).

REFERENCES

1. van Riel D, Munster VJ, de Wit E, Rimmelzwaan GF, Fouchier RA, Osterhaus AD, et al. Human and avian influenza viruses target different cells in the lower respiratory tract of humans and other mammals. *Am J Pathol* (2007) 171(4):1215–23. doi:10.2353/ajpath.2007.070248
2. Lupfer C, Thomas PG, Anand PK, Vogel P, Milasta S, Martinez J, et al. Receptor interacting protein kinase 2-mediated mitophagy regulates inflammasome activation during virus infection. *Nat Immunol* (2013) 14(5):480–8. doi:10.1038/ni.2563
3. Sanders CJ, Doherty PC, Thomas PG. Respiratory epithelial cells in innate immunity to influenza virus infection. *Cell Tissue Res* (2011) 343(1):13–21. doi:10.1007/s00441-010-1043-z
4. Cheong WC, Kang HR, Yoon H, Kang SJ, Ting JP, Song MJ. Influenza A virus NS1 protein inhibits the NLRP3 inflammasome. *PLoS One* (2015) 10(5):e0126456. doi:10.1371/journal.pone.0126456
5. Moriyama M, Chen IY, Kawaguchi A, Koshiba T, Nagata K, Takeyama H, et al. The RNA- and TRIM25-binding domains of influenza virus NS1 protein are essential for suppression of NLRP3 inflammasome-mediated interleukin-1beta secretion. *J Virol* (2016) 90(8):4105–14. doi:10.1128/JVI.00120-16
6. Chakrabarti A, Banerjee S, Franchi L, Loo YM, Gale M Jr, Nunez G, et al. RNase L activates the NLRP3 inflammasome during viral infections. *Cell Host Microbe* (2015) 17(4):466–77. doi:10.1016/j.chom.2015.02.010
7. Schmitz N, Kurrer M, Bachmann MF, Kopf M. Interleukin-1 is responsible for acute lung immunopathology but increases survival of respiratory influenza virus infection. *J Virol* (2005) 79(10):6441–8. doi:10.1128/JVI.79.10.6441-6448.2005
8. Szretter KJ, Gangappa S, Lu X, Smith C, Shieh WJ, Zaki SR, et al. Role of host cytokine responses in the pathogenesis of avian H5N1 influenza viruses in mice. *J Virol* (2007) 81(6):2736–44. doi:10.1128/JVI.02336-06
9. Ichinohe T, Lee HK, Ogura Y, Flavell R, Iwasaki A. Inflammasome recognition of influenza virus is essential for adaptive immune responses. *J Exp Med* (2009) 206(1):79–87. doi:10.1084/jem.20081667
10. Brandes M, Klauschen F, Kuchen S, Germain RN. A systems analysis identifies a feedforward inflammatory circuit leading to lethal influenza infection. *Cell* (2013) 154(1):197–212. doi:10.1016/j.cell.2013.06.013
11. Allen IC, Scull MA, Moore CB, Holl EK, McElvania-TeKippe E, Taxman DJ, et al. The NLRP3 inflammasome mediates *in vivo* innate immunity to influenza A virus through recognition of viral RNA. *Immunity* (2009) 30(4):556–65. doi:10.1016/j.immuni.2009.02.005
12. Breart B, Bousso P. Cellular orchestration of T cell priming in lymph nodes. *Curr Opin Immunol* (2006) 18(4):483–90. doi:10.1016/j.coi.2006.05.006
13. De Silva NS, Klein U. Dynamics of B cells in germinal centres. *Nat Rev Immunol* (2015) 15(3):137–48. doi:10.1038/nri3804
14. van de Pavert SA, Mebius RE. New insights into the development of lymphoid tissues. *Nat Rev Immunol* (2010) 10(9):664–74. doi:10.1038/nri2832
15. Moyron-Quiroz JE, Rangel-Moreno J, Kusser K, Hartson L, Sprague F, Goodrich S, et al. Role of inducible bronchus associated lymphoid tissue (iBALT) in respiratory immunity. *Nat Med* (2004) 10(9):927–34. doi:10.1038/nm1091
16. Halle S, Dujardin HC, Bakocevic N, Fleige H, Danzer H, Willenzon S, et al. Induced bronchus-associated lymphoid tissue serves as a general priming site for T cells and is maintained by dendritic cells. *J Exp Med* (2009) 206(12):2593–601. doi:10.1084/jem.20091472
17. GeurtsvanKessel CH, Willart MA, Bergen IM, van Rijt LS, Muskens F, Elewaut D, et al. Dendritic cells are crucial for maintenance of tertiary lymphoid structures in the lung of influenza virus-infected mice. *J Exp Med* (2009) 206(11) 2339–49. doi:10.1084/jem.20090410
18. Wiley JA, Richert LE, Swain SD, Harmsen A, Barnard DL, Randall TD, et al. Inducible bronchus-associated lymphoid tissue elicited by a protein cage

nanoparticle enhances protection in mice against diverse respiratory viruses. *PLoS One* (2009) 4(9):e7142. doi:10.1371/journal.pone.0007142
19. Kim TS, Hufford MM, Sun J, Fu YX, Braciale TJ. Antigen persistence and the control of local T cell memory by migrant respiratory dendritic cells after acute virus infection. *J Exp Med* (2010) 207(6):1161–72. doi:10.1084/jem.20092017
20. Shinoda K, Hirahara K, Iinuma T, Ichikawa T, Suzuki AS, Sugaya K, et al. Thy1+IL-7+ lymphatic endothelial cells in iBALT provide a survival niche for memory T-helper cells in allergic airway inflammation. *Proc Natl Acad Sci U S A* (2016) 113(20):E2842–51. doi:10.1073/pnas.1512600113
21. Winter S, Loddenkemper C, Aebischer A, Rabel K, Hoffmann K, Meyer TF, et al. The chemokine receptor CXCR5 is pivotal for ectopic mucosa-associated lymphoid tissue neogenesis in chronic *Helicobacter pylori*-induced inflammation. *J Mol Med* (2010) 88(11):1169–80. doi:10.1007/s00109-010-0658-6
22. Henry RA, Kendall PL. CXCL13 blockade disrupts B lymphocyte organization in tertiary lymphoid structures without altering B cell receptor bias or preventing diabetes in nonobese diabetic mice. *J Immunol* (2010) 185(3):1460–5. doi:10.4049/jimmunol.0903710
23. Magliozzi R, Columba-Cabezas S, Serafini B, Aloisi F. Intracerebral expression of CXCL13 and BAFF is accompanied by formation of lymphoid follicle-like structures in the meninges of mice with relapsing experimental autoimmune encephalomyelitis. *J Neuroimmunol* (2004) 148(1–2):11–23. doi:10.1016/j.jneuroim.2003.10.056
24. Litsiou E, Semitekolou M, Galani IE, Morianos I, Tsoutsa A, Kara P, et al. CXCL13 production in B cells via Toll-like receptor/lymphotoxin receptor signaling is involved in lymphoid neogenesis in chronic obstructive pulmonary disease. *Am J Respir Crit Care Med* (2013) 187(11):1194–202. doi:10.1164/rccm.201208-1543OC
25. Rangel-Moreno J, Moyron-Quiroz JE, Hartson L, Kusser K, Randall TD. Pulmonary expression of CXC chemokine ligand 13, CC chemokine ligand 19, and CC chemokine ligand 21 is essential for local immunity to influenza. *Proc Natl Acad Sci U S A* (2007) 104(25):10577–82. doi:10.1073/pnas.0700591104
26. Luther SA, Bidgol A, Hargreaves DC, Schmidt A, Xu Y, Paniyadi J, et al. Differing activities of homeostatic chemokines CCL19, CCL21, and CXCL12 in lymphocyte and dendritic cell recruitment and lymphoid neogenesis. *J Immunol* (2002) 169(1):424–33. doi:10.4049/jimmunol.169.1.424
27. Timmer TC, Baltus B, Vondenhoff M, Huizinga TW, Tak PP, Verweij CL, et al. Inflammation and ectopic lymphoid structures in rheumatoid arthritis synovial tissues dissected by genomics technology: identification of the interleukin-7 signaling pathway in tissues with lymphoid neogenesis. *Arthritis Rheum* (2007) 56(8):2492–502. doi:10.1002/art.22748
28. Takemura S, Braun A, Crowson C, Kurtin PJ, Cofield RH, O'Fallon WM, et al. Lymphoid neogenesis in rheumatoid synovitis. *J Immunol* (2001) 167(2):1072–80. doi:10.4049/jimmunol.167.2.1072
29. van Roon JA, Verweij MC, Wijk MW, Jacobs KM, Bijlsma JW, Lafeber FP. Increased intraarticular interleukin-7 in rheumatoid arthritis patients stimulates cell contact-dependent activation of CD4(+) T cells and macrophages. *Arthritis Rheum* (2005) 52(6):1700–10. doi:10.1002/art.21045
30. Meier D, Bornmann C, Chappaz S, Schmutz S, Otten LA, Ceredig R, et al. Ectopic lymphoid-organ development occurs through interleukin 7-mediated enhanced survival of lymphoid-tissue-inducer cells. *Immunity* (2007) 26(5):643–54. doi:10.1016/j.immuni.2007.04.009
31. Perros F, Dorfmuller P, Montani D, Hammad H, Waelput W, Girerd B, et al. Pulmonary lymphoid neogenesis in idiopathic pulmonary arterial hypertension. *Am J Respir Crit Care Med* (2012) 185(3):311–21. doi:10.1164/rccm.201105-0927OC
32. Ishizuka IE, Chea S, Gudjonson H, Constantinides MG, Dinner AR, Bendelac A, et al. Single-cell analysis defines the divergence between the innate lymphoid cell lineage and lymphoid tissue-inducer cell lineage. *Nat Immunol* (2016) 17(3):269–76. doi:10.1038/ni.3344
33. Baerenwaldt A, von Burg N, Kreuzaler M, Sitte S, Horvath E, Peter A, et al. Flt3 ligand regulates the development of innate lymphoid cells in fetal and adult mice. *J Immunol* (2016) 196(6):2561–71. doi:10.4049/jimmunol.1501380
34. Rangel-Moreno J, Carragher DM, de la Luz Garcia-Hernandez M, Hwang JY, Kusser K, Hartson L, et al. The development of inducible bronchus-associated lymphoid tissue depends on IL-17. *Nat Immunol* (2011) 12(7):639–46. doi:10.1038/ni.2053
35. Lochner M, Ohnmacht C, Presley L, Bruhns P, Si-Tahar M, Sawa S, et al. Microbiota-induced tertiary lymphoid tissues aggravate inflammatory disease in the absence of ROR gamma t and LTi cells. *J Exp Med* (2011) 208(1):125–34. doi:10.1084/jem.20100052
36. Rangel-Moreno J, Moyron-Quiroz JE, Carragher DM, Kusser K, Hartson L, Moquin A, et al. Omental milky spots develop in the absence of lymphoid tissue-inducer cells and support B and T cell responses to peritoneal antigens. *Immunity* (2009) 30(5):731–43. doi:10.1016/j.immuni.2009.03.014
37. Marinkovic T, Garin A, Yokota Y, Fu YX, Ruddle NH, Furtado GC, et al. Interaction of mature CD3+CD4+ T cells with dendritic cells triggers the development of tertiary lymphoid structures in the thyroid. *J Clin Invest* (2006) 116(10):2622–32. doi:10.1172/JCI28993
38. Link A, Hardie DL, Favre S, Britschgi MR, Adams DH, Sixt M, et al. Association of T-zone reticular networks and conduits with ectopic lymphoid tissues in mice and humans. *Am J Pathol* (2011) 178(4):1662–75. doi:10.1016/j.ajpath.2010.12.039
39. Furtado GC, Marinkovic T, Martin AP, Garin A, Hoch B, Hubner W, et al. Lymphotoxin beta receptor signaling is required for inflammatory lymphangiogenesis in the thyroid. *Proc Natl Acad Sci U S A* (2007) 104(12):5026–31. doi:10.1073/pnas.0606697104
40. Endres R, Alimzhanov MB, Plitz T, Futterer A, Kosco-Vilbois MH, Nedospasov SA, et al. Mature follicular dendritic cell networks depend on expression of lymphotoxin beta receptor by radioresistant stromal cells and of lymphotoxin beta and tumor necrosis factor by B cells. *J Exp Med* (1999) 189(1):159–68. doi:10.1084/jem.189.1.159
41. Ansel KM, Ngo VN, Hyman PL, Luther SA, Forster R, Sedgwick JD, et al. A chemokine-driven positive feedback loop organizes lymphoid follicles. *Nature* (2000) 406(6793):309–14. doi:10.1038/35018581
42. Neyt K, Perros F, GeurtsvanKessel CH, Hammad H, Lambrecht BN. Tertiary lymphoid organs in infection and autoimmunity. *Trends Immunol* (2012) 33(6):297–305. doi:10.1016/j.it.2012.04.006
43. Payne RW. Developments from analysis of variance through to generalized linear models and beyond. *Ann Appl Biol* (2014) 164(1):11–7. doi:10.1111/aab.12091
44. Neyt K, Lambrecht BN. The role of lung dendritic cell subsets in immunity to respiratory viruses. *Immunol Rev* (2013) 255(1):57–67. doi:10.1111/imr.12100
45. Lambrecht BN, Hammad H. Lung dendritic cells in respiratory viral infection and asthma: from protection to immunopathology. *Annu Rev Immunol* (2012) 30:243–70. doi:10.1146/annurev-immunol-020711-075021
46. Plantinga M, Guilliams M, Vanheerswynghels M, Deswarte K, Branco Madeira F, Toussaint W, et al. Conventional and monocyte-derived CD11b+ dendritic cells initiate and maintain T helper 2 cell-mediated immunity to house dust mite allergen. *Immunity* (2013) 38:322–35. doi:10.1016/j.immuni.2012.10.016
47. McDonald KG, McDonough JS, Newberry RD. Adaptive immune responses are dispensable for isolated lymphoid follicle formation: antigen-naive, lymphotoxin-sufficient B lymphocytes drive the formation of mature isolated lymphoid follicles. *J Immunol* (2005) 174(9):5720–8. doi:10.4049/jimmunol.174.9.5720
48. Chen CJ, Kono H, Golenbock D, Reed G, Akira S, Rock KL. Identification of a key pathway required for the sterile inflammatory response triggered by dying cells. *Nat Med* (2007) 13(7):851–6. doi:10.1038/nm1603
49. Willart MA, Deswarte K, Pouliot P, Braun H, Beyaert R, Lambrecht BN, et al. Interleukin-1alpha controls allergic sensitization to inhaled house dust mite via the epithelial release of GM-CSF and IL-33. *J Exp Med* (2012) 209:1505–17. doi:10.1084/jem.20112691
50. McAuley JL, Tate MD, MacKenzie-Kludas CJ, Pinar A, Zeng W, Stutz A, et al. Activation of the NLRP3 inflammasome by IAV virulence protein PB1-F2 contributes to severe pathophysiology and disease. *PLoS Pathog* (2013) 9(5):e1003392. doi:10.1371/journal.ppat.1003392
51. Thomas PG, Dash P, Aldridge JR Jr, Ellebedy AH, Reynolds C, Funk AJ, et al. The intracellular sensor NLRP3 mediates key innate and healing responses to influenza A virus via the regulation of caspase-1. *Immunity* (2009) 30(4):566–75. doi:10.1016/j.immuni.2009.02.006
52. Tschernig T, Pabst R. Bronchus-associated lymphoid tissue (BALT) is not present in the normal adult lung but in different diseases. *Pathobiology* (2000) 68(1):1–8. doi:10.1159/000028109
53. Heier I, Malmstrom K, Sajantila A, Lohi J, Makela M, Jahnsen FL. Characterisation of bronchus-associated lymphoid tissue and antigen-presenting cells in central airway mucosa of children. *Thorax* (2011) 66(2):151–6. doi:10.1136/thx.2010.149591

54. Moyron-Quiroz JE, Rangel-Moreno J, Hartson L, Kusser K, Tighe MP, Klonowski KD, et al. Persistence and responsiveness of immunologic memory in the absence of secondary lymphoid organs. *Immunity* (2006) 25(4):643–54. doi:10.1016/j.immuni.2006.08.022
55. Sato M, Hirayama S, Matsuda Y, Wagnetz D, Hwang DM, Guan Z, et al. Stromal activation and formation of lymphoid-like stroma in chronic lung allograft dysfunction. *Transplantation* (2011) 91(12):1398–405. doi:10.1097/TP.0b013e31821b2f7a
56. Van Pottelberge GR, Bracke KR, Van den Broeck S, Reinartz SM, van Drunen CM, Wouters EF, et al. Plasmacytoid dendritic cells in pulmonary lymphoid follicles of patients with COPD. *Eur Respir J* (2010) 36(4):781–91. doi:10.1183/09031936.00140409
57. Morissette MC, Jobse BN, Thayaparan D, Nikota JK, Shen P, Labiris NR, et al. Persistence of pulmonary tertiary lymphoid tissues and anti-nuclear antibodies following cessation of cigarette smoke exposure. *Respir Res* (2014) 15:49. doi:10.1186/1465-9921-15-49
58. van de Pavert SA, Olivier BJ, Goverse G, Vondenhoff MF, Greuter M, Beke P, et al. Chemokine CXCL13 is essential for lymph node initiation and is induced by retinoic acid and neuronal stimulation. *Nat Immunol* (2009) 10(11):1193–9. doi:10.1038/ni.1789
59. Veiga-Fernandes H, Coles MC, Foster KE, Patel A, Williams A, Natarajan D, et al. Tyrosine kinase receptor RET is a key regulator of Peyer's patch organogenesis. *Nature* (2007) 446(7135):547–51. doi:10.1038/nature05597
60. Osborn L, Hession C, Tizard R, Vassallo C, Luhowskyj S, Chi-Rosso G, et al. Direct expression cloning of vascular cell adhesion molecule 1, a cytokine-induced endothelial protein that binds to lymphocytes. *Cell* (1989) 59(6):1203–11. doi:10.1016/0092-8674(89)90775-7
61. Peters A, Pitcher LA, Sullivan JM, Mitsdoerffer M, Acton SE, Franz B, et al. Th17 cells induce ectopic lymphoid follicles in central nervous system tissue inflammation. *Immunity* (2011) 35(6):986–96. doi:10.1016/j.immuni.2011.10.015
62. Fleige H, Haas JD, Stahl FR, Willenzon S, Prinz I, Forster R. Induction of BALT in the absence of IL-17. *Nat Immunol* (2012) 13(1):1. doi:10.1038/ni.2167
63. Sutton C, Brereton C, Keogh B, Mills KH, Lavelle EC. A crucial role for interleukin (IL)-1 in the induction of IL-17-producing T cells that mediate autoimmune encephalomyelitis. *J Exp Med* (2006) 203(7):1685–91. doi:10.1084/jem.20060285
64. Sutton CE, Lalor SJ, Sweeney CM, Brereton CF, Lavelle EC, Mills KH. Interleukin-1 and IL-23 induce innate IL-17 production from gammadelta T cells, amplifying Th17 responses and autoimmunity. *Immunity* (2009) 31(2):331–41. doi:10.1016/j.immuni.2009.08.001
65. Chung Y, Chang SH, Martinez GJ, Yang XO, Nurieva R, Kang HS, et al. Critical regulation of early Th17 cell differentiation by interleukin-1 signaling. *Immunity* (2009) 30(4):576–87. doi:10.1016/j.immuni.2009.02.007
66. Wilson NJ, Boniface K, Chan JR, McKenzie BS, Blumenschein WM, Mattson JD, et al. Development, cytokine profile and function of human interleukin 17-producing helper T cells. *Nat Immunol* (2007) 8(9):950–7. doi:10.1038/ni1497
67. Ludewig B, Odermatt B, Landmann S, Hengartner H, Zinkernagel RM. Dendritic cells induce autoimmune diabetes and maintain disease via de novo formation of local lymphoid tissue. *J Exp Med* (1998) 188(8):1493–501. doi:10.1084/jem.188.8.1493
68. van Rijt LS, Vos N, Willart M, Muskens F, Tak PP, van der Horst C, et al. Persistent activation of dendritic cells after resolution of allergic airway inflammation breaks tolerance to inhaled allergens in mice. *Am J Respir Crit Care Med* (2011) 184(3):303–11. doi:10.1164/rccm.201101-0019OC
69. Muniz LR, Pacer ME, Lira SA, Furtado GC. A critical role for dendritic cells in the formation of lymphatic vessels within tertiary lymphoid structures. *J Immunol* (2011) 187(2):828–34. doi:10.4049/jimmunol.1004233
70. Nacionales DC, Kelly KM, Lee PY, Zhuang H, Li Y, Weinstein JS, et al. Type I interferon production by tertiary lymphoid tissue developing in response to 2,6,10,14-tetramethyl-pentadecane (pristane). *Am J Pathol* (2006) 168(4):1227–40. doi:10.2353/ajpath.2006.050125
71. Pabst R, Tschernig T. Bronchus-associated lymphoid tissue: an entry site for antigens for successful mucosal vaccinations? *Am J Respir Cell Mol Biol* (2010) 43(2):137–41. doi:10.1165/rcmb.2010-0152RT

7

Stromal Fibroblasts in Tertiary Lymphoid Structures: A Novel Target in Chronic Inflammation

Francesca Barone[1], David H. Gardner[1], Saba Nayar[1], Nathalie Steinthal[1], Christopher D. Buckley[1] and Sanjiv A. Luther[2]*

[1] *Rheumatology Research Group, Institute of Inflammation and Ageing, University of Birmingham, Birmingham, UK,*
[2] *Department of Biochemistry, Center for Immunity and Infection, University of Lausanne, Lausanne, Switzerland*

Correspondence:
Francesca Barone
f.barone@bham.ac.uk

Tertiary lymphoid structures (TLS) are organized aggregates of lymphocytes, myeloid, and stromal cells that provide ectopic hubs for acquired immune responses. TLS share phenotypical and functional features with secondary lymphoid organs (SLO); however, they require persistent inflammatory signals to arise and are often observed at target sites of autoimmune disease, chronic infection, cancer, and organ transplantation. Over the past 10 years, important progress has been made in our understanding of the role of stromal fibroblasts in SLO development, organization, and function. A complex and stereotyped series of events regulate fibroblast differentiation from embryonic life in SLOs to lymphoid organ architecture observed in adults. In contrast, TLS-associated fibroblasts differentiate from postnatal, locally activated mesenchyme, predominantly in settings of inflammation and persistent antigen presentation. Therefore, there are critical differences in the cellular and molecular requirements that regulate SLO versus TLS development that ultimately impact on stromal and hematopoietic cell function. These differences may contribute to the pathogenic nature of TLS in the context of chronic inflammation and malignant transformation and offer a window of opportunity for therapeutic interventions in TLS associated pathologies.

Keywords: tertiary lymphoid structures, chemokines, tumor necrosis factor-alpha, lymphotoxin alpha1, beta2 heterotrimer, fibroblasts

INTRODUCTION

Organs are defined as collection of cells, extracellular structures, and fluids, joined into an operational unit to serve a common function. The anatomy of an organ is designed by its structural elements, or resident stromal cells, which provide shape and compartmentalization to the tissues. Secondary lymphoid organs (SLOs), which include spleen, lymph nodes (LN), and Peyer's patches (PP), largely conform to this. SLOs hold a network of fibroblasts, vessels, and nerves that support a large mobile population of leukocyte and which support immune surveillance and response to noxious agents (1, 2). This elegant organization of SLOs develops in a highly conserved and regulated process that largely occurs, both in mice and humans, in embryonic and early postnatal life (3, 4). SLOs evolved simultaneously with the development of an adaptive immune system in vertebrates, with hundreds of LN being distributed at strategic sites, thereby providing a platform for immune cell clustering at well-defined areas. This enables rapid and more efficient adaptive immune responses that outpace pathogen replication, spread, and pathology (5).

Well-developed tertiary or ectopic lymphoid structures (TLS or ELS) resemble SLOs anatomically, as complex aggregates of leukocytes and specialized stromal cells. However, TLS are not capsulated and lack an independent vascular network. TLS form within non-lymphoid tissue in response to specific pathogenic events (6–8) and are commonly found, in adult life, at sites of chronic inflammation and cancer (9–12). It is likely that the capacity to form TLS preceded the development of SLO during evolution, as a tool to accumulate innate immune cells at sites of inflammation in non-vertebrates and lower vertebrates, such as birds, amphibians, and reptiles (13, 14).

Mucosa-associated lymphoid tissues (MALT), such as cryptopatches (CP), fat-associated lymphoid clusters (FALC), and induced nasopharynx-associated lymphoid tissue (iNALT), may be placed, both anatomically and developmentally, between SLOs and TLSs. These are pre-programed in time and space, developing either pre- or postnatally at predetermined sites but are able to expand and accommodate specialized immune responses if required. In CPs, their development into IgA plasma cell-rich isolated lymphoid follicles (ILF) is a classic example of this phenomenon (5). Interestingly, ILF are reversible structures, as indicated by their disaggregation upon antibiotic treatment (15, 16). Similarly, TLS are considered reversible once the antigen source and inflammatory signals are cleared, as will be discussed later.

TLS anatomy is plastic and highly variable, as is its cellular composition. While a certain degree of T/B cell segregation, vascular specialization, and lymphoid tissue chemokine expression is often observed, the level of organization and formation of germinal centers (GC) is dependent on the context, stage, and site of the immune response. Unraveling the mechanisms responsible for the differential maturation of the stromal and leukocyte compartments in TLS and the functional differences between SLO and TLS has provided key information on the biology, clinical relevance, and role of those structures as potential therapeutic targets. In this review, we discuss in detail the contribution of stromal cells, most notably fibroblasts, to both SLO and TLS development and function, and the potential to target therapeutically this specific cell type.

In a "resting state," all organs of the body contain fibroblasts that provide structure and mechanical strength to the tissue. Fibroblast phenotype and function greatly differ between various anatomical sites, as shown by the extensive transcriptional differences detected in fibroblasts isolated from different compartments in diverse locations of the body (17). This specialization is further enhanced by the specific ability of fibroblasts to respond to a series of cytokines and inflammatory stimuli, which increase their proliferative capacity and induce functional adaptations to the environment (18–22). This review will focus on a subset of fibroblasts defined as "lymphoid tissue fibroblasts," which inhabit SLOs and TLS, are characterized by extensive plasticity and specialized functions, and have recently emerged as important regulators of adaptive immunity (8, 23–25).

LYMPHOID STROMAL CELL DIFFERENTIATION IN SLOs AND TLS

In order to understand the TLS development, it is useful to review the development of LN and PP, which is initiated in the sterile environment of the embryo, at approximately E11 and E15, respectively. The locations at which LN develop are predetermined, at least in part, by endothelial expression of the lymphotoxin β receptor (LTβR) (26). Activation of the LTβR signaling pathway enables the clustering of $CD45^{+}CD4^{+}CD3^{-}$ hematopoietic lymphoid tissue inducer (LTi), also known as type 3 innate lymphoid cells (ILC3) expressing LTα1β2, TRANCE, and RORγt (3, 4).

The origin and identity of the signals that induce specification of the mesenchymal progenitor cells prior to LTi arrival remain largely unknown. It is clear that a close anatomical and functional connection between immune cells, mesenchyme, and vascular structures is critical for the establishment of the anlage. At around E13.5, it is possible to identify the nascent LN anlage as small clusters of endothelial cells expressing both podoplanin (gp38) and ICAM-1. The anlage are surrounded by a layer of mesenchymal cells expressing PDGFRα, fibronectin, and ER-TR7 and is separated from the outer layers of fibroblastic cells by a thin $Perlecan^{+}$ basement membrane (27, 28). The early differentiation of the mesenchyme and the initial upregulation of ICAM-1 and VCAM-1, CXCL13 and IL-7, occurs at this stage in the absence of LTα1β2 or LTi cells and is thought to be regulated by retinoic acid signals released by neurons and/or ILC3 (29, 30). Nonetheless, LTα1β2 is required for the further upregulation of adhesion molecules and of lymphoid chemokines. LTα1β2 binds specifically to LTβR and activates the alternative pathway of the NF-κB cascade, while TNFα and LTα3 have TNFR1 and TNFR2 as main receptors and activate the canonical NF-κB pathway (1, 3). The combined activation of TNFR1- and LTβR-signaling pathways not only leads to the activation of both the classical and alternative NF-κB pathways, which act in synergy but also shows complex cross-regulation. In addition, LTβR can be also activated by LIGHT (31). LTβ-receptor regulates in fibroblasts and endothelial cells the expression of various chemokines (CCL19/21, CXCL13) and survival factors (BAFF), while TNF receptor is required for the production of adhesion molecules, such as VCAM-1, ICAM-1, and MAdCAM (32–35). The activation of the alternative pathway, demonstrated by the expression of NIK and the transcription factor RelB, is a specific requirement for the activated mesenchyme to mature in a lymphoid tissue organizer cell (LTo) (1–3). Mature LTo specification facilitates, in turn, further attraction and retention of more LTi cells through the binding of CXCR5, CCR7, α4β1, α4β7, and LTα1β2 with their respective ligands (2, 3). These later steps coincide with the ingrowth of the mesenchymal layer into the endothelial bud (27, 28, 36, 37). The physical interaction between hematopoietic LTi and stromal LTo cells establishes a positive feedback loop that reinforces the formation of the cluster and leads to the stabilization of the anlagen with vascular differentiation, development of high endothelial venules (HEVs), and eventually attraction and compartmentalization of mature lymphoid and myeloid cells (2–4).

Utilizing a CCL19-Cre dependent LTβR ablation (*Ccl19-Cre* × *Ltbr*$^{fl/fl}$ mice), Ludewig and colleagues have recently shown that $CCL19^{+}$ myofibroblastic stromal cell precursor cells can develop the basic LN infrastructure even in absence of LTβR triggering (38). Nonetheless, fibroblastic LTo cells require LTβR signaling to reach full maturation and immunological competence that includes strong expression of ICAM-1, VCAM-1, CCL19, CCL21, IL-7, and RANKL (28, 38, 39). Of note, LTo responsible for the aggregation of different lymphoid tissues are not uniform. This is suggested by the observation that embryonic LTo cells in PP, mesenteric, and peripheral LN display transcriptional differences as well as differential cellular and molecular requirements (40, 41).

Interestingly, LN development is associated with but not fully dependent on a functional lymphatic vasculature network. As a consequence, embryos lacking the major transcriptional regulator for lymphatic cell development, Prox1, either due to full or conditional *Prox1* deletion, fail to form mature LN. Both mutants develop hypoplastic LN anlagen containing small LTi clusters in areas of activated mesenchyme (42). Similarly, Clec-2 knockout mice, which exhibit a defect in lymphatic endothelial cell proliferation late in embryogenesis, form hypoplastic LNs with a mixture of blood and lymphatic flow and reduced LTi and LTo numbers (43).

Evolutionarily more ancient than LNs is the spleen that, together with gut-associated lymphoid tissue (GALT), represents the oldest SLO. The spleen is present in bony fish, amphibians, and reptiles, although in a less complex organization than that observed in mammals (14, 44). The development of the splenic white pulp cords that starts at birth in mice (45–48) and after 15 weeks of gestation in humans (49) does not require LTi cells or LTα1β2 (14, 44, 50, 51). However, as observed in the LN, stromal cell maturation, chemokine expression, and lymphocyte compartmentalization still require LTα1β2 and TNFα (1, 3, 52–56). Those ligands are likely to be provided by B cells and, as a consequence, B cell-deficient mice display smaller spleens, with poorly developed T zones (47). In conclusion, spleen and LN development depend on different types of inducer cells but show a similar hematopoietic–mesenchymal cell interaction, which eventually leads to a similar pathway of fibroblast maturation and lymphoid tissue compartmentalization.

Lymph nodes and PP anlagen formation in the embryo resemble a "sterile inflammation" (5, 13) aimed at forming organs before and independently from the encounter of danger signals. Thereby, these organs collate in a single, highly organized space antigen-presenting cells, naïve lymphocytes, and stromal cells that enable the rapid generation of adaptive immune responses against pathogens.

Tertiary lymphoid structures formation in the adult shares many similarities with SLO development; however, the order of events and molecular mechanisms responsible for TLS development are significantly different from those regulating LN development and partially different from those of the spleen. First, TLS form in the presence of lymphocytes that are absent during embryonic SLO formation. Second, TLS do not develop as separate encapsulated organs but arise as part of highly inflamed tissues, in response to a requirement for lymphocytes to cluster, survive, and generate local, efficient antigen-driven responses. Activation of the resident vascular structures including the upregulation of homing molecules to enable lymphocyte recruitment is therefore a prerequisite of TLS assembly (7, 8). However, while influenced by increased recruitment and defective lymphatic drainage of leukocytes, TLS formation is not simply determined by retention of activated cells in the tissue (57).

Modification of tissue-resident stromal cells into functional lymphoid tissue-like fibroblasts represents another hallmark feature of TLS, specifically, the ectopic and largely segregated expression of chemokines, such as CXCL13, CCL21, CCL19, and CXCL12, and of lymphocyte survival factors, such as IL-7, BAFF, and APRIL (7, 8). Once fully matured, TLS can display a specialized network of follicular dendritic cells (FDCs) capable of driving a functional GC response, and HEVs, differentiated from perivenular capillaries (57). Local upregulation of PNAd, MAdCAM, ICAM-1, and CCL21, first on flat, and later on high endothelial cells, enables the recirculation through the inflamed tissue of naïve T and B lymphocytes, previously excluded by the absence of cognate ligands for CCR7 and L-selectin (8, 57–59).

As opposed to SLO that arise on the backbone of a poorly differentiated mesenchyme, TLS form within organs whose mesenchyme is postnatal and specialized to support local anatomical and functional requirements (8). Accordingly, TLS assembly relies on a larger variety of mesenchymal organizer cells, hematopoietic inducer cells, and cytokines (6–8, 60). TLS preferentially arise in close proximity to vascular or epithelial ductal structures adjacent to pericytes, smooth muscle cells, or myofibroblast-like cells that share many functional and phenotypic features of LTo cells. For example, leukocyte aggregates in the synovium of patients with rheumatoid arthritis (RA) form in close proximity to networks of αSMA^+ fibroblastic cells (61), and $LT\beta R^+$ aortic smooth muscle cells have been observed in vascular TLS that form in murine models of atherosclerosis (62). Focal lymphocytic aggregations that define Sjogren's syndrome (SS) assume a classical periductal structure in close contact to a layer of $gp38^+$ myofibroblastic or pericytic cells that define the ductal basal membrane (63). Similarly, fibroblastic reticular stromal cells that share LTo and lymphoid tissue features have been identified in several murine and human TLS, including SS, primary biliary cirrhosis, insulitis, RA, and lungs infected by *Pseudomonas aeruginosa* (**Table 1**). More recently, a marked increase in the frequency of $PDGFR\alpha^+PDGFR\beta^+$Cadherin-$11^+$ICAM-$1^+$ fibroblasts has also been identified within cerebral lesions of mice that develop experimental autoimmune encephalomyelitis (EAE) (64). Recently, endothelial cells and perivascular fibroblasts of the brain were shown to nucleate local $CD8^+$T cell responses to a neurotropic virus by expressing CCR7 ligands (65). As TLS-associated LTo-like cells are considered resident and long-lived, in comparison to the circulating and short-lived hematopoietic cells, they may hold the key to the reversibility of TLS assembly, providing an interesting therapeutic target for this process.

PRIMING OF FIBROBLASTIC STROMAL CELLS AT SITES OF INFLAMMATION

The cellular and molecular requirement for mesenchymal cell priming, leading to cell differentiation and specialization during TLS establishment, is debated. Transgenic expression of lymphoid tissue chemokines such as CCL21 and CXCL13 overcomes the requirement for LTi cells, but not of LTα1β2 in non–spontaneous models of TLS that form in the eye, thyroid, and pancreas (95–98). The absence of LTi cells, in a CXCL13 transgenic model, leads to the development of smaller and less organized infiltrates suggesting a specific role for those cells in developing larger and more complex infiltrates (63). However, because the aggregates in these

TABLE 1 | Markers associated with fibroblasts found in tertiary lymphoid structures observed in disease settings in mice and human.

Disease	Mouse	Human	Reference
Sjögren's syndrome (salivary glands and lacrimal glands) 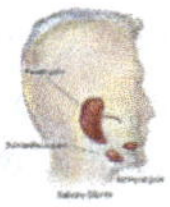	Podoplanin/gp38, CD21, CXCL13, CCL21, VCAM-1, ICAM-1, ER-TR7, FAP	Podoplanin/gp38, CD21, Collagen I, Laminin, CXCL13, CCL21, CXCL12, BAFF, VCAM-1, ICAM-1, ER-TR7, FAP	(63, 66–69)
Primary biliary cirrhosis, primary sclerosis cholangitis (liver) 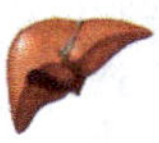	n.d.	Podoplanin/gp38, CD21, Collagen I, Laminin, CCL21, MadCAM-1	(63, 70, 71)
Rheumatoid arthritis (joints) 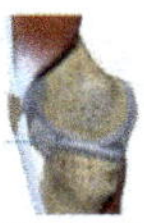	Podoplanin/gp38, VCAM-1, CXCL13, CCL21, FAP, Thy1.1, Cadherin-11	Podoplanin/gp38, VCAM-1, FAP, CD21, CXCL13, CCL21, RANKL	(61, 63, 72–75)
Atherosclerosis (arteries) 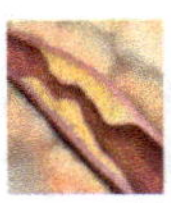	Podoplanin/gp38, VCAM-1, ER-TR7, LTβR, αSMA, CD35, CXCL13, CCL21	n.d.	(76–79)
Autoimmune encephalitis/ multiple sclerosis (central nervous system) 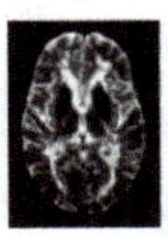	Podoplanin/gp38, PDGFRα, PDGFRβ, VCAM-1, ICAM-1, ER-TR7, Fibronectin, Thy1.1, Cadherin-11	CXCL13, BAFF	(64, 80)
Inflammatory bowel diseases (colon and small intestine) 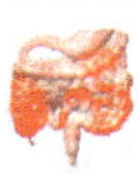	VCAM-1, ICAM-1, CXCL13, CCL21, CXCL12, CD21/35, Podoplanin/gp38, ER-TR7	Podoplanin/gp38, CXCL13, αSMA, FAP, CD21	(81–85)
Mucosal-associated lymphoid tissue (MALT) lymphoma 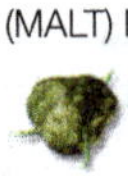	n.d.	Podoplanin/gp38, CXCL13, CCL21, CXCL12	(67, 86)
Helicobacter pylori gastritis (stomach) 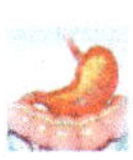	FDC-M1	CD21, CXCL13, CCL21	(86–88)
Inducible bronchus-associated lymphoid tissue (iBALT) (lungs) 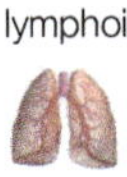	CD21/35, FDC-M1, CXCL13, CXCL12, CCL21, CCL19, CD90, Podoplanin/gp38	CD21, CXCL13, CCL21, CCL19, αSMA	(89–92)
Diabetes (pancreas) 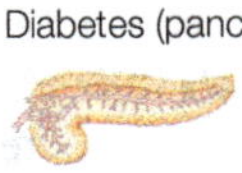	Podoplanin/gp38, FDC-M1, CXCL13, CCL19, CCL21, CXCL12, BAFF	n.d.	(63, 93, 94)

models develop perinatally and in the absence of inflammation, this model cannot be considered a classical model of TLS, and conclusions on its elements should be carefully drawn.

The hierarchy of requirement of TNF family members in physiological lymphoneogenesis is clear, with $LT\alpha^{-/-}$ mice lacking both LTα3 and LTα1β2 expression showing the most severe phenotype, characterized by lack of all LNs and PPs, and a disorganized splenic white pulps (99, 100). In contrast, $LT\beta^{-/-}$ mice, which specifically lack LTα1β2 function, retain MLNs and cervical LNs, and their splenic defects are less pronounced than those of $LT\alpha^{-/-}$ mice (101, 102). A similar phenotype is observed in pregnant mice treated with LTβR–Ig fusion protein, whose progeny lack most PLNs and PP but retain MLNs (103–105). Ruddle and her group have clearly shown that ectopic expression of either TNFα, LTα, or LTα1β2 regulates the assembly of organized TLS, with the formation of MAdCAM+ (in LTα transgenic) and PNAd+ HEV (in LTα1β2 transgenic mice) and a complex network of lymphoid tissue chemokine expression (58, 106). In general, the combined expression of both LTα and β goes along with the formation of better organized lymphoid structures (58).

In spontaneous models of TLS formation, LTα1β2 is not absolutely required to prime the stromal cell compartment. Accordingly, the upregulation of adhesion molecules and the transient expression of lymphoid chemokines can occur in the absence of LTα1β2, or LTi and lymphocytes. Peduto and colleagues first demonstrated that a population of αSMA+ podoplanin+ fibroblasts, which express lymphoid chemokines and survival factors, classically associated with lymphoid stroma in SLOs, can differentiate in non-lymphoid tissue during inflammation and cancer. This phenomenon occurs prior to lymphocyte infiltration in the tissue and is conserved in RORγ-deficient mice (27). Other leukocytes, which are more abundant in the earliest phases of inflammation, such as myeloid cells or granulocytes, might therefore assume a "initiator role" in the formation of TLS by releasing proinflammatory cytokines capable of inducing activation of resident fibroblasts (27, 69, 107–109).

Since, by definition, TLS arise at sites of inflammation, it is virtually impossible to exclude the contribution of one or more of the TNF family members to the early phases of TLS formation. Engagement of TNFR on inflammatory or lymphoid tissue fibroblasts is known to upregulate chemokines, cytokines (including BAFF and IL-6), and adhesion molecules that largely define a primed stroma (110, 111). Moreover, TNF is known to upregulate the receptors for some of the inflammatory cytokines proposed to be involved in TLS establishment (112, 113). One may therefore put forward the hypothesis that the engagement of TNF is key prior to, or synergistically, with the expression of other proinflammatory cytokines to drive the initial priming of resident fibroblasts into functional LTo cells.

Other members of the TNF family have been implicated in lymphoneogenesis. Transgenic expression of LIGHT has been shown to induce TLS formation in models of melanoma and fibrosarcoma (114, 115) and to exacerbate disease in NOD mice (93). Overexpression of RANKL can also support the establishment of lymphoid tissue characterized by stromal cell production of lymphoid chemokines and lymphocyte recruitment (116–118). However, the mechanism by which RANKL regulates TLS assembly is not clear.

Besides TNF and LT family members, the types of cytokines involved in the first phase of stromal cell priming in TLS vary according to the tissues and types of responses (**Figure 1**). IL-6 has been associated with the perivascular accumulation of B cells and mature plasma cells (119). In a model of subcutaneous tumor apoptosis, TGF-β has been demonstrated to induce CXCL13 expression (120), while IL-5 expression has been associated with iBALT development and lung disease (121). IL-4 and IL-13 are known to stimulate, to different extents, the upregulation of adhesion molecules and transient chemokine expression on fibroblasts (122). Finally, IL-4, IL-7, and to a lesser extent IL-15, are known to stimulate expression of LTα1β2 on naïve T lymphocytes that might lead to TLS formation [reviewed in Ref. (95, 123)].

A separate case needs to be made for cytokines belonging to the IL-23 family. IL-17 production by γδ T cells has been demonstrated to provide the trigger for priming of lung fibroblasts in iBALT (92). During EAE, the development of a PDGFRα+PDGFRβ+ podoplanin+CD31− stromal cell network has been shown to be dependent on both IL-17 and IL-22 (64). Within murine salivary glands IL-22, but not IL-17, was deemed a key requirement for stromal cell activation in TLS that form (69). IL-23 expression has been associated with TLS formation in a model of arthritis (124), and the transfer of Th17 cells is sufficient to induce TLS during central nervous system tissue inflammation (109). Interestingly, the production of these cytokines and their relative source appears to be linked to the presence of the transcription factor RORγ that is also required for development and function of ILC3, γδ T cells, and Th17 cells (125–130). Several factors, like IL-23, may act upstream of RORγ, with IL-17 being downstream (131), thus increasing the level of complexity of this system. In some settings, RORγ is deemed dispensable, such as in virus-induced salivary gland infection, where TLS formation and autoantibody generation strongly depend on IL-22 but not IL-17 or RORγ (69). In a model of airway damage and inflammation, it has been shown that IL-17A might regulate both the expression and the proinflammatory properties of IL-22 (132), thus suggesting the possibility that several cytokines can initiate TLS establishment and their relative contribution is likely to be influenced by the site of inflammation and etiological agent.

To date, only one cytokine, IL-27, has been identified that directly inhibits TLS development by negatively regulating the differentiation of Th17 cells, a major driver of TLS development and RA pathogenesis (133).

In summary, multiple pathways and several cell types can act as initiators of TLS assembly and induce activation or priming of the resident fibroblasts in a way that leads to a lymphocyte permissive tissue state (**Figure 1**). The capacity of leukocytes, other than T and B cells, to provide cytokines for stromal cell activation demonstrates a critical uncoupling between stromal cell priming and lymphocyte accumulation in TLS, establishing a model whereby stromal cell priming might occur prior and largely independently from a significant lymphocyte migration into the tissue.

MATURATION AND STABILIZATION OF FIBROBLASTIC STROMAL CELLS ALLOWING TLS FORMATION

Transient activation of stromal cells that often occurs in acute phases of inflammation is not sufficient to support complete lymphoid-like fibroblast maturation associated with TLS formation. Upon resolution of inflammation, the "primed state" of fibroblasts is likely to be lost; alternatively, these activated cells may disappear. Only selected circumstances, such as antigen persistence or severity and length of the inflammatory response, may drive the development of lymphoid tissue-like mesenchyme. Part of this complex phenomenon is also reliant on the dramatic changes that both stromal cells and leukocytes induce in the lymphatic and blood vasculature and that

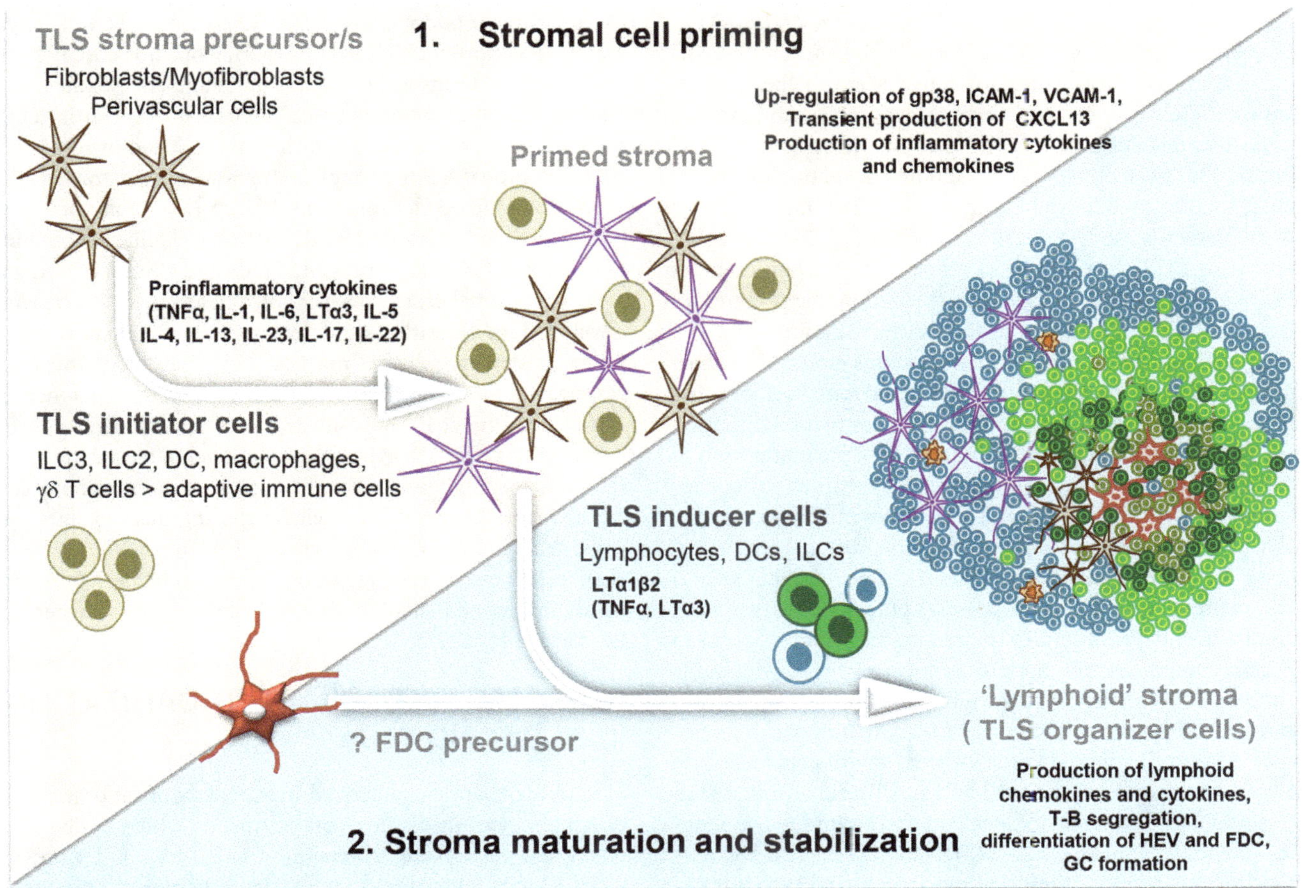

FIGURE 1 | Development and maturation of lymphoid tissue-like stromal fibroblasts in tertiary lymphoid structure (TLS). Multistep model illustrating the priming followed by the stabilization and maturation of the fibroblasts allowing a lymphoid tissue-like organization and function of the lymphocyte infiltrate. Acute inflammation within a tissue results in the localized production of several different proinflammatory cytokines by infiltrating leukocyte populations (initiators) and tissue-resident cells. These signals elicit "priming" of local stromal fibroblasts, which may include the upregulation of gp38, adhesion molecules, and inflammatory cytokines. Prolonged inflammation can lead to local production of LTα1β2, along with TNFα and LTα by hematopoietic inducer cells. This triggers changes in the stromal fibroblast phenotype and function, including the production of chemokines typically expressed in lymphoid organs. FDC differentiation from local fibroblasts might only occur at this stage, when a critical mass of LTα3/LTα1β2/TNFα signals are provided by the co-localizing B cells, possibly inducing a positive feedback loop. Organization of the resident stroma and hematopoietic cells in a T cell (blue cells) and B cell (green cells) rich zone enables priming and activation of T and B cells toward locally displayed antigens. The formation of GC supports affinity maturation and expansion of B cells clones and plasma cells. Not Illustrated: the presence and differentiation of the vascular network [reviewed in Ref. (57)].

occurs as an integral part TLS development (57, 134). In this context, the ability of TLS-associated fibroblasts to secrete pro-angiogenic factors, including VEGF-C and VEGF-D, should also be highlighted (27).

Interestingly, this two-step process of mesenchymal cell priming and maturation is reminiscent of the early phases in the process of lymphoid neogenesis, whereby the early production of CXCL13 and the upregulation of ICAM-1 and VCAM-1 on local mesenchymal cells occur independently of lymphotoxin and LTi. In SLOs, this first phase is followed by the LTα1β2-dependent interaction of LTi cells with the primed mesenchymal cells leading to their specialization as LTo cells capable of inducing HEV development, lymphocyte recruitment, and stromal cell specialization in various subsets (28, 29, 135). Interestingly, in SLOs, the resident mesenchyme is unable to maintain the durable production of survival factors and chemokines if TNFR or LTβR engagement is missing and only a few disorganized LN form in $LT\alpha^{-/-}$ or $LT\beta R^{-/-}$ mice (38, 50). Accordingly, the prolonged treatment of adult wild-type mice with LTβR-Fc leads to dedifferentiation of FDC, HEV, and partially fibroblastic reticular cells (FRC), and as a consequence to reduced lymphocyte recruitment, retention, and compartmentalization (136).

Similarly, in TLS, full differentiation of the lymphoid tissue-like fibroblasts also requires the presence of lymphocytes and LTβR signaling. TLS can form in $LT\alpha^{-/-}$ mice but display a disorganized pattern of lymphocyte aggregation, in absence of clear B/T cell segregation or HEV differentiation (90). LTβR-Fc treatment of established TLS leads to the same outcome, suggesting a continuous need for these signals in order to maintain differentiated HEV and chemokine-expressing fibroblast networks (95, 137, 138). Continuous LTβR and TNFR1 signaling is also required for sustained expression of VCAM-1, CXCL13, and CCL21 in TLS that form in the aorta and in the brain (64, 76, 77). This finding is reminiscent of the requirement for LTα2β1 in order to maintain normal numbers and compartmentalization of lymphocytes in the spleen, PP, and ILFs (47, 53, 137, 139, 140). The combined activation of TNFRI and LTβR is required for the formation of TLS in both inducible and spontaneous models of atherosclerosis (76, 77). However, blockade of LTβR is sufficient to reduce insulitis and diabetes (138) in a NOD mouse model characterized by the presence of podoplanin$^+$ FRC networks and HEV differentiation (63).

All together, these data are consistent with a model of TLS formation in which there is an initial phase of stromal cell priming that occurs independently of LT and precedes tissue infiltration by adaptive immune cells. In the second step, the maturation of resident fibroblasts to a full LTo phenotype appears to be dependent in most settings on LT and TNF, presumably needed to enable dual activation of the NF-κB cascade, with the alternative pathway being maintained over time. Of note, continuous and strong expression of TNF and possibly other NF-kB activating cytokines may bypass this LTα1β2 requirement and still lead to TLS development, though the precise mechanism by which this phenomenon occurs has not been fully clarified. In the context of ectopic lymphoneogenesis, one may therefore propose an extension of the term "lymphoid tissue inducer" to different leukocyte cell types that express sufficient levels of LTα1β2 to induce full differentiation of resident mesenchymal cells into a lymphoid tissue phenotype (96, 108, 141–145). Naïve B cells and DC may qualify for this term, as these cell types on a wild type but not on a LT-deficient background can induce formation of lymphoid tissue structures *in vivo* (47, 146). Evidence is less strong for a LTi like role for T cells although they can express LTα1β2 upon cytokine exposure or activation (147).

Downstream the activation of LTβ receptor is the production of lymphoid tissue chemokines, critically required for lymphocyte recruitment and TLS development. Accordingly, ectopic CCL19 expression under the rat-insulin promoter alone is able to form small infiltrates rich in T cells and dendritic cells; while ectopic CCL21 expression is able to induce the formation of large and better organized infiltrates, characterized by the specific development of T and B zone stroma and HEV differentiation. Similarly, ectopic CXCL13 expression is known to regulate lymphoid tissue neogenesis with T and B cell segregation and complete specialization of the stromal compartment, including FDCs and HEVs (63, 137). These findings in TLS formation are in keeping with the critical role played by CXCL13 and CCL21 in lymphoid organ development during embryogenesis (95).

Interestingly, different functional phenotypes, in terms of chemokine expression, have been observed in fibroblasts isolated from different anatomical sites. In the skin, podoplanin$^+$ inflamed fibroblasts express modest levels of IL-7 and CXCL13, but high quantities of CXCL12 and VEGF-C (27). In contrast, podoplanin$^+$ cells isolated from gut and tumors significantly upregulate the lymphoid chemokines CXCL13, CCL19, CXCL12, and various cytokines, including VEGF-C, connective tissue growth factors, including fibroblast growth factors (27). Stromal cells isolated from iBALT are characterized by CXCL12 expression (92), while the network of podoplanin$^+$ CD31$^-$ cells isolated from salivary gland TLS express CXCL13 and CCL19 but not CXCL12 (69). Differences in terms of TLS organization and chemokine expression can also be observed at different sites or even in TLS at the same anatomical site when they are induced in response to different antigens. For example, intranasal administration of the poxvirus modified vaccinia virus Ankara (MVA) in mice is able to induce highly organized iBALT with B cell follicles containing a network of CXCL13-expressing FDCs and CXCL12-producing follicular stromal cells. However, mice treated with *P. aeruginosa* developed iBALT with B cell follicles that consisted of CXCL12$^+$ follicular stromal cells but not CXCL13$^+$ FDC (92). The signals responsible for these phenotypic and functional differences are unclear and most likely result from an integrated response to different anatomical environments, antigenic stimulations, and inflammatory milieus. While this review focuses on fibroblasts, the ability of hematopoietic cells, including macrophages, dendritic cells, and Th17 cells, to ectopically express CXCL13 should also be acknowledged, suggesting the possibility to consider the cytokine/chemokine, rather than its cellular origin as a therapeutic target (148–152).

STROMAL FIBROBLAST ORGANIZATION IN SLOs AND TLSs

Mature SLOs are characterized by the anatomical organization of lymphocytes in distinct compartments, which is due to the segregated chemokine expression of CCL19/21 in T zones and CXCL13 in B zones. The source of these chemokines are specialized subsets of resident FRC and FDC, which attract and retain specific leukocyte populations, besides providing survival factors.

Fibroblastic reticular cell subsets, including FDC, are defined by their phenotype, anatomical location, and function (2, 24, 153, 154) (**Figure 2**). T zone FRCs or TRC classically inhabit the T cell cortex in LNs and are characterized by the expression of podoplanin and lack of the vascular marker CD31. TRCs are responsible for the recruitment, retention, and movement of naïve T lymphocytes and DCs *via* their expression of CCL19 and CCL21. Besides regulating immune cell trafficking, TRCs produce extracellular matrix, forming a system of microchannels (conduits) that connect the subcapsular sinus with the paracortex and HEVs. TRCs also provide a significant source of IL-7, which in combination with CCL19, sustains naïve T cell survival within the LN T zone, regulating T cell homeostasis (22, 155).

Fibroblastic reticular cells that inhabit the outer B zone, also termed B cell zone FRCs (BRC), are characterized by high levels of BP-3 and podoplanin expression but lack FDC markers like CD21/35. BRC represent an important source of oxysterol chemoattractants, BAFF, CXCL13, and the Notch ligand DL4 (156–158). Marginal reticular cells (MRCs) represent another B zone FRC population that sits underneath the subcapsular sinus and is characterized by RANKL and CXCL13 expression (35, 159). BRC and possibly MRC form conduit networks able to deliver lymph-drained information, including antigens, from the subcapsular sinus to the B cell area and eventually to the FDCs present within the B cell follicles (2, 153, 156–162). Due to their

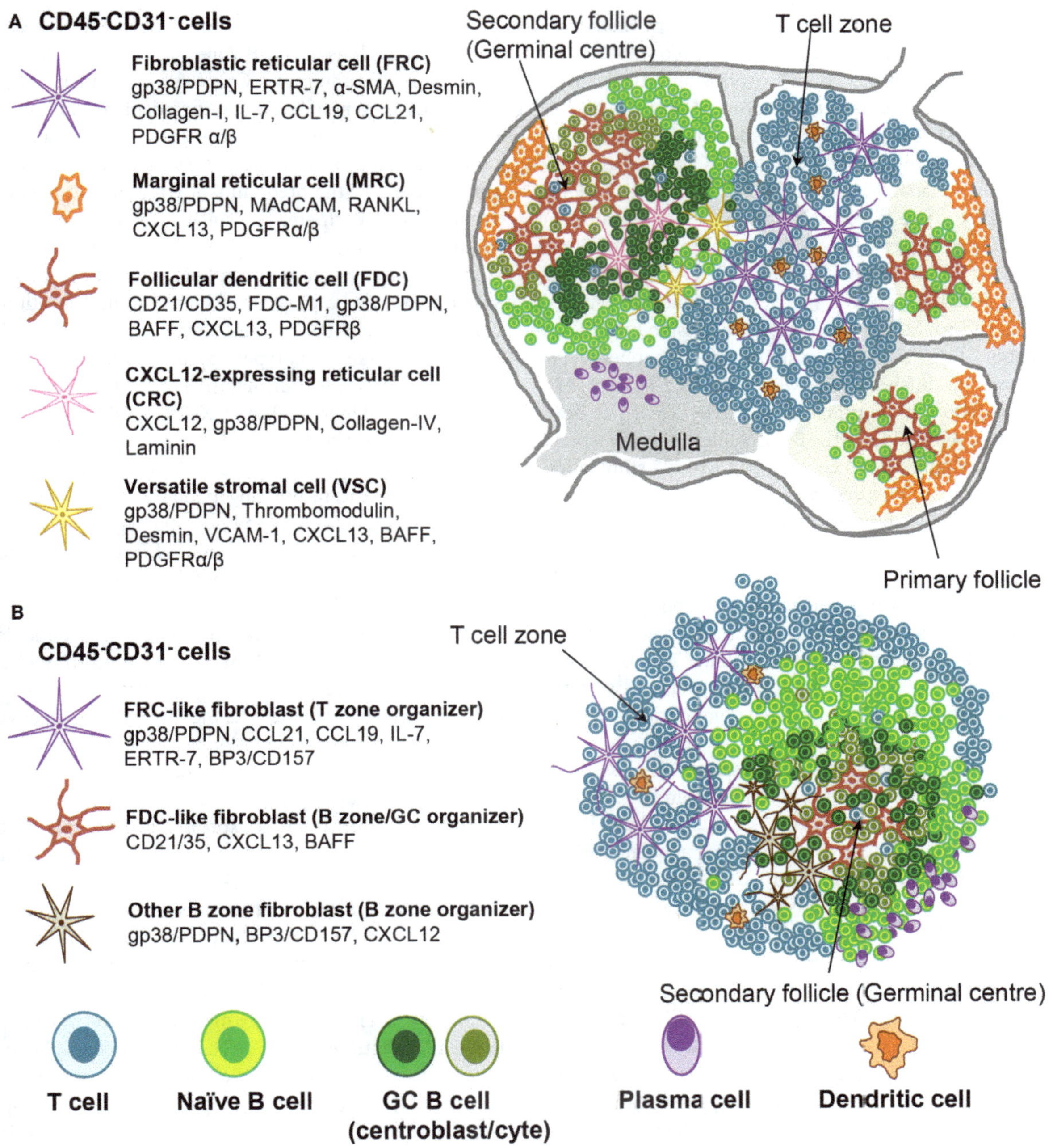

FIGURE 2 | **Stromal fibroblast populations in SLO and TLS. (A)** Fibroblast populations in the lymph node control the organization and survival of lymphocytes in distinct areas. Fibroblastic reticular cells (FRC) produce CCL19 and CCL21 along with the survival factor IL-7 to attract and maintain T cell populations and provide a niche in which their interaction with dendritic cells (DC) can occur. Follicular dendritic cells (FDC) produce CXCL13, which attracts CXCR5+ cells to the B cell follicles. Other stromal cells are thought to play a role during the germinal center reaction (i.e., CRCs) or in antigen delivery (MRC). **(B)** Mature TLS are characterized by segregation into distinct T cell and B cell areas including the presence of germinal center like structures and areas rich in plasma cells. Stromal cell populations that perform comparable functions to those found within SLO can be identified, which underlie this T/B cell segregation within the larger TLS.

phenotypic similarities, MRCs were proposed to represent the adult equivalent of embryonic LTo cells (159). In support of this concept, MRCs were shown to be the precursors of LN FDCs during immune reactions (162).

Follicular dendritic cells are the prominent stromal cell subset found within the central part of primary B cell follicles and localize specifically to the light zone of the GCs in secondary follicles. FDCs are defined by their dendritic appearance and their capacity to retain opsonized antigen *via* Fc and complement receptors. FDCs serve as long-term reservoir of native antigen for the positive selection of affinity matured GC B cells or centrocytes (163). In addition, FDCs are a source of CXCL13 and BAFF, responsible for migration and survival of naïve B cells. TNFR and LTβR signaling are critically required for the maintenance of the

FDC network and in general to support the CXCL13 producing stroma in the follicles (53, 164, 165), as evidenced by their rapid disappearance upon TNFR or LT blockade (45, 166–169).

Recently, a population of CXCL12-expressing reticular cells (CRCs) has been described in the dark zone of the primary follicles and polarized GCs, where they are required for the recruitment of CXCR4$^+$ centroblasts and effective GC responses (170). This subset is fate mapped by both the *Cd21-cre* and *Ccl19-cre* mouse lines with the fate mapping indicating past and/or present expression (171). It lacks most of the classical markers of FDCs [such as CD21/35, VCAM-1, FDC-M2, FDC-M1, M-2, and CD16/32 (FcγRII/III)] or FRCs (such as laminin and type IV collagen association). Moreover, CXCL12 expression on CRCs is independent of LT or TNFα thus establishing critical phenotypic and developmental differences between CRC and FDCs (171). Finally, a population of versatile stromal cells (VSC) has been described at the T zone edges of the B cells follicle, able to respond to inflammatory stimuli, B cell contact, and LTα1β2 stimulation by upregulating CXCL13 expression (172).

Many of the FRC subtypes are fate mapped by the same *Ccl19-Cre* transgenic mouse, suggesting a common precursor in embryonic life for the majority of FRC subsets, at least in the LN (171). In future, mice allowing inducible fate mapping are needed to gather more direct evidence for such a precursor–progeny relationship, both in embryonic and postnatal LN. Currently, very little is known on the specific differentiation and survival signals leading to the complex stromal cell organization observed in adult life.

To study signals regulating FRC function, various FRC lines have been generated from adult murine and human SLO. Murine cell lines constitutively produce CXCL12 and sometimes BAFF but require stimulation of the TNF receptor to upregulate various inflammatory chemokines (e.g., CXCL10, CCL4/5) as well as IL-7 (33, 35). Stimulation of LTβ- or TNF-receptors strongly upregulates matrix production, with the combination of both signals showing synergistic effects. Those signals could be mimicked by CD4$^+$ T cells, physiological neighbors of FRC *in vivo*. Similarly, stimulation of a MAdCAM$^+$ MRC line *via* both LTβ- and TNF-receptors was also able to induce further expression of CXCL13 and CCL19 (33, 35). Interestingly, fluid flow was shown able to induce CCL21 expression in a FRC line (173); while human LN FRC responded to TNFα, IL-6, IL-4, and IL-13 by upregulating various cytokines, adhesion molecules, and metalloproteinases (174). These *in vitro* data support an ability of lymphoid tissue fibroblasts to adopt different functions depending on the signals received from the surrounding environment, and thereby influence neighboring immune or stromal cells.

Our knowledge about stromal fibroblasts within murine and human TLS is still very limited. Current evidence suggests the presence of TRC-like cells within the T cell rich zones, and of FDC-like cells that inhabit B cell rich areas in more organized TLS. MRCs, BRCs, CRCs, or VSCs have not yet been described in TLS. Depending on the size and type of TLS, fibroblasts display a variable degree of the phenotypic and functional features described for their SLO counterparts (**Figure 2**). It is debatable the extent to which TLS stroma reaches a comparable level of polarization and differentiation compared to SLO stroma. The two subsets identified so far in TLS, namely CCL21$^+$ TRC and CXCL13$^+$ FDC, can associate and probably form distinct compartments, such as T and B zones but also allow the formation of functional conduits and GCs (63). These niches appear to be functional in generating a specific adaptive immune response, but it is less clear whether fibroblasts in TLS allow a comparable regulation of immune processes. It is likely that in TLS, similar to SLOs, the predominant lymphocytic population that accumulate in each area imprint locally activated mesenchyme to support an increased requirement for specific survival and chemo-attractive factors. Lymphoid stromal cell differentiation would therefore be programed by anatomical location through contact with neighboring cells. Any polarization toward an FRC-like or FDC-like phenotype may be reenforced as lymphocyte segregation arises within mature TLS by the expression of one or two chemokines, such as CXCL13 and CCL21 (61, 66, 67, 72), thereby restricting stromal cell contact to either T or B cells. It is known that both CXCL13 and CCL21 can induce LTα1β2 expression in the responding lymphocytes, further enhancing chemokine expression by the neighboring fibroblasts (95, 142). The additional factors needed besides LTα1β2 to drive fibroblasts into a differentiation program specific for the B zone or the T zone are currently unknown.

In murine TLS, TRC-like cells expressing podoplanin and other markers (**Figure 2**; **Table 1**) are found throughout T cell rich zones as three-dimensional reticular networks and partly co-localize with dendritic cells thereby forming an environment where cognate T cell stimulation is possible. They associate with matrix fibers that can form functional conduits and connect with HEVs. Often they express CCL21, which is key to the T zone formation. CCL19 and IL-7 expressed by FRC may contribute to local T cell accumulation and possibly to random T cell migration along the TRC network (2, 153, 155, 175).

Follicular dendritic cell networks form only within B zones of large TLSs in mice and are then associated with functional GCs allowing B cell differentiation to affinity matured plasma cells (63, 88, 92, 94, 176, 177). Interestingly, not all tissues, and only a minority of TLSs form fully mature FDC networks, suggesting that while the stimulus for FDC differentiation might be the same as that observed in SLO (TNFα and LT), the threshold required for full FDC differentiation in peripheral tissue is higher. An alternative possibility is that FDC precursors in the periphery are scarce and differentially distributed in different organs. Whether the phenotype, origin, and function of FDCs in peripheral TLSs differ from those of SLO is not known, neither is their differential dependency on LT or LT-inducing pathways. It is important to highlight that even in SLOs, at least two different precursors have been identified for FDCs, which differ between spleen and LNs (162, 178, 179), thus potentially increasing the complexity of signals and progenitors required for FDC differentiation in TLS.

While it is likely that in TLS a single lymphoid tissue-like progenitor gives rise to both FRC and FDC-like cells, it cannot be excluded that FDC might differentiate from FRC-like cells or another precursor later in TLS development. Interestingly, the absence of MRC-like cells and the lack of any anatomical capsule within the TLS appears to exclude the involvement of an "MRC-like progenitor" in FDC differentiation in TLS. Data obtained from parabiosis experiments and fate mapping experiments by Peduto and colleagues suggest that local, rather than circulating, precursors are responsible for the expansion of the stromal network responsible for TLS establishment (27). Proliferation of the resident stroma has been also observed in an inducible model of TLS, both in the vascular and stromal compartments (134) (Nayar et al., manuscript in preparation), which mimics the expansion of the stromal compartment during immunization in SLOs (22, 180–182). Therefore, the most likely scenario is that local differentiation and expansion of tissue-resident mesenchymal cell/s accounts for TLS development.

Even less is known about fibroblasts found in TLS within human pathology, in part due to the lack of markers identifying fibroblasts and distinguishing different cell subsets. Most efforts have concentrated on reporting the presence or absence of CD21$^+$ FDCs or lymphoid tissue chemokines, such as CXCL13, CCL21, CCL19, and CXCL12 (7, 8, 183). Discrete expression of CXCL13, CXCL12, and CCL21 has been described in salivary glands of patients with SS, RA, multiple sclerosis, primary sclerosing cholangitis, atherosclerosis, inflammatory bowel disease, chronic lung diseases, *Helicobacter pylori*-induced gastritis, and lymphoma [reviewed in Ref. (7)]. However, this classical work largely preceded the phenotypic characterization of fibroblast subsets in mice and therefore lacks in-depth characterization of the stromal cell compartment. Nonetheless, the association between the level of organization of TLS with lymphoid chemokine expression (7), together with identification of the source of lymphoid chemokines in the αSMA$^+$ or desmin$^+$ stromal compartment (63), suggests that TLS fibroblast subsets exist in humans. More recently, our laboratories have demonstrated the presence of podoplanin$^+$ FRC-like cells in tonsil, RA synovium, and SS salivary glands, as based on the expression of podoplanin and CCL21 and the association with T cells, DC, and matrix fibers (63). These FRC-like cells were distinct from the CD21$^+$ FDC that organized B cell rich zones, as described previously by several laboratories and summarized in **Table 1**.

While the use of podoplanin to identify "lymphoid tissue stromal cells" in the periphery remains a reasonable approach, podoplanin expression has also been observed on epithelium, lymphatic vessels, Th17 cells, and myeloid cells (184). Its use therefore requires careful analysis of cell morphology and double labeling with cellular markers (absent on fibroblasts) to validate the specificity of the population of cells detected. In future, it will be important to use further markers to discriminate human fibroblast subsets in TLS, in order to improve stromal cell characterization in human TLS histology samples.

EFFECTOR FUNCTIONS OF TLS

Tertiary lymphoid structures are classically defined as lymphoid aggregates forming in organs whose main function is other than the initiation of an adaptive immune response. TLS appear to form there because of an abundance of antigen, either "self" in autoimmune diseases, "self" or "altered self" in cancer, or foreign antigen/s during infections and transplant rejection. At those ectopic sites, TLS can contribute to the generation of an antigen-specific immune response with plasma cell and antibody generation, often maintained by the persistence of the antigen and/or inflammatory signals (6, 8) The local stromal structures needed for naïve cell recruitment and affinity maturation of the B cell compartment are mainly observed in the most organized TLS (66, 185). Interestingly, TLS do not develop in all forms of chronic inflammation and only arise in certain permissive tissues. A classical association with mucosal epithelium has been observed. However, TLS can form in the synovium, a tissue devoid of epithelial structures (7). The factors involved in tissue permissiveness are not clear, and while it is intuitive to suggest the need for proximity to antigen and antigen presenting cells, this is not sufficient as exemplified by the case of the skin, classically considered a "hostile site" for TLS formation.

Aggregation of lymphocytes in small TLS is commonly observed in transient infections where it is considered a positive development, aimed at containing local infections. The development of lung TLS in response to influenza supports the further development of a strong antigen-driven T cell response contributing to viral clearance (186, 187). In these cases, TLS disappear shortly after pathogen clearance leaving the tissue intact (68, 188).

However, in chronic inflammation, the presence of TLS has been associated with poor clinical outcome and disease progression rather than resolution (94, 189). TLS formation correlates with serum autoantibody levels, disease severity, tissue damage, and decreased organ function in several diseases including SS [reviewed in Ref. (7)]. In RA, the formation of subchondral bone TLS supports osteoclast activation and tissue damage (190), and the presence of synovial TLS associates with anti citrullinated antibody production and poor response to anti-TNF antibodies (74, 191). Accordingly, levels of TLS-associated CXCL13 expression correlates with disease severity and persistence of subclinical synovitis (190, 192, 193).

It is arguable that TLS represent a response to and are not *per se* a cause of inflammation. However, a combination of factors, among which excessive cell recruitment, poor lymphatic drainage, disorganized cellular interaction, and excessive survival factors can contribute to TLS persistence in tissue, favoring a pathogenic role in the context of diseases. Interestingly, not all patients with autoimmune disease develop TLS, despite the presence of factors associated with its development, for example, Th17 cells in RA (133). This suggests that the biological relationship between disease progression, clinical features, and TLS formation is more complex. In this context, the detection of GC within salivary glands of patients with SS has been classically associated with increased risk of lymphoma (194), suggesting that chronic antigen stimulation and excess of survival factors might favor the development of malignant B cell clones. However, this proposal is controversial and a strong positive correlation between the two pathogenic entities cannot be identified, leaving the relationship between TLS formation and lymphoma development uncertain (194, 195).

The role of TLS in the context of cancerous growth is also debated. TLS are believed to sustain the antitumor response in solid malignancies that arise in the colon, breast and ovaries as the presence of TLS in the context of cancer has been associated with a favorable prognosis (196). Nonetheless the ability of tumor cells to induce T regulatory cells (T_{reg}) and suppress the host immune response is well known and there is the possibility that cancer cells highjack TLS to exert this immunosuppressive function (197–200).

Classically, the key effector function associated with TLS development has been the formation of GCs and the production of autoantibodies [reviewed in Ref. (7)]. However, more recently a more complex role for TLS in the context of T cell activation and maturation of pathogenic T cell response has been proposed.

While the production of CXCL13 represents a sensitive and powerful readout of stromal cell activation in TLS (69), this is unlikely, in the early phases of TLS establishment, to be restricted to the rather complex events of follicular B cell differentiation, an event that occurs later in TLS (69). It is likely that early CXCL13 production in the context of TLS assembly is aimed at driving the recruitment of $CXCR5^+$ B cells and T follicular helper (T_{fh}) cells (201). Accordingly, interfering with T_{fh} infiltration by ICOS-L blockade results in reduced TLS assembly and progression of vascular disease in a model of TLS associated with atherosclerosis (202). The origin of T_{fh} that arise within TLS is currently not clear. As mentioned, T_{fh} populations have been identified within the circulation in both mice and humans that could be recruited into TLS by newly established CXCL13 gradients (203–205). There is however the possibility that TLS provide a site for local T_{fh} differentiation. In support to this hypothesis, naïve T cell recruitment and priming has been reported within TLS that form in pancreatic tissue in NOD mice (93). However, naïve T cell recruitment requires the upregulation of CCR7 and L-selectin ligands on the vascular endothelium, typically HEVs (59, 206), which is another hallmark of mature TLS. Effector T cells are more likely to be recruited in the earliest phases of TLS assembly, thus suggesting that in TLS, as opposed to SLO, T cell differentiation into T_{fh} might occur from previously activated peripheral T cell populations that already display effector functions. In support of this hypothesis, Th17 cells isolated from TLS of EAE affected mice display features of T_{fh}, including the upregulation of expression of CXCR5, ICOS and Bcl6 (109). Within TLS the activated fibroblast compartment may provide key signals for T cell differentiation, such as IL-6, required for the induction and maintenance of the T_{fh} phenotype (207, 208), thus suggesting an additional role for stromal cells in the context of TLS development.

The presence and function of T_{reg} populations in the context of TLS has been less studied. T_{reg} recruitment into TLS might directly interfere with the activity of TLS associated T_{fh} cells, similarly to what has been described in SLOs (209, 210). Accordingly, in TLS that form in association with atherosclerosis, disruption of $CD8^+$ T_{reg} activity is known to induce an expanded GC B cell response (202). Additionally, in a mouse model of lung adenocarcinoma, T_{reg} that inhabit local TLS, are known to interfere with the antitumor T cell response. In addition to directly inhibiting T cell responses within the TLS, T_{reg} appear to impact upon the recruitment of additional lymphocytes to the TLS by affecting the formation or maintenance of $PNAd^+$ HEVs (211, 212). Interestingly, the tumor microenvironment is conducive to the recruitment, generation, and maintenance of T_{reg} populations (197) and, indeed, T_{reg} infiltration in solid tumors is considered a negative prognostic factor. Whether T_{reg} are less active or abundant in TLS associated with chronic inflammation, as compared to cancer, remains to be answered.

T regulatory and Th17 cell differentiation is promoted by TGF-β; however, Th17 development occurs on a background of proinflammatory cytokines, such IL-6, IL-21, and IL-23 (213–215). It is possible that in TLS that arise in chronic autoimmunity, the inflammatory milieu, partly established by locally activated fibroblasts, positively enforce Th17 over T_{reg} differentiation, favoring the upregulation of the transcription factor RORγ while inhibiting FoxP3 expression (216). Additionally, an environment that is rich in IL-1 and IL-6 and deficient in TGFβ is sufficient to reprogram T_{reg} toward a Th17 phenotype (217, 218), thus suggesting that the inflammatory microenvironment associated with TLS in chronic inflammation may not be able to maintain T_{reg} phenotype cells. Indeed, Th17 differentiation has been observed in RA TLS (133). The differences between diverse T effector populations and the balance between T effector and T_{reg} cells in the different lymphoid niches may therefore explain some of the discrepancies observed between immune responses that occur within TLS associated with cancer and chronic inflammation.

It is not clear to what extent the stromal cell compartment contributes to TLS pathogenicity. In SLOs, FRC are increasingly recognized as active modulators of the immune response. FRCs can interfere with the T cell response through several mechanisms, releasing soluble modulators that negatively regulate T cell proliferation or providing negative co-stimulatory molecules such as PD-L1 (219–221). The ability of FRC to acquire peptide–major histocompatibility (MHC) II complexes from professional antigen presenting cells or to upregulate MHC I and II molecules has also been shown. Moreover, FRC are able to display peripheral tissue antigens mediating the deletion of peripheral autoreactive $CD8^+$ T cells (19, 222, 223) and maintaining the homeostasis of T_{reg} cells (222, 224). Taken together, these studies demonstrate that, while FRCs provide survival niches for lymphocyte homeostasis, they also govern the magnitude of the immune response (19, 221).

The extent to which the regulation of immune responses by stromal cell populations translates from SLOs to TLS has not been explored. Interestingly, fibroblasts isolated from non-inflamed peripheral tissues display a strong propensity to inhibit T cell responses, possibly to protect non-lymphoid tissues from the harmful effects of inflammation (221). In cancer-associated TLS, also characterized by a chronic inflammatory response, stromal fibroblasts are believed to contribute to immune evasion, preventing lymphocyte effector functions and immune cell access to the cancer site (12). However, in contrast with these, most recent findings and the immunosuppressive role described for stromal cells in SLOs and cancer, current evidence strongly suggests a pathogenic role for TLS in autoimmune conditions, sustaining lymphocyte survival and supporting lymphocyte persistence in the tissue (7, 8). The pathogenic, non-immunosuppressive role of lymphoid-like fibroblasts that inhabit TLS found in chronic inflammatory conditions appears therefore unique and requires further characterization. There is the possibility that functional differences exist among fibroblasts that bear a similar phenotype in TLS and SLOs or that functional differences are acquired during disease progression. The different origin of SLO and TLS fibroblasts and the cytokine milieu driving mesenchymal differentiation at ectopic peripheral sites are likely to contribute to this complex phenomenon. A more detailed characterization of the stromal compartment in TLS associated with chronic inflammation in comparison with SLOs might provide key elements to unravel these discrepancies.

STROMAL FIBROBLAST DELETION: A NOVEL STRATEGY TO MANIPULATE THE IMMUNE RESPONSE

Interesting insights into the function of SLO fibroblasts have been derived from cell deletion experiments. Taking advantage of the mouse lines expressing diphtheria toxin receptor (DTR) selectively in fibroblasts by the use of the fibroblast-specific promoters of FAP (fibroblast activation protein α) or CCL19, stromal cell deletion could be obtained in adult LNs. *FAP–DTR* mice treated with DTX showed disrupted LN homeostasis with strongly reduced numbers of T and B lymphocytes and DCs. Upon influenza infection, mice lacking FAP^+ cells mounted a diminished immune response characterized by reduced numbers of GC B cells, plasma B cells, and T_{fh} cells (225). By using a different inducible transgenic model [*Ccl19*-Cre × *Rosa26*-diphtheria toxin receptor (iDTR) mice] Turley, Ludewig, and colleagues demonstrated that selective depletion of FRCs resulted in aberrant localization of T lymphocytes within the LN cortex as well as a reduction in both CD4 and CD8 T cell numbers *via* a mechanism dependent on IL-7. Antigen-specific T cells isolated from these immunized, FRC depleted mice failed to undergo priming and proliferation (157, 226). Humoral responses and B cell homeostasis were also impaired in the absence of FRC, with disorganized B cell accumulation within the GCs and significant reduction of virus-specific antibody production (157). While this defect was largely attributed to the inability of B cells to access homeostatic levels of BAFF once FRC were depleted (157), Acton et al. recently demonstrated that the engagement of CLEC-2 (expressed on DC) by its ligand podoplanin (expressed on FRC) is necessary for DCs to spread, migrate, and provide appropriate Ag presentation to T cells in LNs (227, 228). This suggests that the inability of the DCs to migrate into LNs in FRC-depleted LNs could contribute to the defect in T and B activation observed in this model. It has been reported that ablation of FDC achieved in *Cd21-Cre* × *Rosa26-iDTR* mice results in loss of primary B cell follicles. This effect, partially mediated by BAFF and CXCL13 depletion, is also supported by the decreased levels of IL-6 and integrins present in SLO of transgenic mice treated with DTX (229). All together, these studies indicate that alterations in SLO stromal compartments can alter lymphocyte survival, compartmentalization, and immunological competency, often sequentially linked, which profoundly impact on SLO function.

The impact of stromal cell deletion on TLS has not been addressed as yet and might provide critical clues on the relative immunosuppressive or proinflammatory role of TLS-associated stromal cells, ultimately unveiling whether the role of TLS in different diseases at various anatomic sites is beneficial or detrimental. Whether this approach, using antibody-based therapeutic agents will be feasible in humans is of interest. Deletion of specific subsets of fibroblasts might be problematic due to the anatomical impact related to the apparent overlap of markers between lymphoid stroma in SLOs, TLSs, and non-lymphoid tissues. However, a series of compounds able to interfere with stromal cell activation and functions are available and will present an interesting avenue to target stromal cell activation, alone or in combination with current immunomodulatory agents, such as anti-TNFα, anti-IL-6, anti-CTLA4 and anti-PDL1.

CONCLUSION

The main function of TLS is to maintain lymphocytes populations and provide a level of structural organization that enables the development and regulation of an adaptive immune response within peripheral tissues. This role is largely played by distinct populations of activated mesenchymal cells that acquire features similar to those of the lymphoid fibroblasts that inhabit SLOs. However, fibroblast maturation in TLS is an event, which is highly influenced by the anatomical site, the danger signals, and the inflammatory microenvironment, thus profoundly differing from the stereotypic mesenchyme specification observed during SLO development. Moreover, the organization and size of TLS does not equal that of their highly regulated SLO counterparts. The likely inability to precisely control leukocyte recirculation and cross talk within diseased tissue together with the absence of finely regulated chemokine gradients for lymphocyte positioning and the abundance of lymphocyte survival factors might explain why TLS fail to resolve and thereby contribute to immune-mediated inflammatory disease and its persistence.

AUTHOR CONTRIBUTIONS

All the authors contributed in writing the review.

FUNDING

FB and CB are part of RACE (Arthritis Research UK Rheumatoid Arthritis Pathogenesis Centre of Excellence). RACE was part-funded by Arthritis Research UK (20298); this Centre is a collaboration between the Universities of Glasgow, Newcastle, and Birmingham. FB is an ARUK Senior Fellow.

REFERENCES

1. Mebius RE. Organogenesis of lymphoid tissues. *Nat Rev Immunol* (2003) 3(4):292–303. doi:10.1038/nri1054
2. Roozendaal R, Mebius RE. Stromal cell-immune cell interactions. *Annu Rev Immunol* (2011) 29:23–43. doi:10.1146/annurev-immunol-031210-101357
3. Randall TD, Carragher DM, Rangel-Moreno J. Development of secondary lymphoid organs. *Annu Rev Immunol* (2008) 26:627–50. doi:10.1146/annurev.immunol.26.021607.090257
4. van de Pavert SA, Mebius RE. New insights into the development of lymphoid tissues. *Nat Rev Immunol* (2010) 10(9):664–74. doi:10.1038/nri2832

5. Eberl G. From induced to programmed lymphoid tissues: the long road to preempt pathogens. *Trends Immunol* (2007) 28(10):423–8. doi:10.1016/j.it.2007.07.009
6. Neyt K, Perros F, GeurtsvanKessel CH, Hammad H, Lambrecht BN. Tertiary lymphoid organs in infection and autoimmunity. *Trends Immunol* (2012) 33(6):297–305. doi:10.1016/j.it.2012.04.006
7. Pitzalis C, Jones GW, Bombardieri M, Jones SA. Ectopic lymphoid-like structures in infection, cancer and autoimmunity. *Nat Rev Immunol* (2014) 14(7):447–62. doi:10.1038/nri3700
8. Buckley CD, Barone F, Nayar S, Benezech C, Caamano J. Stromal cells in chronic inflammation and tertiary lymphoid organ formation. *Annu Rev Immunol* (2015) 33:715–45. doi:10.1146/annurev-immunol-032713-120252
9. Noss EH, Brenner MB. The role and therapeutic implications of fibroblast-like synoviocytes in inflammation and cartilage erosion in rheumatoid arthritis. *Immunol Rev* (2008) 223:252–70. doi:10.1111/j.1600-065X.2008.00648.x
10. Dieu-Nosjean MC, Goc J, Giraldo NA, Sautes-Fridman C, Fridman WH. Tertiary lymphoid structures in cancer and beyond. *Trends Immunol* (2014) 35(11):571–80. doi:10.1016/j.it.2014.09.006
11. Ohlund D, Elyada E, Tuveson D. Fibroblast heterogeneity in the cancer wound. *J Exp Med* (2014) 211(8):1503–23. doi:10.1084/jem.20140692
12. Turley SJ, Cremasco V, Astarita JL. Immunological hallmarks of stromal cells in the tumour microenvironment. *Nat Rev Immunol* (2015) 15(11):669–82. doi:10.1038/nri3902
13. Nishikawa SI, Hashi H, Honda K, Fraser S, Yoshida H. Inflammation, a prototype for organogenesis of the lymphopoietic/hematopoietic system. *Curr Opin Immunol* (2000) 12(3):342–5. doi:10.1016/S0952-7915(00)00097-2
14. Boehm T, Hess I, Swann JB. Evolution of lymphoid tissues. *Trends Immunol* (2012) 33(6):315–21. doi:10.1016/j.it.2012.02.005
15. Kweon MN, Yamamoto M, Rennert PD, Park EJ, Lee AY, Chang SY, et al. Prenatal blockage of lymphotoxin beta receptor and TNF receptor p55 signaling cascade resulted in the acceleration of tissue genesis for isolated lymphoid follicles in the large intestine. *J Immunol* (2005) 174(7):4365–72. doi:10.4049/jimmunol.174.7.4365
16. Bouskra D, Brezillon C, Berard M, Werts C, Varona R, Boneca IG, et al. Lymphoid tissue genesis induced by commensals through NOD1 regulates intestinal homeostasis. *Nature* (2008) 456(7221):507–10. doi:10.1038/nature07450
17. Chang HY, Chi JT, Dudoit S, Bondre C, van de Rijn M, Botstein D, et al. Diversity, topographic differentiation, and positional memory in human fibroblasts. *Proc Natl Acad Sci U S A* (2002) 99(20):12877–82. doi:10.1073/pnas.162488599
18. Rinn JL, Kertesz M, Wang JK, Squazzo SL, Xu X, Brugmann SA, et al. Functional demarcation of active and silent chromatin domains in human HOX loci by noncoding RNAs. *Cell* (2007) 129(7):1311–23. doi:10.1016/j.cell.2007.05.022
19. Fletcher AL, Lukacs-Kornek V, Reynoso ED, Pinner SE, Bellemare-Pelletier A, Curry MS, et al. Lymph node fibroblastic reticular cells directly present peripheral tissue antigen under steady-state and inflammatory conditions. *J Exp Med* (2010) 207(4):689–97. doi:10.1084/jem.20092642
20. Buckley CD. Why does chronic inflammation persist: an unexpected role for fibroblasts. *Immunol Lett* (2011) 138(1):12–4. doi:10.1016/j.imlet.2011.02.010
21. Malhotra D, Fletcher AL, Astarita J, Lukacs-Kornek V, Tayalia P, Gonzalez SF, et al. Transcriptional profiling of stroma from inflamed and resting lymph nodes defines immunological hallmarks. *Nat Immunol* (2012) 13(5):499–510. doi:10.1038/ni.2262
22. Yang CY, Vogt TK, Favre S, Scarpellino L, Huang HY, Tacchini-Cottier F, et al. Trapping of naive lymphocytes triggers rapid growth and remodeling of the fibroblast network in reactive murine lymph nodes. *Proc Natl Acad Sci U S A* (2014) 111(1):E109–18. doi:10.1073/pnas.1312585111
23. Siegert S, Luther SA. Positive and negative regulation of T cell responses by fibroblastic reticular cells within paracortical regions of lymph nodes. *Front Immunol* (2012) 3:285. doi:10.3389/fimmu.2012.00285
24. Chang JE, Turley SJ. Stromal infrastructure of the lymph node and coordination of immunity. *Trends Immunol* (2015) 36(1):30–9. doi:10.1016/j.it.2014.11.003
25. Fletcher AL, Acton SE, Knoblich K. Lymph node fibroblastic reticular cells in health and disease. *Nat Rev Immunol* (2015) 15(6):350–61. doi:10.1038/nri3846
26. Onder L, Danuser R, Scandella E, Firner S, Chai Q, Hehlgans T, et al. Endothelial cell-specific lymphotoxin-beta receptor signaling is critical for lymph node and high endothelial venule formation. *J Exp Med* (2013) 210(3):465–73. doi:10.1084/jem.20121462
27. Peduto L, Dulauroy S, Lochner M, Spath GF, Morales MA, Cumano A, et al. Inflammation recapitulates the ontogeny of lymphoid stromal cells. *J Immunol* (2009) 182(9):5789–99. doi:10.4049/jimmunol.0803974
28. Benezech C, White A, Mader E, Serre K, Parnell S, Pfeffer K, et al. Ontogeny of stromal organizer cells during lymph node development. *J Immunol* (2010) 184(8):4521–30. doi:10.4049/jimmunol.0903113
29. van de Pavert SA, Olivier BJ, Goverse G, Vondenhoff MF, Greuter M, Beke P, et al. Chemokine CXCL13 is essential for lymph node initiation and is induced by retinoic acid and neuronal stimulation. *Nat Immunol* (2009) 10(11):1193–9. doi:10.1038/ni.1789
30. van de Pavert SA, Ferreira M, Domingues RG, Ribeiro H, Molenaar R, Moreira-Santos L, et al. Maternal retinoids control type 3 innate lymphoid cells and set the offspring immunity. *Nature* (2014) 508(7494):123–7. doi:10.1038/nature13158
31. Blum KS, Pabst R. Keystones in lymph node development. *J Anat* (2006) 209(5):585–95. doi:10.1111/j.1469-7580.2006.00650.x
32. Dejardin E, Droin NM, Delhase M, Haas E, Cao Y, Makris C, et al. The lymphotoxin-beta receptor induces different patterns of gene expression via two NF-kappaB pathways. *Immunity* (2002) 17(4):525–35. doi:10.1016/S1074-7613(02)00423-5
33. Katakai T, Hara T, Sugai M, Gonda H, Shimizu A. Lymph node fibroblastic reticular cells construct the stromal reticulum via contact with lymphocytes. *J Exp Med* (2004) 200(6):783–95. doi:10.1084/jem.20040254
34. Drayton DL, Liao S, Mounzer RH, Ruddle NH. Lymphoid organ development: from ontogeny to neogenesis. *Nat Immunol* (2006) 7(4):344–53. doi:10.1038/ni1330
35. Katakai T, Suto H, Sugai M, Gonda H, Togawa A, Suematsu S, et al. Organizer-like reticular stromal cell layer common to adult secondary lymphoid organs. *J Immunol* (2008) 181(9):6189–200. doi:10.4049/jimmunol.181.9.6189
36. Cupedo T, Mebius RE. Cellular interactions in lymph node development. *J Immunol* (2005) 174(1):21–5. doi:10.4049/jimmunol.174.1.21
37. White A, Carragher D, Parnell S, Msaki A, Perkins N, Lane P, et al. Lymphotoxin a-dependent and -independent signals regulate stromal organizer cell homeostasis during lymph node organogenesis. *Blood* (2007) 110(6):1950–9. doi:10.1182/blood-2007-01-070003
38. Chai Q, Onder L, Scandella E, Gil-Cruz C, Perez-Shibayama C, Cupovic J, et al. Maturation of lymph node fibroblastic reticular cells from myofibroblastic precursors is critical for antiviral immunity. *Immunity* (2013) 38(5):1013–24. doi:10.1016/j.immuni.2013.03.012
39. Vondenhoff MF, Greuter M, Goverse G, Elewaut D, Dewint P, Ware CF, et al. LTbetaR signaling induces cytokine expression and up-regulates lymphangiogenic factors in lymph node anlagen. *J Immunol* (2009) 182(9):5439–45. doi:10.4049/jimmunol.0801165
40. Yoshida H, Naito A, Inoue J, Satoh M, Santee-Cooper SM, Ware CF, et al. Different cytokines induce surface lymphotoxin-alphabeta on IL-7 receptor-alpha cells that differentially engender lymph nodes and Peyer's patches. *Immunity* (2002) 17(6):823–33. doi:10.1016/S1074-7613(02)00479-X
41. Cupedo T, Vondenhoff MF, Heeregrave EJ, De Weerd AE, Jansen W, Jackson DG, et al. Presumptive lymph node organizers are differentially represented in developing mesenteric and peripheral nodes. *J Immunol* (2004) 173(5):2968–75. doi:10.4049/jimmunol.173.5.2968
42. Vondenhoff MF, van de Pavert SA, Dillard ME, Greuter M, Goverse G, Oliver G, et al. Lymph sacs are not required for the initiation of lymph node formation. *Development* (2008) 136(1):29–34. doi:10.1242/dev.028456
43. Benezech C, Nayar S, Finney BA, Withers DR, Lowe K, Desanti GE, et al. CLEC-2 is required for development and maintenance of lymph nodes. *Blood* (2014) 123(20):3200–7. doi:10.1182/blood-2013-03-489286
44. Brendolan A, Rosado MM, Carsetti R, Selleri L, Dear TN. Development and function of the mammalian spleen. *Bioessays* (2007) 29(2):166–77. doi:10.1002/bies.20528

45. Fu YX, Huang G, Wang Y, Chaplin DD. B lymphocytes induce the formation of follicular dendritic cell clusters in a lymphotoxin alpha-dependent fashion. *J Exp Med* (1998) 187(7):1009–18. doi:10.1084/jem.187.7.1009
46. Endres R, Alimzhanov MB, Plitz T, Futterer A, Kosco-Vilbois MH, Nedospasov SA, et al. Mature follicular dendritic cell networks depend on expression of lymphotoxin beta receptor by radioresistant stromal cells and of lymphotoxin beta and tumor necrosis factor by B cells. *J Exp Med* (1999) 189(1):159–68. doi:10.1084/jem.189.1.159
47. Ngo VN, Cornall RJ, Cyster JG. Splenic T zone development is B cell dependent. *J Exp Med* (2001) 194(11):1649–60. doi:10.1084/jem.194.11.1649
48. Vondenhoff MF, Desanti GE, Cupedo T, Bertrand JY, Cumano A, Kraal G, et al. Separation of splenic red and white pulp occurs before birth in a LTalphabeta-independent manner. *J Leukoc Biol* (2008) 84(1):152–61. doi:10.1189/jlb.0907659
49. Timens W, Rozeboom T, Poppema S. Fetal and neonatal development of human spleen: an immunohistological study. *Immunology* (1987) 60(4):603–9.
50. Futterer A, Mink K, Luz A, Kosco-Vilbois MH, Pfeffer K. The lymphotoxin beta receptor controls organogenesis and affinity maturation in peripheral lymphoid tissues. *Immunity* (1998) 9(1):59–70. doi:10.1016/S1074-7613(00)80588-9
51. Sun Z, Unutmaz D, Zou YR, Sunshine MJ, Pierani A, Brenner-Morton S, et al. Requirement for RORgamma in thymocyte survival and lymphoid organ development. *Science* (2000) 288(5475):2369–73. doi:10.1126/science.288.5475.2369
52. Cook MC, Korner H, Riminton DS, Lemckert FA, Hasbold J, Amesbury M, et al. Generation of splenic follicular structure and B cell movement in tumor necrosis factor-deficient mice. *J Exp Med* (1998) 188(8):1503–10. doi:10.1084/jem.188.8.1503
53. Ngo VN, Korner H, Gunn MD, Schmidt KN, Riminton DS, Cooper MD, et al. Lymphotoxin alpha/beta and tumor necrosis factor are required for stromal cell expression of homing chemokines in B and T cell areas of the spleen. *J Exp Med* (1999) 189(2):403–12. doi:10.1084/jem.189.2.403
54. Cyster JG, Ansel KM, Reif K, Ekland EH, Hyman PL, Tang HL, et al. Follicular stromal cells and lymphocyte homing to follicles. *Immunol Rev* (2000) 176:181–93. doi:10.1034/j.1600-065X.2000.00618.x
55. Coles M, Kioussis D, Veiga-Fernandes H. Cellular and molecular requirements in lymph node and Peyer's patch development. *Prog Mol Biol Transl Sci* (2010) 92:177–205. doi:10.1016/s1877-1173(10)92008-5
56. Coles M, Veiga-Fernandes H. Insight into lymphoid tissue morphogenesis. *Immunol Lett* (2013) 156(1–2):46–53. doi:10.1016/j.imlet.2013.08.001
57. Ruddle NH. Lymphatic vessels and tertiary lymphoid organs. *J Clin Invest* (2014) 124(3):953–9. doi:10.1172/JCI71611
58. Drayton DL, Ying X, Lee J, Lesslauer W, Ruddle NH. Ectopic LT directs lymphoid organ neogenesis with concomitant expression of peripheral node addressin and a HEV-restricted sulfotransferase. *J Exp Med* (2003) 197(9):1153–63. doi:10.1084/jem.20021761
59. Stranford S, Ruddle NH. Follicular dendritic cells, conduits, lymphatic vessels, and high endothelial venules in tertiary lymphoid organs: parallels with lymph node stroma. *Front Immunol* (2012) 3:350. doi:10.3389/fimmu.2012.00350
60. Jones GW, Jones SA. Ectopic lymphoid follicles: inducible centres for generating antigen-specific immune responses within tissues. *Immunology* (2016) 147(2):141–51. doi:10.1111/imm.12554
61. Manzo A, Bugatti S, Caporali R, Prevo R, Jackson DG, Uguccioni M, et al. CCL21 expression pattern of human secondary lymphoid organ stroma is conserved in inflammatory lesions with lymphoid neogenesis. *Am J Pathol* (2007) 171(5):1549–62. doi:10.2353/ajpath.2007.061275
62. Dutertre CA, Clement M, Morvan M, Schakel K, Castier Y, Alsac JM, et al. Deciphering the stromal and hematopoietic cell network of the adventitia from non-aneurysmal and aneurysmal human aorta. *PLoS One* (2014) 9(2):e89983. doi:10.1371/journal.pone.0089983
63. Link A, Hardie DL, Favre S, Britschgi MR, Adams DH, Sixt M, et al. Association of T-Zone reticular networks and conduits with ectopic lymphoid tissues in mice and humans. *Am J Pathol* (2011) 178(4):1662–75. doi:10.1016/j.ajpath.2010.12.039
64. Pikor NB, Astarita JL, Summers-Deluca L, Galicia G, Qu J, Ward LA, et al. Integration of Th17- and lymphotoxin-derived signals initiates meningeal-resident stromal cell remodeling to propagate neuroinflammation. *Immunity* (2015) 43(6):1160–73. doi:10.1016/j.immuni.2015.11.010
65. Cupovic J, Onder L, Gil-Cruz C, Weiler E, Caviezel-Firner S, Perez-Shibayama C, et al. Central nervous system stromal cells control local CD8(+) T cell responses during virus-induced neuroinflammation. *Immunity* (2016) 44(3):622–33. doi:10.1016/j.immuni.2015.12.022
66. Barone F, Bombardieri M, Manzo A, Blades MC, Morgan PR, Challacombe SJ, et al. Association of CXCL13 and CCL21 expression with the progressive organization of lymphoid-like structures in Sjogren's syndrome. *Arthritis Rheum* (2005) 52(6):1773–84. doi:10.1002/art.21062
67. Barone F, Bombardieri M, Rosado MM, Morgan PR, Challacombe SJ, De Vita S, et al. CXCL13, CCL21, and CXCL12 expression in salivary glands of patients with Sjogren's syndrome and MALT lymphoma: association with reactive and malignant areas of lymphoid organization. *J Immunol* (2008) 180(7):5130–40. doi:10.4049/jimmunol.180.7.5130
68. Bombardieri M, Barone F, Lucchesi D, Nayar S, van den Berg WB, Proctor G, et al. Inducible tertiary lymphoid structures, autoimmunity, and exocrine dysfunction in a novel model of salivary gland inflammation in C57BL/6 mice. *J Immunol* (2012) 189(7):3767–76. doi:10.4049/jimmunol.1201216
69. Barone F, Nayar S, Campos J, Cloake T, Withers DR, Toellner KM, et al. IL-22 regulates lymphoid chemokine production and assembly of tertiary lymphoid organs. *Proc Natl Acad Sci U S A* (2015) 112(35):11024–9. doi:10.1073/pnas.1503315112
70. Grant AJ, Lalor PF, Hubscher SG, Briskin M, Adams DH. MAdCAM-1 expressed in chronic inflammatory liver disease supports mucosal lymphocyte adhesion to hepatic endothelium (MAdCAM-1 in chronic inflammatory liver disease). *Hepatology* (2001) 33(5):1065–72. doi:10.1053/jhep.2001.24231
71. Grant AJ, Goddard S, Ahmed-Choudhury J, Reynolds G, Jackson DG, Briskin M, et al. Hepatic expression of secondary lymphoid chemokine (CCL21) promotes the development of portal-associated lymphoid tissue in chronic inflammatory liver disease. *Am J Pathol* (2002) 160(4):1445–55. doi:10.1016/S0002-9440(10)62570-9
72. Manzo A, Paoletti S, Carulli M, Blades MC, Barone F, Yanni G, et al. Systematic microanatomical analysis of CXCL13 and CCL21in situ production and progressive lymphoid organization in rheumatoid synovitis. *Eur J Immunol* (2005) 35(5):1347–59. doi:10.1002/eji.200425830
73. Bauer S, Jendro MC, Wadle A, Kleber S, Stenner F, Dinser R, et al. Fibroblast activation protein is expressed by rheumatoid myofibroblast-like synoviocytes. *Arthritis Res Ther* (2006) 8(6):R171. doi:10.1186/ar2080
74. Humby F, Bombardieri M, Manzo A, Kelly S, Blades MC, Kirkham B, et al. Ectopic lymphoid structures support ongoing production of class-switched autoantibodies in rheumatoid synovium. *PLoS Med* (2009) 6(1):e1. doi:10.1371/journal.pmed.0060001
75. Park YE, Woo YJ, Park SH, Moon YM, Oh HJ, Kim JI, et al. IL-17 increases cadherin-11 expression in a model of autoimmune experimental arthritis and in rheumatoid arthritis. *Immunol Lett* (2011) 140(1–2):97–103. doi:10.1016/j.imlet.2011.07.003
76. Grabner R, Lotzer K, Dopping S, Hildner M, Radke D, Beer M, et al. Lymphotoxin beta receptor signaling promotes tertiary lymphoid organogenesis in the aorta adventitia of aged ApoE-/- mice. *J Exp Med* (2009) 206(1):233–48. doi:10.1084/jem.20080752
77. Lotzer K, Dopping S, Connert S, Grabner R, Spanbroek R, Lemser B, et al. Mouse aorta smooth muscle cells differentiate into lymphoid tissue organizer-like cells on combined tumor necrosis factor receptor-1/lymphotoxin beta-receptor NF-kappaB signaling. *Arterioscler Thromb Vasc Biol* (2010) 30(3):395–402. doi:10.1161/ATVBAHA.109.191395
78. Weih F, Gräbner R, Hu D, Beer M, Habenicht AJ. Control of dichotomic innate and adaptive immune responses by artery tertiary lymphoid organs in atherosclerosis. *Front Physiol* (2012) 3:226. doi:10.3389/fphys.2012.00226
79. Hu D, Mohanta SK, Yin C, Peng L, Ma Z, Srikakulapu P, et al. Artery tertiary lymphoid organs control aorta immunity and protect against atherosclerosis via vascular smooth muscle cell lymphotoxin beta receptors. *Immunity* (2015) 42(6):1100–15. doi:10.1016/j.immuni.2015.05.015
80. Magliozzi R, Columba-Cabezas S, Serafini B, Aloisi F. Intracerebral expression of CXCL13 and BAFF is accompanied by formation of lymphoid follicle-like structures in the meninges of mice with relapsing experimental autoimmune

encephalomyelitis. *J Neuroimmunol* (2004) 148(1–2):11–23. doi:10.1016/j.jneuroim.2003.10.056

81. Powell DW, Pinchuk IV, Saada JI, Chen X, Mifflin RC. Mesenchymal cells of the intestinal lamina propria. *Annu Rev Physiol* (2011) 73:213–37. doi:10.1146/annurev.physiol.70.113006.100646
82. Owens BM, Simmons A. Intestinal stromal cells in mucosal immunity and homeostasis. *Mucosal Immunol* (2013) 6(2):224–34. doi:10.1038/mi.2012.125
83. Owens BM, Steevels TA, Dudek M, Walcott D, Sun MY, Mayer A, et al. CD90(+) stromal cells are non-professional innate immune effectors of the human colonic mucosa. *Front Immunol* (2013) 4:307. doi:10.3389/fimmu.2013.00307
84. Beswick EJ, Johnson JR, Saada JI, Humen M, House J, Dann S, et al. TLR4 activation enhances the PD-L1-mediated tolerogenic capacity of colonic CD90+ stromal cells. *J Immunol* (2014) 193(5):2218–29. doi:10.4049/jimmunol.1203441
85. Owens BM. Inflammation, innate immunity, and the intestinal stromal cell niche: opportunities and challenges. *Front Immunol* (2015) 6:319. doi:10.3389/fimmu.2015.00319
86. Winter S, Loddenkemper C, Aebischer A, Rabel K, Hoffmann K, Meyer TF, et al. The chemokine receptor CXCR5 is pivotal for ectopic mucosa-associated lymphoid tissue neogenesis in chronic *Helicobacter pylori*-induced inflammation. *J Mol Med (Berl)* (2010) 88(11):1169–80. doi:10.1007/00109-010-0658-6
87. Mazzucchelli L, Blaser A, Kappeler A, Scharli P, Laissue JA, Baggiolini M, et al. BCA-1 is highly expressed in *Helicobacter pylori*-induced mucosa-associated lymphoid tissue and gastric lymphoma. *J Clin Invest* (1999) 104(10):R49–54. doi:10.1172/JCI7830
88. Wengner AM, Hopken UE, Petrow PK, Hartmann S, Schurigt U, Brauer R, et al. CXCR5- and CCR7-dependent lymphoid neogenesis in a murine model of chronic antigen-induced arthritis. *Arthritis Rheum* (2007) 56(10):3271–83. doi:10.1002/art.22939
89. Kahnert A, Hopken UE, Stein M, Bandermann S, Lipp M, Kaufmann SH. *Mycobacterium tuberculosis* triggers formation of lymphoid structure in murine lungs. *J Infect Dis* (2007) 195(1):46–54. doi:10.1086/508894
90. Rangel-Moreno J, Carragher DM, de la Luz Garcia-Hernandez M, Hwang JY, Kusser K, Hartson L, et al. The development of inducible bronchus-associated lymphoid tissue depends on IL-17. *Nat Immunol* (2011) 12(7):639–46. doi:10.1038/ni.2053
91. Perros F, Dorfmuller P, Montani D, Hammad H, Waelput W, Girerd B, et al. Pulmonary lymphoid neogenesis in idiopathic pulmonary arterial hypertension. *Am J Respir Crit Care Med* (2012) 185(3):311–21. doi:10.1164/rccm.201105-0927OC
92. Fleige H, Ravens S, Moschovakis GL, Bolter J, Willenzon S, Sutter G, et al. IL-17-induced CXCL12 recruits B cells and induces follicle formation in BALT in the absence of differentiated FDCs. *J Exp Med* (2014) 211(4):643–51. doi:10.1084/jem.20131737
93. Lee Y, Chin RK, Christiansen P, Sun Y, Tumanov AV, Wang J, et al. Recruitment and activation of naive T cells in the islets by lymphotoxin beta receptor-dependent tertiary lymphoid structure. *Immunity* (2006) 25(3):499–509. doi:10.1016/j.immuni.2006.06.016
94. Astorri E, Bombardieri M, Gabba S, Peakman M, Pozzilli P, Pitzalis C. Evolution of ectopic lymphoid neogenesis and in situ autoantibody production in autoimmune nonobese diabetic mice: cellular and molecular characterization of tertiary lymphoid structures in pancreatic islets. *J Immunol* (2010) 185(6):3359–68. doi:10.4049/jimmunol.1001836
95. Luther SA, Bidgol A, Hargreaves DC, Schmidt A, Xu Y, Paniyadi J, et al. Differing activities of homeostatic chemokines CCL19, CCL21, and CXCL12 in lymphocyte and dendritic cell recruitment and lymphoid neogenesis. *J Immunol* (2002) 169(1):424–33. doi:10.4049/jimmunol.169.1.424
96. Marinkovic T, Garin A, Yokota Y, Fu YX, Ruddle NH, Furtado GC, et al. Interaction of mature CD3+CD4+ T cells with dendritic cells triggers the development of tertiary lymphoid structures in the thyroid. *J Clin Invest* (2006) 116(10):2622–32. doi:10.1172/jci28993
97. Nagatake T, Fukuyama S, Kim DY, Goda K, Igarashi O, Sato S, et al. Id2-, RORgammat-, and LTbetaR-independent initiation of lymphoid organogenesis in ocular immunity. *J Exp Med* (2009) 206(11):2351–64. doi:10.1084/jem.20091436
98. Furtado GC, Pacer ME, Bongers G, Benezech C, He Z, Chen L, et al. TNFalpha-dependent development of lymphoid tissue in the absence of RORgammat(+) lymphoid tissue inducer cells. *Mucosal Immunol* (2014) 7(3):602–14. doi:10.1038/mi.2013.79
99. De Togni P, Goellner J, Ruddle NH, Streeter PR, Fick A, Mariathasan S, et al. Abnormal development of peripheral lymphoid organs in mice deficient in lymphotoxin. *Science* (1994) 264(5159):703–7. doi:10.1126/science.8171322
100. Banks TA, Rouse BT, Kerley MK, Blair PJ, Godfrey VL, Kuklin NA, et al. Lymphotoxin-alpha-deficient mice. Effects on secondary lymphoid organ development and humoral immune responsiveness. *J Immunol* (1995) 155(4):1685–93.
101. Alimzhanov MB, Kuprash DV, Kosco-Vilbois MH, Luz A, Turetskaya RL, Tarakhovsky A, et al. Abnormal development of secondary lymphoid tissues in lymphotoxin beta-deficient mice. *Proc Natl Acad Sci U S A* (1997) 94(17):9302–7. doi:10.1073/pnas.94.17.9302
102. Koni PA, Sacca R, Lawton P, Browning JL, Ruddle NH, Flavell RA. Distinct roles in lymphoid organogenesis for lymphotoxins alpha and beta revealed in lymphotoxin beta-deficient mice. *Immunity* (1997) 6(4):491–500. doi:10.1016/S1074-7613(00)80292-7
103. Rennert PD, Browning JL, Mebius R, Mackay F, Hochman PS. Surface lymphotoxin alpha/beta complex is required for the development of peripheral lymphoid organs. *J Exp Med* (1996) 184(5):1999–2006. doi:10.1084/jem.184.5.1999
104. Rennert PD, Browning JL, Hochman PS. Selective disruption of lymphotoxin ligands reveals a novel set of mucosal lymph nodes and unique effects on lymph node cellular organization. *Int Immunol* (1997) 9(11):1627–39. doi:10.1093/intimm/9.11.1627
105. Rennert PD, James D, Mackay F, Browning JL, Hochman PS. Lymph node genesis is induced by signaling through the lymphotoxin beta receptor. *Immunity* (1998) 9(1):71–9. doi:10.1016/S1074-7613(00)80589-0
106. Kratz A, Campos-Neto A, Hanson MS, Ruddle NH. Chronic inflammation caused by lymphotoxin is lymphoid neogenesis. *J Exp Med* (1996) 183(4):1461–72. doi:10.1084/jem.183.4.1461
107. Rangel-Moreno J, Hartson L, Navarro C, Gaxiola M, Selman M, Randall TD. Inducible bronchus-associated lymphoid tissue (iBALT) in patients with pulmonary complications of rheumatoid arthritis. *J Clin Invest* (2006) 116(12):3183–94. doi:10.1172/JCI28756
108. Khader SA, Guglani L, Rangel-Moreno J, Gopal R, Junecko BA, Fountain JJ, et al. IL-23 is required for long-term control of *Mycobacterium tuberculosis* and B cell follicle formation in the infected lung. *J Immunol* (2011) 187(10):5402–7. doi:10.4049/jimmunol.1101377
109. Peters A, Pitcher LA, Sullivan JM, Mitsdoerffer M, Acton SE, Franz B, et al. Th17 cells induce ectopic lymphoid follicles in central nervous system tissue inflammation. *Immunity* (2011) 35(6):986–96. doi:10.1016/j.immuni.2011.10.015
110. Husson H, Lugli SM, Ghia P, Cardoso A, Roth A, Brohmi K, et al. Functional effects of TNF and lymphotoxin alpha1beta2 on FDC-like cells. *Cell Immunol* (2000) 203(2):134–43. doi:10.1006/cimm.2000.1688
111. Hardy R, Juarez M, Naylor A, Tu J, Rabbitt EH, Filer A, et al. Synovial DKK1 expression is regulated by local glucocorticoid metabolism in inflammatory arthritis. *Arthritis Res Ther* (2012) 14(5):R226. doi:10.1186/ar4065
112. Corneth OB, Reijmers RM, Mus AM, Asmawidjaja PS, van Hamburg JP, Papazian N, et al. Loss of IL-22 inhibits autoantibody formation in collagen-induced arthritis in mice. *Eur J Immunol* (2016) 46(6):1404–14. doi:10.1002/eji.201546241
113. Brembilla NC, Dufour AM, Alvarez M, Hugues S, Montanari E, Truchetet ME, et al. IL-22 capacitates dermal fibroblast responses to TNF in scleroderma. *Ann Rheum Dis* (2016) 75(9):1697–705. doi:10.1136/annrheumdis-2015-207477
114. Schrama D, Thor Straten P, Fischer WH, McLellan AD, Brocker EB, Reisfeld RA, et al. Targeting of lymphotoxin-alpha to the tumor elicits an efficient immune response associated with induction of peripheral lymphoid-like tissue. *Immunity* (2001) 14(2):111–21. doi:10.1016/S1074-7613(01)00094-2
115. Yu P, Lee Y, Liu W, Chin RK, Wang J, Wang Y, et al. Priming of naive T cells inside tumors leads to eradication of established tumors. *Nat Immunol* (2004) 5(2):141–9. doi:10.1038/ni1029
116. Hess E, Duheron V, Decossas M, Lezot F, Berdal A, Chea S, et al. RANKL induces organized lymph node growth by stromal cell proliferation. *J Immunol* (2012) 188(3):1245–54. doi:10.4049/jimmunol.1101513

117. Mueller CG, Hess E. Emerging functions of RANKL in lymphoid tissues. *Front Immunol* (2012) 3:261. doi:10.3389/fimmu.2012.00261
118. Cordeiro OG, Chypre M, Brouard N, Rauber S, Alloush F, Romera-Hernandez M, et al. Integrin-alpha IIb identifies murine lymph node lymphatic endothelial cells responsive to RANKL. *PLoS One* (2016) 11(3):e0151848. doi:10.1371/journal.pone.0151848
119. Goya S, Matsuoka H, Mori M, Morishita H, Kida H, Kobashi Y, et al. Sustained interleukin-6 signalling leads to the development of lymphoid organ-like structures in the lung. *J Pathol* (2003) 200(1):82–7. doi:10.1002/path.1321
120. Ammirante M, Shalapour S, Kang Y, Jamieson CA, Karin M. Tissue injury and hypoxia promote malignant progression of prostate cancer by inducing CXCL13 expression in tumor myofibroblasts. *Proc Natl Acad Sci U S A* (2014) 111(41):14776–81. doi:10.1073/pnas.1416498111
121. Lee JJ, McGarry MP, Farmer SC, Denzler KL, Larson KA, Carrigan PE, et al. Interleukin-5 expression in the lung epithelium of transgenic mice leads to pulmonary changes pathognomonic of asthma. *J Exp Med* (1997) 185(12):2143–56. doi:10.1084/jem.185.12.2143
122. Doucet C, Brouty-Boye D, Pottin-Clemenceau C, Canonica GW, Jasmin C, Azzarone B. Interleukin (IL) 4 and IL-13 act on human lung fibroblasts. Implication in asthma. *J Clin Invest* (1998) 101(10):2129–39. doi:10.1172/JCI741
123. Luther SA, Ansel KM, Cyster JG. Overlapping roles of CXCL13, interleukin 7 receptor alpha, and CCR7 ligands in lymph node development. *J Exp Med* (2003) 197(9):1191–8. doi:10.1084/jem.20021294
124. Canete JD, Celis R, Yeremenko N, Sanmarti R, van Duivenvoorde L, Ramirez J, et al. Ectopic lymphoid neogenesis is strongly associated with activation of the IL-23 pathway in rheumatoid synovitis. *Arthritis Res Ther* (2015) 17:173. doi:10.1186/s13075-015-0688-0
125. Ivanov II, McKenzie BS, Zhou L, Tadokoro CE, Lepelley A, Lafaille JJ, et al. The orphan nuclear receptor RORgammat directs the differentiation program of proinflammatory IL-17+ T helper cells. *Cell* (2006) 126(6):1121–33. doi:10.1016/j.cell.2006.07.035
126. Cai Y, Shen X, Ding C, Qi C, Li K, Li X, et al. Pivotal role of dermal IL-17-producing gammadelta T cells in skin inflammation. *Immunity* (2011) 35(4):596–610. doi:10.1016/j.immuni.2011.08.001
127. Mabuchi T, Takekoshi T, Hwang ST. Epidermal CCR6+ gammadelta T cells are major producers of IL-22 and IL-17 in a murine model of psoriasiform dermatitis. *J Immunol* (2011) 187(10):5026–31. doi:10.4049/jimmunol.1101817
128. Pantelyushin S, Haak S, Ingold B, Kulig P, Heppner FL, Navarini AA, et al. Rorgammat+ innate lymphocytes and gammadelta T cells initiate psoriasiform plaque formation in mice. *J Clin Invest* (2012) 122(6):2252–6. doi:10.1172/JCI61862
129. Eberl G, Colonna M, Di Santo JP, McKenzie AN. Innate lymphoid cells. Innate lymphoid cells: a new paradigm in immunology. *Science* (2015) 348(6237):aaa6566. doi:10.1126/science.aaa6566
130. Lee JS, Tato CM, Joyce-Shaikh B, Gulen MF, Cayatte C, Chen Y, et al. Interleukin-23-independent IL-17 production regulates intestinal epithelial permeability. *Immunity* (2015) 43(4):727–38. doi:10.1016/j.immuni.2015.09.003
131. Crome SQ, Wang AY, Levings MK. Translational mini-review series on Th17 cells: function and regulation of human T helper 17 cells in health and disease. *Clin Exp Immunol* (2010) 159(2):109–19. doi:10.1111/j.1365-2249.2009.04037
132. Sonnenberg GF, Nair MG, Kirn TJ, Zaph C, Fouser LA, Artis D. Pathological versus protective functions of IL-22 in airway inflammation are regulated by IL-17A. *J Exp Med* (2010) 207(6):1293–305. doi:10.1084/jem.20092054
133. Jones GW, Bombardieri M, Greenhill CJ, McLeod L, Nerviani A, Rocher-Ros V, et al. Interleukin-27 inhibits ectopic lymphoid-like structure development in early inflammatory arthritis. *J Exp Med* (2015) 212(11):1793–802. doi:10.1084/jem.20132307
134. Nayar S, Campos J, Chung MM, Navarro-Nunez L, Chachlani M, Steinthal N, et al. Bimodal expansion of the lymphatic vessels is regulated by the sequential expression of IL-7 and lymphotoxin alpha1beta2 in newly formed tertiary lymphoid structures. *J Immunol* (2016) 197(5):1957–67. doi:10.4049/jimmunol.1500686
135. Brendolan A, Caamano JH. Mesenchymal cell differentiation during lymph node organogenesis. *Front Immunol* (2012) 3:381. doi:10.3389/fimmu.2012.00381
136. Browning JL, Allaire N, Ngam-Ek A, Notidis E, Hunt J, Perrin S, et al. Lymphotoxin-beta receptor signaling is required for the homeostatic control of HEV differentiation and function. *Immunity* (2005) 23(5):539–50. doi:10.1016/j.immuni.2005.10.002
137. Luther SA, Lopez T, Bai W, Hanahan D, Cyster JG. BLC expression in pancreatic islets causes B cell recruitment and lymphotoxin-dependent lymphoid neogenesis. *Immunity* (2000) 12(5):471–81. doi:10.1016/S1074-7613(00)80199-5
138. Wu Q, Salomon B, Chen M, Wang Y, Hoffman LM, Bluestone JA, et al. Reversal of spontaneous autoimmune insulitis in nonobese diabetic mice by soluble lymphotoxin receptor. *J Exp Med* (2001) 193(11):1327–32. doi:10.1084/jem.193.11.1327
139. Tumanov A, Kuprash D, Lagarkova M, Grivennikov S, Abe K, Shakhov A, et al. Distinct role of surface lymphotoxin expressed by B cells in the organization of secondary lymphoid tissues. *Immunity* (2002) 17(3):239–50. doi:10.1016/S1074-7613(02)00397-7
140. Lochner M, Ohnmacht C, Presley L, Bruhns P, Si-Tahar M, Sawa S, et al. Microbiota-induced tertiary lymphoid tissues aggravate inflammatory disease in the absence of RORgamma t and LTi cells. *J Exp Med* (2011) 208(1):125–34. doi:10.1084/jem.20100052
141. Ware CF, Crowe PD, Grayson MH, Androlewicz MJ, Browning JL. Expression of surface lymphotoxin and tumor necrosis factor on activated T, B, and natural killer cells. *J Immunol* (1992) 149(12):3881–8.
142. Ansel KM, Ngo VN, Hyman PL, Luther SA, Forster R, Sedgwick JD, et al. A chemokine-driven positive feedback loop organizes lymphoid follicles. *Nature* (2000) 406(6793):309–14. doi:10.1038/35018581
143. Suematsu S, Watanabe T. Generation of a synthetic lymphoid tissue-like organoid in mice. *Nat Biotechnol* (2004) 22(12):1539–45. doi:10.1038/nbt1039
144. Furtado GC, Marinkovic T, Martin AP, Garin A, Hoch B, Hubner W, et al. Lymphotoxin beta receptor signaling is required for inflammatory lymphangiogenesis in the thyroid. *Proc Natl Acad Sci U S A* (2007) 104(12):5026–31. doi:10.1073/pnas.0606697104
145. GeurtsvanKessel CH, Willart MA, Bergen IM, van Rijt LS, Muskens F, Elewaut D, et al. Dendritic cells are crucial for maintenance of tertiary lymphoid structures in the lung of influenza virus-infected mice. *J Exp Med* (2009) 206(11):2339–49. doi:10.1084/jem.20090410
146. Moussion C, Girard JP. Dendritic cells control lymphocyte entry to lymph nodes through high endothelial venules. *Nature* (2011) 479(7374):542–6. doi:10.1038/nature10540
147. Muniz LR, Pacer ME, Lira SA, Furtado GC. A critical role for dendritic cells in the formation of lymphatic vessels within tertiary lymphoid structures. *J Immunol* (2011) 187(2):828–34. doi:10.4049/jimmunol.1004233
148. Carlsen HS, Baekkevold ES, Morton HC, Haraldsen G, Brandtzaeg P. Monocyte-like and mature macrophages produce CXCL13 (B cell-attracting chemokine 1) in inflammatory lesions with lymphoid neogenesis. *Blood* (2004) 104(10):3021–7. doi:10.1182/blood-2004-02-0701
149. Perrier P, Martinez FO, Locati M, Bianchi G, Nebuloni M, Vago G, et al. Distinct transcriptional programs activated by interleukin-10 with or without lipopolysaccharide in dendritic cells: induction of the B cell-activating chemokine, CXC chemokine ligand 13 *J Immunol* (2004) 172(11):7031–42. doi:10.4049/jimmunol.172.11.7031
150. Vermi W, Facchetti F, Riboldi E, Heine H, Scutera S, Stornello S, et al. Role of dendritic cell-derived CXCL13 in the pathogenesis of *Bartonella henselae* B-rich granuloma. *Blood* (2006) 107(2):454–62. doi:10.1182/blood-2005-04-1342
151. Manzo A, Vitolo B, Humby F, Caporali R, Jarrossay D, Dell'accio F, et al. Mature antigen-experienced T helper cells synthesize and secrete the B cell chemoattractant CXCL13 in the inflammatory environment of the rheumatoid joint. *Arthritis Rheum* (2008) 58(11):3377–87. doi:10.1002/art.23966
152. McDonald KG, McDonough JS, Dieckgraefe BK, Newberry RD. Dendritic cells produce CXCL13 and participate in the development of murine small intestine lymphoid tissues. *Am J Pathol* (2010) 176(5):2367–77. doi:10.2353/ajpath.2010.090723
153. Mueller SN, Germain RN. Stromal cell contributions to the homeostasis and functionality of the immune system. *Nat Rev Immunol* (2009) 9(9):618–29. doi:10.1038/nri2588

154. Brown FD, Turley SJ. Fibroblastic reticular cells: organization and regulation of the T lymphocyte life cycle. *J Immunol* (2015) 194(4):1389–94. doi:10.4049/jimmunol.1402520
155. Link A, Vogt TK, Favre S, Britschgi MR, Acha-Orbea H, Hinz B, et al. Fibroblastic reticular cells in lymph nodes regulate the homeostasis of naive T cells. *Nat Immunol* (2007) 8(11):1255–65. doi:10.1038/ni1513
156. Yi T, Wang X, Kelly LM, An J, Xu Y, Sailer AW, et al. Oxysterol gradient generation by lymphoid stromal cells guides activated B cell movement during humoral responses. *Immunity* (2012) 37(3):535–48. doi:10.1016/j.immuni.2012.06.015
157. Cremasco V, Woodruff MC, Onder L, Cupovic J, Nieves-Bonilla JM, Schildberg FA, et al. B cell homeostasis and follicle confines are governed by fibroblastic reticular cells. *Nat Immunol* (2014) 15(10):973–81. doi:10.1038/ni.2965
158. Fasnacht N, Huang HY, Koch U, Favre S, Auderset F, Chai Q, et al. Specific fibroblastic niches in secondary lymphoid organs orchestrate distinct Notch-regulated immune responses. *J Exp Med* (2014) 211(11):2265–79. doi:10.1084/jem.20132528
159. Katakai T. Marginal reticular cells: a stromal subset directly descended from the lymphoid tissue organizer. *Front Immunol* (2012) 3:200. doi:10.3389/fimmu.2012.00200
160. Junt T, Moseman EA, Iannacone M, Massberg S, Lang PA, Boes M, et al. Subcapsular sinus macrophages in lymph nodes clear lymph-borne viruses and present them to antiviral B cells. *Nature* (2007) 450(7166):110–4. doi:10.1038/nature06287
161. Roozendaal R, Mempel TR, Pitcher LA, Gonzalez SF, Verschoor A, Mebius RE, et al. Conduits mediate transport of low-molecular-weight antigen to lymph node follicles. *Immunity* (2009) 30(2):264–76. doi:10.1016/j.immuni.2008.12.014
162. Jarjour M, Jorquera A, Mondor I, Wienert S, Narang P, Coles MC, et al. Fate mapping reveals origin and dynamics of lymph node follicular dendritic cells. *J Exp Med* (2014) 211(6):1109–22. doi:10.1084/jem.20132409
163. Allen CD, Cyster JG. Follicular dendritic cell networks of primary follicles and germinal centers: phenotype and function. *Semin Immunol* (2008) 20(1):14–25. doi:10.1016/j.smim.2007.12.001
164. Fu YX, Chaplin DD. Development and maturation of secondary lymphoid tissues. *Annu Rev Immunol* (1999) 17:399–433. doi:10.1146/annurev.immunol.17.1.399
165. Lu TT, Browning JL. Role of the lymphotoxin/LIGHT system in the development and maintenance of reticular networks and vasculature in lymphoid tissues. *Front Immunol* (2014) 5:47. doi:10.3389/fimmu.2014.00047
166. Le Hir M, Bluethmann H, Kosco-Vilbois MH, Muller M, di Padova F, Moore M, et al. Differentiation of follicular dendritic cells and full antibody responses require tumor necrosis factor receptor-1 signaling. *J Exp Med* (1996) 183(5):2367–72. doi:10.1084/jem.183.5.2367
167. Matsumoto M, Mariathasan S, Nahm MH, Baranyay F, Peschon JJ, Chaplin DD. Role of lymphotoxin and the type I TNF receptor in the formation of germinal centers. *Science* (1996) 271(5253):1289–91. doi:10.1126/science.271.5253.1289
168. Fu YX, Molina H, Matsumoto M, Huang G, Min J, Chaplin DD. Lymphotoxin-alpha (LTalpha) supports development of splenic follicular structure that is required for IgG responses. *J Exp Med* (1997) 185(12):2111–20. doi:10.1084/jem.185.12.2111
169. Lorenz RG, Chaplin DD, McDonald KG, McDonough JS, Newberry RD. Isolated lymphoid follicle formation is inducible and dependent upon lymphotoxin-sufficient B lymphocytes, lymphotoxin beta receptor, and TNF receptor I function. *J Immunol* (2003) 170(11):5475–82. doi:10.4049/jimmunol.170.11.5475
170. Bannard O, Horton RM, Allen CD, An J, Nagasawa T, Cyster JG. Germinal center centroblasts transition to a centrocyte phenotype according to a timed program and depend on the dark zone for effective selection. *Immunity* (2013) 39(5):912–24. doi:10.1016/j.immuni.2013.08.038
171. Rodda LB, Bannard O, Ludewig B, Nagasawa T, Cyster JG. Phenotypic and morphological properties of germinal center dark zone Cxcl12-expressing reticular cells. *J Immunol* (2015) 195(10):4781–91. doi:10.4049/jimmunol.1501191
172. Mionnet C, Mondor I, Jorquera A, Loosveld M, Maurizio J, Arcangeli ML, et al. Identification of a new stromal cell type involved in the regulation of inflamed B cell follicles. *PLoS Biol* (2013) 11(10):e1001672. doi:10.1371/journal.pbio.1001672
173. Tomei AA, Siegert S, Britschgi MR, Luther SA, Swartz MA. Fluid flow regulates stromal cell organization and CCL21 expression in a tissue-engineered lymph node microenvironment. *J Immunol* (2009) 183(7):4273–83. doi:10.4049/jimmunol.0900835
174. Vega F, Coombes KR, Thomazy VA, Patel K, Lang W, Jones D. Tissue-specific function of lymph node fibroblastic reticulum cells. *Pathobiology* (2006) 73(2):71–81. doi:10.1159/000094491
175. Fletcher AL, Malhotra D, Acton SE, Lukacs-Kornek V, Bellemare-Pelletier A, Curry M, et al. Reproducible isolation of lymph node stromal cells reveals site-dependent differences in fibroblastic reticular cells. *Front Immunol* (2011) 2:35. doi:10.3389/fimmu.2011.00035
176. Rangel-Moreno J, Moyron-Quiroz JE, Hartson L, Kusser K, Randall TD. Pulmonary expression of CXC chemokine ligand 13, CC chemokine ligand 19, and CC chemokine ligand 21 is essential for local immunity to influenza. *Proc Natl Acad Sci U S A* (2007) 104(25):10577–82. doi:10.1073/pnas.0700591104
177. Rangel-Moreno J, Carragher DM, Misra RS, Kusser K, Hartson L, Moquin A, et al. B cells promote resistance to heterosubtypic strains of influenza via multiple mechanisms. *J Immunol* (2008) 180(1):454–63. doi:10.4049/jimmunol.180.1.454
178. Krautler NJ, Kana V, Kranich J, Tian Y, Perera D, Lemm D, et al. Follicular dendritic cells emerge from ubiquitous perivascular precursors. *Cell* (2012) 150(1):194–206. doi:10.1016/j.cell.2012.05.032
179. Castagnaro L, Lenti E, Maruzzelli S, Spinardi L, Migliori E, Farinello D, et al. Nkx2-5+Islet1+ Mesenchymal precursors generate distinct spleen stromal cell subsets and participate in restoring stromal network integrity. *Immunity* (2013) 38(4):782–91. doi:10.1016/j.immuni.2012.12.005
180. Liao S, Ruddle NH. Synchrony of high endothelial venules and lymphatic vessels revealed by immunization. *J Immunol* (2006) 177(5):3369–79. doi:10.4049/jimmunol.177.5.3369
181. Chyou S, Benahmed F, Chen J, Kumar V, Tian S, Lipp M, et al. Coordinated regulation of lymph node vascular-stromal growth first by CD11c+ cells and then by T and B cells. *J Immunol* (2011) 187(11):5558–67. doi:10.4049/jimmunol.1101724
182. Kumar V, Chyou S, Stein JV, Lu TT. Optical projection tomography reveals dynamics of HEV growth after immunization with protein plus CFA and features shared with HEVs in acute autoinflammatory lymphadenopathy. *Front Immunol* (2012) 3:282. doi:10.3389/fimmu.2012.00282
183. Barone F, Nayar S, Buckley CD. The role of non-hematopoietic stromal cells in the persistence of inflammation. *Front Immunol* (2012) 3:416. doi:10.3389/fimmu.2012.00416
184. Astarita JL, Acton SE, Turley SJ. Podoplanin: emerging functions in development, the immune system, and cancer. *Front Immunol* (2012) 3:283. doi:10.3389/fimmu.2012.00283
185. Bombardieri M, Barone F, Humby F, Kelly S, McGurk M, Morgan P, et al. Activation-induced cytidine deaminase expression in follicular dendritic cell networks and interfollicular large B cells supports functionality of ectopic lymphoid neogenesis in autoimmune sialoadenitis and MALT lymphoma in Sjogren's syndrome. *J Immunol* (2007) 179(7):4929–38. doi:10.4049/jimmunol.179.7.4929
186. Moyron-Quiroz JE, Rangel-Moreno J, Kusser K, Hartson L, Sprague F, Goodrich S, et al. Role of inducible bronchus associated lymphoid tissue (iBALT) in respiratory immunity. *Nat Med* (2004) 10(9):927–34. doi:10.1038/nm1091
187. Moyron-Quiroz JE, Rangel-Moreno J, Hartson L, Kusser K, Tighe MP, Klonowski KD, et al. Persistence and responsiveness of immunologic memory in the absence of secondary lymphoid organs. *Immunity* (2006) 25(4):643–54. doi:10.1016/j.immuni.2006.08.022
188. Wohrer S, Troch M, Raderer M. Therapy of gastric mucosa-associated lymphoid tissue lymphoma. *Expert Opin Pharmacother* (2007) 8(9):1263–73. doi:10.1517/14656566.8.9.1263
189. Salomonsson S, Larsson P, Tengner P, Mellquist E, Hjelmstrom P, Wahren-Herlenius M. Expression of the B cell-attracting chemokine CXCL13 in the target organ and autoantibody production in ectopic lymphoid tissue in the chronic inflammatory disease Sjogren's syndrome. *Scand J Immunol* (2002) 55(4):336–42. doi:10.1046/j.1365-3083.2002.01058.x

190. Bugatti S, Caporali R, Manzo A, Vitolo B, Pitzalis C, Montecucco C. Involvement of subchondral bone marrow in rheumatoid arthritis: lymphoid neogenesis and in situ relationship to subchondral bone marrow osteoclast recruitment. *Arthritis Rheum* (2005) 52(11):3448–59. doi:10.1002/art.21377
191. Canete JD, Celis R, Moll C, Izquierdo E, Marsal S, Sanmarti R, et al. Clinical significance of synovial lymphoid neogenesis and its reversal after anti-tumour necrosis factor alpha therapy in rheumatoid arthritis. *Ann Rheum Dis* (2009) 68(5):751–6. doi:10.1136/ard.2008.089284
192. Bugatti S, Caporali R, Manzo A, Sakellariou G, Rossi S, Montecucco C. Ultrasonographic and MRI characterisation of the palindromic phase of rheumatoid arthritis. *Ann Rheum Dis* (2012) 71(4):625–6. doi:10.1136/annrheumdis-2011-200077
193. Bugatti S, Manzo A, Benaglio F, Klersy C, Vitolo B, Todoerti M, et al. Serum levels of CXCL13 are associated with ultrasonographic synovitis and predict power Doppler persistence in early rheumatoid arthritis treated with non-biological disease-modifying anti-rheumatic drugs. *Arthritis Res Ther* (2012) 14(1):R34. doi:10.1186/ar3742
194. Theander E, Vasaitis L, Baecklund E, Nordmark G, Warfvinge G, Liedholm R, et al. Lymphoid organisation in labial salivary gland biopsies is a possible predictor for the development of malignant lymphoma in primary Sjogren's syndrome. *Ann Rheum Dis* (2011) 70(8):1363–8. doi:10.1136/ard.2010.144782
195. Theander E, Henriksson G, Ljungberg O, Mandl T, Manthorpe R, Jacobsson LT. Lymphoma and other malignancies in primary Sjogren's syndrome: a cohort study on cancer incidence and lymphoma predictors. *Ann Rheum Dis* (2006) 65(6):796–803. doi:10.1136/ard.2005.041186
196. Hiraoka N, Ino Y, Yamazaki-Itoh R. Tertiary lymphoid organs in cancer tissues. *Front Immunol* (2016) 7:244. doi:10.3389/fimmu.2016.00244
197. Ghiringhelli F, Puig PE, Roux S, Parcellier A, Schmitt E, Solary E, et al. Tumor cells convert immature myeloid dendritic cells into TGF-beta-secreting cells inducing CD4+CD25+ regulatory T cell proliferation. *J Exp Med* (2005) 202(7):919–29. doi:10.1084/jem.20050463
198. Valzasina B, Piconese S, Guiducci C, Colombo MP. Tumor-induced expansion of regulatory T cells by conversion of CD4+CD25- lymphocytes is thymus and proliferation independent. *Cancer Res* (2006) 66(8):4488–95. doi:10.1158/0008-5472.CAN-05-4217
199. Liu VC, Wong LY, Jang T, Shah AH, Park I, Yang X, et al. Tumor evasion of the immune system by converting CD4+CD25- T cells into CD4+CD25+ T regulatory cells: role of tumor-derived TGF-beta. *J Immunol* (2007) 178(5):2883–92. doi:10.4049/jimmunol.178.5.2883
200. Joshi NS, Akama-Garren EH, Lu Y, Lee DY, Chang GP, Li A, et al. Regulatory T cells in tumor-associated tertiary lymphoid structures suppress anti-tumor T cell responses. *Immunity* (2015) 43(3):579–90. doi:10.1016/j.immuni.2015.08.006
201. Slight SR, Rangel-Moreno J, Gopal R, Lin Y, Fallert Junecko BA, Mehra S, et al. CXCR5(+) T helper cells mediate protective immunity against tuberculosis. *J Clin Invest* (2013) 123(2):712–26. doi:10.1172/JCI65728
202. Clement M, Guedj K, Andreata F, Morvan M, Bey L, Khallou-Laschet J, et al. Control of the T follicular helper-germinal center B-cell axis by CD8(+) regulatory T cells limits atherosclerosis and tertiary lymphoid organ development. *Circulation* (2015) 131(6):560–70. doi:10.1161/CIRCULATIONAHA.114.010988
203. Chevalier N, Jarrossay D, Ho E, Avery DT, Ma CS, Yu D, et al. CXCR5 expressing human central memory CD4 T cells and their relevance for humoral immune responses. *J Immunol* (2011) 186(10):5556–68. doi:10.4049/jimmunol.1002828
204. Morita R, Schmitt N, Bentebibel SE, Ranganathan R, Bourdery L, Zurawski G, et al. Human blood CXCR5(+)CD4(+) T cells are counterparts of T follicular cells and contain specific subsets that differentially support antibody secretion. *Immunity* (2011) 34(1):108–21. doi:10.1016/j.immuni.2010.12.012
205. Sage PT, Alvarez D, Godec J, von Andrian UH, Sharpe AH. Circulating T follicular regulatory and helper cells have memory-like properties. *J Clin Invest* (2014) 124(12):5191–204. doi:10.1172/JCI76861
206. Ying X, Chan K, Shenoy P, Hill M, Ruddle NH. Lymphotoxin plays a crucial role in the development and function of nasal-associated lymphoid tissue through regulation of chemokines and peripheral node addressin. *Am J Pathol* (2005) 166(1):135–46. doi:10.1016/S0002-9440(10)62239-0
207. Crotty S. T follicular helper cell differentiation, function, and roles in disease. *Immunity* (2014) 41(4):529–42. doi:10.1016/j.immuni.2014.10.004
208. Noss EH, Nguyen HN, Chang SK, Watts GF, Brenner MB. Genetic polymorphism directs IL-6 expression in fibroblasts but not selected other cell types. *Proc Natl Acad Sci U S A* (2015) 112(48):14948–53. doi:10.1073/pnas.1520861112
209. Linterman MA, Pierson W, Lee SK, Kallies A, Kawamoto S, Rayner TF, et al. Foxp3+ follicular regulatory T cells control the germinal center response. *Nat Med* (2011) 17(8):975–82. doi:10.1038/nm.2425
210. Miles B, Miller SM, Folkvord JM, Kimball A, Chamanian M, Meditz AL, et al. Follicular regulatory T cells impair follicular T helper cells in HIV and SIV infection. *Nat Commun* (2015) 6:8608. doi:10.1038/ncomms9608
211. Quezada SA, Peggs KS, Simpson TR, Shen Y, Littman DR, Allison JP. Limited tumor infiltration by activated T effector cells restricts the therapeutic activity of regulatory T cell depletion against established melanoma. *J Exp Med* (2008) 205(9):2125–38. doi:10.1084/jem.20080099
212. Hindley JP, Jones E, Smart K, Bridgeman H, Lauder SN, Ondondo B, et al. T-cell trafficking facilitated by high endothelial venules is required for tumor control after regulatory T-cell depletion. *Cancer Res* (2012) 72(21):5473–82. doi:10.1158/0008-5472.CAN-12-1912
213. Aggarwal S, Ghilardi N, Xie MH, de Sauvage FJ, Gurney AL. Interleukin-23 promotes a distinct CD4 T cell activation state characterized by the production of interleukin-17. *J Biol Chem* (2003) 278(3):1910–4. doi:10.1074/jbc.M207577200
214. Bettelli E, Carrier Y, Gao W, Korn T, Strom TB, Oukka M, et al. Reciprocal developmental pathways for the generation of pathogenic effector TH17 and regulatory T cells. *Nature* (2006) 441(7090):235–8. doi:10.1038/nature04753
215. Korn T, Bettelli E, Gao W, Awasthi A, Jager A, Strom TB, et al. IL-21 initiates an alternative pathway to induce proinflammatory T(H)17 cells. *Nature* (2007) 448(7152):484–7. doi:10.1038/nature05970
216. Korn T, Mitsdoerffer M, Croxford AL, Awasthi A, Dardalhon VA, Galileos G, et al. IL-6 controls Th17 immunity in vivo by inhibiting the conversion of conventional T cells into Foxp3+ regulatory T cells. *Proc Natl Acad Sci U S A* (2008) 105(47):18460–5. doi:10.1073/pnas.0809850105
217. Xu L, Kitani A, Fuss I, Strober W. Cutting edge: regulatory T cells induce CD4+CD25-Foxp3- T cells or are self-induced to become Th17 cells in the absence of exogenous TGF-beta. *J Immunol* (2007) 178(11):6725–9. doi:10.4049/jimmunol.178.11.6725
218. Yang XO, Nurieva R, Martinez GJ, Kang HS, Chung Y, Pappu BP, et al. Molecular antagonism and plasticity of regulatory and inflammatory T cell programs. *Immunity* (2008) 29(1):44–56. doi:10.1016/j.immuni.2008.05.007
219. Mueller SN, Matloubian M, Clemens DM, Sharpe AH, Freeman GJ, Gangappa S, et al. Viral targeting of fibroblastic reticular cells contributes to immunosuppression and persistence during chronic infection. *Proc Natl Acad Sci U S A* (2007) 104(39):15430–5 doi:10.1073/pnas.0702579104
220. Lukacs-Kornek V, Malhotra D, Fletcher AL, Acton SE, Elpek KG, Tayalia P, et al. Regulated release of nitric oxide by nonhematopoietic stroma controls expansion of the activated T cell pool in lymph nodes. *Nat Immunol* (2011) 12(11):1096–104. doi:10.1038/ni.2112
221. Siegert S, Huang HY, Yang CY, Scarpellino L, Carrie L, Essex S, et al. Fibroblastic reticular cells from lymph nodes attenuate T cell expansion by producing nitric oxide. *PLoS One* (2011) 6(11):e27618. doi:10.1371/journal.pone.0027618
222. Baptista AP, Roozendaal R, Reijmers RM, Koning JJ, Unger WW, Greuter M, et al. Lymph node stromal cells constrain immunity via MHC class II self-antigen presentation. *Elife* (2014) 3:3. doi:10.7554/eLife.04433
223. Dubrot J, Duraes FV, Potin L, Capotosti F, Brighouse D, Suter T, et al. Lymph node stromal cells acquire peptide-MHCII complexes from dendritic cells and induce antigen-specific CD4(+) T cell tolerance. *J Exp Med* (2014) 211(6):1153–66. doi:10.1084/jem.20132000
224. Cording S, Wahl B, Kulkarni D, Chopra H, Pezoldt J, Buettner M, et al. The intestinal micro-environment imprints stromal cells to promote efficient Treg induction in gut-draining lymph nodes. *Mucosal Immunol* (2014) 7(2):359–68. doi:10.1038/mi.2013.54

225. Denton AE, Roberts EW, Linterman MA, Fearon DT. Fibroblastic reticular cells of the lymph node are required for retention of resting but not activated CD8+ T cells. *Proc Natl Acad Sci U S A* (2014) 111(33):12139–44. doi:10.1073/pnas.1412910111
226. Novkovic M, Onder L, Cupovic J, Abe J, Bomze D, Cremasco V, et al. Topological small-world organization of the fibroblastic reticular cell network determines lymph node functionality. *PLoS Biol* (2016) 14(7):e1002515. doi:10.1371/journal.pbio.1002515
227. Acton SE, Astarita JL, Malhotra D, Lukacs-Kornek V, Franz B, Hess PR, et al. Podoplanin-rich stromal networks induce dendritic cell motility via activation of the C-type lectin receptor CLEC-2. *Immunity* (2012) 37(2):276–89. doi:10.1016/j.immuni.2012.05.022
228. Astarita JL, Cremasco V, Fu J, Darnell MC, Peck JR, Nieves-Bonilla JM, et al. The CLEC-2-podoplanin axis controls the contractility of fibroblastic reticular cells and lymph node microarchitecture. *Nat Immunol* (2015) 16(1):75–84. doi:10.1038/ni.3035
229. Wang X, Cho B, Suzuki K, Xu Y, Green JA, An J, et al. Follicular dendritic cells help establish follicle identity and promote B cell retention in germinal centers. *J Exp Med* (2011) 208(12):2497–510. doi:10.1084/jem.20111449

8

Understanding Immune Cells in Tertiary Lymphoid Organ Development: It is All Starting to Come Together

Gareth W. Jones, David G. Hill and Simon A. Jones*

Division of Infection and Immunity, Systems Immunity URI, The School of Medicine, Cardiff University, Cardiff, UK

***Correspondence:**
Gareth W. Jones
jonesgw6@cf.ac.uk

Tertiary lymphoid organs (TLOs) are frequently observed in tissues affected by non-resolving inflammation as a result of infection, autoimmunity, cancer, and allograft rejection. These highly ordered structures resemble the cellular composition of lymphoid follicles typically associated with the spleen and lymph node compartments. Although TLOs within tissues show varying degrees of organization, they frequently display evidence of segregated T and B cell zones, follicular dendritic cell networks, a supporting stromal reticulum, and high endothelial venules. In this respect, they mimic the activities of germinal centers and contribute to the local control of adaptive immune responses. Studies in various disease settings have described how these structures contribute to either beneficial or deleterious outcomes. While the development and architectural organization of TLOs within inflamed tissues requires homeostatic chemokines, lymphoid and inflammatory cytokines, and adhesion molecules, our understanding of the cells responsible for triggering these events is still evolving. Over the past 10–15 years, novel immune cell subsets have been discovered that have more recently been implicated in the control of TLO development and function. In this review, we will discuss the contribution of these cell types and consider the potential to develop new therapeutic strategies that target TLOs.

Keywords: tertiary lymphoid organs, ectopic lymphoid structures, lymphoid neogenesis, autoimmunity, infection, rheumatoid arthritis, cancer

INTRODUCTION

Adaptive immune responses are traditionally viewed as reactions that occur in secondary lymphoid organs (SLOs). These include encapsulated SLOs, such as the spleen and lymph nodes, and mucosal-associated lymphoid tissues, such as Peyer's patches, nasal-associated lymphoid tissue, bronchus-associated lymphoid tissue (BALT), and tonsils (1). SLOs develop in pre-determined locations throughout the body to monitor self and non-self antigens as they drain from peripheral tissues. Owing to their highly organized cellular architecture, SLOs provide an optimal environment for cellular communication and the generation of antigen-specific effector cells against foreign antigens. In addition, mucosal-associated lymphoid tissues act as tissue barometers responsible for the maintenance of immune homeostasis and orchestrators of anti-microbial host immunity against invading pathogens. They, therefore, reinforce immunological tolerance within mucosal compartments and support tissue integrity through the maintenance of commensal microbiota (2, 3). However, it is increasingly evident that antigen-specific responses may also be generated at sites separate to those

SLOs. These responses are typically observed in tissues affected by non-resolving inflammation as a result of infection, cancer, autoimmunity, chronic allograft rejection, and environmental irritants, where the local inflammatory environment promotes the organization of lymphoid aggregates that drive adaptive immune reactions (4). These lymphoid organ-like structures are referred to as tertiary lymphoid organs [TLOs; also called ectopic lymphoid-like structures (ELSs); and ectopic lymphoid follicles (ELFs)].

Unlike SLOs that develop during embryogenesis, TLOs are not encapsulated and do not form in pre-determined locations based on developmental signals (1). Rather, TLOs are inducible in response to inflammatory stimuli and, therefore, have the potential to develop in any tissue where persistent inflammation features. Nevertheless studies in human disease, particularly cancer metastases (5), and research using transgenic mice (6) suggest that some tissues are more permissive to TLO development than others. Furthermore, only a fraction of patients with any particular disease develop TLOs in inflamed tissues. This suggests that the local inflammatory microenvironment, including signals provided by stromal tissue cells and resident cells, must provide specific cues conducive to lymphoid neogenesis for TLO development to occur. Importantly, TLOs can influence disease progression, where their effects can either be beneficial or damaging. For example, in certain cancers and infections, TLOs can promote antigen-specific responses that promote anti-tumor and anti-pathogen immunity (5). However, in autoimmune diseases, such as rheumatoid arthritis, TLOs have been shown to support local autoantibody responses (e.g., rheumatoid factor, ACPA/anti-CCP) linked with disease exacerbation and also influence the clinical response to mainstream biologics (e.g., anti-TNF) (4, 7–9). The above highlight key questions that need addressing: *What are the stromal and immune cell signals that drive TLO development? What determines why some patients develop TLOs during chronic inflammation and others not? What are the most suitable biologics for the treatment of TLO-associated autoimmune diseases? Do TLOs hold promise for establishing anti-tumour immunity to improve cancer therapy? Do signatures of TLO development and activity constitute biomarkers capable of patient stratification that aid clinical decision-making?*

While TLOs borrow developmental cues from secondary lymphoid organogenesis, there are also distinct immune cells, stromal cells, and effector cytokines implicated in TLO development (1, 4). This suggests that during TLO development, immune cells, and their effector molecules can substitute for the traditional players involved in lymphoid organ development. Here, we review recent discoveries relating to the immune cells involved in TLO development, their functions that influence disease progression, and the potential of TLOs as therapeutic targets.

SECONDARY LYMPHOID ORGANOGENESIS AS A MODEL FOR TLO DEVELOPMENT

Secondary lymphoid organs display a highly organized cellular architecture, including segregated T cell zones and B cell follicles comprising active germinal centers (GCs); follicular dendritic cell (fDC) networks; PNAd$^+$ high endothelial venules (HEVs) that allow naïve and central memory T and B cell homing; and stromal reticular networks. While TLOs display many of these features, in human diseases they can often present as less ordered structures ranging from simple T and B cell aggregates through to highly organized and segregated structures featuring HEVs and active GCs. This heterogeneity likely reflects the stage at which tissue biopsies are taken and may represent developing TLOs that have not fully matured. Similarly, TLOs can often be "transient" and regress upon successful antigen clearance or resolution of inflammation. Therefore, regression of TLOs may also contribute to the heterogeneity seen in tissues biopsied from human diseases. While TLOs exhibit more heterogeneity than SLOs, much of our understanding of TLO development stems from studies of secondary lymphoid organogenesis [comprehensively reviewed elsewhere (1, 10)].

Secondary lymphoid organ development is initiated when CD3$^-$ CD4$^+$ CD45$^+$ lymphoid tissue inducer (LTi) cells of hematopoietic origin interact with mesenchymal-derived lymphoid tissue organizer (LTo) cells (**Figure 1**). LTi cells express the chemokine receptor CXCR5 and IL-7R (CD127), which results in their accumulation at sites of lymph node development in response to the local production of CXCL13 and IL-7. Recruited LTi cells express lymphotoxin (LT)$\alpha_1\beta_2$, which stimulates stromal LTo cells to produce the homeostatic chemokines CXCL13, CCL19, and CCL21 initiating the recruitment of hematopoietic cells. The retention of cells is further supported by the expression of adhesion molecules, including intracellular adhesion molecule 1 (ICAM-1) and vascular cell adhesion molecule 1 (VCAM-1) by LTo cells (11). The secretion of growth factors, such as vascular endothelial growth factor-C (VEGF-C), fibroblast growth factor-2 (FGF2), and hepatocyte growth factor (HGF) also promotes lymphangiogenesis (the formation of lymphatic vessels from pre-existing lymphatic vessels) and HEV development (1, 12). Finally, LTo cells differentiate into fDCs, and fibroblastic and marginal reticular cells, which form stromal cell networks that provide a structural scaffold that supports cellular migration (13–15). Once initiated, the expression of homeostatic chemokines (CXCL13, CCL19, CCL21, and CXCL12) by LTo cells perpetuates the recruitment of further LTi cells and lymphocytes. This provides a sustained source of LTo cell stimulation through the LTβ receptor (LTβR), thus ensuring the maintenance of lymphoid organ development.

The mechanisms of TLO development share many similarities with those of lymph node development (**Figure 1**). Perhaps the most prominent example is the establishment of a chemokine-directed positive feedback loop that orchestrates lymphocyte recruitment and organization (4, 5). However, TLOs can form in the absence of LTi cells. For example, mice deficient in the nuclear hormone receptor retinoic acid-related orphan receptor-γt (RORγt) and the transcriptional repressor Id2 still retain the capacity to develop TLOs at inflammatory sites, despite lacking LTi cells (16–19). This highlights one of the most striking differences between TLO and SLO development. While both rely on homeostatic chemokines (e.g., CXCL13, CCL19, CCL21, and CXCL12) and lymphoneogenic cytokines (e.g., LTαβ) for

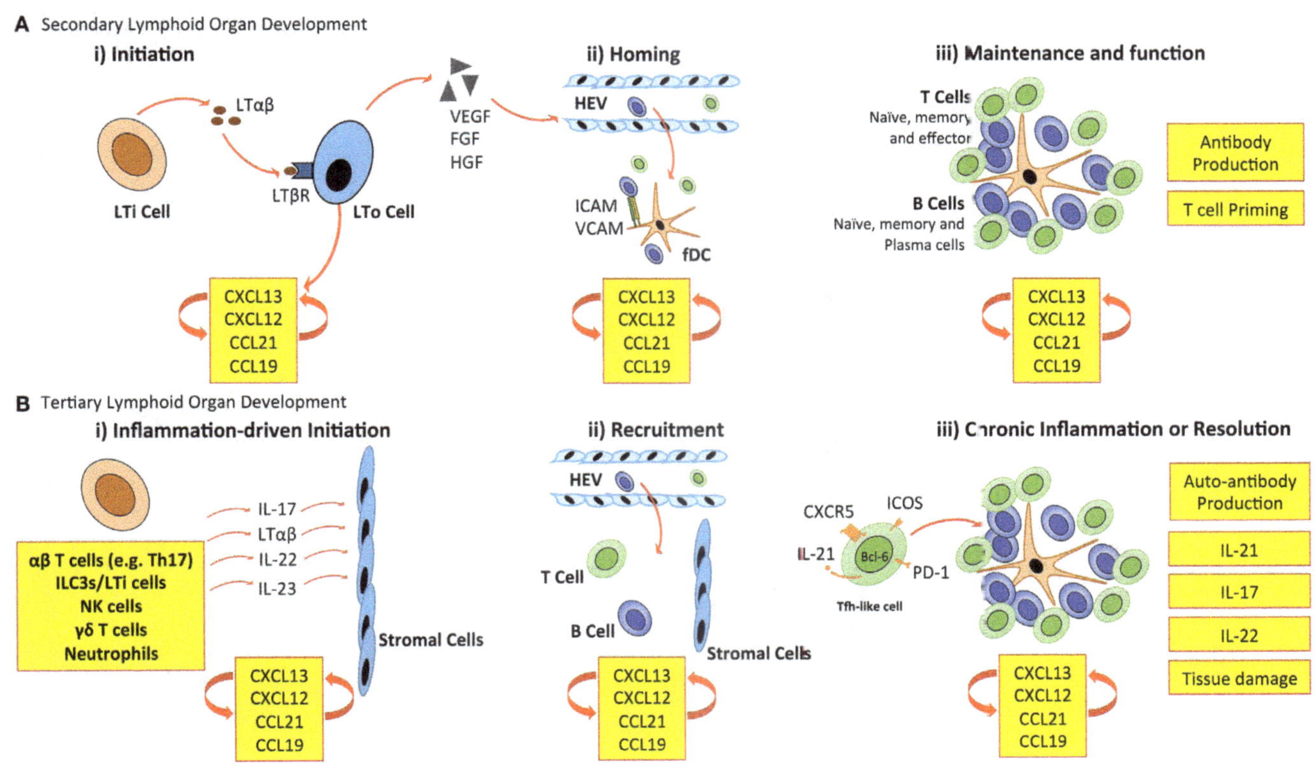

FIGURE 1 | Cellular control of lymphoid organ development. (A) LTi cells accumulate at sites of SLO development and secrete lymphotoxin (LT) αβ, which engages the LTβ receptor (LTβR) expressed on stromal LTo cells. LTo cells respond by releasing homeostatic chemokines (CXCL13, CXCL12, CCL21, and CCL19), further recruiting and spatially organizing hematopoietic cells into lymphoid organs. Release of vascular endothelial growth factor (VEGF), fibroblast growth factor (FGF), and hepatocyte growth factor (HGF) by stromal LTo cells promotes the development of high endothelial venules (HEVs). Expression of ICAM and VCAM on fDCs and resident stromal cells further supports leukocyte recruitment. Stromal LTo cells are also capable of differentiating into cell lineages (e.g., follicular DCs) that support SLO development. SLOs are sites for T cell activation and differentiation (e.g., into Th1, Th2, Th17, and Tfh cells). Tfh cells promote the development and maintenance of germinal centers and interact with B cells to generate high-affinity antibodies. **(B)** In TLO development, immune cells can substitute for conventional cells involved in lymphoid organogenesis. The accumulation of TLO-initiating immune cells at sites of inflammation, and their interaction with tissue resident and stromal cells initiates release of homeostatic chemokines (CXCL13, CXCL12, CCL21, and CCL19) that are involved in the recruitment and spatial organization of cells into TLOs. The plasticity of T cells may contribute to TLO development through the acquisition of Tfh-like effector characteristics that promote B cell activities and antibody generation. As in SLOs, fDCs may support TLO development and maintenance through chemokine production and provide a cellular network for B cell migration. LTi, lymphoid tissue inducer; LTo, lymphoid tissue organizer; ICAM, intracellular adhesion molecule; VCAM, vascular cell adhesion molecule; fDC, follicular dendritic cell.

their development, the initiation of TLO development relies on an inducible inflammatory trigger, while SLOs are developmentally pre-programed. In this regard, immune cells may substitute for LTi cells and act as primary orchestrators of tertiary lymphoneogenesis.

T HELPER 17 TYPE RESPONSES AND PLASTICITY DRIVE TLO DEVELOPMENT IN CHRONIC INFLAMMATION

T helper cells and their effector cytokines, particularly IL-17-secreting CD4$^+$ (Th17) cells have recently emerged as key initiators of TLO development in inflammatory diseases (**Figure 2**) (20). For example, in a model of lipopolysaccharide (LPS)-driven pulmonary inflammation, neonatal mice developed inducible (i) BALT associated with heightened CXCL13 and CCL19 expression (19). Despite the presence of CD3$^-$CD4$^+$ LTi cells, iBALT development was dependent on IL-17 production by CD4$^+$ T cells. Interestingly, antibody blockade revealed that IL-17 was important for initiation of iBALT development, but was dispensable for the maintenance of established lymphoid clusters. The development of iBALT has previously been shown in response to viral challenge (21, 22), bacterial infection (23), cigarette smoke (24), and protein nanoparticles (25). Notably, in response to infection with a replication-deficient poxvirus modified vaccinia virus Ankara, iBALT development was independent of both IL-17A and another Th17 effector cytokine, IL-17F (26). Therefore, while common mechanisms involving IL-17 may promote pulmonary TLO development in response to various inflammatory stimuli, it is also important to note that iBALT formation can occur independently of IL-17/Th17 involvement.

Recent studies have also highlighted roles for Th17 cells in TLO development in the central nervous system (CNS), inflamed joint tissues, and salivary glands. Peters et al. demonstrated a role for Th17 cells in promoting TLOs in an experimental model of

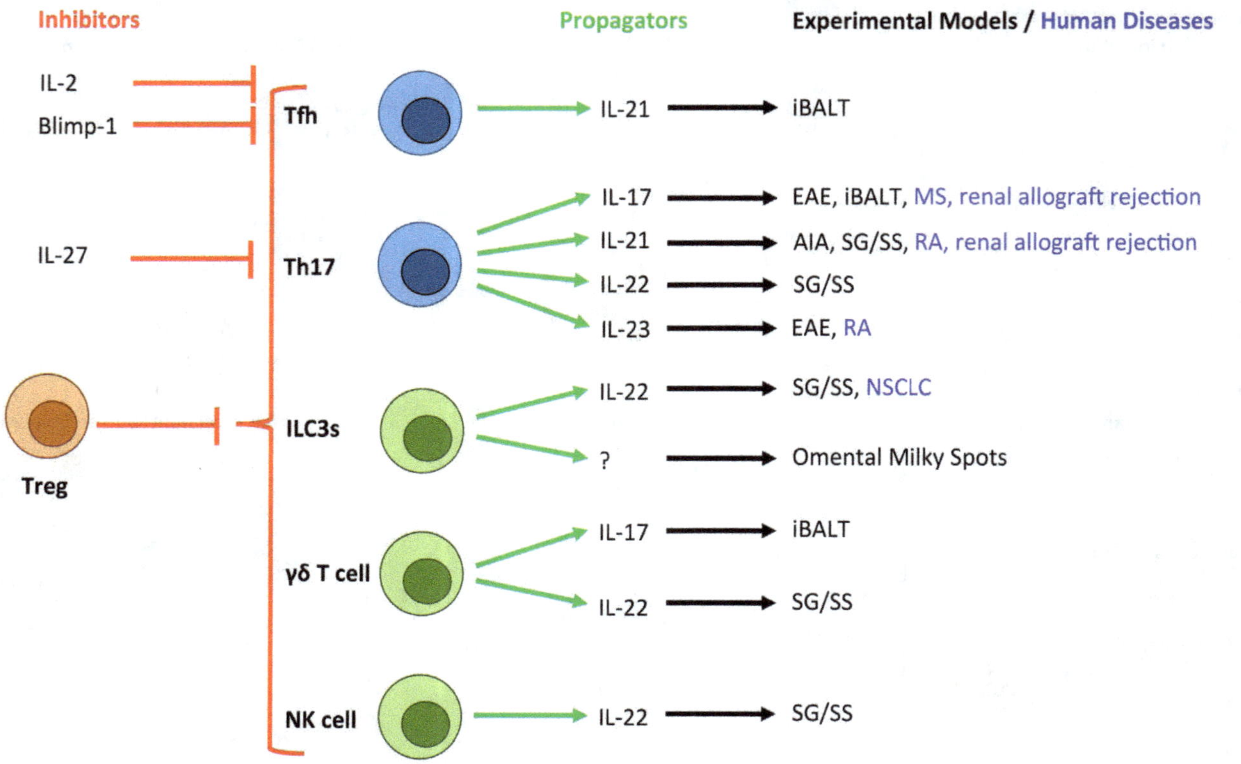

FIGURE 2 | Novel T cell and innate lymphocyte-derived cytokines associated with TLOs in experimental and human diseases. Due to the crucial role that T cells (blue) and innate lymphocyte populations (green) play in the development of TLOs, a number of their secretory cytokines have been associated with tertiary lymphoneogenesis. Here, we show the cytokines and transcription factors associated with positive (green arrows) and negative (red arrows) control of TLOs. T cell-derived IL-2 and activation of Blimp-1 result in suppression of Bcl-6 expression and inhibition of Tfh differentiation. IL-27 is produced by activated antigen-presenting cells and potently inhibits the development of Th17 cells, which have been linked with TLO development. Experimental and human diseases where these cells have been linked with TLO development are shown. Tfh, T follicular helper cell; Th17, T helper 17 cell; ILC3s, group 3 innate lymphoid cells; NK cell, Natural Killer cell; Treg, regulatory T cell; EAE, experimental autoimmune encephalomyelitis; AIA, antigen-induced arthritis; iBALT, inducible bronchus-associated lymphoid tissue; RA, rheumatoid arthritis; MS, multiple sclerosis; NSCLC, non-small cell lung carcinoma; SG/SS, salivary gland infection displaying Sjögren's syndrome-like characteristics.

multiple sclerosis (27). Here, adoptive transfer of *in vitro* generated Th17 cells induced TLOs, which was partly IL-17 dependent. Only Th17 cells differentiated in the presence of IL-23, which maintains Th17 effector function (28, 29), were capable of inducing TLOs. Notably, the adoptive transfer of Th1, Th2, and Th9 cells failed to induce this phenotype. Interestingly, the development of TLOs in this model was also partly dependent on the expression of podoplanin (gp38) on transferred Th17 cells. While an appreciation of a role for podoplanin in regulating T cell responses is only now emerging (30), there is significant evidence for a role in regulating tertiary lymphoneogenesis. For example, we recently described IL-27 as a negative regulator of TLO development in experimental inflammatory arthritis (31). Here, synovial TLO development in IL-27R-deficient mice was associated with an increased number of peripheral podoplanin-expressing Th17 cells and the local recruitment of podoplanin-positive T cells to synovial lymphoid aggregates. The Th17 axis and podoplanin have also been linked with TLO development in human diseases, including rheumatoid arthritis, multiple sclerosis, renal allograft rejection, and giant-cell arteritis (31–35). Therefore, consistent with a key role for podoplanin and its ligand CLEC-2 in lymph node development (11, 27, 36), podoplanin expression on T cells may support the recruitment and retention of leukocytes within TLOs.

While IL-17 stands as the "signature" cytokine for Th17 cells, these cells also produce IL-17F, IL-22, and IL-21. Recently, IL-17 and IL-22 have been shown to induce stromal production of homeostatic chemokines resulting in TLO development in mucosal tissues (37, 38). For example, IL-22 promotes TLO development in salivary glands following local adenovirus delivery (37). Here, the major source of IL-22 was $\alpha\beta^+$ T cells and $\gamma\delta^+$ T cells, which induced the expression of CXCL13 in podoplanin$^+$ stromal cells and CXCL12 in epithelial cells. Therapeutic blockade of IL-22 activity inhibited TLO development and maintenance, thus highlighting IL-22-targeted therapies as a novel approach for the treatment of conditions featuring TLOs and autoantibody-driven disease.

IL-21 plays a central role in Th17 and T follicular helper (Tfh) cell differentiation, the development of naïve B cells into plasma cells or GC B cells, and the generation of high-affinity antibodies (39). Therefore Th17 or Tfh cell-derived IL-21 has potential to play an important role in TLO development and function. Elevated expression of IL-21 has been observed in tissues containing TLOs in experimental and clinical rheumatoid arthritis (31, 32), a model of salivary gland inflammation with Sjögren's syndrome-like characteristics (40) and in human renal grafts undergoing terminal failure (34). A recent study also described the development of TLOs in the retina during experimental uveitis, where TLOs were associated with heightened expression of Tfh cell markers (41). Interestingly, T helper cell plasticity may contribute to the development of TLOs, where T cells may transiently or fully acquire effector characteristics that support tertiary lymphoneogenesis. For example, Th17 cells that migrate and support the development of IgA-producing GC B cells in Peyer's patches acquire a Tfh-like phenotype, including the expression of IL-21, Bcl-6, CXCR5, and PD-1 (42). Similarly, Th17 cells that promote TLO development in the CNS during experimental autoimmune encephalomyelitis develop Tfh-like effector characteristics (27). While the development of TLOs in this latter model was independent of IL-21, the contribution of other Tfh effector characteristics cannot be excluded. Therefore, plasticity among T helper cell subsets may allow for the acquisition of Tfh-like effector characteristics (43, 44) that can support GC reactions and the development of TLOs.

REGULATORY T CELLS AS SUPPRESSORS OF TLO DEVELOPMENT AND FUNCTION

In chronic inflammatory disorders, TLOs are generally considered perpetuators of adaptive immune responses that contribute to pathology. A recent study describing a protective role for TLOs in atherosclerosis (45) raises an interesting question: *How can TLOs in the majority of chronic inflammatory disorders be damaging, yet in some be protective?*

In aged apolipoprotein E (ApoE)-deficient mice with atherosclerosis, smooth muscle cells beneath intimal plaques take on LTo-like properties and secrete CXCL13 and CCL21 to drive tertiary lymphoneogenesis (46). Engagement of the LTβR on smooth muscle cells played a central role in the induction of lymphoneogenic chemokines and the development of aortic TLOs, which were atheroprotective. These TLOs represent principal sites for the regulation of atherosclerotic T cell responses, including the development and activation of anti-inflammatory regulatory T (Treg) cells (45). In these aged mice, highly activated Treg cells within aortic TLOs may skew the local immune response toward anti-atherogenic outcomes by restricting the activation of effector and central memory T cells. Here, communication between aortic TLOs and vascular smooth muscle cells expressing the LTβR may be important in maintaining the structure, size, and composition of TLOs associated with protection from atherosclerosis (45). Notably, another recent study in ApoE-deficient mice outlines a role for regulatory CD8$^+$ T cells in limiting the development of aortic TLOs during atherosclerosis (47). However, this study described a pro-atherogenic role for TLOs in both mouse and human atherosclerosis, where Tfh cells support GC reactions and the local maturation of potentially pathogenic B cells. Therefore, while Treg cells can prevent the development of aortic TLOs, further investigation is needed to determine the precise role played by TLOs during atherogenesis. The relative proportions of pro-inflammatory and Treg cell populations within aortic TLOs may be influenced by factors, such as age, stage of disease, and environmental factors, and may ultimately determine the impact of TLOs on disease progression.

Immunotherapies that inhibit Treg cell development or functionality have the potential of supporting antigen-specific responses against tumor antigens and prevent immune evasion by cancer cells. In this regard, many cancer immunotherapies focus on counteracting the immunosuppressive tumor environment to support tumor-specific T cell responses. The presence of tumor-infiltrating Treg cells is linked with immunosuppression and often correlates with poor patient prognosis (48), while TLOs have been associated with improved patient outcomes in certain cancers (5). This raises an interesting question: *Do therapies targeting Treg activities hold potential for supporting local anti-cancer responses at tumour-associated TLOs?* TLO's have been described in melanoma, mucosal-associated lymphoid tissue lymphoma, and non-small cell lung carcinoma (NSCLC), as well as breast, colorectal, rectal, ovarian, and germ cell cancers [see Dieu-Nosjean et al. (5) for a comprehensive review of TLOs in cancer]. Studies have reported a correlation between the number of TLOs, T/B cell infiltration into tumors and improved patient survival (49–52). In experimental mouse models and human cancers, there is significant evidence that TLOs are functional. For example, in a mouse model of melanoma, tumor-infiltrating lymphocytes developed TLOs and displayed clonal expansion of T cells that are reactive to tumor antigens on melanoma cells and inhibit tumor growth through the release of IFNγ (53, 54). Similar activities were also observed in LTα-deficient mice that lack peripheral lymph nodes, suggesting that T cell responses are primed locally within the tissue (54). In human NSCLC, TLOs are associated with improved patient survival. Here, enhanced anti-tumor immunity is associated with an increased frequency of follicular B cells and plasma cells that display antibody specificity to tumor-associated antigens (50). Therefore, TLO and HEV development in tumors may allow the recruitment of T and B cells that promote GC reactions and anti-tumor immunity.

Some recent studies support the hypothesis that targeting Treg cells can help establish anti-tumor immune responses locally at tumor-associated TLOs. In a mouse model of lung adenocarcinoma, TLOs that included activated Treg cells were observed in ~90% of tumors, where Treg cells suppressed anti-tumor responses (55). In this study, depletion of Treg cells resulted in enhanced expression of costimulatory molecules on dendritic cells (DCs), T cell proliferation, and anti-tumor responses leading to tumor destruction. The development of HEVs, a common feature of TLOs, is also linked with longer remission, reduced metastasis and improved patient survival (5, 56, 57). Here, HEVs allow for the infiltration of naïve, central memory and effector Th1 cells that support the local priming of antigen-specific tumor responses (53, 58, 59). In a model of carcinogen-induced fibrosarcoma, Treg cell depletion resulted in the formation of HEVs and reduced tumor growth associated with an increase in T cell infiltration into tumors (60). Similarly improved outcomes were seen in a murine model of pancreatic cancer following TGFβ blockade, a cytokine involved in both Treg cell development and effector function (61).

In cancerous tissues, Treg cell populations suppress the proliferative expansion of $CD8^+$ T cells responsible for delivering anti-tumor immunity. For example, studies have revealed that depletion of Treg cells contributes to $CD8^+$ T cell proliferation and the development of enhanced anti-tumor responses (55, 60). These findings are highly relevant to human forms of cancer where $CD8^+$ T cells, which are often found in tumor-associated TLOs, are linked with improved patient outcomes. Interestingly, NSCLC patients with a high frequency of $CD8^+$ T cell infiltrates together with a high density of TLOs are associated with significantly improved survival compared to patients with high cytotoxic T cell infiltration without TLOs (51). Thus, tumor-associated TLOs enhance the prognostic value of tumor-infiltrating $CD8^+$ T cells. While such studies demonstrate a correlation between $CD8^+$ T cell infiltration, TLO densities, and patient survival, they also raise an interesting question regarding the function of cytotoxic T cells: *Are tumour infiltrating $CD8^+$ T cells better equipped to control cancer due to their education within tumour-associated TLOs?* While further research is still needed in this area, a recent study of ovarian cancer showed that $CD8^+$ tumor-infiltrating lymphocyte responses were increased in the presence of TLOs containing dense accumulations of plasma cells (62). Here, plasma cells expressed markers of active antigen-specific responses and were associated with heightened expression of cytotoxicity-related genes in tumors. TLOs may, therefore, support robust anti-tumor responses, where cytotoxic T cell activity and antibody-secreting plasma cells cooperate to improve patient survival.

Therapeutic strategies that support the development of tumor-associated TLOs and cytotoxic T cell responses may, therefore, prove beneficial for patient treatment. These may include antagonists of Treg cell development, maintenance, or activity. Blockade of TGFβ has been shown to inhibit Treg cells in experimental cancer and autoimmunity (61, 63). Treg cells can also be selectively depleted by metronomic low-dose cyclophosphamide, which improved tumor-specific T cell responses in cancer patients (64, 65). Further strategies may include antibodies, such as ipilimumab that target the CTLA-4 immune-checkpoint receptor, which has been shown to effectively deplete intratumoural Treg cells (66–68). Novel concepts currently in pre-clinical development may also inform next-generation approaches for inducing TLOs in cancer. For example, engineered adjuvant vector cells have been shown to promote the development of TLOs resulting in enhanced antigen-specific T cell responses in pre-clinical cancer models (69). While the majority of studies relating to Treg cells in TLOs are in the cancer field, these cells have also been implicated in suppressing iBALT development in LPS-challenged mice (70) and TLOs in atherosclerosis (45, 47). Where TLOs offer the potential of disease protection, interventions that block Treg cell activities or target their selective depletion may support the development of TLOs and promote anti-cancer or anti-pathogen responses. Such approaches may represent novel routes to patient treatment. However, such immunotherapeutic strategies must delicately balance establishing strong anti-cancer responses with minimizing the development of autoimmunity. This highlights the need to identify approaches for targeting Treg cells within the tumor microenvironment without compromising their role in maintaining immune tolerance.

INNATE IMMUNE CELLS ASSOCIATED WITH THE DEVELOPMENT OF TLOs

Innate leukocyte subsets have also been implicated in TLO regulation (**Figure 2**). These include roles for neutrophils (70) and innate lymphoid cells (ILCs) (71–73). Innate lymphocytes have recently emerged as important effector cells with roles in host defense and chronic inflammatory diseases. These cells have been termed ILCs and include cytotoxic ILCs represented by conventional NK cells and three new ILC groups that parallel T helper cell subsets in their cytokine-producing capacity and transcriptional programs (ILC1, ILC2, and ILC3) (74). Of these, ILC3s (which includes both prenatal and adult $CCR6^+$ LTi cells) mirror Th17 cells in their expression of the master transcriptional regulator RORγt; the chemokine receptor CCR6; secretion of IL-17, IL-22, and granulocyte-macrophage colony-stimulating factor (GM-CSF); and responsiveness to IL-23 and aryl hydrocarbon receptor (Ahr) ligands (18, 75–77). It is perhaps these similarities in effector characteristics with Th17 cells that result in ILC3s being involved in TLO development (78). For example, adoptive transfer of adult $CD4^+CD3^-$ LTi cells into newborn *Cxcr5*$^{-/-}$ mice, which phenotypically lack Peyer's patches and isolated lymphoid follicles (ILFs), promoted the development of intestinal lymphoid tissues (73). Here, IL-7 supported the *de novo* generation, proliferation, and survival of LTi cells. In another study, the same group demonstrated that transgenic overexpression of IL-7 supported the development of LTi cells that formed Peyer's patches, cecal patches and TLOs that displayed functional T cell-dependent B cell responses and GC reactions (72).

Recently, ILC3s have also been associated with tumor-associated TLOs (71). In NSCLC, natural cytotoxicity receptor (NCR)-expressing ILC3s localized to the edge of TLOs and produced IL-22, TNF, IL-8, and IL-2. These NCR^+ ILC3s interacted with tumor cells and tumor-associated fibroblasts via their NKp44 receptor to trigger production of LTαβ, which resulted in the activation of endothelial cells and mesenchymal stem cells, including upregulation of ICAM-1 and VCAM-1. Thus, ILC3s correlate with the presence of TLOs in NSCLC and may drive the development of lymphoid structures linked with improved patient survival (49).

Innate lymphoid cells have now been associated with TLO development in a number of experimental models of inflammation or infection. While their presence and generation of pro-lymphoneogenic cytokines at TLOs is undisputed, their precise role in tertiary lymphoneogenesis remains to be fully elucidated. For example, ILCs and NK cells contribute to an early production of IL-22 that supports TLO development in salivary glands (37). However, while ILCs may contribute to TLO development in this context, the predominant source of IL-22 in this model were αβ and γδ T cells. Likewise, LTi cells have been found in inflamed lungs that develop iBALT. However, development of these lymphoid aggregates was not reliant on LTi cell activity (19). Intestinal TLOs also develop in response to microbiota in RORγt-deficient mice that lack LTi cells (17). Thus, despite mounting evidence for the presence of ILC3s at TLOs, further research is required to determine a precise role in the initiation of tertiary lymphoneogenesis, where tissue- and disease-specific factors may affect their input. Nevertheless given their presence at TLOs, ILC3s may contribute to the function of TLOs where crosstalk with LTβR-expressing stromal cells and the stimulation of B cells *via* B cell-activation factor (BAFF) and the ligand of costimulatory receptor CD40 (CD40L) has been shown to support antibody production (79–81).

In a similar fashion to ILC3s, γδ T cells can also share effector characteristics with activated Th17 cells, including the secretion of IL-17A, IL-17F, IL-22, IL-21, and GM-CSF (78). While the precise role of γδ T cells in TLO development is also unclear, there is evidence that they contribute to early tertiary lymphoneogenesis. In mice displaying iBALT in response to *Pseudomonas aeruginosa* infection, IL-17 triggered stromal cell differentiation into podoplanin$^+$ follicular cells that express CXCL12 (38). Here, γδ T cells were the main source of IL-17. Similarly, development of iBALT in LPS-challenged neonatal mice is also IL-17 dependent, where both γδ and αβ T cells secrete IL-17 (19). Adoptive transfer experiments revealed that while γδ T cells facilitated the development of iBALT, αβ T cells formed larger areas of lymphoid aggregates. It has, therefore, been proposed that an early innate γδ T cell response initiates the development of iBALT, which is later maintained by infiltrating αβ T cells (19, 82). A similar role for γδ T cells in TLO development may occur in salivary glands, where an early prominent IL-22-producing γδ T cell response is later replaced by αβ T cells (37).

Fat-associated lymphoid clusters (FALCs) are TLO-like structures that develop within adipose tissues, including the mesentery, pericardial fat, and milky spots of the omentum (3). Interestingly, milky spots of the omentum increase in number and size during peritoneal dialysis (83, 84). During treatment, catheter insertion, exposure to peritoneal dialysis solution and particularly peritonitis associated with infection results in the expansion and alteration of the cellular composition of milky spots. This suggests an active role for milky spots in peritoneal immunity. Studies in mice demonstrate that the omentum senses peritoneal antigens and represents a site for generating adaptive T cell (CD4$^+$ and CD8$^+$) and B cell responses, including antibody class switching and somatic hypermutation (85, 86). In these studies, the development of milky spots was independent of LTi/ILC3s and LTαβ, but required stromal CXCL13 for the recruitment of B-1 cells. Interestingly, TNF-expressing myeloid cells, NKT cells, and IL-4R signaling were required for FALC formation following inflammatory challenge (86). This study and others have also demonstrated that FALCs can contain ILC2 cells. For example, during helminth infection, Lin$^-$c-Kit$^+$Sca-1$^+$ cells produce Th2-type cytokines that support B-1 cell proliferation and drive goblet cell hyperplasia (87). Therefore, FALCs, including milky spots, play a role in regulating local immune responses. However, while they display similarities to TLOs, they are often less organized structures with fewer T cells and fDCs and are highly enriched for B-1 cells (3, 85).

Dendritic cells prime adaptive immune responses via antigen processing and presentation to T cells. While DCs are a common feature of TLOs, relatively little is known regarding their precise role in tertiary lymphoneogenesis. This gap in knowledge was addressed by two investigations. First, CD11c^{hi} DCs were identified as being essential for the long-term maintenance and function of iBALT following influenza virus infection (22). Here, depletion of DCs resulted in a loss of LTβ, CXCL13, CCL21, CCL19, and CXCL12 expression that disrupted the structural integrity and cellular organization of iBALT. This was associated with a reduced number of class-switched plasma cells in the lung and a lowering of antiviral serum IgG titers. In a similar approach, Halle et al. used a replication-deficient modified vaccinia virus Ankara to demonstrate that antigen-loaded DCs migrate into iBALT to support the activation of antigen-specific T cells (21). Thus, TLO-associated DCs are a major source of homeostatic chemokines and lymphoid cytokines that support the long-term maintenance of TLOs and encourage the generation of adaptive immune responses through local T cell priming and control of GC reactions.

FOLLICULAR B CELLS DRIVE AUTOANTIBODY-MEDIATED DISEASES AT TLOs

For TLOs to fully recapitulate the function of SLOs they must provide an environment for B cells to undergo affinity maturation and differentiation into memory B cells and antibody-secreting plasma cells (**Figure 3**). Active GCs express activation-induced cytidine deaminase (AID; also known as AICDA), which promotes somatic hypermutation and class-switch recombination to fine-tune antibody specificity and expand antibody-mediated effector functions (88, 89). In support of TLOs being factories for the development of adaptive immune responses, AID is expressed at TLOs in autoimmunity (7, 90–92), infection (93), and transplant rejection (34). Indeed, analysis of the variable (V)-gene repertoires in TLOs from inflamed tissues reveals a restricted profile of encoded sequences, indicating a clonal expansion of antigen-specific B cells within these lymphoid aggregates (91, 94–96). Furthermore, analysis of Iγ–Cμ and Iα–Cμ circular transcript expression reveals on-going class-switch recombination from IgM to IgG and IgA respectively at TLOs (7, 91, 97). Therefore, significant evidence exists to demonstrate that TLOs can contain functional GCs.

While TLOs may generally be considered protective in infection and cancer, GC activity at TLOs in autoimmunity can result in the local generation of disease-specific autoantibodies that perpetuate disease progression. For example, autoreactive plasma cells release autoantibodies, such as anti-citrullinated protein antibodies (ACPA/anti-CCP) in rheumatoid arthritis (7); antibodies targeting ribonucleoproteins Ro (Sjögren's syndrome antigen A; SSA) and La (Sjögren's syndrome antigen B; SSB) in Sjögren's syndrome (98); anti-thyroglobulin and thyroperoxidase antibodies in Hashimoto's thyroiditis (99); and nicotinic acetylcholine receptor-specific antibodies in myasthenia gravis (100). The mechanisms that allow autoreactive B cells to accumulate

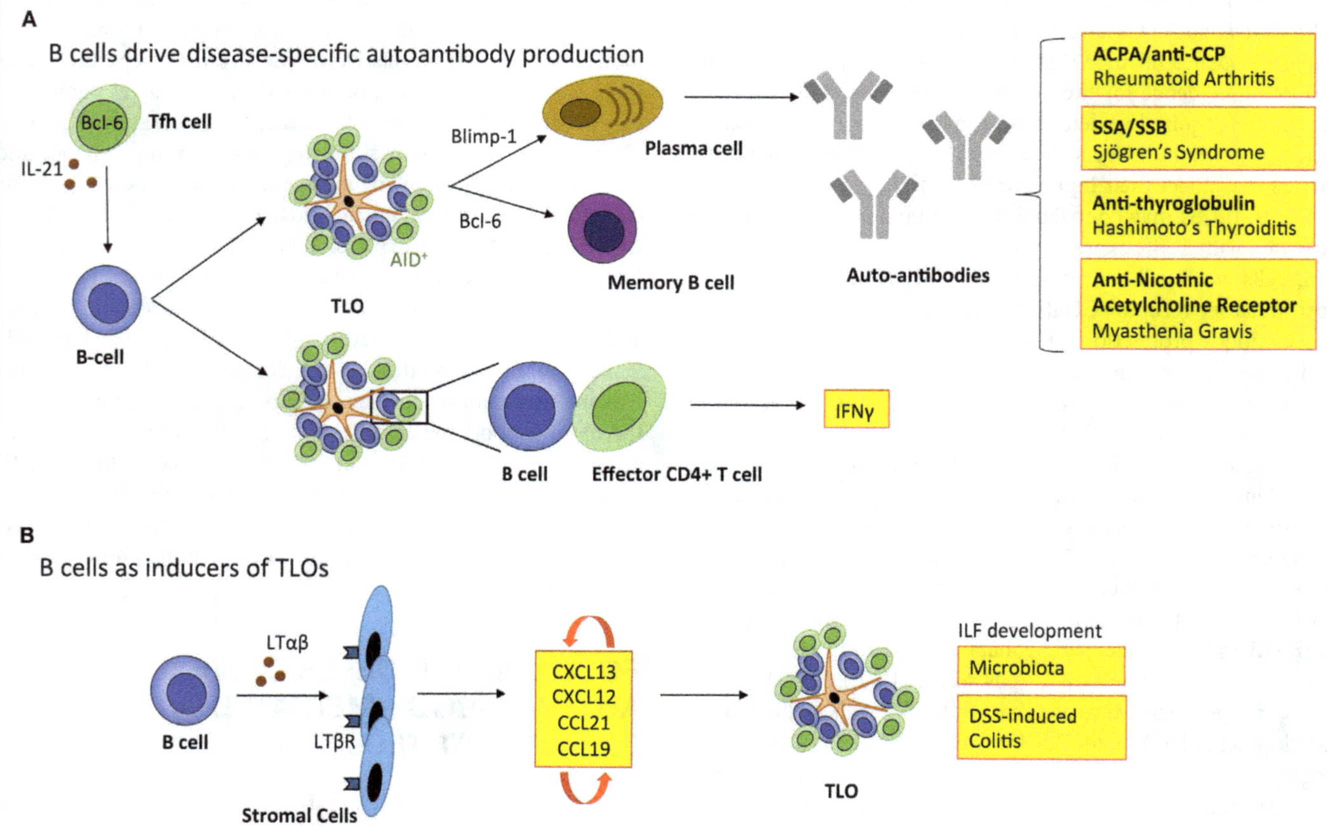

FIGURE 3 | B cells regulate tertiary lymphoid organ development and function. **(A)** B cells enable TLOs to recapitulate the function of SLOs. Tfh cells support B cell responses in lymphoid organs. The inverse relationship between Blimp-1 and Bcl-6 governs B cell differentiation into memory B cells or immunoglobulin producing plasma cells. In TLOs, the local generation of disease-specific autoantibodies contributes to disease progression. The expression of activation-induced cytidine deaminase (AID) within TLOs marks active class switching and somatic hypermutation that fine-tunes antibody specificity and effector functions. Also, B cells within TLOs can support T cell effector function, including the secretion of IFNγ. **(B)** B cells can also adopt LTi-like characteristics to promote the development of isolated lymphoid follicles (ILFs) in the small intestine in response to microbiota and dextran sulfate sodium (DSS)-induced colitis. Here, the interaction between B cells and resident stromal cells leads to the production of homeostatic chemokines (CXCL13, CXCL12, CCL21, and CCL19) triggering the recruitment of lymphocytes that initiate lymphoid organ development. Tfh, T follicular helper cell; ACPA/anti-CCP, anti-citrullinated protein antibodies; SSA, Sjögrens syndrome antigen A; SSB, Sjögrens syndrome antigen B; LTαβ, lymphotoxin αβ; LTβR, lymphotoxin β receptor; IFNγ, interferon-γ.

within TLOs (101), when they are efficiently eliminated from GCs in SLOs are currently unclear. In SLOs autoreactive B cells become anergic and are excluded from follicular entry through downregulation of CXCR5, the receptor for CXCL13 (102). Emerging evidence points to a potential role for latent Epstein–Barr virus (EBV) in the development of autoimmunity at TLOs. EBV is a life-long infection, and infected B cells display increased proliferation and survival (103). EBV-infected cells are often observed within TLOs in the inflamed tissues of patients affected by autoimmunity, including rheumatoid arthritis, Sjögren's syndrome, multiple sclerosis, and myasthenia gravis (92, 104–106). For example, infected B cells display autoreactivity toward citrullinated fibrinogen and ribonucleoprotein Ro, the disease-specific autoantigens for rheumatoid arthritis and Sjögren's syndrome, respectively (105, 106). Therefore, EBV-infected autoreactive B cells may migrate to target tissues where they differentiate into autoantibody secreting plasma cells and perpetuate autoimmunity.

In addition to their classical role in generating antibody responses, B cells also support local immune cell activation within inflamed tissues. Using an experimental model where synovial biopsies comprising TLOs from rheumatoid arthritis patients are transplanted into severe combined immunodeficient mice (the HuRA-SCID model), Takemura and co-workers demonstrated that depletion of B cells from grafted synovial tissue resulted in a reduction in T cell derived IFNγ production and IL-1β secretion (107). Hence, synovial B cells contribute to T helper cell effector responses in rheumatoid synovitis to influence disease progression.

Typically when addressing the role of B cells in TLOs, the development of antigen-specific antibody responses is the primary consideration. However, B cells have long been known to produce LTαβ, which suggested a potential role in lymphoid neogenesis or the maintenance of lymphoid organs (108). More recently, a role for B cells in promoting the development of ILFs in the small intestine was described (109). Studies using bone marrow chimeric mice demonstrated that LTαβ-producing B cells were required for the development of these TLO-like structures. Similarly, Lochner et al. describe a LTαβ-dependent LTi-like role for B cells in the development of TLOs in dextran sulfate sodium (DSS)-induced colitis (17). This suggests that deploying B cell targeted therapies for the treatment of TLO-associated autoimmune diseases, such as rheumatoid arthritis has the potential to interfere with both early initiation of TLO development and the long-term maintenance of autoantibody responses and local T cell priming. However, in this context, an improved understanding of B cell targeted therapies (e.g., rituximab) is needed, where studies evaluate the peripheral effect on SLOs as well as the local impact on TLOs in inflamed tissues.

IMMUNE CELL–STROMAL CELL CROSSTALK IS CENTRAL TO TLO DEVELOPMENT AND FUNCTION

Our understanding of immune cells in the development, function, and maintenance of TLOs has greatly expanded in recent years. While this review is primarily focused on the role of immune cells, it is also important to emphasize the importance of immune cell–stromal cell crosstalk in the development and function of TLOs [comprehensively reviewed elsewhere (110)]. While immune cells adopt LTi-like functions to drive the development of TLOs during inflammation, activated resident stromal cells must phenotypically respond like LTo cells. For example, lung inflammation resulting in the development of iBALT in mice is dependent on immune cell derived IL-17, which triggers CXCL13 and CCL19 expression to recruit and organize lymphocytes (19). While early induction of CXCL13 and CCL19 expression was LTα-independent, once established, homeostatic chemokines and engagement of the LTβR was required for the maintenance of iBALT. Such observations suggest that the dual targeting of both IL-17 and LT signaling may be beneficial for the management of diseases where TLOs are a feature of local pathology. Similar studies using an influenza infection model revealed PNAd^{+} HEVs and stromal cells are the primary source of CXCL13, CCL21, and CCL19 during iBALT development (111). In other infection models that feature TLOs, effector cytokines, such as IL-17 and IL-22, have been shown to drive stromal cell differentiation toward podoplanin-positive CXCL12 and CXCL13 expressing cells (37, 38). Such experimental observations also translate into human disease, where the stromal cell response to inflammation contributes to TLO development. For example, in rheumatoid arthritis patients who display TLOs in inflamed joint tissue, synovial fibroblasts display LTo-like properties including the production of homeostatic chemokines and the induction of BAFF, which supports synovial B cell responses (112–114). Recently, several illustrative examples have further emphasized the significance of immune cell–stromal cell interactions. A highly novel role for TLOs as niches for the maturation of malignant hepatocellular carcinoma progenitor cells was recently described (115). Here, carcinoma progenitor cells exiting TLOs supported tumor growth and outline a detrimental role for TLOs in cancer. Consequently, further work is required to establish the context in which TLOs contribute to the tumor microenvironment. Crosstalk between Th17 cells and stromal cells was also recently shown to be important in an experimental model of multiple sclerosis, where stromal LTβR signaling promoted extracellular matrix deposition, T cell effector cytokine responses, and chemokine production that supported leukocyte retention in the meninges (116). Similarly, in experimental atherosclerosis, vascular smooth muscle cells provided LTo-like function within atherosclerotic aortas to support the development and maintenance of protective TLOs (45). Thus, while immune cells provide a trigger for the development of TLOs in inflamed tissues, the response of stromal cells is equally important in providing an environment conducive to lymphoid neogenesis.

CONCLUDING REMARKS

Studies in recent years have increasingly highlighted potent roles for TLOs in regulating local immune responses in conditions featuring chronic inflammation. Experimental models of disease have provided mechanistic insight and identified novel immune cell subsets involved in TLO regulation, as well as verifying a role for TLOs in pathologic processes. Similarly, studies in human diseases have clearly demonstrated the presence, function, and correlative associations of TLOs with disease severity. However, further research is required to better define the precise role of TLOs in these clinical conditions. Here, it will be important to evaluate the prognostic and diagnostic potential of TLOs in specific diseases, their potential as novel therapeutic targets, as well as to determine how diseases with significant TLO involvement respond to the current arsenal of biologic interventions used in routine clinical practice. In this regard, research into the impact of TLOs in rheumatoid arthritis has provided valuable insight. For example, evidence suggests that rheumatoid arthritis patients with TLOs in inflamed joint tissues display an inferior response to frontline biological therapies that target TNF (8). Therefore, patients with synovial TLOs may be managed better using alternative biological therapies. Given the central role played by TLO B cells in the production of disease-specific autoantibodies, rituximab (an anti-CD20 B cell depleting antibody) may be a better alternative. While further research is needed in this area, two studies oppose this prediction. The first demonstrates that while rituximab treatment results in a reduction of disease-specific autoantibodies (rheumatoid factor and ACPA/anti-CCP) in patient serum, this treatment failed to reduce the local production of these autoantibodies in lymphoid aggregate-containing joint tissue (9). The second study in chronic renal allograft rejection similarly demonstrates that while rituximab treatment depleted peripheral B cells, surprisingly, intragraft B cells in TLOs evaded depletion (117). Thus, B cells residing within the TLO microenvironment may receive signals that allow them to survive rituximab treatment (117). Given the recent emergence of IL-17, and Th17- and Tfh-associated cytokines in the development of TLOs, it will now be interesting to see how targeting these axes fares in the management of TLO-associated diseases. While IL-17-targeted modalities have shown limited clinical efficacy in inflammatory arthritis (118, 119), these clinical trials did not stratify patients for the presence of synovial TLOs. In inflammatory arthritis, sampling of synovial tissue through ultrasound-directed biopsies has become more common in clinical trial design, and have provided new insight into the impact of intervention on TLOs (120). Such approaches may pave the way to identifying optimal strategies for the clinical management of TLO-associated diseases. The success of such approaches may prove important is shaping how clinicians evaluate the diagnosis and treatment of other chronic conditions.

AUTHOR CONTRIBUTIONS

GJ, DH, and SJ co-wrote the manuscript and prepared the figures.

FUNDING

GJ and SJ are supported by career development fellowship and programme grant funding from Arthritis Research UK (20305, 20770). DH is funded by a Medical Research Council Ph.D. studentship.

REFERENCES

1. van de Pavert SA, Mebius RE. New insights into the development of lymphoid tissues. *Nat Rev Immunol* (2010) 10(9):664–74. doi:10.1038/nri2832
2. Kurashima Y, Goto Y, Kiyono H. Mucosal innate immune cells regulate both gut homeostasis and intestinal inflammation. *Eur J Immunol* (2013) 43(12):3108–15. doi:10.1002/eji.201343782
3. Randall TD, Mebius RE. The development and function of mucosal lymphoid tissues: a balancing act with micro-organisms. *Mucosal Immunol* (2014) 7(3):455–66. doi:10.1038/mi.2014.11
4. Pitzalis C, Jones GW, Bombardieri M, Jones SA. Ectopic lymphoid-like structures in infection, cancer and autoimmunity. *Nat Rev Immunol* (2014) 14(7):447–62. doi:10.1038/nri3700
5. Dieu-Nosjean MC, Goc J, Giraldo NA, Sautes-Fridman C, Fridman WH. Tertiary lymphoid structures in cancer and beyond. *Trends Immunol* (2014) 35(11):571–80. doi:10.1016/j.it.2014.09.006
6. Chen SC, Vassileva G, Kinsley D, Holzmann S, Manfra D, Wiekowski MT, et al. Ectopic expression of the murine chemokines CCL21a and CCL21b induces the formation of lymph node-like structures in pancreas, but not skin, of transgenic mice. *J Immunol* (2002) 168(3):1001–8. doi:10.4049/jimmunol.168.3.1001
7. Humby F, Bombardieri M, Manzo A, Kelly S, Blades MC, Kirkham B, et al. Ectopic lymphoid structures support ongoing production of class-switched autoantibodies in rheumatoid synovium. *PLoS Med* (2009) 6(1):e1. doi:10.1371/journal.pmed.0060001
8. Canete JD, Celis R, Moll C, Izquierdo E, Marsal S, Sanmarti R, et al. Clinical significance of synovial lymphoid neogenesis and its reversal after anti-tumour necrosis factor alpha therapy in rheumatoid arthritis. *Ann Rheum Dis* (2009) 68(5):751–6. doi:10.1136/ard.2008.089284
9. Rosengren S, Wei N, Kalunian KC, Zvaifler NJ, Kavanaugh A, Boyle DL. Elevated autoantibody content in rheumatoid arthritis synovia with lymphoid aggregates and the effect of rituximab. *Arthritis Res Ther* (2008) 10(5):R105. doi:10.1186/ar2497
10. Drayton DL, Liao S, Mounzer RH, Ruddle NH. Lymphoid organ development: from ontogeny to neogenesis. *Nat Immunol* (2006) 7(4):344–53. doi:10.1038/ni1330
11. Peduto L, Dulauroy S, Lochner M, Spath GF, Morales MA, Cumano A, et al. Inflammation recapitulates the ontogeny of lymphoid stromal cells. *J Immunol* (2009) 182(9):5789–99. doi:10.4049/jimmunol.0803974
12. Vondenhoff MF, Greuter M, Goverse G, Elewaut D, Dewint P, Ware CF, et al. LTbetaR signaling induces cytokine expression and up-regulates lymphangiogenic factors in lymph node anlagen. *J Immunol* (2009) 182(9):5439–45. doi:10.4049/jimmunol.0801165
13. Bajenoff M, Egen JG, Koo LY, Laugier JP, Brau F, Glaichenhaus N, et al. Stromal cell networks regulate lymphocyte entry, migration, and territoriality in lymph nodes. *Immunity* (2006) 25(6):989–1001. doi:10.1016/j.immuni.2006.10.011
14. Jarjour M, Jorquera A, Mondor I, Wienert S, Narang P, Coles MC, et al. Fate mapping reveals origin and dynamics of lymph node follicular dendritic cells. *J Exp Med* (2014) 211(6):1109–22. doi:10.1084/jem.20132409
15. Katakai T. Marginal reticular cells: a stromal subset directly descended from the lymphoid tissue organizer. *Front Immunol* (2012) 3:200. doi:10.3389/fimmu.2012.00200
16. Cherrier M, Sawa S, Eberl G. Notch, Id2, and RORgammat sequentially orchestrate the fetal development of lymphoid tissue inducer cells. *J Exp Med* (2012) 209(4):729–40. doi:10.1084/jem.20111594
17. Lochner M, Ohnmacht C, Presley L, Bruhns P, Si-Tahar M, Sawa S, et al. Microbiota-induced tertiary lymphoid tissues aggravate inflammatory disease in the absence of RORgamma t and LTi cells. *J Exp Med* (2011) 208(1):125–34. doi:10.1084/jem.20100052
18. Sawa S, Cherrier M, Lochner M, Satoh-Takayama N, Fehling HJ, Langa F, et al. Lineage relationship analysis of RORgammat+ innate lymphoid cells. *Science* (2010) 330(6004):665–9. doi:10.1126/science.1194597
19. Rangel-Moreno J, Carragher DM, de la Luz Garcia-Hernandez M, Hwang JY, Kusser K, Hartson L, et al. The development of inducible bronchus-associated lymphoid tissue depends on IL-17. *Nat Immunol* (2011) 12(7):639–46. doi:10.1038/ni.2053
20. Grogan JL, Ouyang W. A role for Th17 cells in the regulation of tertiary lymphoid follicles. *Eur J Immunol* (2012) 42(9):2255–62. doi:10.1002/eji.201242656
21. Halle S, Dujardin HC, Bakocevic N, Fleige H, Danzer H, Willenzon S, et al. Induced bronchus-associated lymphoid tissue serves as a general priming site for T cells and is maintained by dendritic cells. *J Exp Med* (2009) 206(12):2593–601. doi:10.1084/jem.20091472
22. GeurtsvanKessel CH, Willart MA, Bergen IM, van Rijt LS, Muskens F, Elewaut D, et al. Dendritic cells are crucial for maintenance of tertiary lymphoid structures in the lung of influenza virus-infected mice. *J Exp Med* (2009) 206(11):2339–49. doi:10.1084/jem.20090410
23. Kahnert A, Hopken UE, Stein M, Bandermann S, Lipp M, Kaufmann SH. Mycobacterium tuberculosis triggers formation of lymphoid structure in murine lungs. *J Infect Dis* (2007) 195(1):46–54. doi:10.1086/508894
24. Escolar Castellon JD, Escolar Castellon A, Roche Roche PA, Minana Amada C. Bronchial-associated lymphoid tissue (BALT) response to airway challenge with cigarette smoke, bovine antigen and anti-pulmonary serum. *Histol Histopathol* (1992) 7(3):321–8.
25. Wiley JA, Richert LE, Swain SD, Harmsen A, Barnard DL, Randall TD, et al. Inducible bronchus-associated lymphoid tissue elicited by a protein cage nanoparticle enhances protection in mice against diverse respiratory viruses. *PLoS One* (2009) 4(9):e7142. doi:10.1371/journal.pone.0007142
26. Fleige H, Haas JD, Stahl FR, Willenzon S, Prinz I, Forster R. Induction of BALT in the absence of IL-17. *Nat Immunol* (2012) 13(1):1. doi:10.1038/ni.2167 author reply 2
27. Peters A, Pitcher LA, Sullivan JM, Mitsdoerffer M, Acton SE, Franz B, et al. Th17 cells induce ectopic lymphoid follicles in central nervous system tissue inflammation. *Immunity* (2011) 35(6):986–96. doi:10.1016/j.immuni.2011.10.015
28. McGeachy MJ, Chen Y, Tato CM, Laurence A, Joyce-Shaikh B, Blumenschein WM, et al. The interleukin 23 receptor is essential for the terminal differentiation of interleukin 17-producing effector T helper cells in vivo. *Nat Immunol* (2009) 10(3):314–24. doi:10.1038/ni.1698
29. Stritesky GL, Yeh N, Kaplan MH. IL-23 promotes maintenance but not commitment to the Th17 lineage. *J Immunol* (2008) 181(9):5948–55. doi:10.4049/jimmunol.181.9.5948
30. Peters A, Burkett PR, Sobel RA, Buckley CD, Watson SP, Bettelli E, et al. Podoplanin negatively regulates CD4+ effector T cell responses. *J Clin Invest* (2015) 125(1):129–40. doi:10.1172/JCI74685

31. Jones GW, Bombardieri M, Greenhill CJ, McLeod L, Nerviani A, Rocher-Ros V, et al. Interleukin-27 inhibits ectopic lymphoid-like structure development in early inflammatory arthritis. *J Exp Med* (2015) 212(11):1793–802. doi:10.1084/jem.20132307
32. Canete JD, Celis R, Yeremenko N, Sanmarti R, van Duivenvoorde L, Ramirez J, et al. Ectopic lymphoid neogenesis is strongly associated with activation of the IL-23 pathway in rheumatoid synovitis. *Arthritis Res Ther* (2015) 17:173. doi:10.1186/s13075-015-0688-0
33. Chaitanya GV, Omura S, Sato F, Martinez NE, Minagar A, Ramanathan M, et al. Inflammation induces neuro-lymphatic protein expression in multiple sclerosis brain neurovasculature. *J Neuroinflammation* (2013) 10:125. doi:10.1186/1742-2094-10-125
34. Deteix C, Attuil-Audenis V, Duthey A, Patey N, McGregor B, Dubois V, et al. Intragraft Th17 infiltrate promotes lymphoid neogenesis and hastens clinical chronic rejection. *J Immunol* (2010) 184(9):5344–51. doi:10.4049/jimmunol.0902999
35. Ciccia F, Rizzo A, Maugeri R, Alessandro R, Croci S, Guggino G, et al. Ectopic expression of CXCL13, BAFF, APRIL and LT-beta is associated with artery tertiary lymphoid organs in giant cell arteritis. *Ann Rheum Dis* (2016). doi:10.1136/annrheumdis-2016-209217
36. Benezech C, Nayar S, Finney BA, Withers DR, Lowe K, Desanti GE, et al. CLEC-2 is required for development and maintenance of lymph nodes. *Blood* (2014) 123(20):3200–7. doi:10.1182/blood-2013-03-489286
37. Barone F, Nayar S, Campos J, Cloake T, Withers DR, Toellner KM, et al. IL-22 regulates lymphoid chemokine production and assembly of tertiary lymphoid organs. *Proc Natl Acad Sci U S A* (2015) 112(35):11024–9. doi:10.1073/pnas.1503315112
38. Fleige H, Ravens S, Moschovakis GL, Bolter J, Willenzon S, Sutter G, et al. IL-17-induced CXCL12 recruits B cells and induces follicle formation in BALT in the absence of differentiated FDCs. *J Exp Med* (2014) 211(4):643–51. doi:10.1084/jem.20131737
39. Spolski R, Leonard WJ. Interleukin-21: a double-edged sword with therapeutic potential. *Nat Rev Drug Discov* (2014) 13(5):379–95. doi:10.1038/nrd4296
40. Bombardieri M, Barone F, Lucchesi D, Nayar S, van den Berg WB, Proctor G, et al. Inducible tertiary lymphoid structures, autoimmunity, and exocrine dysfunction in a novel model of salivary gland inflammation in C57BL/6 mice. *J Immunol* (2012) 189(7):3767–76. doi:10.4049/jimmunol.1201216
41. Kielczewski JL, Horai R, Jittayasothorn Y, Chan CC, Caspi RR. Tertiary lymphoid tissue forms in retinas of mice with spontaneous autoimmune uveitis and has consequences on visual function. *J Immunol* (2016) 196(3):1013–25. doi:10.4049/jimmunol.1501570
42. Hirota K, Turner JE, Villa M, Duarte JH, Demengeot J, Steinmetz OM, et al. Plasticity of Th17 cells in Peyer's patches is responsible for the induction of T cell-dependent IgA responses. *Nat Immunol* (2013) 14(4):372–9. doi:10.1038/ni.2552
43. Lu KT, Kanno Y, Cannons JL, Handon R, Bible P, Elkahloun AG, et al. Functional and epigenetic studies reveal multistep differentiation and plasticity of in vitro-generated and in vivo-derived follicular T helper cells. *Immunity* (2011) 35(4):622–32. doi:10.1016/j.immuni.2011.07.015
44. Nakayamada S, Kanno Y, Takahashi H, Jankovic D, Lu KT, Johnson TA, et al. Early Th1 cell differentiation is marked by a Tfh cell-like transition. *Immunity* (2011) 35(6):919–31. doi:10.1016/j.immuni.2011.11.012
45. Hu D, Mohanta SK, Yin C, Peng L, Ma Z, Srikakulapu P, et al. Artery tertiary lymphoid organs control aorta immunity and protect against atherosclerosis via vascular smooth muscle cell lymphotoxin beta receptors. *Immunity* (2015) 42(6):1100–15. doi:10.1016/j.immuni.2015.05.015
46. Grabner R, Lotzer K, Dopping S, Hildner M, Radke D, Beer M, et al. Lymphotoxin beta receptor signaling promotes tertiary lymphoid organogenesis in the aorta adventitia of aged ApoE-/- mice. *J Exp Med* (2009) 206(1):233–48. doi:10.1084/jem.20080752
47. Clement M, Guedj K, Andreata F, Morvan M, Bey L, Khallou-Laschet J, et al. Control of the T follicular helper-germinal center B-cell axis by CD8(+) regulatory T cells limits atherosclerosis and tertiary lymphoid organ development. *Circulation* (2015) 131(6):560–70. doi:10.1161/CIRCULATIONAHA.114.010988
48. Fridman WH, Pages F, Sautes-Fridman C, Galon J. The immune contexture in human tumours: impact on clinical outcome. *Nat Rev Cancer* (2012) 12(4):298–306. doi:10.1038/nrc3245
49. Dieu-Nosjean MC, Antoine M, Danel C, Heudes D, Wislez M, Poulot V, et al. Long-term survival for patients with non-small-cell lung cancer with intratumoral lymphoid structures. *J Clin Oncol* (2008) 26(27):4410–7. doi:10.1200/JCO.2007.15.0284
50. Germain C, Gnjatic S, Tamzalit F, Knockaert S, Remark R, Goc J, et al. Presence of B cells in tertiary lymphoid structures is associated with a protective immunity in patients with lung cancer. *Am J Respir Crit Care Med* (2014) 189(7):832–44. doi:10.1164/rccm.201309-1611OC
51. Goc J, Germain C, Vo-Bourgais TK, Lupo A, Klein C, Knockaert S, et al. Dendritic cells in tumor-associated tertiary lymphoid structures signal a Th1 cytotoxic immune contexture and license the positive prognostic value of infiltrating CD8+ T cells. *Cancer Res* (2014) 74(3):705–15. doi:10.1158/0008-5472.CAN-13-1342
52. Ladanyi A, Kiss J, Somlai B, Gilde K, Fejos Z, Mohos A, et al. Density of DC-LAMP(+) mature dendritic cells in combination with activated T lymphocytes infiltrating primary cutaneous melanoma is a strong independent prognostic factor. *Cancer Immunol Immunother* (2007) 56(9):1459–69. doi:10.1007/s00262-007-0286-3
53. Schrama D, thor Straten P, Fischer WH, McLellan AD, Brocker EB, Reisfeld RA, et al. Targeting of lymphotoxin-alpha to the tumor elicits an efficient immune response associated with induction of peripheral lymphoid-like tissue. *Immunity* (2001) 14(2):111–21. doi:10.1016/S1074-7613(01)00094-2
54. Kirk CJ, Hartigan-O'Connor D, Mule JJ. The dynamics of the T-cell antitumor response: chemokine-secreting dendritic cells can prime tumor-reactive T cells extranodally. *Cancer Res* (2001) 61(24):8794–802.
55. Joshi NS, Akama-Garren EH, Lu Y, Lee DY, Chang GP, Li A, et al. Regulatory T cells in tumor-associated tertiary lymphoid structures suppress anti-tumor T cell responses. *Immunity* (2015) 43(3):579–90. doi:10.1016/j.immuni.2015.08.006
56. Martinet L, Filleron T, Le Guellec S, Rochaix P, Garrido I, Girard JP. High endothelial venule blood vessels for tumor-infiltrating lymphocytes are associated with lymphotoxin beta-producing dendritic cells in human breast cancer. *J Immunol* (2013) 191(4):2001–8. doi:10.4049/jimmunol.1300872
57. Martinet L, Garrido I, Filleron T, Le Guellec S, Bellard E, Fournie JJ, et al. Human solid tumors contain high endothelial venules: association with T- and B-lymphocyte infiltration and favorable prognosis in breast cancer. *Cancer Res* (2011) 71(17):5678–87. doi:10.1158/0008-5472.CAN-11-0431
58. Martinet L, Le Guellec S, Filleron T, Lamant L, Meyer N, Rochaix P, et al. High endothelial venules (HEVs) in human melanoma lesions: major gateways for tumor-infiltrating lymphocytes. *Oncoimmunology* (2012) 1(6):829–39. doi:10.4161/onci.20492
59. Schrama D, Voigt H, Eggert AO, Xiang R, Zhou H, Schumacher TN, et al. Immunological tumor destruction in a murine melanoma model by targeted LTalpha independent of secondary lymphoid tissue. *Cancer Immunol Immunother* (2008) 57(1):85–95. doi:10.1007/s00262-007-0352-x
60. Hindley JP, Jones E, Smart K, Bridgeman H, Lauder SN, Ondondo B, et al. T-cell trafficking facilitated by high endothelial venules is required for tumor control after regulatory T-cell depletion. *Cancer Res* (2012) 72(21):5473–82. doi:10.1158/0008-5472.CAN-12-1912
61. Soares KC, Rucki AA, Kim V, Foley K, Solt S, Wolfgang CL, et al. TGF-beta blockade depletes T regulatory cells from metastatic pancreatic tumors in a vaccine dependent manner. *Oncotarget* (2015) 6(40):43005–15. doi:10.18632/oncotarget.5656
62. Kroeger DR, Milne K, Nelson BH. Tumor-infiltrating plasma cells are associated with tertiary lymphoid structures, cytolytic t-cell responses, and superior prognosis in ovarian cancer. *Clin Cancer Res* (2016) 22(12):3005–15. doi:10.1158/1078-0432.CCR-15-2762
63. Powrie F, Carlino J, Leach MW, Mauze S, Coffman RL. A critical role for transforming growth factor-beta but not interleukin 4 in the suppression of T helper type 1-mediated colitis by CD45RB(low) CD4+ T cells. *J Exp Med* (1996) 183(6):2669–74. doi:10.1084/jem.183.6.2669
64. Ghiringhelli F, Menard C, Puig PE, Ladoire S, Roux S, Martin F, et al. Metronomic cyclophosphamide regimen selectively depletes CD4+CD25+ regulatory T cells and restores T and NK effector functions in end stage cancer patients. *Cancer Immunol Immunother* (2007) 56(5):641–8. doi:10.1007/s00262-006-0225-8
65. Scurr M, Bloom A, Pembroke T, Srinivasan R, Brown C, Smart K, et al. Escalating regulation of 5T4-specific IFN-gamma+ CD4+ T cells

distinguishes colorectal cancer patients from healthy controls and provides a target for *in vivo* therapy. *Cancer Immunol Res* (2013) 1(6):416–25. doi:10.1158/2326-6066.CIR-13-0035
66. Marabelle A, Kohrt H, Sagiv-Barfi I, Ajami B, Axtell RC, Zhou G, et al. Depleting tumor-specific Tregs at a single site eradicates disseminated tumors. *J Clin Invest* (2013) 123(6):2447–63. doi:10.1172/JCI64859
67. Selby MJ, Engelhardt JJ, Quigley M, Henning KA, Chen T, Srinivasan M, et al. Anti-CTLA-4 antibodies of IgG2a isotype enhance antitumor activity through reduction of intratumoral regulatory T cells. *Cancer Immunol Res* (2013) 1(1):32–42. doi:10.1158/2326-6066.CIR-13-0013
68. Simpson TR, Li F, Montalvo-Ortiz W, Sepulveda MA, Bergerhoff K, Arce F, et al. Fc-dependent depletion of tumor-infiltrating regulatory T cells co-defines the efficacy of anti-CTLA-4 therapy against melanoma. *J Exp Med* (2013) 210(9):1695–710. doi:10.1084/jem.20130579
69. Shimizu K, Yamasaki S, Shinga J, Sato Y, Watanabe T, Ohara O, et al. Systemic DC activation modulates the tumor microenvironment and shapes the long-lived tumor-specific memory mediated by CD8+ T cells. *Cancer Res* (2016) 76(13):3756–66. doi:10.1158/0008-5472.CAN-15-3219
70. Foo SY, Zhang V, Lalwani A, Lynch JP, Zhuang A, Lam CE, et al. Regulatory T cells prevent inducible BALT formation by dampening neutrophilic inflammation. *J Immunol* (2015) 194(9):4567–76. doi:10.4049/jimmunol.1400909
71. Carrega P, Loiacono F, Di Carlo E, Scaramuccia A, Mora M, Conte R, et al. NCR(+)ILC3 concentrate in human lung cancer and associate with intratumoral lymphoid structures. *Nat Commun* (2015) 6:8280. doi:10.1038/ncomms9280
72. Meier D, Bornmann C, Chappaz S, Schmutz S, Otten LA, Ceredig R, et al. Ectopic lymphoid-organ development occurs through interleukin 7-mediated enhanced survival of lymphoid-tissue-inducer cells. *Immunity* (2007) 26(5):643–54. doi:10.1016/j.immuni.2007.04.009
73. Schmutz S, Bosco N, Chappaz S, Boyman O, Acha-Orbea H, Ceredig R, et al. Cutting edge: IL-7 regulates the peripheral pool of adult ROR gamma+ lymphoid tissue inducer cells. *J Immunol* (2009) 183(4):2217–21. doi:10.4049/jimmunol.0802911
74. Klose CS, Artis D. Innate lymphoid cells as regulators of immunity, inflammation and tissue homeostasis. *Nat Immunol* (2016) 17(7):765–74. doi:10.1038/ni.3489
75. Takatori H, Kanno Y, Watford WT, Tato CM, Weiss G, Ivanov II, et al. Lymphoid tissue inducer-like cells are an innate source of IL-17 and IL-22. *J Exp Med* (2009) 206(1):35–41. doi:10.1084/jem.20072713
76. Kirchberger S, Royston DJ, Boulard O, Thornton E, Franchini F, Szabady RL, et al. Innate lymphoid cells sustain colon cancer through production of interleukin-22 in a mouse model. *J Exp Med* (2013) 210(5):917–31. doi:10.1084/jem.20122308
77. Sonnenberg GF, Monticelli LA, Elloso MM, Fouser LA, Artis D. CD4(+) lymphoid tissue-inducer cells promote innate immunity in the gut. *Immunity* (2011) 34(1):122–34. doi:10.1016/j.immuni.2010.12.009
78. Jones GW, Jones SA. Ectopic lymphoid follicles: inducible centres for generating antigen-specific immune responses within tissues. *Immunology* (2016) 147(2):141–51. doi:10.1111/imm.12554
79. Kruglov AA, Grivennikov SI, Kuprash DV, Winsauer C, Prepens S, Seleznik GM, et al. Nonredundant function of soluble LTalpha3 produced by innate lymphoid cells in intestinal homeostasis. *Science* (2013) 342(6163):1243–6. doi:10.1126/science.1243364
80. Magri G, Miyajima M, Bascones S, Mortha A, Puga I, Cassis L, et al. Innate lymphoid cells integrate stromal and immunological signals to enhance antibody production by splenic marginal zone B cells. *Nat Immunol* (2014) 15(4):354–64. doi:10.1038/ni.2830
81. Tsuji M, Suzuki K, Kitamura H, Maruya M, Kinoshita K, Ivanov II, et al. Requirement for lymphoid tissue-inducer cells in isolated follicle formation and T cell-independent immunoglobulin A generation in the gut. *Immunity* (2008) 29(2):261–71. doi:10.1016/j.immuni.2008.05.014
82. Zhu M, Fu Y. Proinflammatory IL-17 induces iBALT development. *Cell Mol Immunol* (2012) 9(2):101–2. doi:10.1038/cmi.2011.46
83. Beelen RH, Oosterling SJ, van Egmond M, van den Born J, Zareie M. Omental milky spots in peritoneal pathophysiology (spots before your eyes). *Perit Dial Int* (2005) 25(1):30–2.
84. Di Paolo N, Sacchi G, Garosi G, Sansoni E, Bargagli L, Ponzo P, et al. Omental milky spots and peritoneal dialysis – review and personal experience. *Perit Dial Int* (2005) 25(1):48–57.
85. Rangel-Moreno J, Moyron-Quiroz JE, Carragher DM, Kusser K, Hartson L, Moquin A, et al. Omental milky spots develop in the absence of lymphoid tissue-inducer cells and support B and T cell responses to peritoneal antigens. *Immunity* (2009) 30(5):731–43. doi:10.1016/j.immuni.2009.03.014
86. Benezech C, Luu NT, Walker JA, Kruglov AA, Loo Y, Nakamura K, et al. Inflammation-induced formation of fat-associated lymphoid clusters. *Nat Immunol* (2015) 16(8):819–28. doi:10.1038/ni.3215
87. Moro K, Yamada T, Tanabe M, Takeuchi T, Ikawa T, Kawamoto H, et al. Innate production of T(H)2 cytokines by adipose tissue-associated c-Kit(+) Sca-1(+) lymphoid cells. *Nature* (2010) 463(7280):540–4. doi:10.1038/nature08636
88. Muramatsu M, Kinoshita K, Fagarasan S, Yamada S, Shinkai Y, Honjo T. Class switch recombination and hypermutation require activation-induced cytidine deaminase (AID), a potential RNA editing enzyme. *Cell* (2000) 102(5):553–63. doi:10.1016/S0092-8674(00)00078-7
89. Stavnezer J, Guikema JE, Schrader CE. Mechanism and regulation of class switch recombination. *Annu Rev Immunol* (2008) 26:261–92. doi:10.1146/annurev.immunol.26.021607.090248
90. Bombardieri M, Barone F, Humby F, Kelly S, McGurk M, Morgan P, et al. Activation-induced cytidine deaminase expression in follicular dendritic cell networks and interfollicular large B cells supports functionality of ectopic lymphoid neogenesis in autoimmune sialoadenitis and MALT lymphoma in Sjogren's syndrome. *J Immunol* (2007) 179(7):4929–38. doi:10.4049/jimmunol.179.7.4929
91. Nacionales DC, Weinstein JS, Yan XJ, Albesiano E, Lee PY, Kelly-Scumpia KM, et al. B cell proliferation, somatic hypermutation, class switch recombination, and autoantibody production in ectopic lymphoid tissue in murine lupus. *J Immunol* (2009) 182(7):4226–36. doi:10.4049/jimmunol.0800771
92. Serafini B, Rosicarelli B, Franciotta D, Magliozzi R, Reynolds R, Cinque P, et al. Dysregulated Epstein-Barr virus infection in the multiple sclerosis brain. *J Exp Med* (2007) 204(12):2899–912. doi:10.1084/jem.20071030
93. Takahashi E, Kataoka K, Indalao IL, Konoha K, Fujii K, Chida J, et al. Oral clarithromycin enhances airway immunoglobulin A (IgA) immunity through induction of IgA class switching recombination and B-cell-activating factor of the tumor necrosis factor family molecule on mucosal dendritic cells in mice infected with influenza A virus. *J Virol* (2012) 86(20):10924–34. doi:10.1128/JVI.01207-12
94. Cheng J, Torkamani A, Grover RK, Jones TM, Ruiz DI, Schork NJ, et al. Ectopic B-cell clusters that infiltrate transplanted human kidneys are clonal. *Proc Natl Acad Sci U S A* (2011) 108(14):5560–5. doi:10.1073/pnas.1101148108
95. Scheel T, Gursche A, Zacher J, Haupl T, Berek C. V-region gene analysis of locally defined synovial B and plasma cells reveals selected B cell expansion and accumulation of plasma cell clones in rheumatoid arthritis. *Arthritis Rheum* (2011) 63(1):63–72. doi:10.1002/art.27767
96. Stott DI, Hiepe F, Hummel M, Steinhauser G, Berek C. Antigen-driven clonal proliferation of B cells within the target tissue of an autoimmune disease. The salivary glands of patients with Sjogren's syndrome. *J Clin Invest* (1998) 102(5):938–46. doi:10.1172/JCI3234
97. Grewal JS, Pilgrim MJ, Grewal S, Kasman L, Werner P, Bruorton ME, et al. Salivary glands act as mucosal inductive sites via the formation of ectopic germinal centers after site-restricted MCMV infection. *FASEB J* (2011) 25(5):1680–96. doi:10.1096/fj.10-174656
98. Salomonsson S, Jonsson MV, Skarstein K, Brokstad KA, Hjelmstrom P, Wahren-Herlenius M, et al. Cellular basis of ectopic germinal center formation and autoantibody production in the target organ of patients with Sjogren's syndrome. *Arthritis Rheum* (2003) 48(11):3187–201. doi:10.1002/art.11311
99. Armengol MP, Juan M, Lucas-Martin A, Fernandez-Figueras MT, Jaraquemada D, Gallart T, et al. Thyroid autoimmune disease: demonstration of thyroid antigen-specific B cells and recombination-activating gene expression in chemokine-containing active intrathyroidal germinal centers. *Am J Pathol* (2001) 159(3):861–73. doi:10.1016/S0002-9440(10)61762-2
100. Berrih-Aknin S, Ragheb S, Le Panse R, Lisak RP. Ectopic germinal centers, BAFF and anti-B-cell therapy in myasthenia gravis. *Autoimmun Rev* (2013) 12(9):885–93. doi:10.1016/j.autrev.2013.03.011
101. Le Pottier L, Devauchelle V, Fautrel A, Daridon C, Saraux A, Youinou P, et al. Ectopic germinal centers are rare in Sjogren's syndrome salivary glands and do not exclude autoreactive B cells. *J Immunol* (2009) 182(6):3540–7. doi:10.4049/jimmunol.0803588

102. Ekland EH, Forster R, Lipp M, Cyster JG. Requirements for follicular exclusion and competitive elimination of autoantigen-binding B cells. *J Immunol* (2004) 172(8):4700–8. doi:10.4049/jimmunol.172.8.4700
103. Pender MP. Infection of autoreactive B lymphocytes with EBV, causing chronic autoimmune diseases. *Trends Immunol* (2003) 24(11):584–8. doi:10.1016/j.it.2003.09.005
104. Cavalcante P, Serafini B, Rosicarelli B, Maggi L, Barberis M, Antozzi C, et al. Epstein-Barr virus persistence and reactivation in myasthenia gravis thymus. *Ann Neurol* (2010) 67(6):726–38. doi:10.1002/ana.21902
105. Croia C, Astorri E, Murray-Brown W, Willis A, Brokstad KA, Sutcliffe W, et al. Implication of Epstein-Barr virus infection in disease-specific autoreactive B cell activation in ectopic lymphoid structures of Sjogren's syndrome. *Arthritis Rheumatol* (2014) 66(9):2545–57. doi:10.1002/art.38726
106. Croia C, Serafini B, Bombardieri M, Kelly S, Humby F, Severa M, et al. Epstein-Barr virus persistence and infection of autoreactive plasma cells in synovial lymphoid structures in rheumatoid arthritis. *Ann Rheum Dis* (2013) 72(9):1559–68. doi:10.1136/annrheumdis-2012-202352
107. Takemura S, Klimiuk PA, Braun A, Goronzy JJ, Weyand CM. T cell activation in rheumatoid synovium is B cell dependent. *J Immunol* (2001) 167(8):4710–8. doi:10.4049/jimmunol.167.8.4710
108. Laskov R, Lancz G, Ruddle NH, McGrath KM, Specter S, Klein T, et al. Production of tumor necrosis factor (TNF-alpha) and lymphotoxin (TNF-beta) by murine pre-B and B cell lymphomas. *J Immunol* (1990) 144(9):3424–30.
109. Lorenz RG, Chaplin DD, McDonald KG, McDonough JS, Newberry RD. Isolated lymphoid follicle formation is inducible and dependent upon lymphotoxin-sufficient B lymphocytes, lymphotoxin beta receptor, and TNF receptor I function. *J Immunol* (2003) 170(11):5475–82. doi:10.4049/jimmunol.170.11.5475
110. Buckley CD, Barone F, Nayar S, Benezech C, Caamano J. Stromal cells in chronic inflammation and tertiary lymphoid organ formation. *Annu Rev Immunol* (2015) 33:715–45. doi:10.1146/annurev-immunol-032713-120252
111. Rangel-Moreno J, Moyron-Quiroz JE, Hartson L, Kusser K, Randall TD. Pulmonary expression of CXC chemokine ligand 13, CC chemokine ligand 19, and CC chemokine ligand 21 is essential for local immunity to influenza. *Proc Natl Acad Sci U S A* (2007) 104(25):10577–82. doi:10.1073/pnas.0700591104
112. Takemura S, Braun A, Crowson C, Kurtin PJ, Cofield RH, O'Fallon WM, et al. Lymphoid neogenesis in rheumatoid synovitis. *J Immunol* (2001) 167(2):1072–80. doi:10.4049/jimmunol.167.2.1072
113. Bombardieri M, Kam NW, Brentano F, Choi K, Filer A, Kyburz D, et al. A BAFF/APRIL-dependent TLR3-stimulated pathway enhances the capacity of rheumatoid synovial fibroblasts to induce AID expression and Ig class-switching in B cells. *Ann Rheum Dis* (2011) 70(10):1857–65. doi:10.1136/ard.2011.150219
114. Timmer TC, Baltus B, Vondenhoff M, Huizinga TW, Tak PP, Verweij CL, et al. Inflammation and ectopic lymphoid structures in rheumatoid arthritis synovial tissues dissected by genomics technology: identification of the interleukin-7 signaling pathway in tissues with lymphoid neogenesis. *Arthritis Rheum* (2007) 56(8):2492–502. doi:10.1002/art.22748
115. Finkin S, Yuan D, Stein I, Taniguchi K, Weber A, Unger K, et al. Ectopic lymphoid structures function as microniches for tumor progenitor cells in hepatocellular carcinoma. *Nat Immunol* (2015) 16(12):1235–44. doi:10.1038/ni.3290
116. Pikor NB, Astarita JL, Summers-Deluca L, Galicia G, Qu J, Ward LA, et al. Integration of Th17- and lymphotoxin-derived signals initiates meningeal-resident stromal cell remodeling to propagate neuroinflammation. *Immunity* (2015) 43(6):1160–73. doi:10.1016/j.immuni.2015.11.010
117. Thaunat O, Patey N, Gautreau C, Lechaton S, Fremeaux-Bacchi V, Dieu-Nosjean MC, et al. B cell survival in intragraft tertiary lymphoid organs after rituximab therapy. *Transplantation* (2008) 85(11):1648–53. doi:10.1097/TP.0b013e3181735723
118. Genovese MC, Durez P, Richards HB, Supronik J, Dokoupilova E, Mazurov V, et al. Efficacy and safety of secukinumab in patients with rheumatoid arthritis: a phase II, dose-finding, double-blind, randomised, placebo controlled study. *Ann Rheum Dis* (2013) 72(6):863–9. doi:10.1136/annrheumdis-2012-201601
119. McInnes IB, Sieper J, Braun J, Emery P, van der Heijde D, Isaacs JD, et al. Efficacy and safety of secukinumab, a fully human anti-interleukin-17A monoclonal antibody, in patients with moderate-to-severe psoriatic arthritis: a 24-week, randomised, double-blind, placebo-controlled, phase II proof-of-concept trial. *Ann Rheum Dis* (2014) 73(2):349–56. doi:10.1136/annrheumdis-2012-202646
120. Pitzalis C, Kelly S, Humby F. New learnings on the pathophysiology of RA from synovial biopsies. *Curr Opin Rheumatol* (2013) 25(3):334–44. doi:10.1097/BOR.0b013e32835fd8eb

9

Ectopic Lymphoid Structures: Powerhouse of Autoimmunity

*Elisa Corsiero, Alessandra Nerviani, Michele Bombardieri and Costantino Pitzalis**

Centre for Experimental Medicine and Rheumatology, William Harvey Research Institute, Barts and The London School of Medicine and Dentistry, Queen Mary University of London, London, UK

Correspondence:
Costantino Pitzalis
c.pitzalis@qmul.ac.uk

Ectopic lymphoid structures (ELS) often develop at sites of inflammation in target tissues of autoimmune diseases, such as rheumatoid arthritis, Sjögren's syndrome, multiple sclerosis, myasthenia gravis, and systemic lupus erythematosus. ELS are characterized by the formation of organized T/B cells aggregates, which can acquire follicular dendritic cells network supporting an ectopic germinal center response. In this review, we shall summarize the mechanisms that regulate the formation of ELS in tertiary lymphoid organs, with particular emphasis on the role of lymphoid chemokines in both formation and maintenance of ELS, the role of emerging positive and negative regulators of ELS development and function, including T follicular helper cells and IL-27, respectively. Finally, we shall discuss the main functions of ELS in supporting the affinity maturation, clonal selection, and differentiation of autoreactive B cells contributing to the maintenance and perpetuation of humoral autoimmunity.

Keywords: tertiary lymphoid structures, autoimmunity, lymphoid chemokines, autoimmune diseases, ectopic germinal center

INTRODUCTION

It is now well appreciated that ectopic (or tertiary) lymphoid structures (ELS) can develop in target organs of several autoimmune diseases, which are sites of chronic inflammation, although they can also develop in association with cancer, infection, and graft rejection, as previously discussed (1). At particular mucosal sites, ELS can be named based on the site of inflammation where they occur, e.g., inducible bronchus-associated or gut-associated lymphoid tissue or iGALT and iBALT, respectively (2). ELS are characterized by aggregates of T and B cells often showing T/B segregation (i.e., separated areas within the aggregates densely populated by T or B cells only), development of high endothelial venules (HEVs), and, in the majority of cases, follicular dendritic cell (FDC) networks. Compared to lymphoid aggregates forming in secondary lymphoid organs (SLOs), ELS are transient structures that can be triggered by immunization or infection (3) and often resolve after antigen clearance (2). However, in autoimmune diseases, ELS mostly develop in the context of a chronic inflammation, contribute to maintain the disease process, and are often associated with a more severe disease course (1, 4). As we shall discuss later in this review, ELS developing in chronic autoimmune conditions are capable of activating the molecular machinery to sustain *in situ* antibody diversification, isotype switching, B cell differentiation, and oligoclonal expansion, which are in keeping with their ability to function as active ectopic germinal centers (GCs), which can also support the production of autoreactive plasma cells at the local site of inflammation.

The biological events that bring to ELS formation in disease tissues show numerous similarities with the signaling pathways involved in secondary lymphoid tissue organogenesis; nevertheless, there are site-specific differences, particularly regarding the cellular sources of the key factors regulating lymphoid neogenesis, which depend, at least in part, on the nature of the site of inflammation (1, 2).

In this review, we shall first focus on the mechanisms regulating ELS formation and functions, including the well-established role of lymphoid chemokines and lymphotoxins (LTs) in ELS formation, together with the emerging importance of cytokines as positive (i.e., IL-21, IL-22) and negative (i.e., IL-27) regulators in ELS development, maintenance, and function. In the second part of this review, we shall discuss the evidence supporting the concept that ELS in autoimmune diseases contribute to the perpetuation and spreading of autoimmunity *via* the differentiation autoantibody-producing cells selected for disease-specific antigens within ectopic GCs. We will mostly focus on rheumatic autoimmune diseases, such as rheumatoid arthritis (RA) and Sjögren's syndrome (SS), but we will also refer to other organ-specific autoimmune conditions to highlight differences in the antigen-driven process underlying ELS formation.

DEVELOPMENT AND ORGANIZATION OF ELS: THE ROLE OF LYMPHOTOXINS AND LYMPHOID CHEMOKINES

The signals regulating ELS formation and perpetuation, mostly referred as lymphoid neogenesis, largely overlap with those regulating the same events in SLOs during embryonic life, known as lymphoid organogenesis, but with notable differences in the cellular sources of these factors in ELS development (5). Either in SLOs and ELS formation and perpetuation, the chemoattractant signaling pathway involves several homeostatic lymphoid chemokines, such as CXCL13, CCL19, CCL21, and CXCL12, and their specific receptors CXCR5 (for CXCL13), CCR7 (for CCL19 and CCL21), and CXCR4 (for CXCL12). In classic models of lymphoid organogenesis, the interaction between hematopoietic lymphoid tissue inducer cells ($CD3^{-}CD4^{+}IL\text{-}7Ra^{+}RANK^{+}$) and VCAM-1 + ICAM-1 + $LTBR^{+}$ mesenchymal organizer cells drives the establishment of a $LT\alpha1\beta2$ (also known as $LT\beta$)/lymphoid chemokine feedback loop, which is required for SLOs development including early B/T cell clustering and segregation as well as the differentiation of HEVs, as reviewed extensively elsewhere (1, 6, 7). Conversely, the early stages of lymphoid neogenesis in adult life are not fully understood, although recent evidence suggests an important role for inflammatory cytokines, such as IL-22 and IL-17, as early contributors in ELS formation, as discussed later. Regardless, once ELS are established, additional and/or alternative cell types can express lymphoid chemokines and LTs during chronic inflammation in autoimmune conditions. In ELS, myofibroblast-like stromal cells support the production of CCL21 around HEVs in the T cell-rich area of the lymphoid aggregate, whereas CXCL13 can be produced by infiltrating cells (i.e. $CD14^{+}$ inflammatory monocytes, $CD68^{+}$ macrophages, and memory $CD3^{+}CD4^{+}$ T cells) but also resident tissue cells such as activated stromal and epithelial cells (6). Therefore, it is believed that the immune cells recruited at the site of inflammation, in cross-talk with resident cells which are tissue-specific, exert an active role in the initiation of ELS development (2). Another example of the importance of the site-specific inflammatory milieu in ELS development and/or maintenance in autoimmune diseases is represented by TNF-α, which is abundantly expressed in the synovium of RA patients. In this regard, evidence that TNF-blockade can reverse ELS formation in the joints, at least in a subset of patients, would suggest that in some conditions, TNF-α can play a non-redundant role in ELS maintenance over and above LT-β (8).

Once ELS are established, lymphoid chemokines CCL19, CCL21, and CXCL13 are critical for their perpetuation and function by controlling the homing and tissue localization of immune cells subsets, which are crucial in adaptive immune responses. The concomitant presence of CCL19/CCL21 and peripheral node addressin (PNAd-positive) HEVs allows the homing of $CCR7^{+}$ T cells (i.e., naïve and central memory) and mature $CCR7^{+}$ dendritic cells (DCs) from the systemic circulation upon binding to $PNAd^{+}$ HEVs through L-selectin (6, 9). Naïve B cells can also express at lower level CCR7, and together with CXCR4 and CXCR5, they use these receptors to enter ELS from the systemic circulation (6, 10), although B cell positioning into ectopic follicles is mainly controlled by CXCR5 in response to a CXCL13 gradient. B cells can actively contribute to ELS maintenance as they become strong producers of $LT\beta$.

Lymphoid chemokines CXCL13 and CXCL12 are also critical in the function of ELS as ectopic GCs by regulating the shuttling of B cells between the dark and light zones. Inside the GC, CXCL13, mostly produced by FDCs, mainly directs GC B cells to the light zone of the GC where antigen selection occurs. Within the GC, CXCL12, mostly produced by tingible body macrophages in ELS (11), is critically involved in the migration of $CXCR4^{high}$ centroblasts to the dark zone, where somatic hypermutation of the B cell receptor takes place (6). As discussed later in this review, in the target organs of autoimmune diseases, the formation of functional GCs as a result of the lymphoid neogenesis process is critical in the selection and differentiation of autoantibody-producing B cells.

THE EMERGING ROLE OF CYTOKINES AS POSITIVE AND NEGATIVE REGULATORS OF ELS FORMATION, PERPETUATION, AND FUNCTION

As mentioned earlier, besides the classic LT/lymphoid chemokines feedback loop, there is strong emerging evidence that cytokines produced in the context of the inflammatory process are also critically involved in the lymphoid neogenesis in autoimmune diseases. These include, not exhaustively, IL-17, IL-21, IL-22, IL-23, and TNF (2). For instance, IL-17 produced by a subset of podoplanin-expressing CD4 T cells has been strongly linked with ELS formation in animal models of inducible ELS, and the IL-23/IL-17 axis has been recently associated with ELS formation in RA (12, 13). Because the role of IL-17 in ELS has been recently reviewed extensively (1, 2), here we will focus on the emerging role of positive and negative regulators of ELS formation and function such as IL-21/IL-22 and IL-27, respectively.

Using a model of inducible ELS formation, autoimmunity and exocrine dysfunction resembling SS that we recently developed and which is triggered by local viral infection in the salivary glands of C57BL/6 mice (3), Barone et al. demonstrated that the early production (i.e., within few hours from viral infection) of IL-22, a cytokine belonging to the IL-10 family, by γδT-cells first and by conventional CD4 T cells thereafter, was directly responsible for the induction of CXCL13 by a subset of resident stromal cells expressing gp38. Although IL-22 was able to induce CXCL13 *in vitro* in a LT-β-independent manner, it is yet to be established whether IL-22 is sufficient to induce ELS *in vivo* in the absence of lymphotoxins (12). These findings seem applicable to ELS forming in human autoimmune diseases, as IL-22 has been associated with the formation of inflammatory aggregates both in RA and SS (13, 14).

While IL-22 appears critical in the early phase of ELS development, another cytokine, IL-21, a member of the common cytokine receptor γ chain-binding family, has been shown to play a fundamental role in the function of ELS as ectopic GCs. This cytokine is primarily produced by T follicular helper (Tfh) cells, a highly specialized subset of $CD4^+$ memory T cells expressing high amount of CXCR5 (15) and thus able to migrate toward B cell follicles in response to CXCL13 production by FDCs.

In the last decade, Tfh cells have emerged as essential players in the regulation of B cell activation, antibody affinity maturation, and the GC reaction *via* the expression of surface receptors such as inducible T-cell costimulator (ICOS) and programed cell death protein 1 (PD1). They also express the transcription factor B cell lymphoma protein 6 (Bcl-6), which promotes the expression of CXCR5 and represses other T-cell subset-specific transcription factors (16–18). IL-21 is the main soluble factor released by Tfh and binds a receptor complex consisting of the common γ chain and a unique IL-21R. On B cells, IL-21/IL-21R interactions provide potent signaling for B-cell survival, proliferation, and differentiation (19). Indeed, the absence of Tfh cells impairs GC formation and the generation of long-lived plasma cells, resulting in impaired high affinity antibody responses (20).

Among autoimmune diseases, elevated frequencies of Tfh cells in the peripheral blood have been demonstrated in RA, SS, multiple sclerosis (MS), myasthenia gravis (MG), and systemic lupus erythematosus (SLE) (21). Not surprisingly, IL-21 directly correlated with the frequency of Tfh-like cells. Both IL-21 level and number of Tfh-like cells were associated with higher titer of anti-CCP antibodies and disease activity score in RA (22). In the context of ELS, IL-21 and IL-21R expression are upregulated in the synovial tissue of RA patients, whereby IL-21 strictly segregates with the formation of ELS (23–25). Moreover, blocking IL-21/IL-21R in animal models of RA and SS has a beneficial effect on the disease progression (26, 27).

Interestingly, plasticity between Th17 cells (but also Th1 and Th2) with Tfh cells has been observed (28) and may play an important role in autoimmune diseases, including models of experimental MS, whereby Th17 cells crossing the blood–brain barrier can acquire a Tfh-like cells phenotype, thus supporting ELS development and function in the central nervous system (2, 4). However, and of likely relevance to ELS and ectopic GC, Tfh2 and Tfh17, but not Tfh1, are able to secrete IL-21 and induce naïve B cells to secrete class-switched immunoglobulin (Ig) (28).

Together with positive regulators of ELS formation, the existence of cytokines exerting a negative role on lymphoid neogenesis, such as IL-27, has been recently described. IL-27 is a heterodimeric cytokine belonging to the IL-12 family and is composed of EBI3 and IL-27p28 (29). IL-27 signals through a receptor were composed of IL-27Rα and gp130, the latter used also by other cytokines such as IL-6 (29). IL-27 seems to be able to limit antibody production since overexpression of IL-27Rα in the MLR/lpr mouse model of lupus can ameliorate the antibody response (29). Moreover, it has been recently shown that $IL27R\alpha^{-/-}$ mice developed a more severe form of arthritis after immunization with methylated bovine serum albumin (mBSA), which was also characterized by multiple lymphoid aggregates forming in the inflamed synovial tissue (25). IL-27 can also restrict the expansion of Th17 cells and suppress secretion of IL-17, a cytokine associated also with survival and proliferation of B cells (25, 29, 30). In regard to ELS development, e.g., in human synovium, it has been observed that IL-27 is inversely correlated with the degree of lymphocytic infiltration in the inflamed tissue as well as with the expression of IL-17 and IL-21 at mRNA level (25). However, further experimental and mechanistic data will be required before exploiting the role of IL-27 as a negative regulator of ELS formation and function for therapeutic purposes in autoimmune diseases.

THE ROLE OF ELS AS PERPETUATORS OF AUTOIMMUNITY IN THE TARGET ORGANS OF AUTOIMMUNE DISEASES

Ectopic lymphoid structures arise in the target organs of patients affected by autoimmune diseases, such as salivary glands in SS (6), synovial tissue in RA (31), kidneys in SLE (32), thymuses in MG (33), meninges in MS (34), and thyroids in Hashimoto's thyroiditis (35) (**Figure 1A**). However, for reasons that are currently not clear, the frequency of ELS in these conditions varies significantly, from a minority of patients with SLE to virtually 100% of patients with thyroiditis (36). For instance, in the RA synovium, the immune infiltrates can be arranged into three main microstructural levels of organization including (i) follicular synovitis with ELS (lymphoid pathotype, 40% of RA patients) (31, 37, 38); (ii) diffuse pattern of infiltration with a predominant macrophages component (myeloid pathotype); and (iii) pauci-immune synovitis, characterized by a virtual absence of immune cells (fibroid pathotype) (39). Similarly, around 30–40% of patients with SS show ELS in the affected salivary glands (40, 41), and patients with ELS are significantly more likely to develop B-cell lymphomas of the mucosal-associated lymphoid tissue (MALT-L) (42, 43). In lupus nephritis, B/T cells aggregates can be found in up to 50% of patients in the tubulo-interstitium, but fully organized ectopic GC follicles are detectable in <10% of patients (44). As previously mentioned, ELS in autoimmune conditions are not only structurally reminiscent of SLOs but also functionally active as ectopic GC. There is now conclusive evidence that ELS in autoimmune diseases favor the affinity maturation of B-cells *via*

A

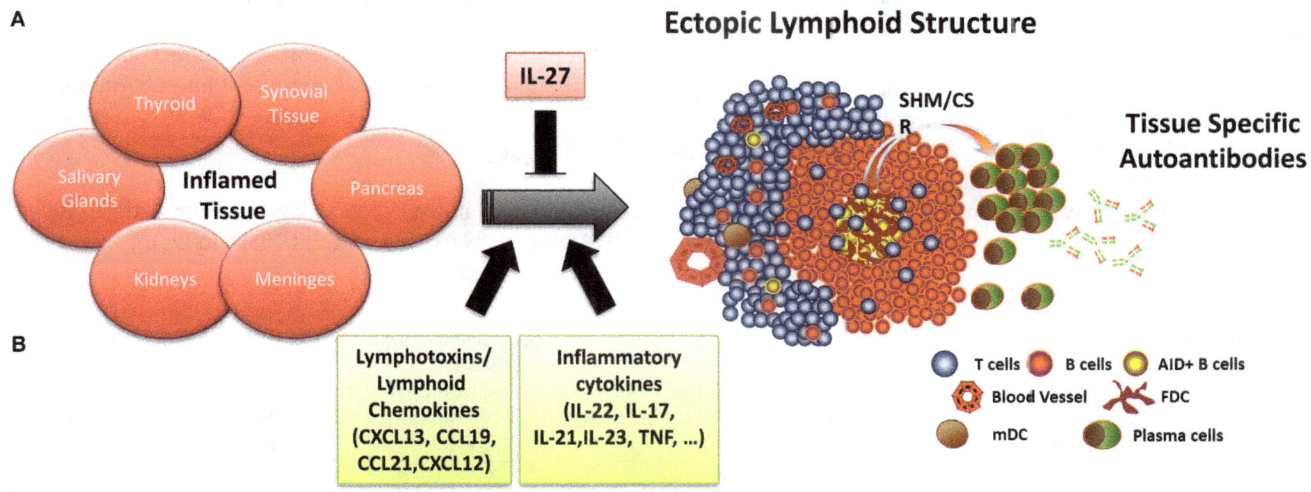

B

Disease Specific Autoantigens	Disease/Tissue-related ELS
Citrullinated proteins	Rheumatoid Arthritis/Synovial Tissue
Ribonucleoproteins Ro/SSA and La/SSB	Sjogren's syndrome/Salivary Glands
Thyroglobulin/Thyroperoxidase	Hashimoto's thyroiditis/Thyroids
Insulin ?	Type 1 Diabetis/Pancreas
Acetylcholine receptor	Myasthenia Gravis/Thymus
Double stranded DNA	Systemic Lupus Erythematosus/Kidneys
?	Multiple sclerosis/Meninges

FIGURE 1 | Ectopic lymphoid structure (ELS) formation in autoimmune disease tissue. (A) Importance of lymphotoxins/lymphoid chemokines and inflammatory cytokines in the formation and maintenance of ELS in the target organs of patients with autoimmune diseases, where ELS preferentially drives the affinity maturation and clonal selection of autoantibodies toward specific autoantigens. **(B)** Summary table listing the main disease-specific autoantigens and the associated autoimmune disease where ELS formation has been observed.

an antigen-driven selection process and their differentiation to plasma cells. B cell isolated from ELS in autoimmune conditions display highly somatically hypermutated Ig VH and VL regions in line with a local antigen-driven process (45–47). Furthermore, lineage tree analysis of the Ig gene repertoire of B-cells and plasma cells infiltrating ELS + tissues in autoimmune diseases proved that clonal diversification and differentiation to antibody-producing cells take place within ELS (45, 47, 48). In keeping with the above evidence, B cells within ELS display detectable activation-induced cytidine deaminase (49), the enzyme which regulates both somatic hypermutation and isotype class switching of the Ig genes (50).

Accumulating experimental data indicate that ELS in autoimmune diseases preferentially favor affinity maturation and clonal selection toward autoantigens, which are frequently the target of autoantibodies detectable in the patients' circulation (**Figure 1B**). Specifically, ELS allow the selection and differentiation of autoreactive B cells into high-affinity plasma cells reacting against citrullinated antigens in RA (49), anti-ribonucleoproteins Ro/SSA and La/SSB in SS (40), thyroglobulin and thyroperoxidase in Hashimoto's thyroiditis (35), and insulin in type 1 diabetes (51, 52). More in details, we and other provided evidence that (i) perifollicular CD138^{+} plasma cells frequently bind biotinylated citrullinated fibrinogen and the Ro52 antigen in synovial and salivary gland ELS of RA and SS patients, respectively, but not vice versa, using double immunofluorescence experiments (40, 49, 53, 54); (ii) the engraftment of ELS + tissue from the RA synovium, SS salivary gland, and MG thymus in SCID mice in a series of chimeric human/murine models resulted in the release and detection of human autoantibodies against disease-specific autoantigens in the mouse circulation (54–56). More recently, (iii) by combining single B-cell sorting, Ig VH and VL gene cloning, and recombinant monoclonal antibody production from ELS + RA synovia or from ACPA + RA synovial fluid, we and others demonstrated that around 30% of the synovial humoral response is directed toward citrullinated antigens (36, 48).

Thus, in conclusion, although the processes underlying ELS formation in autoimmune diseases largely follow a stereotyped lymphoid neogenesis process, the autoantigens driving the autoimmune response within ELS in the respective target organs appear to be disease specific. An important consequence of this phenomenon is that a better understanding of the fine specificity of the autoantigens driving the autoimmune response within ELS would strongly enhance our knowledge of the underlying processes perpetuating autoimmunity and chronic inflammation in the different autoimmune diseases. Furthermore, and perhaps more importantly, the identification of dominant autoantigens driving B and T cell responses, as recently suggested by large throughput sequencing studies in the RA synovium, could pave the way for future vaccination and tolerogenic therapeutic strategies (57, 58).

AUTHOR CONTRIBUTIONS

All authors listed have made substantial, direct, and intellectual contribution to the work and approved it for publication.

FUNDING

This work was funded by research grants from Arthritis Research UK (grant 20089 to MB and grant 20858 to EC).

REFERENCES

1. Pitzalis C, Jones GW, Bombardieri M, Jones SA. Ectopic lymphoid-like structures in infection, cancer and autoimmunity. *Nat Rev Immunol* (2014) 14:447–62. doi:10.1038/nri3700
2. Jones GW, Jones SA. Ectopic lymphoid follicles: inducible centres for generating antigen-specific immune responses within tissues. *Immunology* (2016) 147:141–51. doi:10.1111/imm.12554
3. Bombardieri M, Barone F, Lucchesi D, Nayar S, Van Den Berg WB, Proctor G, et al. Inducible tertiary lymphoid structures, autoimmunity, and exocrine dysfunction in a novel model of salivary gland inflammation in C57BL/6 mice. *J Immunol* (2012) 189:3767–76. doi:10.4049/jimmunol.1201216
4. Peters A, Pitcher LA, Sullivan JM, Mitsdoerffer M, Acton SE, Franz B, et al. Th17 cells induce ectopic lymphoid follicles in central nervous system tissue inflammation. *Immunity* (2011) 35:986–96. doi:10.1016/j.immuni.2011.10.015
5. Germain C, Gnjatic S, Dieu-Nosjean MC. Tertiary lymphoid structure-associated B cells are key players in anti-tumor immunity. *Front Immunol* (2015) 6:67. doi:10.3389/fimmu.2015.00067
6. Corsiero E, Bombardieri M, Manzo A, Bugatti S, Uguccioni M, Pitzalis C. Role of lymphoid chemokines in the development of functional ectopic lymphoid structures in rheumatic autoimmune diseases. *Immunol Lett* (2012) 145:62–7. doi:10.1016/j.imlet.2012.04.013
7. Randall TD, Mebius RE. The development and function of mucosal lymphoid tissues: a balancing act with micro-organisms. *Mucosal Immunol* (2014) 7:455–66. doi:10.1038/mi.2014.11
8. Canete JD, Celis R, Moll C, Izquierdo E, Marsal S, Sanmarti R, et al. Clinical significance of synovial lymphoid neogenesis and its reversal after anti-tumour necrosis factor alpha therapy in rheumatoid arthritis. *Ann Rheum Dis* (2009) 68:751–6. doi:10.1136/ard.2008.089284
9. Link A, Vogt TK, Favre S, Britschgi MR, Acha-Orbea H, Hinz B, et al. Fibroblastic reticular cells in lymph nodes regulate the homeostasis of naive T cells. *Nat Immunol* (2007) 8:1255–65. doi:10.1038/ni1513
10. Pereira JP, Kelly LM, Cyster JG. Finding the right niche: B-cell migration in the early phases of T-dependent antibody responses. *Int Immunol* (2010) 22:413–9. doi:10.1093/intimm/dxq047
11. Barone F, Bombardieri M, Rosado MM, Morgan PR, Challacombe SJ, De Vita S, et al. CXCL13, CCL21, and CXCL12 expression in salivary glands of patients with Sjogren's syndrome and MALT lymphoma: association with reactive and malignant areas of lymphoid organization. *J Immunol* (2008) 180:5130–40. doi:10.4049/jimmunol.180.7.5130
12. Barone F, Nayar S, Campos J, Cloake T, Withers DR, Toellner KM, et al. IL-22 regulates lymphoid chemokine production and assembly of tertiary lymphoid organs. *Proc Natl Acad Sci U S A* (2015) 112:11024–9. doi:10.1073/pnas.1503315112
13. Canete JD, Celis R, Yeremenko N, Sanmarti R, Van Duivenvoorde L, Ramirez J, et al. Ectopic lymphoid neogenesis is strongly associated with activation of the IL-23 pathway in rheumatoid synovitis. *Arthritis Res Ther* (2015) 17:173. doi:10.1186/s13075-015-0688-0
14. Ciccia F, Guggino G, Rizzo A, Ferrante A, Raimondo S, Giardina A, et al. Potential involvement of IL-22 and IL-22-producing cells in the inflamed salivary glands of patients with Sjogren's syndrome. *Ann Rheum Dis* (2012) 71:295–301. doi:10.1136/ard.2011.154013
15. Breitfeld D, Ohl L, Kremmer E, Ellwart J, Sallusto F, Lipp M, et al. Follicular B helper T cells express CXC chemokine receptor 5, localize to B cell follicles, and support immunoglobulin production. *J Exp Med* (2000) 192:1545–52. doi:10.1084/jem.192.11.1545
16. Zotos D, Coquet JM, Zhang Y, Light A, D'Costa K, Kallies A, et al. IL-21 regulates germinal center B cell differentiation and proliferation through a B cell-intrinsic mechanism. *J Exp Med* (2010) 207:365–78. doi:10.1084/jem.20091777
17. Shulman Z, Gitlin AD, Weinstein JS, Lainez B, Esplugues E, Flavell RA, et al. Dynamic signaling by T follicular helper cells during germinal center B cell selection. *Science* (2014) 345:1058–62. doi:10.1126/science.1257861
18. Liu D, Xu H, Shih C, Wan Z, Ma X, Ma W, et al. T-B-cell entanglement and ICOSL-driven feed-forward regulation of germinal centre reaction. *Nature* (2015) 517:214–8. doi:10.1038/nature13803
19. Karnell JL, Ettinger R. The interplay of IL-21 and BAFF in the formation and maintenance of human B cell memory. *Front Immunol* (2012) 3:2. doi:10.3389/fimmu.2012.00002
20. Ballesteros-Tato A, Randall TD. Priming of T follicular helper cells by dendritic cells. *Immunol Cell Biol* (2014) 92:22–7. doi:10.1038/icb.2013.62
21. Ueno H, Banchereau J, Vinuesa CG. Pathophysiology of T follicular helper cells in humans and mice. *Nat Immunol* (2015) 16:142–52. doi:10.1038/ni.3054
22. Ma J, Zhu C, Ma B, Tian J, Baidoo SE, Mao C, et al. Increased frequency of circulating follicular helper T cells in patients with rheumatoid arthritis. *Clin Dev Immunol* (2012) 2012:827480. doi:10.1155/2012/827480
23. Jungel A, Distler JH, Kurowska-Stolarska M, Seemayer CA, Seibl R, Forster A, et al. Expression of interleukin-21 receptor, but not interleukin-21, in synovial fibroblasts and synovial macrophages of patients with rheumatoid arthritis. *Arthritis Rheum* (2004) 50:1468–76. doi:10.1002/art.20218
24. Kwok SK, Cho ML, Park MK, Oh HJ, Park JS, Her YM, et al. Interleukin-21 promotes osteoclastogenesis in humans with rheumatoid arthritis and in mice with collagen-induced arthritis. *Arthritis Rheum* (2012) 64:740–51. doi:10.1002/art.33390
25. Jones GW, Bombardieri M, Greenhill CJ, Mcleod L, Nerviani A, Rocher-Ros V, et al. Interleukin-27 inhibits ectopic lymphoid-like structure development in early inflammatory arthritis. *J Exp Med* (2015) 212:1793–802. doi:10.1084/jem.20132307
26. Young DA, Hegen M, Ma HL, Whitters MJ, Albert LM, Lowe L, et al. Blockade of the interleukin-21/interleukin-21 receptor pathway ameliorates disease in animal models of rheumatoid arthritis. *Arthritis Rheum* (2007) 56:1152–63. doi:10.1002/art.22452
27. Liu H, Liu G, Gong L, Zhang Y, Jiang G. Local suppression of IL-21 in submandibular glands retards the development of Sjogren's syndrome in non-obese diabetic mice. *J Oral Pathol Med* (2012) 41:728–35. doi:10.1111/j.1600-0714.2012.01175.x
28. Morita R, Schmitt N, Bentebibel SE, Ranganathan R, Bourdery L, Zurawski G, et al. Human blood CXCR5(+)CD4(+) T cells are counterparts of T follicular cells and contain specific subsets that differentially support antibody secretion. *Immunity* (2011) 34:108–21. doi:10.1016/j.immuni.2010.12.012
29. Yoshida H, Hunter CA. The immunobiology of interleukin-27. *Annu Rev Immunol* (2015) 33:417–43. doi:10.1146/annurev-immunol-032414-112134
30. Stumhofer JS, Laurence A, Wilson EH, Huang E, Tato CM, Johnson LM, et al. Interleukin 27 negatively regulates the development of interleukin 17-producing T helper cells during chronic inflammation of the central nervous system. *Nat Immunol* (2006) 7:937–45. doi:10.1038/ni1376
31. Manzo A, Bombardieri M, Humby F, Pitzalis C. Secondary and ectopic lymphoid tissue responses in rheumatoid arthritis: from inflammation

to autoimmunity and tissue damage/remodeling. *Immunol Rev* (2010) 233:267–85. doi:10.1111/j.0105-2896.2009.00861.x

32. Bird AK, Meednu N, Anolik JH. New insights into B cell biology in systemic lupus erythematosus and Sjogren's syndrome. *Curr Opin Rheumatol* (2015) 27:461–7. doi:10.1097/BOR.0000000000000201
33. Berrih-Aknin S, Ragheb S, Le Panse R, Lisak RP. Ectopic germinal centers, BAFF and anti-B-cell therapy in myasthenia gravis. *Autoimmun Rev* (2013) 12:885–93. doi:10.1016/j.autrev.2013.03.011
34. Magliozzi R, Howell O, Vora A, Serafini B, Nicholas R, Puopolo M, et al. Meningeal B-cell follicles in secondary progressive multiple sclerosis associate with early onset of disease and severe cortical pathology. *Brain* (2007) 130:1089–104. doi:10.1093/brain/awm038
35. Armengol MP, Juan M, Lucas-Martin A, Fernandez-Figueras MT, Jaraquemada D, Gallart T, et al. Thyroid autoimmune disease: demonstration of thyroid antigen-specific B cells and recombination-activating gene expression in chemokine-containing active intrathyroidal germinal centers. *Am J Pathol* (2001) 159:861–73. doi:10.1016/S0002-9440(10)61762-2
36. Aloisi F, Pujol-Borrell R. Lymphoid neogenesis in chronic inflammatory diseases. *Nat Rev Immunol* (2006) 6:205–17. doi:10.1038/nri1786
37. Takemura S, Braun A, Crowson C, Kurtin PJ, Cofield RH, O'Fallon WM, et al. Lymphoid neogenesis in rheumatoid synovitis. *J Immunol* (2001) 167:1072–80. doi:10.4049/jimmunol.167.2.1072
38. Dennis G Jr, Holweg CT, Kummerfeld SK, Choy DF, Setiadi AF, Hackney JA, et al. Synovial phenotypes in rheumatoid arthritis correlate with response to biologic therapeutics. *Arthritis Res Ther* (2014) 16:R90. doi:10.1186/ar4555
39. Pitzalis C, Kelly S, Humby F. New learnings on the pathophysiology of RA from synovial biopsies. *Curr Opin Rheumatol* (2013) 25:334–44. doi:10.1097/BOR.0b013e32835fd8eb
40. Salomonsson S, Jonsson MV, Skarstein K, Brokstad KA, Hjelmstrom P, Wahren-Herlenius M, et al. Cellular basis of ectopic germinal center formation and autoantibody production in the target organ of patients with Sjogren's syndrome. *Arthritis Rheum* (2003) 48:3187–201. doi:10.1002/art.11311
41. Barone F, Bombardieri M, Manzo A, Blades MC, Morgan PR, Challacombe SJ, et al. Association of CXCL13 and CCL21 expression with the progressive organization of lymphoid-like structures in Sjogren's syndrome. *Arthritis Rheum* (2005) 52:1773–84. doi:10.1002/art.21062
42. Bombardieri M, Barone F, Humby F, Kelly S, Mcgurk M, Morgan P, et al. Activation-induced cytidine deaminase expression in follicular dendritic cell networks and interfollicular large B cells supports functionality of ectopic lymphoid neogenesis in autoimmune sialoadenitis and MALT lymphoma in Sjogren's syndrome. *J Immunol* (2007) 179:4929–38. doi:10.4049/jimmunol.179.7.4929
43. Theander E, Vasaitis L, Baecklund E, Nordmark G, Warfvinge G, Liedholm R, et al. Lymphoid organisation in labial salivary gland biopsies is a possible predictor for the development of malignant lymphoma in primary Sjogren's syndrome. *Ann Rheum Dis* (2011) 70:1363–8. doi:10.1136/ard.2010.144782
44. Chang A, Henderson SG, Brandt D, Liu N, Guttikonda R, Hsieh C, et al. In situ B cell-mediated immune responses and tubulointerstitial inflammation in human lupus nephritis. *J Immunol* (2011) 186:1849–60. doi:10.4049/jimmunol.1001983
45. Stott DI, Hiepe F, Hummel M, Steinhauser G, Berek C. Antigen-driven clonal proliferation of B cells within the target tissue of an autoimmune disease. The salivary glands of patients with Sjogren's syndrome. *J Clin Invest* (1998) 102:938–46. doi:10.1172/JCI3234
46. Cheng J, Torkamani A, Grover RK, Jones TM, Ruiz DI, Schork NJ, et al. Ectopic B-cell clusters that infiltrate transplanted human kidneys are clonal. *Proc Natl Acad Sci U S A* (2011) 108:5560–5. doi:10.1073/pnas.1101148108
47. Scheel T, Gursche A, Zacher J, Haupl T, Berek C. V-region gene analysis of locally defined synovial B and plasma cells reveals selected B cell expansion and accumulation of plasma cell clones in rheumatoid arthritis. *Arthritis Rheum* (2011) 63:63–72. doi:10.1002/art.27767
48. Corsiero E, Bombardieri M, Carlotti E, Pratesi F, Robinson W, Migliorini P, et al. Single cell cloning and recombinant monoclonal antibodies generation from RA synovial B cells reveal frequent targeting of citrullinated histones of NETs. *Ann Rheum Dis* (2016) 75(10):1866–75. doi:10.1136/annrheumdis-2015-208356
49. Humby F, Bombardieri M, Manzo A, Kelly S, Blades MC, Kirkham B, et al. Ectopic lymphoid structures support ongoing production of class-switched autoantibodies in rheumatoid synovium. *PLoS Med* (2009) 6:e1. doi:10.1371/journal.pmed.0060001
50. Muramatsu M, Kinoshita K, Fagarasan S, Yamada S, Shinkai Y, Honjo T. Class switch recombination and hypermutation require activation-induced cytidine deaminase (AID), a potential RNA editing enzyme. *Cell* (2000) 102:553–63. doi:10.1016/S0092-8674(00)00078-7
51. Kendall PL, Yu G, Woodward EJ, Thomas JW. Tertiary lymphoid structures in the pancreas promote selection of B lymphocytes in autoimmune diabetes. *J Immunol* (2007) 178:5643–51. doi:10.4049/jimmunol.178.9.5643
52. Astorri E, Bombardieri M, Gabba S, Peakman M, Pozzilli P, Pitzalis C. Evolution of ectopic lymphoid neogenesis and in situ autoantibody production in autoimmune nonobese diabetic mice: cellular and molecular characterization of tertiary lymphoid structures in pancreatic islets. *J Immunol* (2010) 185:3359–68. doi:10.4049/jimmunol.1001836
53. Rangel-Moreno J, Hartson L, Navarro C, Gaxiola M, Selman M, Randall TD. Inducible bronchus-associated lymphoid tissue (iBALT) in patients with pulmonary complications of rheumatoid arthritis. *J Clin Invest* (2006) 116:3183–94. doi:10.1172/JCI28756
54. Croia C, Astorri E, Murray-Brown W, Willis A, Brokstad KA, Sutcliffe N, et al. Implication of Epstein-Barr virus infection in disease-specific autoreactive B cell activation in ectopic lymphoid structures of Sjogren's syndrome. *Arthritis Rheumatol* (2014) 66:2545–57. doi:10.1002/art.38726
55. Yoshikawa H, Lennon VA. ACh receptor protein drives primary and memory autoantibody responses in chimeric human-SCID mice. *Clin Immunol* (2002) 104:128–37. doi:10.1006/clim.2002.5251
56. Croia C, Serafini B, Bombardieri M, Kelly S, Humby F, Severa M, et al. Epstein-Barr virus persistence and infection of autoreactive plasma cells in synovial lymphoid structures in rheumatoid arthritis. *Ann Rheum Dis* (2013) 72:1559–68. doi:10.1136/annrheumdis-2012-202352
57. Klarenbeek PL, De Hair MJ, Doorenspleet ME, Van Schaik BD, Esveldt RE, Van De Sande MG, et al. Inflamed target tissue provides a specific niche for highly expanded T-cell clones in early human autoimmune disease. *Ann Rheum Dis* (2012) 71:1088–93. doi:10.1136/annrheumdis-2011-200612
58. Doorenspleet ME, Klarenbeek PL, De Hair MJ, Van Schaik BD, Esveldt RE, Van Kampen AH, et al. Rheumatoid arthritis synovial tissue harbours dominant B-cell and plasma-cell clones associated with autoreactivity. *Ann Rheum Dis* (2014) 73:756–62. doi:10.1136/annrheumdis-2012-202861

10

Fat-Associated Lymphoid Clusters in Inflammation and Immunity

Sara Cruz-Migoni and Jorge Caamaño**

College of Medical and Dental Sciences, Institute of Immunology and Immunotherapy, University of Birmingham, Birmingham, UK

***Correspondence:**
Sara Cruz-Migoni
s.b.cruzmigoni@bham.ac.uk;
Jorge Caamaño
j.caamano@bham.ac.uk

Fat-associated lymphoid clusters (FALCs) are atypical lymphoid tissues that were originally identified in mouse and human mesenteries due to that they contain a high number of type 2 innate lymphoid cells/nuocytes/natural helper cells. FALCs are located on adipose tissues in mucosal surfaces such as the mediastinum, pericardium, and gonadal fat. Importantly, these clusters contain B1, B2 and T lymphocytes as well as myeloid and other innate immune cell populations. The developmental cues of FALC formation have started to emerge, showing that these clusters depend on a different set of molecules and cells than secondary lymphoid tissues for their formation. Here, we review the current knowledge on FALC formation, and we compare FALCs and omental milky spots and their responses to inflammation.

Keywords: lymphoid tissues, fat-associated lymphoid clusters, peritoneal inflammation, peritoneal immune responses, tertiary lymphoid structures

INTRODUCTION

The interactions between different types of immune cells are essential for both innate and adaptive immune responses to pathogens. Such interactions require strategically situated microenvironments to increase the chances that rare antigen-specific lymphocytes become activated. These specialized microenvironments are found in secondary lymphoid organs (SLOs) such as lymph nodes and Peyer's patches. Specialized populations of $CD45^-$ fibroblastic and endothelial cells express an arrangement of cell adhesion molecules, chemokines, and survival factors that guide the recruitment, co-localization and interactions of bone marrow-derived cells to their specific areas being T cells and dendritic cells (DCs) to the T cell area while B cells and follicular T helper cells to the B cell follicles. The development and organization of secondary lymphoid tissues is dependent on signals by the tumor necrosis factor (TNF) family of proteins such as lymphotoxin αβ (LTαβ), lymphotoxin β receptor (LTβR), and TNF-TNF receptor I and the downstream pathways such as activation of the nuclear factor kappa B family of transcription factors. The target genes of these pathways include the cell adhesion molecules VCAM-1, ICAM-1, MAdCAM-1, and the chemokines CXCL13, CCL19, and CCL21. Several detailed reviews of the processes that mediate lymph node development have been published (1–3).

Lymph nodes are characterized by well-defined B and T cell areas. B cell areas contain follicles that are organized by a specific population of reticular cell expressing the B cell-attracting chemokine

CXCL13. Paracortical T cell areas are organized by a different type of stromal cells named T zone reticular cells that express CCL21 and CCL19, which attract T cells, and DCs to facilitate their interactions (4).

In addition to secondary lymphoid tissues such as lymph nodes, there are a series of inducible lymphoid tissues present in mucosal surfaces such as bronchial-associated lymphoid tissues (BALT) in the lung (5–9), gut-associated lymphoid tissues that comprise the isolated lymphoid follicles in the intestine (ILFs) (10–12), tear duct-associated lymphoid tissues (13, 14), nasopharyngeal-associated lymphoid tissues (NALT) (15, 16) and portal tract-associated lymphoid tissues (17, 18) to cite a few examples (see **Table 1**). Recently a novel type of lymphoid tissue called fat-associated lymphoid clusters (FALCs) has been identified in the mesenteries of humans and mice (19).

THE STRUCTURE OF FALCs

Fat-associated lymphoid clusters are non-classical lymphoid tissues associated to adipocytes in mucosal surfaces, including omental, mesenteric, mediastinal, gonadal, and pericardial fat (19, 24, 25).

The frequency of FALCs varies among different adipose tissues (AT) in mice. Whereas gonadal AT has as little as 1–2 clusters, the omentum can harbor up to 80 clusters per depot in homeostatic conditions (24). This heterogeneity is also reflected in FALC size, which ranges from 100 to 500 μm in diameter (19).

Unlike lymph nodes, FALCs are not encapsulated and are in direct contact with surrounding adipocytes (19). The arrangement of leukocytes found in FALCs also differs from the organization of conventional SLOs. For instance, no discernible B and T cell compartmentalization areas are evident. Instead, FALCs from mesenteric AT are composed of a tight cluster of B220$^+$ or IgM$^+$ B cells, with variable numbers of CD4$^+$ T cells and CD11b$^+$ myeloid cells (19, 24). Both myeloid cell precursors (CD31/ER-MP58$^+$) and mature macrophages (F4/80$^+$) have been detected in omental FALCs, suggesting that these lymphoid clusters form permissive microenvironments where the former cells can proliferate locally to be a source of free macrophages within the peritoneal cavity (32). A similar process is likely to take place in FALCs in the mediastinum and pericardium (33, 34). Importantly, FALCs contain type 2 innate lymphoid cells (ILC2) that can support the proliferation of B1 cells through the expression of IL-5 (19).

B cell recruitment to mesenteric FALCs requires the presence of a network of stromal cells expressing the chemokine CXCL13 (24). These cells are found scattered along the lymphoid clusters and are thought to be different from follicular dendritic cells (FDCs), which require signaling through LTβR to induce CXCL13 expression (35). Importantly, FALCs are present in *Cxcl13*$^{-/-}$ mice although they are devoid of B cells and their size is smaller than in their wild type littermates.

Fat-associated lymphoid clusters are highly vascularized as shown by their close association to blood vessels (19, 24). Moreover, lymphoid clusters in the omentum have also been found to contain high endothelial venules (HEVs), a specialized type of post-capillary venules essential for lymphocyte trafficking (30, 36). In contrast, FALCs connection with lymphatic vessels remains to be further investigated (24, 25, 27, 37). Earlier evidence has shown that FALCs in the omentum can collect antigens and particles directly from fluids within the peritoneal cavity (27).

TABLE 1 | Main characteristics of mucosal lymphoid tissues.

Lymphoid structure	Location	Structural organization	Ontogeny	Developmental requirements	Reference
Bronchial-associated lymphoid tissue (BALT)	Near the basal side of the bronchial epithelium of the lungs	Arranged in a B cell follicle with clusters of IgD$^+$ cells, grouped around follicular dendritic cells (FDCs). They also contain a discrete T cell zone	Formation after birth, following antigen exposure or inflammatory challenge. High frequency in the neonatal stage	Defective architecture in *Lta*$^{-/-}$ mice. Defective number in *Il7ra*$^{-/-}$ mice. Absent in mice lacking *Cxcl13*, *Ccl19*, and *Ccl21a*	Fleige et al. (5), Kocks et al. (8), Moyron-Quiroz et al. (20), Rangel-Moreno et al. (9)
Isolated lymphoid follicles	Along the anti-mesenteric wall of the small intestine	Composed of a B cell area (germinal center) and few T cells	Formation after birth in response to inflammation or infection	Absent in *Lta*$^{-/-}$, *Ltbr*$^{-/-}$ *Aly/aly*, *Cxcr5*$^{-/-}$, and *Rorc*$^{-/-}$ mice. Requirement of commensal flora for maturation	Baptista et al. (10), Hamada et al. (11), Lorenz et al. (12), Velaga et al. (21)
Nasopharyngeal-associated lymphoid tissue (NALT)	Nasal passages of the nasal cavity	Composed of B and T cell areas	Formation after birth, first detected at postnatal day 7 in mouse	Defective formation in *Lta*$^{-/-}$, *Ltbr*$^{-/-}$, *Il7ra*$^{-/-}$, *Aly/aly*, *Cxcr5*$^{-/-}$, and *Cxcl13*$^{-/-}$ mice. Absent in *Id2*$^{-/-}$ mice. Requirement of microbiota for maturation	Asanuma et al. (15), Fukuyama et al. (16), Harmsen et al. (22), Rangel-Moreno et al. (23)
Tear duct-associated lymphoid tissue (TALT)	Lacrimal sac and tear duct of the eye	Composed of B cell aggregates, DCs and T cells	Formation after birth, between postnatal days 5 and 10 in mouse	Defective size and number in *Lta*$^{-/-}$, *Il7ra*$^{-/-}$, and *Cxcl13*$^{-/-}$ mice. TALT formation is preserved in *Id2*$^{-/-}$ and *Rorc*$^{-/-}$ mice	Nagatake et al. (13), Paulsen et al. (14)
Portal tract-associated lymphoid tissue	Portal triad of the liver	Composed of B cell aggregates, FDCs and T cells	Formation after birth, triggered in response to bacterial and viral infections	Formation may be dependent on CCL21 expression	Grant et al. (17), Yoneyama et al. (18)

DEVELOPMENTAL REQUIREMENTS FOR FALC FORMATION

Conventional SLOs such as lymph nodes and Peyer's patches develop in a timely manner during embryogenesis, independently of pathogen-induced inflammation (38). In contrast, FALCs develop postnatally and could be identified at around 2–3 weeks after birth, reaching a plateau at around 18 weeks of age in mice (24). Unlike classical SLOs, FALC formation is not dependent on LTβR signaling as shown by the occurrence of these clusters in *Ltβr*$^{-/-}$ and *Ltα*$^{-/-}$ mice (24). Furthermore, FALCs also form in *Rag2*$^{-/-}$ and *Rorc*$^{-/-}$ mice, which lack B and T cells and LTi/ILC3 cells, respectively. FALCs are not the only lymphoid structures that develop independently of LTi cells and LTβR signaling, as other mucosal-associated lymphoid tissues, but also follow these developmental requirements (see **Table 1**) (9, 13, 16, 39).

Fat-associated lymphoid clusters are absent in *Rag2*$^{-/-}$*Il2rg*$^{-/-}$ mice, which lack lymphocytes and ILCs, indicating a requirement of the latter for their development (24). Moreover, FALC formation is defective in *Tnfrsf1a*$^{-/-}$*Tnfrsf1b*$^{-/-}$ mice, which lack TNF receptors (TNFR1 and TNFR2) (24). Further analysis has shown that AT macrophages are the main source of TNF and that stromal cells respond to this cytokine *via* TNFR, leading to FALC formation (**Figure 1**) (24).

Fat-associated lymphoid cluster numbers are also greatly reduced in germ-free (GF) mice, suggesting a potential role of commensal flora in the formation of these structures (24). Interestingly, other lymphoid structures such as ILFs, which are found in the wall of the small intestine, are reduced or immature in GF mice (10). This suggests that similar to ILFs, the presence of commensal microbes or their by-products results in an inflammatory stimulus that induces the formation of FALCs. It will be interesting to test whether disruption of the intestinal epithelial barrier has an effect in the number and/or cellular composition of mesenteric FALCs (29).

ARE FALCs SIMILAR TO MILKY SPOTS (MS) OF THE OMENTUM?

Milky spots were first described by von Recklinghausen in 1863 as white spots in the omentum of rabbits (40). These structures were later characterized as highly vascularized accumulations of macrophages, B and T lymphocytes, and mast cells within the stroma of the greater omentum (41, 42). The omentum is generally divided in two parts, the greater and lesser omentum, depending on its position within the peritoneal cavity. Moreover, the omentum contains two distinguishable regions: a translucent collagenous membrane-like region and an adipose-rich region

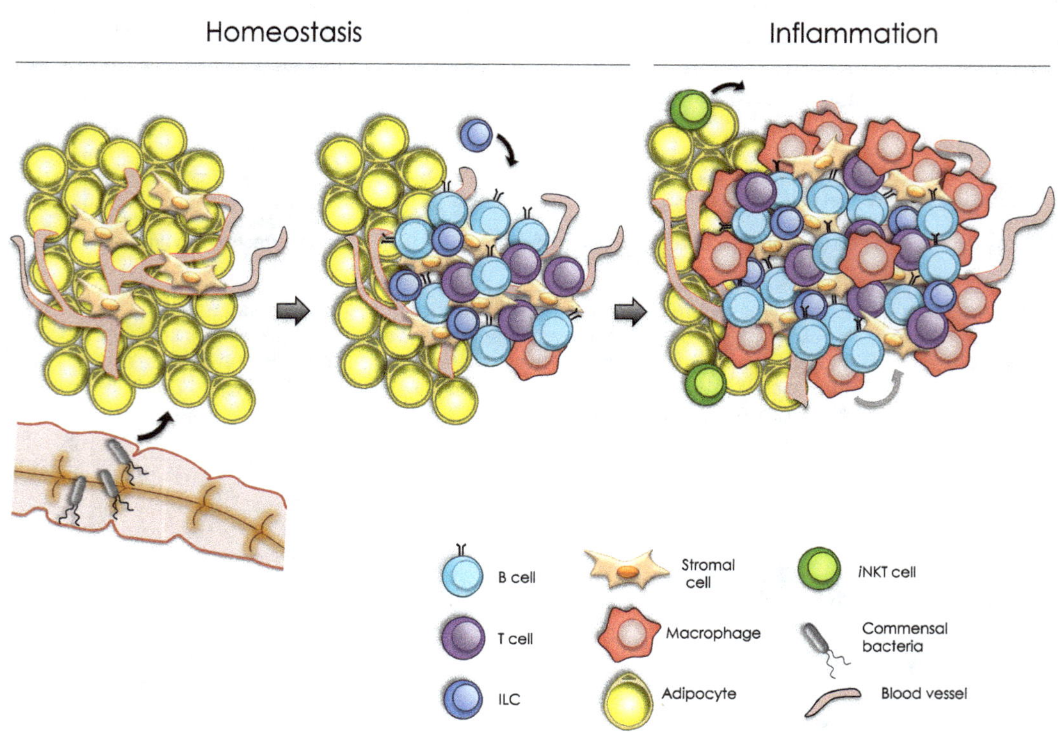

FIGURE 1 | Model of fat associated lymphoid cluster (FALC) formation. In homeostasis, FALC formation can be modulated by different signals, including colonization by commensal microbiota, tumor necrosis factor (TNF) signaling, and type 2 innate lymphoid cells function. These signals may trigger cytokine production from local cells within the adipose tissue. For instance, CXCL13-expressing stromal cells can promote the recruitment of B cells into arranged lymphoid clusters. Following an inflammatory challenge, FALCs increase in number and size. Under these conditions, infiltrating macrophages are able to secrete TNF, which upon signaling through TNF receptors in stromal cells, promoting FALC growth. Moreover, invariant natural killer T cells stimulate FALC formation through the production of T helper type 2 cytokines, including IL-4 and IL-13, which may also promote the resolution of inflammation.

TABLE 2 | Comparison of milky spots (MS) and fat-associated lymphoid clusters (FALCs).

Feature	MS	FALCs
Location	Greater omentum	Mesenteric, mediastinal gonadal, and pericardial fat (19, 24, 25)
Size	349–756 μm in diameter in humans (26). 850 μm in diameter in healthy rabbits (27)	100–500 μm in diameter in mice (19). Size tends to increase with age (28)
Cell composition	Macrophages (47.5%) B lymphocytes (29.1%) T lymphocytes (11.7%) Mast cells (6.1%) (26) Type 2 innate lymphoid cells (ILC2) (19) CXCL13$^+$ and FDCM1$^+$ stromal cells (29, 30)	B lymphocytes T lymphocytes Macrophages ILC2 (20–40%) (19) CXCL13$^+$ stromal cells (24)
Developmental requirements	MS develop independently of ILC3/LTi cells and the chemokines CCL19 and CCL21. On the other hand, MS are defective or absent in *Cxcl13*$^{-/-}$ and *Lta*$^{-/-}$ mice (30)	FALCs develop independently of ILC3/LTi cells and LTβR signaling. In contrast, their development is dependent on TNF signaling on stromal cells. IL-4R signaling and the presence of invariant natural killer T cells are also required. The requirement for type 2 ILCs in FALC development remains to be investigated (24)
Ontogeny	Accumulation of myeloid cells in the greater omentum has been observed at 20 weeks of gestation. True MS are observed at 35 weeks of gestation in humans (31)	Mesenteric FALCs are formed after birth, with visible clusters at 2–3 weeks of age in mice (24)

containing blood and lymphatic vessels, stromal cells, and clusters of immune cells (43). In mice and humans, MS have been found in the adipose region of the omentum, whereas in dogs, the aggregates of lymphoid cells are only found scattered in the translucent area (43, 44). However, no clear distinction in the exact location of MS within the omentum has been established. Interestingly, some authors have divided MS in two categories: vascularized and non-vascularized MS. Vascularized MS are supplied with blood vessels and are found in the omental fat region. On the other hand, non-vascularized MS do not have blood supply and are located in the omental membrane (45). Whether these features that translate into functional differences remain to be investigated.

A close examination showed no discernible differences between MS and the FALCs in mesenteries, mediastinum, and gonadal fat (see **Table 2**). In light of their similar characteristics but distinct locations and for clarity, we will be calling the omental MS as omFALCs while mesFALCs correspond to the clusters in the mesenteries, medFALCs the structures in the mediastinum, perFALC for the structures in the pericardium, and gonFALC the clusters present in gonadal fat.

FALC RESPOND TO INFLAMMATION AND IMMUNIZATION

MesFALCs and omFALCs increase in number and size in response to acute or chronic peritoneal inflammation (24, 27, 37). For instance, upon intraperitoneal (IP) injection of Zymosan, a yeast-derived ligand of Toll-like receptor 2, the abundance and size of mesFALCs increased significantly (24). *Rag2*$^{-/-}$ and *Cd1d*$^{-/-}$ mice failed to induce FALC formation in response to Zymosan-induced inflammation. Interestingly, IP injection of invariant natural killer T (iNKT) cells into *Rag2*$^{-/-}$ mice was able to restore mesFALC formation following Zymosan challenge, indicating a role of iNKT cells in this process (24). More specifically, activated iNKT cells can produce T helper type 2 (T_H2) cytokines, including IL-4 and IL-13, which may have redundant roles in the formation of FALCs following peritoneal inflammation in the BALB/c strain background (**Figure 1**) (24).

Likewise, IP injection of lipid A, a component of bacterial lipopolysaccharide, leads to an increase in the number of B1 cells and macrophages in the omentum (29). Moreover, IP injection of polydextran particles or polyacrylamide beads increases the number and size of omFALC (37, 46). Different models of inflammation including TNF injection, *Escherichia coli* infection, and cecal ligation lead to the influx of neutrophils to the omFALC *via* HEVs (36).

Earlier evidence of the mechanisms by which FALCs respond to immunization comes from studies on immune responses in the omentum. Using an elegant mouse model that lacks spleen, lymph nodes, and Peyer's patches (SLP mice), Rangel-Moreno, Randall, and colleagues have shown that omFALC are sufficient to respond to an immunological challenge and support T cell responses, immunoglobulin switching, and moderate affinity maturation (30). It is possible that the antigen-specific immune response shown in serum in SLP mice upon IP immunization that had been attributed to the omFALC may have a relative contribution from mesFALCs. Peritoneal immunization resulted in a marked recruitment of macrophages to the omFALC similar to what has been shown in mesFALCs (24). OmFALCs were shown to collect IP injected fluorophore-labeled antigens or GFP-labeled tumor cells. Peritoneal cell migration to the omentum is mediated by mechanisms that are both dependent and independent of chemokines, but clustering of B and T lymphocytes is dependent on the latter.

Macrophages are the most important cell type to engulf and eliminate bacteria in omFALCs (30). Indeed, it has been shown in a diet-induced obesity model that macrophages in gonFALC are able to proteolytically process antigen and present it in the context of MHC II complexes, indicating that they can function as antigen-presenting cells to induce T cell proliferation (47). Furthermore, IP immunizations with T-cell-dependent antigens showed that antigen-specific B cells undergo expansion, Ig switching, and acquired markers of GC reaction further indicating that adaptive immune responses take place in mesFALCs (24).

Mesenteric FALCs are also able to respond to intestinal helminth infection (*Nippostrongylus brasiliensis*) *via* ILC2 activation and expression of the T_H2 cytokines IL-5 and IL-13. These cytokines are produced in response to IL-33 and IL-25 and promote goblet cell hyperplasia and helminth expulsion (19, 48). Likewise, a recent report has shown that medFALCs and perFALCs respond to both lung infection with the nematode *Litomosoides sigmodontis* and lung inflammation *via* fungal allergen inhalation (33). Under these conditions, medFALC stromal cells produce IL-33, which leads to ILC2 activation and IL-5 secretion. This in turn promotes the recruitment and activation of B cells and culminates in the production of natural IgM antibodies (Ab) for local protection (33).

A recent report has shown that medFALC are present in large numbers in two animal models of autoimmunity that develop a phenotype similar to human systemic lupus erythematosus (SLE) (49). The MRL/MpJ-lpr mouse model carries a mutation in the gene encoding Fas, a cell membrane receptor that induces caspase activation and apoptosis. This mutant strain develops a severe autoimmune syndrome with lymphadenopathy, splenomegaly, and the production of anti-double strand DNA (dsDNA) Ab as well as immune complex deposition in several organs including kidney, resembling human SLE. The BXSB/MpJ-Yaa mice developed systemic autoimmunity, with males being more affected due to a locus called autoimmune accelerator located in the Y chromosome. Both strains showed large medFALCs size that correlated with a significant increased level of immune cell infiltration in the lungs with respect to their control strains (49). It will be interesting to assess whether medFALCs in the MRL/MpJ-lpr model contained anti dsDNA Ab-forming B cells.

Several reports indicate a link between FALCs and cancer metastasis in the peritoneum. A study has shown a direct correlation between the presence and number of FALCs and the colonization of the clusters by ovarian cancer cells, with the omentum containing the largest number of FALCs and metastasis/foci of tumor cells (50). The foci formation by tumor cells in FALCs is not affected by the absence of lymphocytes, indicating a role for specialized stromal cells, endothelium, and adipocytes in the clusters that facilitate malignant cell recruitment. Similarly, IP injection of gastric and colon cancer cells resulted in their rapid migration and survival in omental and mesFALCs (51–53). These reports together with the evidence of metastasis formation in the omentum and peritoneal cavity for some human cancers (54) indicate the presence of a favorable microenvironment in FALCs that allows the tumor cells to thrive and form micrometastasis in these tissues. Along this line, some reports have shown that gastric, colon, and some liver cancer cells express the chemokine receptors CCR4 and CXCR4, whereas cell populations from omFALCs and mesenteries can express their ligands (CCL22 and CXCL12), which may favor their migration to these structures (51, 52, 55).

CONCLUSION

The rapid formation of FALCs following inflammation or infection, the changes in cellular composition and the presence of innate immune cells and B cells undergoing a germinal center reaction indicate a central role for these clusters in the formation of local immune responses.

Understanding what signals and cells are essential to FALC formation in homeostasis and following infection will allow inducing their formation to support antitumor responses. Conversely, it may be possible to reduce or preclude FALC formation during aberrant immune responses or peritoneal inflammation.

The physiological significance of the close association of FALCs with visceral AT remains to be further investigated. It is tempting to hypothesize that FALCs have an additional function in supporting type 2 ILCs and other immune cells that ultimately maintain the homeostasis of AT and whole body metabolism. Ultimately, understanding FALC formation in the mesenteries, omentum, and gonadal fat may facilitate the design of therapies to target low-grade chronic inflammation and other symptoms associated with obesity and metabolic syndrome.

AUTHOR CONTRIBUTIONS

SC-M prepared the tables and figure. SC-M and JC wrote the manuscript.

FUNDING

This work was supported by a grant from the Biotechnology and Biological Sciences Research Council (BB/K009400/1) to JC and the College of Medical and Dental Sciences of the University of Birmingham.

REFERENCES

1. Randall TD, Carragher DM, Rangel-Moreno J. Development of secondary lymphoid organs. *Annu Rev Immunol* (2008) 26:627–50. doi:10.1146/annurev.immunol.26.021607.090257
2. Ruddle NH, Akirav EM. Secondary lymphoid organs: responding to genetic and environmental cues in ontogeny and the immune response. *J Immunol* (2009) 183:2205–12. doi:10.4049/jimmunol.0804324
3. van de Pavert SA, Mebius RE. New insights into the development of lymphoid tissues. *Nat Rev Immunol* (2010) 10:664–74. doi:10.1038/nri2832
4. Fletcher AL, Acton SE, Knoblich K. Lymph node fibroblastic reticular cells in health and disease. *Nat Rev Immunol* (2015) 15:350–61. doi:10.1038/nri3846
5. Fleige H, Haas JD, Stahl FR, Willenzon S, Prinz I, Forster R. Induction of BALT in the absence of IL-17. *Nat Immunol* (2011) 13(1):1. doi:10.1038/ni.2167
6. Fleige H, Ravens S, Moschovakis GL, Bölter J, Willenzon S, Sutter G, et al. IL-17-induced CXCL12 recruits B cells and induces follicle formation in BALT in the absence of differentiated FDCs. *J Exp Med* (2014) 211(4):643–51. doi:10.1084/jem.20131737

7. Hwang JY, Randall TD, Silva-Sanchez A. Inducible bronchus-associated lymphoid tissue: taming inflammation in the lung. *Front Immunol* (2016) 7:258. doi:10.3389/fimmu.2016.00258
8. Kocks JR, Davalos-Misslitz AC, Hintzen G, Ohl L, Forster R. Regulatory T cells interfere with the development of bronchus-associated lymphoid tissue. *J Exp Med* (2007) 204:723–34. doi:10.1084/jem.20061424
9. Rangel-Moreno J, Carragher DM, de la Luz Garcia-Hernandez M, Hwang JY, Kusser K, Hartson L, et al. The development of inducible bronchus-associated lymphoid tissue depends on IL-17. *Nat Immunol* (2011) 12:639–46. doi:10.1038/ni.2053
10. Baptista AP, Olivier BJ, Goverse G, Greuter M, Knippenberg M, Kusser K, et al. Colonic patch and colonic SILT development are independent and differentially regulated events. *Mucosal Immunol* (2013) 6:511–21. doi:10.1038/mi.2012.90
11. Hamada H, Hiroi T, Nishiyama Y, Takahashi H, Masunaga Y, Hachimura S, et al. Identification of multiple isolated lymphoid follicles on the antimesenteric wall of the mouse small intestine. *J Immunol* (2002) 168:57–64. doi:10.4049/jimmunol.168.1.57
12. Lorenz RG, Chaplin DD, McDonald KG, McDonough JS, Newberry RD. Isolated lymphoid follicle formation is inducible and dependent upon lymphotoxin-sufficient B lymphocytes, lymphotoxin beta receptor, and TNF receptor I function. *J Immunol* (2003) 170:5475–82. doi:10.4049/jimmunol.170.11.5475
13. Nagatake T, Fukuyama S, Kim DY, Goda K, Igarashi O, Sato S, et al. Id2-, RORgammat-, and LTbetaR-independent initiation of lymphoid organogenesis in ocular immunity. *J Exp Med* (2009) 206:2351–64. doi:10.1084/jem.20091436
14. Paulsen FP, Paulsen JI, Thale AB, Tillmann BN. Mucosa-associated lymphoid tissue in human efferent tear ducts. *Virchows Arch* (2000) 437:185–9. doi:10.1007/s004280000248
15. Asanuma H, Thompson AH, Iwasaki T, Sato Y, Inaba Y, Aizawa C, et al. Isolation and characterization of mouse nasal-associated lymphoid tissue. *J Immunol Methods* (1997) 202:123–31. doi:10.1016/S0022-1759(96)00243-8
16. Fukuyama S, Hiroi T, Yokota Y, Rennert PD, Yanagita M, Kinoshita N, et al. Initiation of NALT organogenesis is independent of the IL-7R, LTbetaR, and NIK signaling pathways but requires the Id2 gene and CD3- CD4+ CD45+ cells. *Immunity* (2002) 17:31–40. doi:10.1016/S1074-7613(02)00339-4
17. Grant AJ, Goddard S, Ahmed-Choudhury J, Reynolds G, Jackson DG, Briskin M, et al. Hepatic expression of secondary lymphoid chemokine (CCL21) promotes the development of portal-associated lymphoid tissue in chronic inflammatory liver disease. *Am J Pathol* (2002) 160:1445–55. doi:10.1016/S0002-9440(10)62570-9
18. Yoneyama H, Matsuno K, Zhang Y, Murai M, Itakura M, Ishikawa S, et al. Regulation by chemokines of circulating dendritic cell precursors, and the formation of portal tract–associated lymphoid tissue, in a granulomatous liver disease. *J Exp Med* (2000) 193:35–49. doi:10.1084/jem.193.1.35
19. Moro K, Yamada T, Tanabe M, Takeuchi T, Ikawa T, Kawamoto H, et al. Innate production of T(H)2 cytokines by adipose tissue-associated c-Kit(+)Sca-1(+) lymphoid cells. *Nature* (2010) 463:540–4. doi:10.1038/nature08636
20. Moyron-Quiroz JE, Rangel-Moreno J, Kusser K, Hartson L, Sprague F, Goodrich S, et al. Role of inducible bronchus associated lymphoid tissue (iBALT) in respiratory immunity. *Nat Med* (2004) 10:927–34. doi:10.1038/nm1091
21. Velaga S, Herbrand H, Friedrichsen M, Jiong T, Dorsch M, Hoffmann MW, et al. Chemokine receptor CXCR5 supports solitary intestinal lymphoid tissue formation, B cell homing, and induction of intestinal IgA responses. *J Immunol* (2009) 182:2610–9. doi:10.4049/jimmunol.0801141
22. Harmsen A, Kusser K, Hartson L, Tighe M, Sunshine MJ, Sedgwick JD, et al. Cutting edge: organogenesis of nasal-associated lymphoid tissue (NALT) occurs independently of lymphotoxin-alpha (LT alpha) and retinoic acid receptor-related orphan receptor-gamma, but the organization of NALT is LT alpha dependent. *J Immunol* (2002) 168:986–90. doi:10.4049/jimmunol.168.3.986
23. Rangel-Moreno J, Moyron-Quiroz J, Kusser K, Hartson L, Nakano H, Randall TD. Role of CXC chemokine ligand 13, CC chemokine ligand (CCL) 19, and CCL21 in the organization and function of nasal-associated lymphoid tissue. *J Immunol* (2005) 175:4904–13. doi:10.4049/jimmunol.175.8.4904
24. Bénézech CC, Luu N-T, Walker JA, Kruglov AA, Loo Y, Nakamura K, et al. Inflammation-induced formation of fat-associated lymphoid clusters. *Nat Immunol* (2015) 16:819–28. doi:10.1038/ni.3215
25. Elewa YH, Ichii O, Otsuka S, Hashimoto Y, Kon Y. Characterization of mouse mediastinal fat-associated lymphoid clusters. *Cell Tissue Res* (2014) 357:731–41. doi:10.1007/s00441-014-1889-6
26. Shimotsuma M, Takahashi T, Kawata M, Dux K. Cellular subsets of the milky spots in the human greater omentum. *Cell Tissue Res* (1991) 264:599–601. doi:10.1007/BF00319049
27. DiPaolo N, Sacchi G, Garosi G, Sansoni E, Bargagli L, Ponzo P, et al. Omental milky spots and peritoneal dialysis – review and personal experience. *Perit Dial Int* (2005) 25:48–57.
28. Lumeng CN, Liu J, Geletka L, Delaney C, Delproposto J, Desai A, et al. Aging is associated with an increase in T cells and inflammatory macrophages in visceral adipose tissue. *J Immunol* (2011) 187:6208–16. doi:10.4049/jimmunol.1102188
29. Ha SA, Tsuji M, Suzuki K, Meek B, Yasuda N, Kaisho T, et al. Regulation of B1 cell migration by signals through Toll-like receptors. *J Exp Med* (2006) 203:2541–50. doi:10.1084/jem.20061041
30. Rangel-Moreno J, Moyron-Quiroz JE, Carragher DM, Kusser K, Hartson L, Moquin A, et al. Omental milky spots develop in the absence of lymphoid tissue-inducer cells and support B and T cell responses to peritoneal antigens. *Immunity* (2009) 30:731–43. doi:10.1016/j.immuni.2009.03.014
31. Krist LFG, Koenen H, Calame W, van der Harten JJ, van der Linden JC, Eestermans IL, et al. Ontogeny of milky spots in the human greater omentum – an immunochemical study. *Anat Rec* (1997) 249:399–404. doi:10.1002/(SICI)1097-0185(199711)249:3<399::AID-AR11>3.0.CO;2-J
32. Wijffels JF, Hendrickx RJ, Steenbergen JJ, Eestermans IL, Beelen RH. Milky spots in the mouse omentum may play an important role in the origin of peritoneal macrophages. *Res Immunol* (1992) 143:401–9. doi:10.1016/S0923-2494(05)80072-0
33. Jackson-Jones LH, Duncan SM, Magalhaes MS, Campbell SM, Maizels RM, McSorley HJ, et al. Fat-associated lymphoid clusters control local IgM secretion during pleural infection and lung inflammation. *Nat Commun* (2016) 7:12651. doi:10.1038/ncomms12651
34. Jenkins SJ, Ruckerl D, Cook PC, Jones LH, Finkelman FD, van Rooijen N, et al. Local macrophage proliferation, rather than recruitment from the blood, is a signature of TH2 inflammation. *Science* (2011) 332:1284–8. doi:10.1126/science.1204351
35. Ngo VN, Korner H, Gunn MD, Schmidt KN, Riminton DS, Cooper MD, et al. Lymphotoxin a/b and tumor necrosis factor are required for stromal cell expression of homing chemokines in B and T cell areas of the spleen. *J Exp Med* (1999) 189:403–12. doi:10.1084/jem.189.2.403
36. Buscher K, Wang H, Zhang X, Striewski P, Wirth B, Saggu G, et al. Protection from septic peritonitis by rapid neutrophil recruitment through omental high endothelial venules. *Nat Commun* (2016) 7:10828. doi:10.1038/ncomms10828
37. Litbarg NO, Gudehithlu KP, Sethupathi P, Arruda JA, Dunea G, Singh AK. Activated omentum becomes rich in factors that promote healing and tissue regeneration. *Cell Tissue Res* (2007) 328:487–97. doi:10.1007/s00441-006-0356-4
38. Carragher DM, Rangel-Moreno J, Randall TD. Ectopic lymphoid tissues and local immunity. *Semin Immunol* (2008) 20:26–42. doi:10.1016/j.smim.2007.12.004
39. Randall TD, Mebius RE. The development and function of mucosal lymphoid tissues: a balancing act with micro-organisms. *Mucosal Immunol* (2014) 7:455–66. doi:10.1038/mi.2014.11
40. Recklinghausen FV. Uber Eiter und Bindesgewebs-korperchen. *Vir Arch Pathol Anat* (1863) 28:157–66. doi:10.1007/BF01930779
41. Krist LFG, Eestermans IL, Steenbergen JJE, Hoefsmit ECM, Cuesta MA, Meyer S, et al. Cellular composition of milky spots in the human greater omentum: an immunochemical and ultrastructural study. *Anat Rec* (1995) 241:163–74. doi:10.1002/ar.1092410204
42. Yildirim A, Aktas A, Nergiz Y, Akkus M. Analysis of human omentum-associated lymphoid tissue components with S-100 – an immunohistochemical study. *Rom J Morphol Embryol* (2010) 51:759–64.
43. Wilkosz S, Ireland G, Khwaja N, Walker M, Butt R, Giorgio-Miller AD, et al. A comparative study of the structure of human and murine greater omentum. *Anat Embryol* (2005) 209:251–61. doi:10.1007/s00429-004-0446-6

44. Huyghe S, de Rooster H, Doom M, Van den Broeck W. The microscopic structure of the omentum in healthy dogs: the mystery unravelled. *Anat Histol Embryol* (2016) 45:209–18. doi:10.1111/ahe.12189
45. Takemori N, Hirai K, Onodera R, Saito N, Namiki M. Light and electron microscopic study of omental milky spots in New Zealand Black mice, with special reference to the extramedullary hematopoiesis. *Anat Embryol* (1994) 189:215–26. doi:10.1007/BF00239009
46. Shah S, Lowery E, Braun RK, Martin A, Huang N, Medina M, et al. Cellular basis of tissue regeneration by omentum. *PLoS One* (2012) 7:e38368. doi:10.1371/journal.pone.0038368
47. Morris DL, Cho KW, Delproposto JL, Oatmen KE, Geletka LM, Martinez-Santibanez G, et al. Adipose tissue macrophages function as antigen-presenting cells and regulate adipose tissue CD4+ T cells in mice. *Diabetes* (2013) 62:2762–72. doi:10.2337/db12-1404
48. von Moltke J, Ji M, Liang HE, Locksley RM. Tuft-cell-derived IL-25 regulates an intestinal ILC2-epithelial response circuit. *Nature* (2016) 529:221–5. doi:10.1038/nature16161
49. Elewa YH, Ichii O, Kon Y. Comparative analysis of mediastinal fat-associated lymphoid cluster development and lung cellular infiltration in murine autoimmune disease models and the corresponding normal control strains. *Immunology* (2016) 147:30–40. doi:10.1111/imm.12539
50. Clark R, Krishnan V, Schoof M, Rodriguez I, Theriault B, Chekmareva M, et al. Milky spots promote ovarian cancer metastatic colonization of peritoneal adipose in experimental models. *Am J Pathol* (2013) 183:576–91. doi:10.1016/j.ajpath.2013.04.023
51. Cao L, Cao X, Zhang Y, Sun XT. Omental milky spots in screening gastric cancer stem cells. *Neoplasma* (2011) 58:20–6. doi:10.4149/neo_2011_01_20
52. Kasagi Y, Harada Y, Morodomi Y, Iwai T, Saito S, Yoshida K, et al. Peritoneal dissemination requires an Sp1-dependent CXCR4/CXCL12 signaling axis and extracellular matrix-directed spheroid formation. *Cancer Res* (2016) 76:347–57. doi:10.1158/0008-5472.CAN-15-1563
53. Sedlacek AL, Gerber SA, Randall TD, van Rooijen N, Frelinger JG, Lord EM. Generation of a dual-functioning antitumor immune response in the peritoneal cavity. *Am J Pathol* (2013) 183:1318–28. doi:10.1016/j.ajpath.2013.06.030
54. Koppe MJ, Nagtegaal ID, de Wilt JH, Ceelen WP. Recent insights into the pathophysiology of omental metastases. *J Surg Oncol* (2014) 110:670–5. doi:10.1002/jso.23681
55. Abe H, Ina K, Kitamura H, Sumiyoshi H, Tatsukawa S, Yoshioka H, et al. Role of the CXCL12/CXCR4 axis in milky spots of rats bearing ascitic-type hepatoma. *Anat Sci Int* (2009) 84:226–36. doi:10.1007/s12565-009-0028-z

Biosynthesis and Functional Significance of Peripheral Node Addressin in Cancer-Associated TLO

*Aliyah M. Weinstein[1] and Walter J. Storkus[1,2,3]**

[1] Department of Immunology, University of Pittsburgh School of Medicine, Pittsburgh, PA, USA, [2] Department of Dermatology, University of Pittsburgh School of Medicine, Pittsburgh, PA, USA, [3] University of Pittsburgh Cancer Institute, Pittsburgh, PA, USA

***Correspondence:**
Walter J. Storkus
storkuswj@upmc.edu

Peripheral node addressin (PNAd) marks high endothelial venules (HEV), which are crucial for the recruitment of lymphocytes into lymphoid organs in non-mucosal tissue sites. PNAd is a sulfated and fucosylated glycoprotein recognized by the prototypic monoclonal antibody, MECA-79. PNAd is the ligand for L-selectin, which is expressed on the surface of naive and central memory T cells, where it mediates leukocyte rolling on vascular endothelial surfaces. Although PNAd was first identified in the HEV of peripheral lymph nodes, recent work suggests a critical role for PNAd in the context of chronic inflammatory diseases, where it can be used as a marker for the formation of tertiary lymphoid organs (TLOs). TLO form in tissues impacted by sustained inflammation, such as the tumor microenvironment where they function as local sites of adaptive immune cell priming. This allows for specific B- and T-cell responses to be initiated or reactivated in inflamed tissues without dependency on secondary lymphoid organs. Recent studies of cancer in mice and humans have identified PNAd as a biomarker of improved disease prognosis. Blockade of PNAd or its ligand, L-selectin, can abrogate protective antitumor immunity in murine models. This review examines pathways regulating PNAd biosynthesis by the endothelial cells integral to HEV and the formation and maintenance of lymphoid structures throughout the body, particularly in the setting of cancer.

Keywords: high endothelial venule, L-selectin, peripheral node addressin, tertiary lymphoid organ, tumor

PATHWAYS REGULATING PNAd EXPRESSION

Signaling Through the Lymphotoxin Beta Receptor Is Required for HEV Differentiation

Lymphotoxin beta receptor (LTβR) signaling drives expression of adhesion molecules and chemokines involved in the recruitment of circulating lymphocytes into lymphoid organs, including CCL21, CXCL13, MAdCAM-1, and peripheral node addressin (PNAd) (1). Specifically, expression of LTβR on endothelial cells in peripheral lymph nodes is required for their development into high

---

Abbreviations: BGC, germinal center B cell; BV, blood vessel; cDC, conventional dendritic cell; fDC, follicular dendritic cell; Gal, galactose; GalNAc, *N*-acetylgalactosamine; GlcNAc, *N*-acetylglucosamine; HEC, high endothelial cell; HEV, high endothelial venule; HVEM, herpes virus entry mediator; PNAd, peripheral node addressin; SA, sialic acid; SLO, secondary lymphoid organ; TLO, tertiary lymphoid structure; TME, tumor microenvironment; TNFR, tumor necrosis factor receptor; VSMC, vascular smooth muscle cell.

endothelial venules (HEV), with high endothelial cells (HEC) functioning as lymphoid tissue organizer (LTo) cells. Endothelial cell-specific deletion of LTβR leads to a reduction in: (i) MECA-79 staining, (ii) CCL19, CCL21, and GlyCAM-1 expression, and (iii) the ability to assume cuboidal morphology by endothelial cells in peripheral lymphoid organs [**Figure 1A**; (2)]. *In vivo* work using bone marrow chimeric mice deficient in LTα in their hematopoietic compartment also implicates a role for LTβR-mediated signaling in the maintenance of HEV, as these mice exhibit profoundly reduced lymph node cellularity (3).

$LT\alpha_1\beta_2$ and LIGHT can bind and signal through the LTβR, while a related ligand, $LT\alpha_3$, can signal through TNFRI, TNFRII, and HVEM. All three ligands can be produced by $CD11c^+$ DC (3). However, each ligand appears to have a distinct role in regulating PNAd expression. In secondary lymphoid organs (SLO), LIGHT appears to have little impact on PNAd expression (4). Using a transgenic model of lymphotoxin overexpression in the pancreas, it was observed that LTα and LTβ play distinct roles in the formation of tertiary lymphoid organs (TLOs). $LT\alpha_1\beta_2$ controls luminal PNAd expression, while $LT\alpha_3$ controls abluminal PNAd expression (1). These differences in ligand function appear to relate to their impact on the level of GlcNAc6ST expression by endothelial cells. GlcNAc6ST-2 expression was reduced if only LTα, but not LTβ, was present, with HEV in $LT\beta^{-/-}$ animals (that retained GlcNAc6ST-2) expressing PNAd (1). $LT\alpha^{-/-}$ animals were deficient in GlcNAc6ST-2 expression on HEV, although they retained PNAd expression (5). Blockade of LTβR signaling also decreases transcription of GlcNAc6ST-2 in lymph nodes by 10-fold, with GlcNAc6ST-1, FucT-VII, and FucT-IV levels also coordinately reduced, thereby limiting posttranslational modification of PNAd and inhibiting its ability to be recognized by L-selectin (4).

Lymphocytes are also able to secrete lymphotoxin ligands (2, 4). Interestingly, the requirement for T or B cells themselves in HEV activation in SLO is equivocal. Reports suggest that neither cell type is required for HEV differentiation (4), although it has also been observed that *Rag*$^{-}$/$^{-}$ mice exhibit decreased expression of GlcNAc6ST-2 compared to WT mice (6).

Posttranslational Modifications Are Required for L-Selectin Recognition of PNAd

Members of the PNAd family of addressins include GlyCAM-1, CD34, sgp200, podocalyxin, endomucin, and nepmucin: however, not all PNAd ligands appear to be required for lymphocyte trafficking (7, 8). For example, lymphocyte trafficking to peripheral lymph nodes remains unaltered in $CD34^{-/-}$ (9) or $GlyCAM1^{-/-}$ (10) mice, suggesting redundancy in the functional roles of PNAd family members. In order for PNAd to be recognized by MECA-79 as well as its receptor, L-selectin, a series of posttranslational modifications must first occur (**Figure 1**). Specifically, while PNAd undergoes sulfation and glycosylation (11), it is sulfation of the 6 sialyl Lewis X motif that renders these molecules recognizable by the MECA-79 antibody (12). Fucosylation of the Core 2 branched *O*-glycan serves as the recognition site of PNAd by L-selectin (**Figure 1B**) (13, 14).

Sulfation

GlcNAc6ST-1 and GlcNAc6ST-2 are members of the GalNAc6ST-6-*O*-sulfotransferase subfamily of glycosyl sulfotransferases that are critical to the transfer of sulfate groups to galactose or GlcNAc at the sixth position, with this sulfation of carbohydrate motifs on PNAd required for it to be presented at the cell surface and to be recognized by the MECA-79 antibody and by its natural ligand, L-selectin (15).

Though related, GlcNAc6ST-1 and GlcNAc6ST-2 have different roles in the sulfation of PNAd. Using mice deficient in either single sulfotransferase, it was shown that GlcNAc6ST-2 controls luminal expression of PNAd while GlcNAc6ST-1 controls expression of PNAd on the abluminal vascular surface (16, 17).

GlcNAc6ST-2 is expressed by mature, but not immature, HEV. Using a Cre-recombinase model, Kawashima and colleagues observed that expression of GlcNAc6ST-2 is activated in HEV cells recognized by the MECA-79 antibody (i.e., expressing PNAd), but not in cells reactive only with the MECA-367 antibody (recognizing MAdCAM-1) (18). This is consistent with observations that GlNAc6ST-1 and -2 have little impact on cellular expression of MAdCAM-1, a canonical marker of immature HEV in SLO within non-mucosal tissue sites (19).

Glycosylation

A family of α-(1,3)-fucosyltransferases control the fucosulation of E-, P-, and L-selectin ligands (20). In particular, FucT-VII and FucT-IV play distinct roles in the generation of L-selectin ligands on the surface of HEV. FucT-IV is required for the expression of L-selectin ligands on the surface of HEV, whereas the primary role of FucT-VII appears to be in its contribution to enhancing GlyCAM-1-mediated tethering of rolling lymphocytes. The specific role of FucT-VII temporally follows glycosylation and sulfation of the glycoprotein and is involved in capping the molecule to produce the preferred ligand recognized by L-selectin. Double knockout of both FucT-VII and FucT-IV in mice reduced lymphocyte recruitment to SLO by over 80% when compared to $FucT\text{-}VII^{-/-}$ mice (21).

MARKERS OF HIGH ENDOTHELIAL VENULES

Two sets of adhesion molecules dominantly modulate lymphocyte recruitment to SLO/TLO depending upon which site in the body the cells are trafficking to: recruitment to peripheral lymph nodes is dependent upon the L-selectin–PNAd interaction, while recruitment to mucosal sites requires the $\alpha_4\beta_7$ integrin–MAdCAM-1 interaction (22). The same HEC that express PNAd or MAdCAM-1 also express CCL21, a CCR7 ligand. Supporting the importance of PNAd- and CCL21-expressing HEV for the recruitment of lymphocytes, the majority of lymphocytes in HEV-expressing tissues are spatially located within approximately 20 μm of HEV (23). CCL21 preferentially recruits $CCR7^+$ $CD4^+$ L-selectin$^+$ (naive) T cells, which can interact with PNAd on the cells of the HEV. CCL21, like PNAd, is under the control of intrinsic LTβR-mediated signaling during HEV development (but not in mature lymphoid tissues) (1, 4).

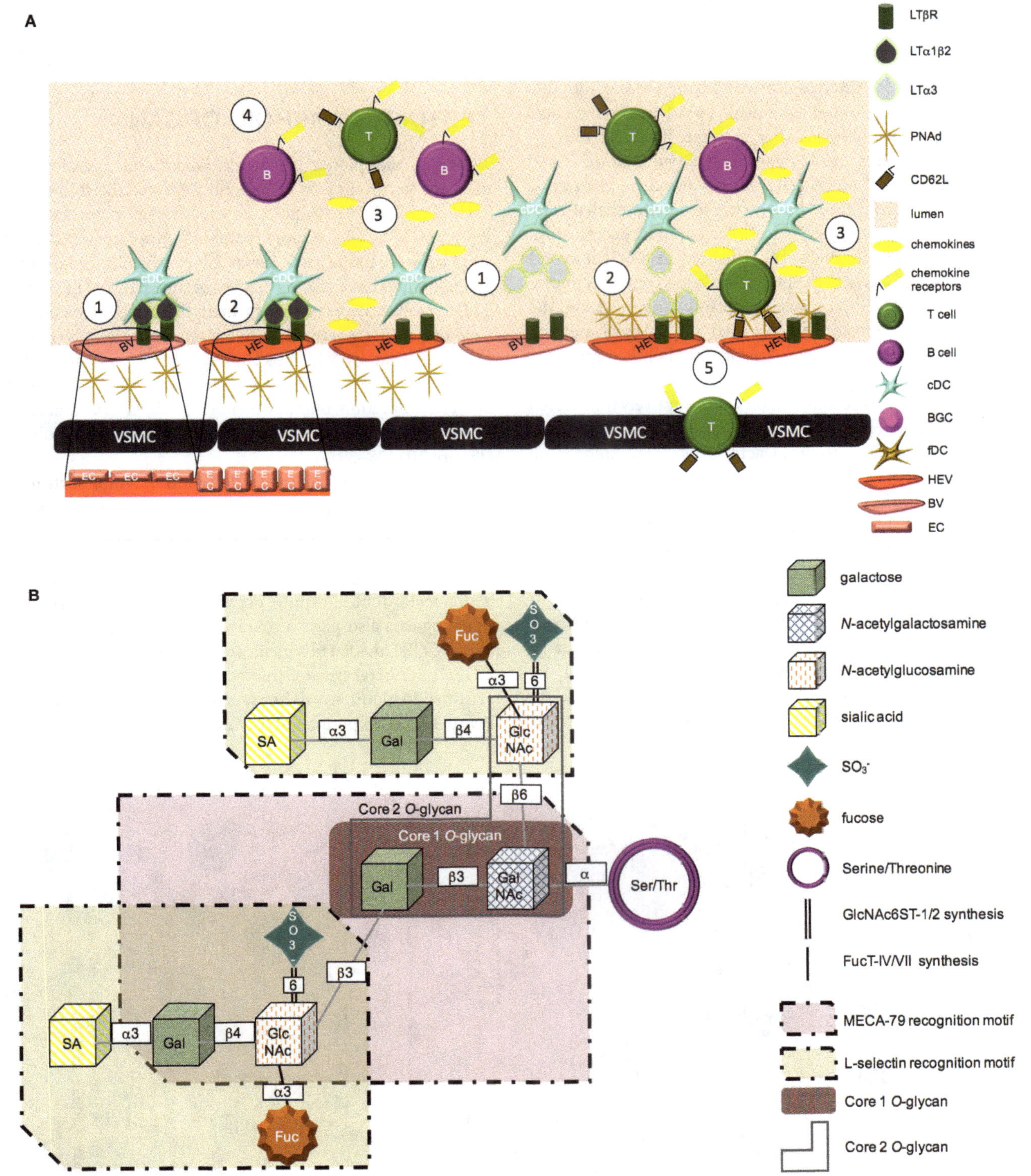

FIGURE 1 | PNAd biosynthesis. (A) (1) LTβR is expressed on blood vessel endothelial cells. Membrane-bound LTα1β2 or secreted LTα3 secreted from cDC can signal through this receptor. (2) LTβR-mediated signaling promotes a physical change in vascular endothelial cells from a flat to cuboidal morphology. This signaling cascade also leads to the expression of PNAd on the surface of vascular endothelial cells, promoting HEV status. (3) LTβR signaling further induces HEV secreted chemokines, including CCL19, CCL21, and CXCL13. (4) Chemokines form gradients and "decorate" the blood vessel wall, initiating the recruitment of CCR7+ T cells or CXCR5+ B lymphocytes from the peripheral blood circulation into chronically inflamed tissues. (5) L-selectin on the surface of T cells is able to bind PNAd on the surface of HEV. These cells are then able to adhere to the vessel wall and extravasate into the tissue. **(B)** PNAd is synthesized from a Core 1 *O*-glycan. The extended Core 1 *O*-glycan serves as the MECA-79 recognition motif. The fucosylated Core 2 *O*-glycans are able to be recognized by L-selectin. Sulfation of the extended Core 1 and Core 2 *O*-glycans at the sixth position is mediated by GlcNAc6ST-1 and -2; α3 fucosylation is added by FucT-IV and -VII.

IMMUNE CELL RECRUITMENT BY HEV

Peripheral node addressin binds L-selectin (aka CD62L or LECAM-1) expressed on the surface of lymphocytes. This interaction is required for the recruitment of lymphocytes into SLO (24). Posttranslational modifications of PNAd family members are critical for this interaction. For example, B cell recruitment to peripheral lymph nodes is dependent on sulfation of PNAd (19). The velocity of T and B cell rolling is also dependent upon sulfation of L-selectin ligands on lymph node endothelial cells, with adherence of lymphocytes to the vessel wall decreased in GlcNAc6ST-deficient animals (19). This may also be controlled by the presence of DC within SLO, as the velocity of lymphocyte rolling in CD11c-DTR mice was significantly increased, and the percentage of lymphocytes able to adhere to the vessel wall was decreased, in these mice after treatment with diphtheria toxin to delete DC. The HEV of DC-depleted mice regained expression of MAdCAM-1, and after reconstitution with adoptively transferred CD11c$^+$ DC, these HEV recovered classical cuboidal morphology, suggesting that DC-produced factor(s) is/are required for the maturation of HEV (3).

The CCR7–CCL21 axis is also important for lymphocyte recruitment into lymphoid organs. Mice deficient in CCR7 have impaired migration of B and T cells, as well as DC, to SLO including lymph nodes and Peyer's patches. This limits primary immune responses against infectious agents (25). Expression of CCL21 by HEC is controlled by a pathway unique to these cells versus HEC expressing alternate addressins. Specifically, heparan sulfate, a glycosaminoglycan primarily found on the surface of vascular endothelial cells, is required for CCL21 expression on HEV (26). Using an *Ext1*-flox/flox mouse crossed with a GlcNAc6ST-2-cre transgenic mouse to delete a glycosyltransferase necessary for the synthesis of heparan sulfate in PNAd-expressing cells, expression of CCL21 on the surface of HEV was abrogated (23).

TERTIARY LYMPHOID ORGANS

Although the pioneering work identifying PNAd and the pathways controlling its expression were initially studied in the context of SLO, recent literature supports an important role for PNAd in TLO (aka ectopic lymphoid structures) that develop in peripheral tissue sites impacted by chronic inflammation. Overall, TLOs have varying degrees of similarity to SLO. Classical TLO closely resembles SLO in their cellular composition, with TLO containing a network of follicular dendritic cells (fDC) and germinal centers in which B cells reside, proliferate, and differentiate (**Figure 2A**). Non-classical TLO also contain some degree of B cell infiltration, but they do not exhibit an fDC "framework" (27), with only diffuse, sparse B cell distributions being observed (**Figure 2B**) (28–30).

The L-selectin–PNAd interaction controls lymphocyte recruitment to TLOs. In particular, PNAd upregulation in affected tissues is observed in the settings of allergic contact dermatitis, lymphoid hyperplasia, and a variety of types of skin lesions and cutaneous lymphomas, i.e., diseases characterized by robust lymphocytic infiltrates into peripheral tissues (31). The CCR7 signaling axis also plays a role in TLO formation. Most importantly, CCR7-mediated signals are required for the clustering of DC in peripheral tissues. Interactions between DC and T cells proximal to blood vessels appears required for the acquisition of PNAd + HEV in peripheral tissues (5).

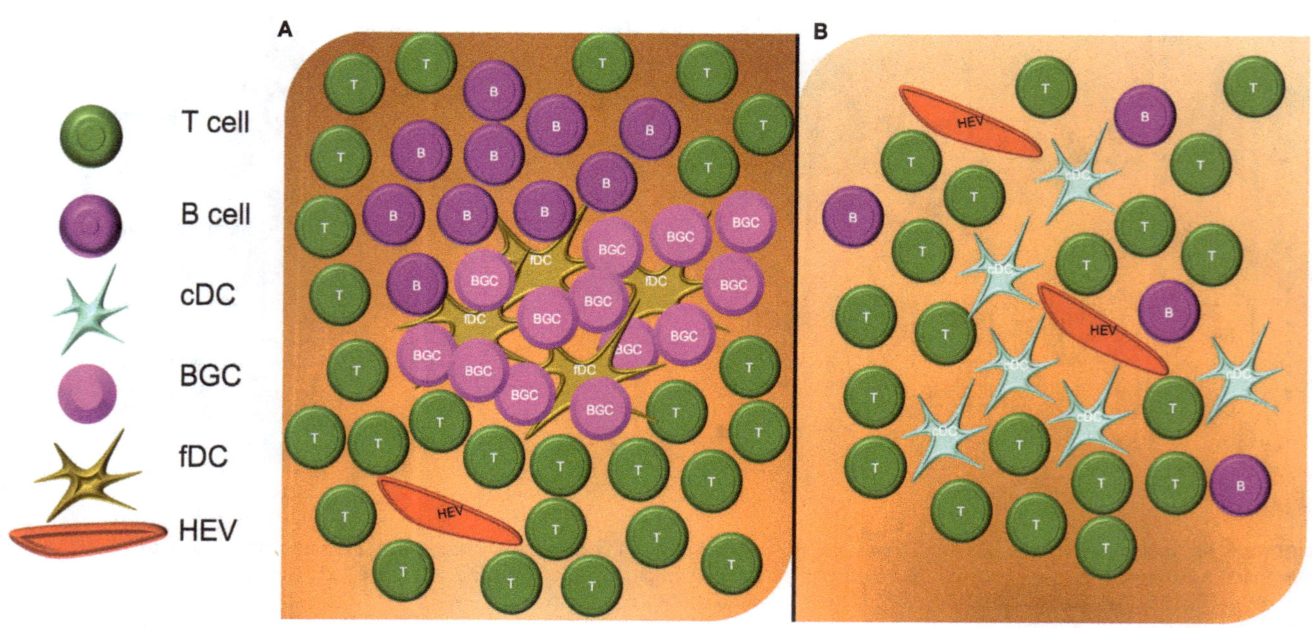

FIGURE 2 | Structure of classical and non-classical tertiary lymphoid organs. (A) Classical TLO contain a nucleated core of fDC and germinal center B cells (BGC), surrounded by an HEV-containing T cell zone. **(B)** Non-classical TLO do not contain fDC or BGC, but may contain sparse B cell, T cell, and DC infiltrates surrounding HEV.

Notably, LTβR-mediated signaling controls the formation of HEV in peripheral tissues (5, 32). Akin to the roles that lymphotoxin signaling plays in the control of PNAd expression in SLO, LTα3-dependent signaling has been reported to dominantly control PNAd expression on HEV within the tumor microenvironment (TME) in murine melanoma models (32), while in human breast cancer, LTβ (produced by DC-LAMP + DC) appears to play a comparable dominant role (33).

Tertiary lymphoid organs have been observed in a variety of chronic inflammatory diseases, including arthritis (34), gastritis and ulcerative colitis (13, 35), atherosclerosis (36), and cancer (37). As the development of TLO in chronic/autoimmune diseases has been well-reviewed (38, 39), we will now focus on the emerging field of TLO formation in solid tumors.

TLO in Cancer

Cancer-associated TLO characteristically contain $PNAd^+$ vessels and are commonly localized to the outer margin (versus the core) of the tumor lesion (40). With the exception of reports for TLO predicting a worse prognosis in patients with renal cell carcinoma (RCC) (41) and some cases of colorectal cancer (42), the vast weight of the literature has correlated the presence of TLOs in human solid tumors with better clinical prognoses (43). Both classical and non-classical TLO have been reported within the TME (**Figure 2**). Of these two forms of TLO, however, the presence of classical TLO in tumors may provide a superior index for improved prognosis when compared to the presence of only non-classical TLO in the TME (27). These results suggest that systematic analysis of PNAd expression and TLO status in tumor biopsies may be a useful in addition to current clinical criteria used to predict patient outcomes.

Lung Cancer

In non-small-cell lung cancer (NSCLC), $PNAd^+$ vessels have been identified exclusively within TLO (44). In these tumors, the composition of cells within the TLO specifically correlates with patient prognosis. While T cells (all tumor-infiltrating L-selectin$^+$ T cells, comprised of both naive and central memory $CD4^+$ and $CD8^+$ cells) are localized to TLO (44, 45), overall T cell infiltrate and density appears to play a minor role in patient outcome when evaluated independently of other prognostic markers. Instead, the density and proximity of mature DC to TLO within the tumor may be most important, and patients with high DC-LAMP$^+$ mDC infiltrates exhibit markedly extended overall survival (45). These findings are further supported by gene array data indicating that *CXCR4*, a gene associated with DC migration toward CXCL12 gradients, is strongly correlated with increased overall survival in NSCLC patients (46). Unlike T cells, B cells do appear to play a significant protective role against lung cancer, and their presence can be used as a positive prognostic marker of overall survival. Interestingly, DC and B cell density in TLO can be used as a coordinate prognostic marker for patients with greatest overall survival. In NSCLC, B cells organize into germinal center-like structures containing $CD21^+$ fDC. These B cells proliferate and differentiate *in situ*, leading to locoregional secretion of IgG and IgA antibodies reactive against tumor-associated antigens (47).

Skin Cancers

Tertiary lymphoid organs have been identified in both primary and metastatic melanoma, where they have been observed to contain $PNAd^+$ vessels (48, 49). TLO in primary melanomas can be either classical or non-classical TLO. In metastatic melanoma, these structures are primarily composed of $CD3^+$ T cells and mature (DC-LAMP$^+$) DC proximal to $PNAd^+$ HEV (50). Plasma B cells may also be present in such TLO, with these cells producing Th-dependent IgG and IgA antibodies specific for tumor-associated antigens (48, 50). In primary cutaneous melanoma, the presence of intratumoral HEV has been correlated with robust lymphocytic infiltration and tumor regression. Furthermore, if the HEC making up HEV have a cuboidal morphology, indicative of functional HEV, a positive correlation with CCR7, CCL19, and CCL21 expression within the tumor has also been observed (51).

The presence of TLO also portends better clinical outcome (recurrence free and overall survival) in the setting of Merkel cell carcinoma. These structures are also characterized by an increased $CD8^+/CD4^+$ T cell ratio at the tumor periphery and by a co-clustering of T and B cells within these anatomic sites (52).

Colon Cancer

Tertiary lymphoid organs in human colon cancer have been detected in both the colon crypt and at the invasive front of the tumor, as well as in the peritumoral region (53, 54). They contain immune cell types typically observed in SLO, including B cells, $CD21^+$ fDC, T cells, and mature DC marked by DC-LAMP$^+$, with $CD31^+$ vascular endothelial cells and LYVE-1$^+$ lymphatic vessels also noted (53, 54). T cells and mature DC represent positive prognostic markers in both primary (43) and metastatic (41) colorectal cancer. In such tumors, the B cells may not organize into germinal center-like structures (53, 54). These TLO appear to function as local sites for the priming and expansion of both B and T cells, based on the expression of the Ki-67 marker in *de facto* germinal centers in these diseased tissues (54).

Therapeutic Induction of TLO

Recent work from our group suggests that intratumoral TLO can be induced therapeutically *via* adoptive transfer of gene-modified DC, leading to reduced tumor progression. Following intratumoral injection of Type 1-polarized DC (DC engineered to overexpress Tbet, i.e., DC.Tbet) into established murine sarcomas or colon carcinomas, $CD4^+$ and $CD8^+$ T cell recruitment to the TME is observed within 2 days, with an upregulation of PNAd expression detected by 5 days after treatment. This suggests that PNAd-independent events control early T cell recruitment to the TME, and that T cell-dependent factors may consequently result in PNAd upregulation on tumor-associated VEC (28, 29). Once established, $PNAd^+$ vessels become surrounded by dense infiltrates of both $CD11c^+$ DC and $CD3^+$ T cells, with these non-classical TLO principally localized near the tumor periphery for at least 2 weeks following initial therapeutic intervention (28, 29). The presence of DC in TLO is consistent with prior studies of SLO demonstrating that DC accumulation proximal to HEV is required for the subsequent optimal homing of lymphocytes into SLO (3).

FUTURE PERSPECTIVES

Although there appears to be some variability in the cellular composition across tumor types, TLO in the TME contain PNAd$^+$ HEV typically surrounded by dense B cell and/or DC infiltrates. Importantly, the presence of intratumoral or peritumoral TLO has been almost universally linked with superior clinical prognosis in patients with solid forms of cancer. Though T cells are also present in intratumoral TLO, their presence has thus far proven equivocal as a prognostic biomarker. The spontaneous formation of TLO has been observed in a variety of human cancers, including those reviewed above as well as oral squamous cell carcinoma (27, 55), gastric cancer (40, 56), bladder cancer (57), breast cancer (30, 58, 59), and others (37, 60). Thus, it may ultimately be best to employ PNAd as well as B cell and DC infiltration in the TME as biomarkers to stratify patients based on TLO status, i.e., to differentiate individuals that may respond better to treatment intervention, including immunotherapies (based on superior locoregional immune competency). Furthermore, because TLO may be induced therapeutically (at least in murine models), it is also intriguing to speculate on the possibility that protective TLO may be conditionally sponsored in patients receiving chemo- or immunotherapies (61), and that such structures may be used to monitor/predict the patient's outcome and prospective treatment management.

AUTHOR CONTRIBUTIONS

Both authors contributed to the design, writing, and editing of the submitted manuscript.

ACKNOWLEDGMENTS

The authors wish to thank Ms. Subhara Raveendran for her thoughtful review of this manuscript. This work was supported by NIH R01 CA204419 (to WJS) and NIH T32 AI089443 (to AMW).

REFERENCES

1. Drayton DL, Ying X, Lee J, Lesslauer W, Ruddle NH. Ectopic LT alpha beta directs lymphoid organ neogenesis with concomitant expression of peripheral node addressin and a HEV-restricted sulfotransferase. *J Exp Med* (2003) 197(9):1153–63. doi:10.1084/jem.20021761
2. Onder L, Danuser R, Scandella E, Firner S, Chai Q, Hehlgans T, et al. Endothelial cell-specific lymphotoxin-β receptor signaling is critical for lymph node and high endothelial venule formation. *J Exp Med* (2013) 210(3):465–73. doi:10.1084/jem.20121462
3. Moussion C, Girard J-P. Dendritic cells control lymphocyte entry to lymph nodes through high endothelial venules. *Nature* (2011) 479(7374):542–6. doi:10.1038/nature10540
4. Browning JL, Allaire N, Ngam-Ek A, Notidis E, Hunt J, Perrin S, et al. Lymphotoxin-beta receptor signaling is required for the homeostatic control of HEV differentiation and function. *Immunity* (2005) 23(5):539–50. doi:10.1016/j.immuni.2005.10.002
5. Marinkovic T, Garin A, Yokota Y, Fu Y-X, Ruddle NH, Furtado GC, et al. Interaction of mature CD3+CD4+ T cells with dendritic cells triggers the development of tertiary lymphoid structures in the thyroid. *J Clin Invest* (2006) 116(10):2622–32. doi:10.1172/JCI28993
6. Liao S, Ruddle NH. Synchrony of high endothelial venules and lymphatic vessels revealed by immunization. *J Immunol* (2006) 177(5):3369–79. doi:10.4049/jimmunol.177.5.3369
7. Sperandio M, Gleissner CA, Ley K. Glycosylation in immune cell trafficking. *Immunol Rev* (2009) 230(1):97–113. doi:10.1111/j.1600-065X.2009.00795.x
8. Umemoto E, Tanaka T, Kanda H, Jin S, Tohya K, Otani K, et al. Nepmucin, a novel HEV sialomucin, mediates L-selectin–dependent lymphocyte rolling and promotes lymphocyte adhesion under flow. *J Exp Med* (2006) 203(6):1603–14. doi:10.1084/jem.20052543
9. Suzuki A, Andrew DP, Gonzalo JA, Fukumoto M, Spellberg J, Hashiyama M, et al. CD34-deficient mice have reduced eosinophil accumulation after allergen exposure and show a novel crossreactive 90-kD protein. *Blood* (1996) 87(9):3550–62.
10. Rosen SD. Ligands for L-selectin: homing, inflammation, and beyond. *Annu Rev Immunol* (2004) 22:129–56. doi:10.1146/annurev.immunol.21.090501.080131
11. Arata-Kawai H, Singer MS, Bistrup A, Zante AV, Wang YQ, Ito Y, et al. Functional contributions of N- and O-glycans to L-selectin ligands in murine and human lymphoid organs. *Am J Pathol* (2011) 178(1):423–33. doi:10.1016/j.ajpath.2010.11.009
12. Hemmerich S, Butcher EC, Rosen SD. Sulfation-dependent recognition of high endothelial venules (HEV)-ligands by L-selectin and MECA 79, and adhesion-blocking monoclonal antibody. *J Exp Med* (1994) 180(6):2219–26. doi:10.1084/jem.180.6.2219
13. Kobayashi M, Fukuda M, Nakayama J. Role of sulfated O-glycans expressed by high endothelial venule-like vessels in pathogenesis of chronic inflammatory gastrointestinal diseases. *Biol Pharm Bull* (2009) 32(5):774–9. doi:10.1248/bpb.32.774
14. Lowe JB. Glycosylation, immunity, and autoimmunity. *Cell* (2001) 104(6):809–12. doi:10.1016/S0092-8674(01)00277-X
15. Grunwell JR, Bertozzi CR. Carbohydrate sulfotransferases of the GalNAc/Gal/GlcNAc6ST family. *Biochemistry* (2002) 41(44):13117–26. doi:10.1021/bi020507h
16. Hemmerich S, Bistrup A, Singer MS, van Zante A, Lee JK, Tsay D, et al. Sulfation of L-selectin ligands by an HEV-restricted sulfotransferase regulates lymphocyte homing to lymph nodes. *Immunity* (2001) 15(2):237–47. doi:10.1016/S1074-7613(01)00188-1
17. Uchimura K, Kadomatsu K, El-Fasakhany FM, Singer MS, Izawa M, Kannagi R, et al. N-acetylglucosamine 6-O-sulfotransferase-1 regulates expression of L-selectin ligands and lymphocyte homing. *J Biol Chem* (2004) 279(33):35001–8. doi:10.1074/jbc.M404456200
18. Kawashima H, Hirakawa J, Tobisawa Y, Fukuda M, Saga Y. Conditional gene targeting in mouse high endothelial venules. *J Immunol* (2009) 182(9):5461–8. doi:10.4049/jimmunol.0802327
19. Uchimura K, Gauguet J-M, Singer MS, Tsay D, Kannagi R, Muramatsu T, et al. A major class of L-selectin ligands is eliminated in mice deficient in two sulfotransferases expressed in high endothelial venules. *Nat Immunol* (2005) 6(11):1105–13. doi:10.1038/ni1258
20. Malý P, Thall AD, Petryniak B, Rogers CE, Smith PL, Marks RM, et al. The α(1,3)Fucosyltransferase Fuc-TVII controls leukocyte trafficking through an essential role in L-, E-, and P-selectin ligand biosynthesis. *Cell* (1996) 86(4):643–53. doi:10.1016/S0092-8674(00)80137-3
21. Homeister JW, Thall AD, Petryniak B, Malý P, Rogers CE, Smith PL, et al. The α(1,3)fucosyltransferases FucT-IV and FucT-VII exert collaborative control over selectin-dependent leukocyte recruitment and lymphocyte homing. *Immunity* (2001) 15(1):115–26. doi:10.1016/S1074-7613(01)00166-2

22. Miyasaka M, Tanaka T. Lymphocyte trafficking across high endothelial venules: dogmas and enigmas. *Nat Rev Immunol* (2004) 4(5):360–70. doi:10.1038/nri1354
23. Tsuboi K, Hirakawa J, Seki E, Imai Y, Yamaguchi Y, Fukuda M, et al. Role of high endothelial venule-expressed heparan sulfate in chemokine presentation and lymphocyte homing. *J Immunol* (2013) 191(1):448–55. doi:10.4049/jimmunol.1203061
24. Berg EL, Robinson MK, Warnock RA, Butcher EC. The human peripheral lymph node vascular addressin is a ligand for LECAM-1, the peripheral lymph node homing receptor. *J Cell Biol* (1991) 114(2):343–9. doi:10.1083/jcb.114.2.343
25. Förster R, Schubel A, Breitfeld D, Kremmer E, Renner-Müller I, Wolf E, et al. CCR7 coordinates the primary immune response by establishing functional microenvironments in secondary lymphoid organs. *Cell* (1999) 99(1):23–33. doi:10.1016/S0092-8674(00)80059-8
26. Nelson RM, Cecconi O, Roberts WG, Aruffo A, Linhardt RJ, Bevilacqua MP. Heparin oligosaccharides bind L- and P-selectin and inhibit acute inflammation. *Blood* (1993) 82(11):3253–8.
27. Wirsing AM, Rikardsen OG, Steigen SE, Uhlin-Hansen L, Hadler-Olsen E. Characterisation and prognostic value of tertiary lymphoid structures in oral squamous cell carcinoma. *BMC Clin Pathol* (2014) 14:38. doi:10.1186/1472-6890-14-38
28. Chen L, Fabian KL, Taylor JL, Storkus WJ. Therapeutic use of dendritic cells to promote the extranodal priming of anti-tumor immunity. *Front Immunol* (2013) 4:388. doi:10.3389/fimmu.2013.00388
29. Chen L, Taylor JL, Sabins NC, Lowe DB, Qu Y, You Z, et al. Extranodal induction of therapeutic immunity in the tumor microenvironment after intratumoral delivery of Tbet gene-modified dendritic cells. *Cancer Gene Ther* (2013) 20(8):469–77. doi:10.1038/cgt.2013.42
30. Mahmoud SMA, Lee AHS, Paish EC, Macmillan RD, Ellis IO, Green AR. The prognostic significance of B lymphocytes in invasive carcinoma of the breast. *Breast Cancer Res Treat* (2012) 132(2):545–53. doi:10.1007/s10549-011-1620-1
31. Michie SA, Streeter PR, Bolt PA, Butcher EC, Picker LJ. The human peripheral lymph node vascular addressin. An inducible endothelial antigen involved in lymphocyte homing. *Am J Pathol* (1993) 143(6):1688–98.
32. Peske JD, Thompson ED, Gemta L, Baylis RA, Fu Y-X, Engelhard VH. Effector lymphocyte-induced lymph node-like vasculature enables naive T-cell entry into tumours and enhanced anti-tumour immunity. *Nat Commun* (2015) 6:7114. doi:10.1038/ncomms8114
33. Martinet L, Filleron T, Le Guellec S, Rochaix P, Garrido I, Girard J-P. High endothelial venule blood vessels for tumor-infiltrating lymphocytes are associated with lymphotoxin-producing dendritic cells in human breast cancer. *J Immunol* (2013) 191(4):2001–8. doi:10.4049/jimmunol.1300872
34. Yang J, Rosen SD, Bendele P, Hemmerich S. Induction of PNAd and N-acetylglucosamine 6-O-sulfotransferases 1 and 2 in mouse collagen-induced arthritis. *BMC Immunol* (2006) 7:12. doi:10.1186/1471-2172-7-12
35. Kobayashi M, Hoshino H, Masumoto J, Fukushima M, Suzawa K, Kageyama S, et al. GlcNAc6ST-1-mediated decoration of MAdCAM-1 protein with L-selectin ligand carbohydrates directs disease activity of ulcerative colitis. *Inflamm Bowel Dis* (2009) 15(5):697–706. doi:10.1002/ibd.20827
36. Hu D, Mohanta SK, Yin C, Peng L, Ma Z, Srikakulapu P, et al. Artery tertiary lymphoid organs control aorta immunity and protect against atherosclerosis via vascular smooth muscle cell lymphotoxin β receptors. *Immunity* (2015) 42(6):1100–15. doi:10.1016/j.immuni.2015.05.015
37. Pimenta EM, Barnes BJ. Role of tertiary lymphoid structures (TLS) in anti-tumor immunity: potential tumor-induced cytokines/chemokines that regulate TLS formation in epithelial-derived cancers. *Cancers (Basel)* (2014) 6(2):969–97. doi:10.3390/cancers6020969
38. Neyt K, Perros F, GeurtsvanKessel CH, Hammad H, Lambrecht BN. Tertiary lymphoid organs in infection and autoimmunity. *Trends Immunol* (2012) 33(6):297–305. doi:10.1016/j.it.2012.04.006
39. Pitzalis C, Jones GW, Bombardieri M, Jones SA. Ectopic lymphoid-like structures in infection, cancer and autoimmunity. *Nat Rev Immunol* (2014) 14(7):447–62. doi:10.1038/nri3700
40. Enarsson K, Johnsson E, Lindholm C, Lundgren A, Pan-Hammarström Q, Strömberg E, et al. Differential mechanisms for T lymphocyte recruitment in normal and neoplastic human gastric mucosa. *Clin Immunol* (2006) 118(1):24–34. doi:10.1016/j.clim.2005.08.001
41. Remark R, Alifano M, Cremer I, Lupo A, Dieu-Nosjean M-C, Riquet M, et al. Characteristics and clinical impacts of the immune environments in colorectal and renal cell carcinoma lung metastases: influence of tumor origin. *Clin Cancer Res* (2013) 19(15):4079–91. doi:10.1158/1078-0432.CCR-12-3847
42. Bento DC, Jones E, Junaid S, Tull J, Williams GT, Godkin A, et al. High endothelial venules are rare in colorectal cancers but accumulate in extra-tumoral areas with disease progression. *Oncoimmunology* (2015) 4(3):e974374. doi:10.4161/2162402X.2014.974374
43. Fridman WH, Pagès F, Sautès-Fridman C, Galon J. The immune contexture in human tumours: impact on clinical outcome. *Nat Rev Cancer* (2012) 12(4):298–306. doi:10.1038/nrc3245
44. de Chaisemartin L, Goc J, Damotte D, Validire P, Magdeleinat P, Alifano M, et al. Characterization of chemokines and adhesion molecules associated with T cell presence in tertiary lymphoid structures in human lung cancer. *Cancer Res* (2011) 71(20):6391–9. doi:10.1158/0008-5472.CAN-11-0952
45. Goc J, Germain C, Vo-Bourgais TKD, Lupo A, Klein C, Knockaert S, et al. Dendritic cells in tumor-associated tertiary lymphoid structures signal a Th1 cytotoxic immune contexture and license the positive prognostic value of infiltrating CD8– T cells. *Cancer Res* (2014) 74(3):705–15. doi:10.1158/0008-5472.CAN-13-1342
46. Kossenkov AV, Dawany N, Evans TL, Kucharczuk JC, Albelda SM, Showe LC, et al. Peripheral immune cell gene expression predicts survival of patients with non-small cell lung cancer. *PLoS One* (2012) 7(3):e34392. doi:10.1371/journal.pone.0034392
47. Germain C, Gnjatic S, Tamzalit F, Knockaert S, Remark R, Goc J, et al. Presence of B cells in tertiary lymphoid structures is associated with a protective immunity in patients with lung cancer. *Am J Respir Crit Care Med* (2014) 189(7):832–44. doi:10.1164/rccm.201309-1611OC
48. Cipponi A, Mercier M, Seremet T, Baurain J-F, Théate I, van den Oord J, et al. Neogenesis of lymphoid structures and antibody responses occur in human melanoma metastases. *Cancer Res* (2012) 72(16):3997–4007. doi:10.1158/0008-5472.CAN-12-1377
49. Martinet L, Garrido I, Filleron T, Le Guellec S, Bellard E, Fournie J-J, et al. Human solid tumors contain high endothelial venules: association with T- and B-lymphocyte infiltration and favorable prognosis in breast cancer. *Cancer Res* (2011) 71(17):5678–87. doi:10.1158/0008-5472.CAN-11-0431
50. van Baren N, Baurain J-F, Coulie PG. Lymphoid neogenesis in melanoma: what does it tell us? *Oncoimmunology* (2013) 2(1):e22505. doi:10.4161/onci.22505
51. Avram G, Sánchez-Sendra B, Martín JM, Terrádez L, Ramos D, Monteagudo C. The density and type of MECA-79-positive high endothelial venules correlate with lymphocytic infiltration and tumour regression in primary cutaneous melanoma. *Histopathology* (2013) 63(6):852–61. doi:10.1111/his.12235
52. Behr DS, Peitsch WK, Hametner C, Lasitschka F, Houben R, Schönhaar K, et al. Prognostic value of immune cell infiltration, tertiary lymphoid structures and PD-L1 expression in Merkel cell carcinomas. *Int J Clin Exp Pathol* (2014) 7(11):7610–21.
53. Bergomas F, Grizzi F, Doni A, Pesce S, Laghi L, Allavena P, et al. Tertiary intratumor lymphoid tissue in colo-rectal cancer. *Cancers (Basel)* (2011) 4(1):1–10. doi:10.3390/cancers4010001
54. Coppola D, Nebozhyn M, Khalil F, Dai H, Yeatman T, Loboda A, et al. Unique ectopic lymph node-like structures present in human primary colorectal carcinoma are identified by immune gene array profiling. *Am J Pathol* (2011) 179(1):37–45. doi:10.1016/j.ajpath.2011.03.007
55. Shen H, Wang X, Shao Z, Liu K, Xia X-Y, Zhang H-Z, et al. Alterations of high endothelial venules in primary and metastatic tumors are correlated with lymph node metastasis of oral and pharyngeal carcinoma. *Cancer Biol Ther* (2014) 15(3):342–9. doi:10.4161/cbt.27328
56. Kobayashi M, Mitoma J, Hoshino H, Yu S-Y, Shimojo Y, Suzawa K, et al. Prominent expression of sialyl Lewis X-capped core 2-branched O-glycans on high endothelial venule-like vessels in gastric MALT lymphoma. *J Pathol* (2011) 224(1):67–77. doi:10.1002/path.2851
57. Taga M, Hoshino H, Low S, Imamura Y, Ito H, Yokoyama O, et al. A potential role for 6-sulfo sialyl Lewis X in metastasis of bladder urothelial carcinoma. *Urol Oncol* (2015) 33(11):e1–9. doi:10.1016/j.urolonc.2015.05.026
58. Denkert C, Loibl S, Noske A, Roller M, Müller BM, Komor M, et al. Tumor-associated lymphocytes as an independent predictor of response to neoadjuvant chemotherapy in breast cancer. *J Clin Oncol* (2010) 28(1):105–13. doi:10.1200/JCO.2009.23.7370

59. Nzula S, Going JJ, Stott DI. Antigen-driven clonal proliferation, somatic hypermutation, and selection of B lymphocytes infiltrating human ductal breast carcinomas. *Cancer Res* (2003) 63(12):3275–80. doi:10.4049/jimmunol.169.5.2701
60. Weinstein AM, Storkus WJ. Therapeutic lymphoid organogenesis in the tumor microenvironment. *Adv Cancer Res* (2015) 128:197–233. doi:10.1016/bs.acr.2015.04.003
61. Stoll G, Enot D, Mlecnik B, Galon J, Zitvogel L, Kroemer G. Immune-related gene signatures predict the outcome of neoadjuvant chemotherapy. *Oncoimmunology* (2014) 3(1):e27884. doi:10.4161/onci.27884

12

Tertiary Lymphoid Structures in Cancers: Prognostic Value, Regulation and Manipulation for Therapeutic Intervention

*Catherine Sautès-Fridman[1,2,3], Myriam Lawand[1,2,3], Nicolas A. Giraldo[1,2,3], Hélène Kaplon[1,2,3], Claire Germain[1,2,3], Wolf Herman Fridman[1,2,3] and Marie-Caroline Dieu-Nosjean[1,2,3]**

[1] INSERM, UMR_S 1138, Team "Cancer, Immune Control and Escape", Cordeliers Research Center, Paris, France, [2] UMR_S 1138, Centre de Recherche des Cordeliers, University Paris Descartes, Paris, France, [3] UMR_S 1138, Centre de Recherche des Cordeliers, Sorbonne University, UPMC University Paris 06, Paris, France

***Correspondence:**
Marie-Caroline Dieu-Nosjean
mc.dieu-nosjean@crc.jussieu.fr

Tertiary lymphoid structures (TLS) are ectopic lymphoid aggregates that reflect lymphoid neogenesis occurring in tissues at sites of inflammation. They are detected in tumors where they orchestrate local and systemic anti-tumor responses. A correlation has been found between high densities of TLS and prolonged patient's survival in more than 10 different types of cancer. TLS can be regulated by the same set of chemokines and cytokines that orchestrate lymphoid organogenesis and by regulatory T cells. Thus, TLS offer a series of putative new targets that could be used to develop therapies aiming to increase the anti-tumor immune response.

Keywords: cancer, tertiary lymphoid structure, tumor microenvironment, chemokine, adaptive immune response

INTRODUCTION

Tertiary lymphoid structures (TLS) are transient ectopic lymphoid organizations that develop after birth in non-lymphoid tissues, in situations of chronic inflammation. They display an overall organization similar to that observed in canonical secondary lymphoid organs (SLOs), such as lymph nodes (LNs), with a T cell-rich area characterized by a T cell and mature DC-Lamp$^+$ dendritic cell (DCs) cluster, a B-cell-rich area composed of a mantle of naïve B cells surrounding an active germinal center (GC) (1–3), the presence of high endothelial venules (HEVs), a particular type of blood vessels expressing peripheral node addressins (PNAd) and specialized in the extravasation of circulating immune cells, and the secretion of chemokines (CCL19, CCL21, CXCL10, CXCL12, and CXCL13) that are crucial for lymphocyte recruitment and entry into the LN (4–8). TLS have been detected in the tumor invasive margin and/or in the stroma of most cancers and their densities correlate with a favorable clinical outcome for the patients (**Table 1**). A series of studies performed by our group in non-small-cell lung cancer (NSCLC) demonstrated that TLS are important sites for the initiation and/or maintenance of the local and systemic T- and B-cell responses against tumors, in accordance with a specific signature of genes related to T and B cell lineage, chemotaxis, Th1 polarization, lymphocyte activation, and effector function associated with TLS presence (**Table 2**). They represent a privileged area for the recruitment of lymphocytes into tumors and the generation of central-memory T and B cells that circulate and limit cancer progression (5, 9, 10).

TABLE 1 | Prognostic value of TLS in primary and metastatic tumors.

Criteria	Cancer type	Stages of the disease	No. of patients	TLS detection IHC	TLS detection gene expression	Prognostic value	Reference
Primary tumors	Breast carcinoma	I–III	146	PNAd	–	Positive	(8)
		I–III	146	DC-Lamp	–	Positive	(11)
		I–III	794	–	T_{FH}, CXCL13	Positive	(12)
	Breast carcinoma (triple negative)	I–III	769	H&S	–	Positive	(13)
	Colorectal cancer	I–IV	350	H&S	–	Positive	(14)
		ND	25	DC-Lamp	–	Positive	(15)
		I–IV	40	CD3, CD83	–	Positive	(16)
		II	185	CD3	–	Positive	(17)
		III	166	CD3	–	No value	(17)
		0–IV-A	21	–	12-chemokine genes	Positive	(3)
		I–IV	125	–	CXCL13 and CD20	Positive	(18)
	Gastric cancer	All without chemo	82	CD20	–	Positive	(19)
		I–III	365	–	both Th1 and B	Positive	(19)
	NSCLC	I–II	74	DC-Lamp	–	Positive	(1)
		I–IV	362	DC-Lamp	–	Positive	(9)
		III with neo-adj. chemo	122	DC-Lamp, CD20	–	Positive	(2)
	Melanoma	I-A–III-A	82	DC-Lamp	–	Positive	(20)
		IV	21	–	12-chemokine genes	Positive	(21)
	Oral SCC	All	80	CD3, CD20, CD21, BCL6, PNAd	–	Positive	(22)
	Pancreatic cancer	All	308 + 226	H&E	–	Positive	(23)
	RCC	All	135	DC-Lamp	–	Positive	(24)
	Hepatocellular Cancer	All	82	H&S	11-chemokine genes	Negative	(25)
	Biliary tract cancer	All	335	CD20 (TMA)	–	No value	(26)
Metastatic tumors	Colorectal cancer (liver)	All	14 + 51	CD20	–	Positive	(27)
	Colorectal cancer (lung)	ND	140	DC-Lamp	–	Positive	(15)

In this mini review, we summarize the available data in the literature regarding the prognostic value of TLS in human cancers, and discuss how these structures are controlled and could be manipulated in order to increase anti-tumor immune responses.

TLS AND PROGNOSIS IN CANCERS

In recent years, numerous publications have assessed the prognosis associated with the presence of TLS in different types of tumors. Several strategies for their quantification have been used. Historically, the first method to measure the densities of TLS was the quantification of mature DCs (DC-Lamp$^+$) within CD3$^+$ T cell aggregates (1, 20). Although relatively challenging due to the relative low number of DC-Lamp$^+$ DCs in some tumors (as compared to other immune populations), our group has described it as the most accurate marker for quantifying TLS (28, 29). Up-to-date, eight publications have found a positive association between increased densities of DC-Lamp$^+$ DCs and prognosis, in several types of tumors, including NSCLC (1, 2, 9), melanoma (20), renal cell carcinoma [RCC (24)], breast (11), and colorectal cancer (15) (**Table 1** and **Figure 1**).

The analysis of expression levels of TLS-related genes gives the possibility to rapidly assess the prognostic impact of these immune aggregates in large retrospective cohorts of tumors. So far, six studies have evaluated the prognostic impact of increased expression of TLS-related genes in cancer. Despite heterogeneity in the TLS-signatures, a significant correlation with good prognosis has been found in melanoma (21), colorectal (3, 18), and gastric (19) cancers (**Table 1**). Interestingly, TLS found in inflammatory zones from hepatocellular carcinoma (HCC) correlate with increased risk for late recurrence and a trend toward decreased overall survival after HCC resection. This result could reflect an unexpected role for TLS, serving as niche for HCC progenitor cells *via* local production of Lymphotoxin (LT)-β (25, 30).

Another approach that has been used to estimate the densities of TLS in cancers is the quantification of B-cell aggregates by immunohistochemistry (IHC) (CD20$^+$ B-cell aggregates or islets). The majority of publications measuring CD20$^+$ aggregates (four out of five), accounting for more than 349 analyzed tumors, has determined that increased densities of this population correlate with good prognosis in several neoplasias, such as NSCLC (2), colorectal cancer liver metastasis (27), gastric (19), and oral (22) cancer (**Table 1** and **Figure 1**). Most of the studies quantifying the CD3$^+$ T cell aggregates and immune-cell aggregates (after hematoxylin counterstaining) have also found a positive impact on patient's prognosis. However, high numbers of B cell or T cell aggregates were found to have no impact on prognosis in biliary tract cancer and in stage III colorectal cancer, respectively. Further studies are needed to investigate whether it reflects that cell aggregates counting is not an accurate method to quantify TLS, or a functional impairment of TLS in these two cancer types (**Table 1** and **Figure 1**).

Overall, despite the heterogeneity of methods used for quantifying TLS, most of the studies have consistently found a correlation between high densities of TLS and prolonged patient's survival in more than 10 different types of cancer (**Table 1**).

TABLE 2 | Expression of genes associated with TLS presence in human cancers.

Name of the gene	Main names of the protein	Main immune functions and process	Cluster of gene related to TLS presence	Reference
CCL2	CCL2, MCP-1, MCAF	Monocyte, immature DC and T cell chemotaxis, G-protein-coupled receptor signaling pathway, cell adhesion, JAK-STAT cascade, MAPK cascade, cellular calcium ion homeostasis, cellular response to IFN-γ, IL-1, and IL-6	Chemotaxis	(3)
CCL3	CCL3, MIP-1α	Monocyte and T cell chemotaxis, G-protein-coupled receptor signaling pathway, cell adhesion, MAPK cascade, calcium-mediated signaling, cell activation, cellular response to IFN-γ, TNF-α, and IL-1, eosinophil degranulation, inflammatory response	Chemotaxis	(3)
CCL4	CCL4, MIP-1β, LAG1	Monocyte and neutrophil and T cell chemotaxis, G-protein-coupled receptor signaling pathway, cell adhesion, calcium-mediated signaling, cell activation, cellular response to IFN-γ, TNF-α, and IL-1, inflammatory response, positive regulation of ERK1 and ERK2 cascade, positive regulation of GTPase activity	Chemotaxis	(3)
CCL5	CCL5, RANTES	Monocyte, neutrophil and T cell chemotaxis, G-protein-coupled receptor signaling pathway, calcium-mediated signaling, cellular response to IFN-γ, TNF-α, and IL-1, inflammatory response	Chemotaxis	(3, 9)
CCL8	CCL8, MCP-2, HC14	Monocyte, neutrophil and T cell chemotaxis, G-protein-coupled receptor signaling pathway, cellular response to IFN-γ, TNF-α, and IL-1, chronic inflammatory response, positive regulation of ERK1 and ERK2 cascade, positive regulation of GTPase activity, negative regulation of leukocyte proliferation	Chemotaxis	(3)
CCL17	CCL17, TARC, ABCD-2	Monocyte and T cell chemotaxis, G-protein-coupled receptor signaling pathway, cellular response to IFN-γ, TNF-α, and IL-1, inflammatory response, positive regulation of ERK1 and ERK2 cascade, positive regulation of GTPase activity	Chemotaxis/T cells	(5)
CCL18	CCL18, PARC, MIP-4, AMAC-1, DC-CK1	Monocyte, neutrophil and T cell chemotaxis, G-protein-coupled receptor signaling pathway, cellular response to IFN-γ, TNF-α, and IL-1, inflammatory response, positive regulation of ERK1 and ERK2 cascade, positive regulation of GTPase activity	Chemotaxis	(3)
CCL19	CCL19, MIP-3β, ELC	Mature DC and T cell chemotaxis, G-protein-coupled receptor signaling pathway, T cell costimulation, cell maturation, cellular response to IFN-γ, TNF-α, and IL-1, inflammatory response, activation of JUN kinase activity, establishment of T cell polarty, immunological synapse formation, inflammatory response, positive regulation of IL-1β, IL-12, and TNF-α secretion, positive regulation of ERK1 ERK2 JNK cascade, response to PGE	Chemotaxis, chemotaxis/T cells	(3, 5)
CCL20	MIP-3α, LARC, Exodus	Immature DC monocyte neutrophil and T cell chemotaxis, G-protein-coupled receptor signaling pathway, cellular response to IL-1, TNF-α, and LPS, inflammatory response, positive regulation of ERK1 and ERK2 cascade	Th1/B cells	(19)
CCL21	CCL21, SLC, 6Ckine, TCA4	Mature DC neutrophil and T cell chemotaxis, G-protein-coupled receptor signaling pathway, T cell costimulation, cell maturation, cellular response to IFN-γ, TNF-α, and IL-1, inflammatory response, cell maturation, establishment of T cell polarity, negative regulation of DC dendrite assembly, positive regulation of DC APC function, immunological synapse formation, inflammatory response, activation of GTPase activity, cellular response to IL-1 and TNF-α, positive regulation of ERK1 ERK2 JNK cascade, response to PGE	Chemotaxis, chemotaxis/T cells	(3, 5)
CCL22	CCL22, MDC, ABCD-1, DC/B-CK	Monocyte and T cell chemotaxis, G-protein-coupled receptor signaling pathway, cellular response to IFN-γ, TNF-α, and IL-1, inflammatory response, positive regulation of ERK1 and ERK2 cascade, positive regulation of GTPase activity	Chemotaxis/T cells	(5)
CCR2	CCR2, CD192, CC-CKR2	Monocyte, immature DC and lymphocyte chemotaxis, G-protein-coupled receptor signaling pathway, positive regulation of inflammatory response, JAK–STAT cascade, negative regulation of eosinophil degranulation, positive regulation of Th1 immune response, negative regulation of Th2 immune response, positive regulation of IL-1β, IL-2, IL-6, and TNF production	Chemotaxis/Th1/cytotoxicity/activation	(9)
CCR4	CCR4, CD194, ChemR13, CC-CKR4	Monocyte and lymphocyte chemotaxis, G-protein-coupled receptor signaling pathway, inflammatory response, tolerance induction	Chemotaxis/Th1/cytotoxicity/activation	(9)
CCR5	CCR5, CD195	Myeloid and lymphocyte chemotaxis, G-protein-coupled receptor signaling pathway, inflammatory response, negative regulation of macrophage apoptotic process, positive regulation of IL-1, IL-6, and TNF production, co-receptor of HIV	Chemotaxis/Th1/cytotoxicity/activation, Th1/B cells	(9, 19)
CCR7	CCR7, CD197, CMKBR7, CC-CKR7, BLR2, EBI1	Monocyte mature DC and lymphocyte chemotaxis, G-protein-coupled receptor signaling pathway, inflammatory response, positive regulation of ERK1 and ERK2 cascade, positive regulation of GTPase activity, establishment of T cell polarity, negative thymic T cell selection, positive regulation of JNK cascade, positive regulation of T cell costimulation and TCR signaling pathway, positive regulation of APC function, positive regulation of humoral immunity, regulation of IFN-γ, IL-1β, and IL-12 production	Chemotaxis/Th1/cytotoxicity/activation	(9)

(Continued)

TABLE 2 | Continued

Name of the gene	Main names of the protein	Main immune functions and process	Cluster of gene related to TLS presence	Reference
CD3e	CD3, TCRE, IMD18	T cell activation and costimulation, TCR signaling pathway, negative thymic T cell selection, positive regulation of T cell proliferation and anergy, positive regulation of IFN-γ, IL-2, and IL-4 production	Chemotaxis/T cells, chemotaxis/Th1/cytotoxicity/activation	(5, 9)
CD4	CD4	T cell activation, T cell differentiation, T cell selection, cytokine production	Chemotaxis/Th1/cytotoxicity/activation, Th1/B cells	(9, 19)
CD5	CD5, LEU1	T cell costimulation, apoptotic signaling pathway, cell proliferation, cell recognition, receptor-mediated endocytosis	Th1/B cells	(19)
CD8A	CD8A, Leu2, p32	T cell activation, T cell-mediated immunity, cell surface receptor signaling pathway, cytotoxic T cell differentiation, defense response to virus	Chemotaxis/Th1/cytotoxicity/activation	(9)
CD19	CD19, B4, CVID3	B-cell receptor signaling pathway, cell surface receptor signaling pathway, cellular defense response, phosphatidylinositol-mediated signaling, regulation of immune response	Chemotaxis/Th1/cytotoxicity/activation	(9)
CD20	CD20, MS4A1, LEU-16	B-cell lineage, B-cell proliferation, humoral immune response	Th1/B cells	(18, 19)
CD28	CD28, Tp44	T cell costimulation, TCR signaling pathway, negative thymic T cell selection, positive regulation of T cell proliferation, positive regulation of IL-2, IL-4, and IL-10 production, immunological synapse, positive regulation of isotype switching to IgG, humoral immune response	Chemotaxis/Th1/cytotoxicity/activation	(9)
CD38	CD38, ADPRC1	T cell activation, positive regulation of B-cell proliferation, B-cell receptor signaling pathway, negative regulation of apoptotic process, cell adhesion, calcium signaling, response to IL-1	Chemotaxis/Th1/cytotoxicity/activation, Th1/B cells	(9, 19)
CD40	CD40, TNFRSF5	B-cell proliferation, inflammatory response, positive regulation of B-cell proliferation, positive regulation of MAP kinase activity, positive regulation of IL-12 production, positive regulation of isotype switching to IgG, regulation of Ig secretion, TNF-mediated signaling pathway	Chemotaxis/Th1/cytotoxicity/activation, Th1/B cells	(9, 19)
CD40L	CD40 ligand, TRAP, CD154, HIGM1, TNFSF5, IGM	B-cell differentiation and proliferation, T cell costimulation, Ig secretion, isotype switching, negative regulation of apoptotic process, inflammatory response, positive regulation of NF-kappaB transcription factor activity, positive regulation of T cell proliferation, positive regulation of IL-4, IL-10, and IL-12 production, TNF-mediated signaling pathway	Chemotaxis/Th1/cytotoxicity/activation	(9)
CD62L	CD62L, L-selectin, LECAM1, LAM1	Cell adhesion, leukocyte migration, regulation of immune response	Chemotaxis/Th1/cytotoxicity/activation	(9)
CD68	CD68, LAMP4, GP110, SCARD1	Cellular response to organic substance	Chemotaxis/Th1/cytotoxicity/activation	(9)
CD80	CD80, B7, BB1, B7-1, CD28LG1	T cell activation, T cell costimulation, intracellular signal transduction, phosphatidylinositol-mediated signaling, positive regulation of Th1 cell differentiation, positive regulation of αβT cell proliferation, positive regulation of IL-2	Chemotaxis/Th1/cytotoxicity/activation	(9)
CD86	CD86, B7-2, B70, CD28LG2	B and T cell activation, T cell costimulation, cellular response to cytokine stimulus, DC activation, negative regulation of T cell anergy, phosphatidylinositol-mediated signaling, positive regulation of Th2 differentiation and T cell proliferation, positive regulation of IL-2 and IL-4 biosynthetic process, positive regulation of transcription and DNA-templated, response to IFN-γ, TLR3 signaling pathway	Chemotaxis/Th1/cytotoxicity/activation	(9)
CD200	CD200, OX-2	Regulation of immune response, negative regulation of macrophage activation, cell recognition	Tfh cells	(12)
CSF2	CSF2, GM-CSF	DC differentiation, macrophage activation, MAPK cascade, negative regulation of cytolysis, positive regulation of cell proliferation, positive regulation of IL-23 production, positive regulation of gene expression	Th1/B cells	(19)
CTLA-4	CTLA-4, CD152, IDDM12, ALPS5, GSE	T cell costimulation, negative regulation of Treg differentiation, negative regulator of B-cell proliferation, B-cell receptor signaling pathway, positive regulation of apoptotic process	Chemotaxis/Th1/cytotoxicity/activation	(9)
CXCL9	CXCL9, MIG, CMK	Neutrophil and T cell chemotaxis, Th1 polarization, G-protein-coupled receptor signaling pathway, inflammatory response, regulation of cell proliferation	Chemotaxis, Th1 orientation	(3)
CXCL10	CXCL10, IP10	Neutrophil monocyte and T cell chemotaxis, Th1 polarization, G-protein-coupled receptor signaling pathway, inflammatory response, positive regulation of cell proliferation	Chemotaxis, chemotaxis/Th1/cytotoxicity/activation	(3, 9)

(Continued)

TABLE 2 | Continued

Name of the gene	Main names of the protein	Main immune functions and process	Cluster of gene related to TLS presence	Reference
CXCL11	CXCL11, IP9, I-TAC	T cell chemotaxis, Th1 polarization, G-protein-coupled receptor signaling pathway, inflammatory response, positive regulation of cell proliferation	Chemotaxis, chemotaxis/ Th1/cytotoxicity/ activation	(3, 9)
CXCL13	CXCL13, BLC, BCA1, SCYB13	B and Tfh cell chemotaxis, germinal center formation, lymph node development, regulation of humoral immunity, regulation of cell proliferation	Chemotaxis, chemotaxis/ T cells, Tfh cells	(3, 5, 12, 18, 19)
CXCR3	CXCR3, CD182, CD183, GPR9	Neutrophil and T cell chemotaxis, Th1 polarization, G-protein-coupled receptor signaling pathway, inflammatory response, apoptotic process, cell adhesion, calcium-mediated signaling	Chemotaxis/Th1/ cytotoxicity/activation	(9)
FasLG	Fas ligand, FASL, APTL, CD178, CD95L, TNFSF6, TNLG1A	T cell apoptotic process, activation of cysteine-type endopeptidase activity involved in apoptotic process, inflammatory cell apoptotic process, necroptotic signaling pathway, positive regulation of I-kappaB kinase/NK-kappaB signaling, positive regulation of cell proliferation, response to growth factor, transcription and DNA-templated	Chemotaxis/Th1/ cytotoxicity/activation	(9)
FBLN7	FBLN7, Fibulin-7, TM14	Cell adhesion	Tfh cells	(12)
GF11	GF11	Regulation of transcription	Th1/B cells	(19)
GNLY	Granulysin, LAG2, NKG5	Cellular defense response, defense response to bacterium fungus, killing of cells of other organism	Chemotaxis/Th1/ cytotoxicity/activation	(9)
HLA-DRA	HLA-DRA	T cell costimulation, TCR signaling pathway, antigen processing and presentation of exogenous peptide or polysaccharide antigen via MHC class II, IFN-γ-mediated signaling pathway, immune response	Chemotaxis/Th1/ cytotoxicity/activation	(9)
ICAM-3	ICAM-3, CD50, ICAM-R	Cell adhesion, extracellular matrix organization, phagocytosis, regulation of immune response, stimulatory C-type lectin receptor signaling pathway	Chemotaxis/T cells	(5)
ICOS	ICOS, CD278	T cell costimulation, T cell tolerance induction, immune response	Chemotaxis/Th1/ cytotoxicity/activation, Tfh cells	(9, 12)
IFN-γ	IFN-γ	T cell receptor signaling pathway, Th1-related cytokine	Chemotaxis/Th1/ cytotoxicity/activation	(9)
IGSF6	IGSF6, DORA	Cell surface receptor signaling pathway, immune response	Th1/B cells	(19)
IL1R1	IL1RA, IL1R, CD121A	Cell surface receptor signaling pathway, IL-1-mediated signaling pathway, regulation of inflammatory response, response to TGF-β	Th1/B cells	(19)
IL1R2	IL1R2, CD121b, IL1RB	Inflammatory response, cytokine-mediated signaling pathway	Th1/B cells	(19)
IL-2	IL-2, lymphokine, TCGF	MAPK cascade, T cell differentiation, adaptive immune response, extrinsic apoptosis signaling pathway in absence of ligand, NK cell activation, negative regulation of B-cell apoptotic process, positive regulation of B and activated T cell proliferation, positive regulation of Ig secretion, positive regulation of IFN-γ and IL-17 production, positive regulation of isotype switching to IgG, positive regulation of Treg differentiation, regulation of T cell homeostatic proliferation	Chemotaxis/Th1/ cytotoxicity/activation	(9)
IL2RA	IL2RA, CD25, IL2R, p55	Activation-induced cell death of T cells, positive regulation of activated T cell proliferation, positive regulation of T cell differentiation, inflammatory response, IL-2-mediated signaling pathway, regulation of T cell tolerance induction	Th1/B cells	(19)
IL-10	IL-10, TGIF, GVHDS, CSIF	B-cell differentiation, inflammatory response, negative regulation of T- and B-cell proliferation, negative regulation of apoptotic process, negative regulation of cytokine activity, negative regulation of IFN-γ, IL-1, IL-12, IL-18, IL-6, IL-8, and TNF production, negative regulation of myeloid DC activation, positive regulation of JAK-STAT cascade, regulation of isotype switching, Th3/Tr1/regulatory immune responses	Chemotaxis/Th1/ cytotoxicity/activation, Th1/B cells	(9, 19)
IL-12B	IL12B, CLMF, NKSF, IMD28, IMD29	Positive regulation of Th1 and Th17 immune responses, Th differentiation, cellular response to IFN-γ, defense response to virus, positive regulation of NK and T cell activation, positive regulation of memory T cell differentiation, regulation of IL-10, IL-12, IL-17, TNF-α, and GM-CSF production, positive regulation of NK T cell activation and proliferation, positive regulation of T cell-mediated cytotoxicity, regulation of tyrosine phosphorylation of STAT1	Chemotaxis/Th1/ cytotoxicity/activation	(9)
IL-15	IL-15	NK T cell proliferation, extra-thymic T cell selection, inflammatory response, LN development, positive regulation of NK and T cell proliferation, positive regulation of IL-17 production, signal transduction, tyrosine phosphorylation of STAT5	Chemotaxis/Th1/ cytotoxicity/activation	(9)

(Continued)

TABLE 2 | Continued

Name of the gene	Main names of the protein	Main immune functions and process	Cluster of gene related to TLS presence	Reference
IL-16	IL-16, LCF, NIL16	Immune response, induction of positive chemotaxis, regulation of transcription and DNA-templated	Chemotaxis/T cells	(5)
IL-18	IL-18, IGIF, IL1γ, IL1F4	MAPK cascade, Th1/Th2 immune response, GM-CSF biosynthetic process, inflammatory response, IFN-γ, IL-2, and IL-13 biosynthetic process, NK cell activation and proliferation, positive regulation of IL-17 and IFN-γ production, positive regulation of tyrosine phosphorylation of STAT3	Chemotaxis/Th1/ cytotoxicity/activation	(9)
IRF4	IRF4, MUM1, LSIRF	T cell activation, Th17 cell lineage commitment, IFN-γ-mediated signaling pathway, positive regulation of IL-10, IL-13, IL-2, and IL-4 biosynthetic process, regulation of Th cell differentiation, Type-I IFN signaling pathway, positive regulation of transcription	Th1/B cells	(19)
ITGAL	ITGAL, CD11A, LFA-1	Extracellular matrix organization, T cell activation via TCR contact with antigen bound to MHC molecule on APC, leukocyte migration, heterotypic cell–cell adhesion, immune response, integrin-mediated signaling pathway, inflammatory response, phagocytosis, regulation of immune response	Chemotaxis/T cells	(5)
ITGAD	ITGAD, ADB2, CD11D	Extracellular matrix organization, heterotypic cell–cell adhesion, immune response, integrin-mediated signaling pathway	Chemotaxis/T cells	(5)
ITGA4	ITGA4, CD49D	B-cell differentiation, cell-matrix adhesion, diapedesis, extracellular matrix organization, heterotypic cell–cell adhesion, integrin-mediated signaling pathway, leukocyte migration tethering or rolling, regulation of immune response	Chemotaxis/T cells	(5)
LTA	LTA, Lymphotoxin α, TNFB, TNFSF1	Positive regulation of apoptotic process, cell–cell signaling, positive regulation of humoral immune response mediated by circulating Ig, LN development, positive regulation of IFN-γ production, TNF-mediated signaling pathway	Chemotaxis/Th1/ cytotoxicity/activation	(9)
MADCAM1	MADCAM1	Cell–matrix adhesion, extracellular matrix organization, heterotypic cell–cell adhesion, integrin-mediated signaling pathway, leukocyte tethering or rolling, receptor clustering, regulation of immune response, signal transduction	Chemotaxis/T cells	(5)
PDCD1	PD-1	T cell costimulation, humoral immune response, positive regulator of T cell apoptotic process	Tfh cells	(12)
PRF1	Perforin, PFP, FLH2, PFN1	Apoptotic process, cellular defense response, cytolysis, defense response to tumor cell, immunological synapse formation, transmembrane transport	Chemotaxis/Th1/ cytotoxicity/activation	(9)
SDC1	SDC, CD138, syndecan	Cell migration, inflammatory response, canonical Wnt signaling pathway	Th1/B cells	(19)
SGPP2	SGPP2, Spp2, SPPase2	Regulation of immune response, positive regulation of signal transduction, positive regulation of NK-mediated cytotoxicity	Tfh cells	(12)
SH2D1A		Signal transduction of T- and B-cell activation	Tfh cells	(12)
STAT5A	STAT5A, MGF	JAK–STAT cascade, peptidyl-tyrosine phosphorylation, regulator of transcription	Th1/B cells	(19)
TBX21	T-Bet, TBLYM	T cell differentiation, lymphocyte migration, positive regulation of transcription and DNA-templated, positive regulation of isotype switching to IgG	Chemotaxis/Th1/ cytotoxicity/activation	(9)
TIGIT	TIGIT, VSTM3, VSIG9	T cell co-inhibitory receptor, negative regulation of IL-12 production, positive regulation of IL-10 production	Tfh cells	(12)
TNF-α	TNF-α, DIF, TNFSF2	I-kappaB kinase/NF-kappaB signaling, JNK cascade, MAPK cascade, activation of MAPK and MAPKKK activities, humoral immune response, inflammatory response, necroptotic signaling pathway, negative regulation of cytokine secretion, negative regulation of cytokine and chemokine production, negative regulation of transcription and DNA-templated, positive regulation of ERK1 and ERK2 cascade, positive regulation of I-kappaB kinase/NF-kappaB signaling, positive regulation of JUN and MAP kinase activity, positive regulation of apoptotic process, positive regulation of humoral response and Ig secretion	Chemotaxis/Th1/ cytotoxicity/activation	(9)
TRAF6	TRAF6, RNF85	FcE receptor signaling pathway, JNK cascade, MyD88-dependent TLR signaling pathway, MyD88-independent TLR signaling pathway, TCR signaling pathway, Th1 immune response, activation of MAPK activity, Ag processing and presentation of exogenous peptide Ag, myeloid DC differentiation, positive regulation of T cell activation proliferation and cytokine production, positive regulation of IL-12 production, response to IL-1, TLR signaling pathway	Th1/B cells	(19)
VCAM-1	VCAM-1, CD106	B-cell differentiation, acute inflammatory response, cell–matrix adhesion, cellular response to TNF-α and VEGF, IFN-γ-mediated signaling pathway, leukocyte tethering or rolling, positive regulation of T cell proliferation, regulation of immune response, response to hypoxia	Chemotaxis/T cells	(5)

Genes selectively overexpressed in tumors having high density of TLS in cancer patients.

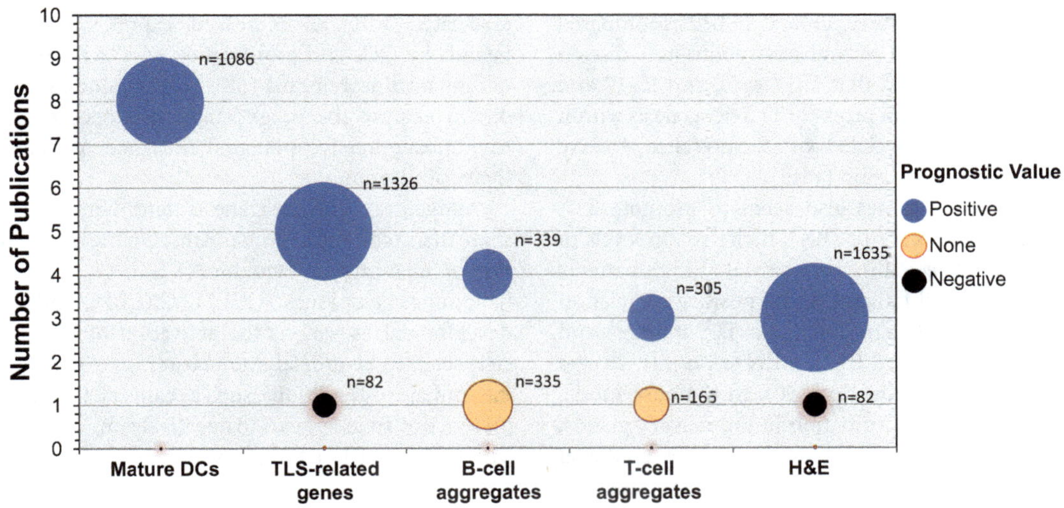

FIGURE 1 | Prognostic value of TLS-associated biomarkers in primary and metastatic cancers. The number of publications studying the impact of mature DCs, TLS-related gene signatures, B-cell aggregates, T cell aggregates, or H&E with regard to prognosis in human cancers is represented (12 cancer types have been included). Blue, orange, and red circles represent an association with good, none, and poor prognosis, respectively. The diameter of the circles represents the total number of tumors (*n*) that have been analyzed on these studies.

Further efforts should be made to optimize TLS-quantifying methods. Indeed the use of multicolor IHC will facilitate their characterization, by allowing the simultaneous detection of all major cell types and providing an extensive analysis of their cellular complexity.

TLS NEOGENESIS

The cellular composition and spatial organization of TLS share many similarities with those of SLO. Indeed, an increasing number of studies performed in a large variety of inflammatory disorders, in mice and in humans, suggest that their formation and regulation involve the same set of chemokines than those acting in lymphoid organogenesis.

Positive Regulators

Lymphotoxin, CCL21, and CXCL13 were shown to play a major role during TLS neogenesis, and are related to TLS presence in human tumors (**Table 2**). In a mouse model of atherosclerosis, the activation of LTβR$^+$ medial smooth muscle cells in the abdominal aorta by LT produced by CD11c$^+$ CD68$^+$ Ly6C^{lo} monocytes leads to the expression of CCL19, CCL21, CXCL13, and CXCL16 chemokines, which in turn trigger the recruitment of lymphocytes to the adventitia and the development of TLS (31). The same observation was made by Thaunat et al. in a rat model of chronic allograft rejection, in which M1-macrophages behaved as LTi cells in diseased arteries by expressing high levels of LTα and TNF-α (32). In human NSCLC, a TLS-related gene signature was identified, including CCL19, CCL21, IL-16, and CXCL13 (5) (**Table 2**). Interestingly, Matsuda et al. recently suggested in a mouse intrapulmonary tracheal transplant model that lymphoid neogenesis was dependent on spleen tyrosine kinase (Syk)-signaling. Decreased expression of CXCL12, CXCL13, and VEGF-α, lower B-cell recruitment into allograft, and smaller lymphoid aggregate area were observed in Syk-deficient recipient mice as compared to controls (33).

The generation of HEVs is also a critical step in TLS neogenesis. HEV endothelial cells express LTβR, and the continuous engagement of LTβR on HEVs by LT$^+$ CD11c$^+$ DCs is critical for the induction and maintenance of the mature HEV phenotype required for the extravasation of blood lymphocyte into LNs (34–37). In addition, CD11c$^+$ DCs can be sources of proangiogenic factors, such as VEGF, favoring the development of HEVs, and ultimately lymphocyte entry into LN (38–41). Consistently, LTβ expression correlates with that of HEV-associated chemokines in human breast cancer, and DC-Lamp$^+$ DC density correlates with HEV density, lymphocyte infiltration, and favorable clinical outcome (11). Other cell types were shown to favor the development of HEV. For instance, ectopic expression of CCL21 in the thyroid gives rise first to the recruitment of CD3$^+$ CD4$^+$ T cells followed by DC, and this DC-T cross-talk is required for the local development of both TLS and mature HEV (42). Tumor-infiltrating CD8$^+$ T cells and NK cells were also shown to drive the *de novo* development of PNAd$^+$ TNFR1$^+$ CCL21$^+$ HEV-like blood vessels through the production of LT and IFN-γ (43).

Th17 cells share many developmental and effector markers with LTi cells, including the nuclear hormone receptor retinoic acid-related orphan receptor γt (RORγt), which promotes not only the production of IL-17 and IL-22 by Th17 cells, LTi cells, and other RORγt$^+$ innate lymphoid cells (ILCs), but also cell membrane expression of LT [reviewed in Ref. (44)]. In mice lungs, the formation of TLS [called here induced-bronchus-associated lymphoid tissues (i-BALT)] following LPS sensitization was dependent of IL-17 production by T cells, including Th17 and γδ T cells (45). This observation was also observed in a mouse experimental autoimmune encephalomyelitis (EAE) model of multiple sclerosis (46). Similarly, IL-17α-deficient mice exposed to cigarette smoke displayed decreased number of ectopic lymphoid follicles and decreased expression of CXCL12 as compared to wild-type mice in a model of chronic obstructive lung disease (47). It has also been suggested that Th17 cells, and IL-17 and IL-21 secretion by these cells can promote TLS neogenesis within human renal grafts, and are associated with the presence of active GC B cells and fast chronic rejection (48).

Other inflammatory cytokines also seem to promote TLS neogenesis. In rheumatoid arthritis (RA), high protein levels of IL-23 and IL-17F were detected in the synovial fluid of patients displaying ectopic lymphoid follicles, and a positive correlation was observed between CD21L mRNA (as a TLS marker) and IL-23 but also IL-17F, IL-21, and IL-22 mRNAs (49). IL-22 was also proposed to favor TLS induction (50). In a mouse model of virus-induced autoantibody formation in the salivary glands, it was shown that the ligation of IL-22R expressed by epithelial cells and fibroblasts leads to CXCL12 and CXCL13 production, allowing B-cell recruitment and TLS organization. In that case, IL-22 was mainly produced by γδ T cells and to a lesser extent by ILCs and NK cells during the early phase post-infection, and then by αβ T cells later after infection.

Negative Regulators

On the opposite, IL-27, a cytokine known to inhibit effector Th17 responses was recently suggested to negatively regulate the development of ectopic lymphoid-like structures in the synovial tissues of RA patients. While patients having a high density of TLS displayed high synovial levels of IL-17 and IL-21, high levels of IL-27 were observed in patients devoid of any TLS, and IL-27 expression was inversely correlated with $CD3^+$ and $CD20^+$ infiltrates and with synovitis. This observation was confirmed in a mouse model of RA (51).

Among the immune cells infiltrating tumors are regulatory T cells (Tregs), which have been considered in many reports as a marker of poor prognosis in cancer (52, 53). Tregs have been reported to negatively interfere with BALT development. Indeed in CCR7-deficient mice, BALTs developed spontaneously in the absence of infection, an event that is directly reverted by the adoptive transfer of wild-type Tregs but not $CCR7^{-/-}$ Tregs (54). In human breast cancer, Tregs were detected in lymphoid aggregates surrounding tumor nests, and their presence was linked with the poor clinical outcome of patients (55). In mice bearing breast tumors, Treg depletion led to an increased density of HEV within the tumor, facilitated T cell recruitment from the blood, and ultimately induced tumor destruction (56). This observation is in accordance with a human study showing that HEV^{high} breast tumors correlated with a high LT-β expression, a high density of tumor-infiltrating mature DC, and a decreased $FoxP3^+/CD3^+$ T cell ratio (11).

More recently, a new mechanism involving regulation of TLS formation by Tregs was found, by dampening neutrophilic inflammation (57). The presence of neutrophils seemed to be critical for the neogenesis and the humoral immune function of i-BALT by enhancing B-cell activation and survival, Ig class switching to IgA as well as plasma cell survival (57).

Regulatory T cells have been shown to dampen the effector T cell response promoted within tumor-associated TLS. Treg depletion causes immune-mediated tumor destruction associated with an increased expression of co-stimulatory ligands by DCs and proliferation of T cells in a murine model of lung adenocarcinoma (58). Further studies should be carried out to analyze the prognostic importance of Tregs and their immunosuppressive potential in cancer patients according to their localization.

Altogether, TLS neogenesis and lymphoid organogenesis share many common mechanisms. On the one hand, the production of inflammatory cytokines (LT, IL-17, IL-22, and IL-23) and lymphoid chemokines (CCL21, CXCL12, and CXCL13), HEV development as well as the activation of DCs, B, and effector cells seem to be crucial events leading to TLS neogenesis under inflammatory conditions, such as cancers. On the other hand, the presence of Tregs appears to negatively impact TLS formation and TLS-associated T cell responses.

MANIPULATION OF TLS FOR A THERAPEUTIC INTERVENTION IN CANCER

A series of studies suggest that TLS are sites for generation and maintenance of adaptive anti-tumor responses (10). Therefore, TLS induction could be used as a therapeutic intervention for a better tumor control and prolonged survival of cancer patients. Since LN and TLS share many similarities in terms of cellular composition and organization, deciphering the mechanisms of lymphoid organogenesis enables to first highlight some putative key molecules that can support TLS neogenesis.

Targeting Molecules Involved in Lymphoid Organogenesis

The key cross-talk between LTi cells and lymphoid tissue organizer cells (LTo cells that are cells of mesenchymal origin) occurring during LN development involves several molecules along with RANK and its ligand, which lead to LTβR signaling (59). Therefore, targeting RANK/LT pathway may modulate TLS development through the activation of LTo cells. Currently, antagonists of LTα (Pateclizumab NCT01225393), LTβR (Baminercept, NCT01552681) and RANK signaling (NCT01973569) are under investigation in several inflammatory situations. A special attention should be made in cancer setting where these antagonists might block TLS formation and, hence, reduce survival. The use of agonists might rather present a benefit to cancer patients but no drugs have been developed so far.

Activation of LTβR signaling pathway in LTo cells induces VCAM-1 and ICAM-1 upregulation, and ultimately leukocyte infiltration (60). Because both molecules are known to be induced by inflammation, an ICAM-1 antagonist called Alicaforsen has been tested in autoimmune diseases (NCT00048113, NCT00063830). We can speculate that the development of VCAM-1/ICAM-1 agonists would promote LTi-like cells-LTo clusterings and improve the leukocyte recruitment in order to generate cancer-associated TLS.

IL-7 receptor (CD127) signaling has been reported as a key pathway for TLS neogenesis (61). IL-7 is not only crucial for the survival and proliferation of LTi cells but also for GC formation and Tfh differentiation (62). To date, only one pharmacologic agent (IL-7R) is under investigation in NOD mice to deplete autoreactive T cells and to regulate pro-inflammatory mediators (63).

Altogether, as a counterpart of autoimmune diseases, development of agonist molecules targeting lymphoid organogenesis might be a promising strategy for the initiation and the maintenance of TLS in cancers.

Modulation of Chemokine and Cytokine Networks

Lymphoid chemokines represent a good therapeutic target for the modulation of TLS (**Table 2**). The CCL19–CCL21/CCR7 and CXCL13/CXCR5 couples are induced after LT-βR signaling during lymphoid genesis (60). They are overexpressed in TLS of melanoma (21), colorectal (3), and lung (5) cancer patients. Using lymphoid chemokines or their agonists could be a promising strategy to induce TLS neogenesis in cancers. For example, CCL21 has been shown to attract circulating naïve T cells and DCs in tumors, and contribute to the control of tumor growth (64–66). A Phase I clinical trial is currently under investigation in NSCLC patients receiving intra-tumoral injections of CCL21-transduced autologous DCs (NCT00601094, NCT01574222). It is tempting to speculate that this vaccine therapy would boost TLS formation in tumors associated with an influx of lymphocytes, an effective anti-tumor immune response, and a reduction of tumor burden.

IL-21, which is mainly secreted by Th17 cells and neutrophils, represents also an interesting molecular target. First, this cytokine has been shown to promote TLS neogenesis in lungs after acute LPS exposure and IL-$21^{-/-}$ mice exhibit fewer TLS in allografts than the control group (57). Second, IL-21 can enhance B and plasma cell survival as well as B-cell-dependent immunity, and induce conventional T cells to become refractory to Treg immunosuppression (48, 57, 67). Even if IL-21 can block IL-2 production with deleterious consequences in terms of Treg differentiation, IL-21 can substitute for IL-2 as a T cell growth factor (68). Recombinant IL-21 is currently tested in many clinical trials, alone or in combination with chemotherapy, therapeutic antibodies or tyrosine kinase inhibitors (e.g., NCT00617253, NCT00389285, NCT00095108, NCT01629758, NCT00336986, and NCT01489059). Altogether, it is likely that IL-21 could promote a robust anti-tumor immunity in a TLS-dependent manner.

CONCLUSION AND PERSPECTIVES

By facilitating the direct entry of CCR7$^+$ naïve T cells and CXCR5$^+$ B cells into tumors through HEVs, TLS allow T cells to differentiate into effector cells upon contact with mature DCs and B cells to form GC, protected from the immunosuppressive milieu of the tumor microenvironment. Therefore, TLS represent sites for the induction and maintenance of the local and systemic anti-tumor responses, which confer long-term protection against metastasis and, hence, correlate with good prognosis for the patients. Indeed, therapies aiming to increase TLS formation may allow generating anti-tumor responses directly *in situ* and would be beneficial in patients with high mutational load. TLS may also constitute biomarkers of anti-tumor response in patients undergoing immunotherapies. Thus, TLS induction was observed in cervical cancer patients vaccinated with HPV DNA (69) or with G-VAX (70), and one may speculate that TLS signature could be used to evidence response to therapies that unlock the adaptive immune responses.

AUTHOR CONTRIBUTIONS

ML, NG, HK, CG, and CSF wrote and revised the paper. WF and MCDN revised the paper.

ACKNOWLEDGMENTS

We thank all members of the Laboratory "Cancer, Immune control and Escape," pathologists and clinicians who have participated in these studies, for their help and valuable discussions, as well as cancer patients.

FUNDING

This work was supported by Institut National de la Santé et de la Recherche Médicale (INSERM), University Paris Descartes, University Pierre et Marie Curie, the Institut National du Cancer (2009-1-PLBIO07-INSERM6-, 2010-1-PLBIO03-INSERM 6-1, 2011-1-PLBIO-06-INSERM 6-1, PLBIO09-088-IDF-KROEMER), CARPEM (CAncer Research for PErsonalized Medicine), the Labex Immuno-Oncology (LAXE62_9UMS872 FRIDMAN), foundation ARC pour la recherche sur le cancer (SL220110603483), Ligue Nationale contre le Cancer (GB/MA/CD/EP-12003), and MedImmune (Gaithersburg, USA, n°11796A10). HK was supported by a grant from La Ligue contre le Cancer.

REFERENCES

1. Dieu-Nosjean MC, Antoine M, Danel C, Heudes D, Wislez M, Poulot V, et al. Long-term survival for patients with non-small-cell lung cancer with intratumoral lymphoid structures. *J Clin Oncol* (2008) 26(27):4410–7. doi:10.1200/JCO.2007.15.0284
2. Germain C, Gnjatic S, Tamzalit F, Knockaert S, Remark R, Goc J, et al. Presence of B cells in tertiary lymphoid structures is associated with a protective immunity in patients with lung cancer. *Am J Respir Crit Care Med* (2014) 189(7):832–44. doi:10.1164/rccm.201309-1611OC
3. Coppola D, Nebozhyn M, Khalil F, Dai H, Yeatman T, Loboda A, et al. Unique ectopic lymph node-like structures present in human primary colorectal carcinoma are identified by immune gene array profiling. *Am J Pathol* (2011) 179(1):37–45. doi:10.1016/j.ajpath.2011.03.007
4. Cipponi A, Mercier M, Seremet T, Baurain JF, Théate I, van den Oord J, et al. Neogenesis of lymphoid structures and antibody responses occur in human melanoma metastases. *Cancer Res* (2012) 72(16):3997–4007. doi:10.1158/0008-5472.CAN-12-1377
5. de Chaisemartin L, Goc J, Damotte D, Validire P, Magdeleinat P, Alifano M, et al. Characterization of chemokines and adhesion molecules associated with T cell presence in tertiary lymphoid structures in human lung cancer. *Cancer Res* (2011) 71(20):6391–9. doi:10.1158/0008-5472.CAN-11-0952
6. Martinet L, Garrido I, Girard JP. Tumor high endothelial venules (HEVs) predict lymphocyte infiltration and favorable prognosis in breast cancer. *Oncoimmunology* (2012) 1(5):789–90. doi:10.4161/onci.19787

7. Martinet L, Le Guellec S, Filleron T, Lamant L, Meyer N, Rochaix P, et al. High endothelial venules (HEVs) in human melanoma lesions: major gateways for tumor-infiltrating lymphocytes. *Oncoimmunology* (2012) 1(6):829–39. doi:10.4161/onci.20492
8. Martinet L, Garrido I, Filleron T, Le Guellec S, Bellard E, Fournie JJ, et al. Human solid tumors contain high endothelial venules: association with T- and B-lymphocyte infiltration and favorable prognosis in breast cancer. *Cancer Res* (2011) 71(17):5678–87. doi:10.1158/0008-5472.CAN-11-0431
9. Goc J, Germain C, Vo-Bourgais TK, Lupo A, Klein C, Knockaert S, et al. Dendritic cells in tumor-associated tertiary lymphoid structures signal a Th1 cytotoxic immune contexture and license the positive prognostic value of infiltrating CD8 + T cells. *Cancer Res* (2014) 74(3):705–15. doi:10.1158/0008-5472.CAN-13-1342
10. Hosmalin A, Sautès-Fridman C, Fougereau M, Yssel H, Fischer A. 50(th) Anniversary of the French Society for Immunology (SFI). *Eur J Immunol* (2016) 46(7):1545–7. doi:10.1002/eji.201670073
11. Martinet L, Filleron T, Le Guellec S, Rochaix P, Garrido I, Girard JP. High endothelial venule blood vessels for tumor-infiltrating lymphocytes are associated with lymphotoxin β-producing dendritic cells in human breast cancer. *J Immunol* (2013) 191(4):2001–8. doi:10.4049/jimmunol.1300872
12. Gu-Trantien C, Loi S, Garaud S, Equeter C, Libin M, de Wind A, et al. $CD4^+$ follicular helper T cell infiltration predicts breast cancer survival. *J Clin Invest* (2013) 123(7):2873–92. doi:10.1172/JCI67428
13. Lee HJ, Park IA, Song IH, Shin SJ, Kim JY, Yu JH, et al. Tertiary lymphoid structures: prognostic significance and relationship with tumour-infiltrating lymphocytes in triple-negative breast cancer. *J Clin Pathol* (2016) 69(5):422–30. doi:10.1136/jclinpath-2015-203089
14. Väyrynen JP, Sajanti SA, Klintrup K, Mäkelä J, Herzig KH, Karttunen TJ, et al. Characteristics and significance of colorectal cancer associated lymphoid reaction. *Int J Cancer* (2014) 134(9):2126–35. doi:10.1002/ijc.28533
15. Remark R, Alifano M, Cremer I, Lupo A, Dieu-Nosjean MC, Riquet M, et al. Characteristics and clinical impacts of the immune environments in colorectal and renal cell carcinoma lung metastases: influence of tumor origin. *Clin Cancer Res* (2013) 19(15):4079–91. doi:10.1158/1078-0432.CCR-12-3847
16. McMullen TPW, Lai R, Dabbagh L, Wallace TM, de Gara CJ. Survival in rectal cancer is predicted by T cell infiltration of tumour-associated lymphoid nodules. *Clin Exp Immunol* (2010) 161(1):81–8. doi:10.1111/j.1365-2249.2010.04147.x
17. Di Caro G, Bergomas F, Grizzi F, Doni A, Bianchi P, Malesci A, et al. Occurrence of tertiary lymphoid tissue is associated with T-cell infiltration and predicts better prognosis in early-stage colorectal cancers. *Clin Cancer Res* (2014) 20(8):2147–58. doi:10.1158/1078-0432.CCR-13-2590
18. Bindea G, Mlecnik B, Tosolini M, Kirilovsky A, Waldner M, Obenauf AC, et al. Spatiotemporal dynamics of intratumoral immune cells reveal the immune landscape in human cancer. *Immunity* (2013) 39(4):782–95. doi:10.1016/j.immuni.2013.10.003
19. Hennequin A, Derangère V, Boidot R, Apetoh L, Vincent J, Orry D, et al. Tumor infiltration by Tbet + effector T cells and CD20 + B cells is associated with survival in gastric cancer patients. *Oncoimmunology* (2016) 5(2):e1054598. doi:10.1080/2162402X.2015.1054598
20. Ladányi A, Kiss J, Somlai B, Gilde K, Fejos Z, Mohos A, et al. Density of DC-LAMP(+) mature dendritic cells in combination with activated T lymphocytes infiltrating primary cutaneous melanoma is a strong independent prognostic factor. *Cancer Immunol Immunother* (2007) 56(9):1459–69. doi:10.1007/s00262-007-0286-3
21. Messina JL, Fenstermacher DA, Eschrich S, Qu X, Berglund AE, Lloyd MC, et al. 12-chemokine gene signature identifies lymph node-like structures in melanoma: potential for patient selection for immunotherapy? *Sci Rep* (2012) 2:765. doi:10.1038/srep00765
22. Wirsing AM, Rikardsen OG, Steigen SE, Uhlin-Hansen L, Hadler-Olsen E. Characterisation and prognostic value of tertiary lymphoid structures in oral squamous cell carcinoma. *BMC Clin Pathol* (2014) 14:38. doi:10.1186/1472-6890-14-38
23. Hiraoka N, Ino Y, Yamazaki-Itoh R, Kanai Y, Kosuge T, Shimada K. Intratumoral tertiary lymphoid organ is a favourable prognosticator in patients with pancreatic cancer. *Br J Cancer* (2015) 112(11):1782–90. doi:10.1038/bjc.2015.145
24. Giraldo NA, Becht E, Pagès F, Skliris G, Verkarre V, Vano Y, et al. Orchestration and prognostic significance of immune checkpoints in the microenvironment of primary and metastatic renal cell cancer. *Clin Cancer Res* (2015) 21(13):3031–40. doi:10.1158/1078-0432.CCR-14-2926
25. Finkin S, Yuan D, Stein I, Taniguchi K, Weber A, Unger K, et al. Ectopic lymphoid structures function as microniches for tumor progenitor cells in hepatocellular carcinoma. *Nat Immunol* (2015) 16(12):1235–44. doi:10.1038/ni.3290
26. Goeppert B, Frauenschuh L, Zucknick M, Stenzinger A, Andrulis M, Klauschen F, et al. Prognostic impact of tumour-infiltrating immune cells on biliary tract cancer. *Br J Cancer* (2013) 109(10):2665–74. doi:10.1038/bjc.2013.610
27. Meshcheryakova A, Tamandl D, Bajna E, Stift J, Mittlboeck M, Svoboda M, et al. B cells and ectopic follicular structures: novel players in anti-tumor programming with prognostic power for patients with metastatic colorectal cancer. *PLoS One* (2014) 9(6):e99008. doi:10.1371/journal.pone.0099008
28. Dieu-Nosjean MC, Giraldo NA, Kaplon H, Germain C, Fridman WH, Sautès-Fridman C. Tertiary lymphoid structures, drivers of the anti-tumor responses in human cancers. *Immunol Rev* (2016) 271(1):260–75. doi:10.1111/imr.12405
29. Dieu-Nosjean MC, Goc J, Giraldo NA, Sautès-Fridman C, Fridman WH. Tertiary lymphoid structures in cancer and beyond. *Trends Immunol* (2014) 35(11):571–80. doi:10.1016/j.it.2014.09.006
30. Sautès-Fridman C, Fridman WH. TLS in tumors: what lies within. *Trends Immunol* (2016) 37(1):1–2. doi:10.1016/j.it.2015.12.001
31. Gräbner R, Lötzer K, Döpping S, Hildner M, Radke D, Beer M, et al. Lymphotoxin beta receptor signaling promotes tertiary lymphoid organogenesis in the aorta adventitia of aged ApoE-/- Mice. *J Exp Med* (2009) 206(1):233–48. doi:10.1084/jem.20080752
32. Thaunat O, Field AC, Dai J, Louedec L, Patey N, Bloch MF, et al. Lymphoid neogenesis in chronic rejection: evidence for a local humoral alloimmune response. *Proc Natl Acad Sci U S A* (2005) 102(41):14723–8. doi:10.1073/pnas.0507223102
33. Matsuda Y, Wang X, Oishi H, Guan Z, Saito M, Liu M, et al. Spleen tyrosine kinase modulates fibrous airway obliteration and associated lymphoid neogenesis after transplantation. *Am J Transplant* (2016) 16(1):342–52. doi:10.1111/ajt.13442
34. Browning JL, Allaire N, Ngam-Ek A, Notidis E, Hunt J, Perrin S, et al. Lymphotoxin-beta receptor signaling is required for the homeostatic control of HEV differentiation and function. *Immunity* (2005) 23(5):539–50. doi:10.1016/j.immuni.2005.10.002
35. Liao S, Ruddle NH. Synchrony of high endothelial venules and lymphatic vessels revealed by immunization. *J Immunol* (2006) 177(5):3369–79. doi:10.4049/jimmunol.177.5.3369
36. Kumar V, Scandella E, Danuser R, Onder L, Nitschké M, Fukui Y, et al. Global lymphoid tissue remodeling during a viral infection is orchestrated by a B cell-lymphotoxin-dependent pathway. *Blood* (2010) 115(23):4725–33. doi:10.1182/blood-2009-10-250118
37. Moussion C, Girard JP. Dendritic cells control lymphocyte entry to lymph nodes through high endothelial venules. *Nature* (2011) 479(7374):542–6. doi:10.1038/nature10540
38. Wendland M, Willenzon S, Kocks J, Davalos-Misslitz AC, Hammerschmidt SI, Schumann K, et al. Lymph node T cell homeostasis relies on steady state homing of dendritic cells. *Immunity* (2011) 35(6):945–57. doi:10.1016/j.immuni.2011.10.017
39. Sozzani S, Rusnati M, Riboldi E, Mitola S, Presta M. Dendritic cell-endothelial cell cross-talk in angiogenesis. *Trends Immunol* (2007) 28(9):385–92. doi:10.1016/j.it.2007.07.006
40. Webster B, Ekland EH, Agle LM, Chyou S, Ruggieri R, Lu TT. Regulation of lymph node vascular growth by dendritic cells. *J Exp Med* (2006) 203(8):1903–13. doi:10.1084/jem.20052272
41. Benahmed F, Chyou S, Dasoveanu D, Chen J, Kumar V, Iwakura Y, et al. Multiple CD11c + cells collaboratively express IL-1β to modulate stromal vascular endothelial growth factor and lymph node vascular-stromal growth. *J Immunol* (2014) 192(9):4153–63. doi:10.4049/jimmunol.1301765
42. Marinkovic T, Garin A, Yokota Y, Fu YX, Ruddle NH, Furtado GC, et al. Interaction of mature CD3 + CD4 + T cells with dendritic cells triggers the development of tertiary lymphoid structures in the thyroid. *J Clin Invest* (2006) 116(10):2622–32. doi:10.1172/JCI28993

43. Peske JD, Thompson ED, Gemta L, Baylis RA, Fu YX, Engelhard VH. Effector lymphocyte-induced lymph node-like vasculature enables naive T-cell entry into tumours and enhanced anti-tumour immunity. *Nat Commun* (2015) 6:7114. doi:10.1038/ncomms8114
44. Grogan JL, Ouyang W. A role for Th17 cells in the regulation of tertiary lymphoid follicles. *Eur J Immunol* (2012) 42(9):2255–62. doi:10.1002/eji.201242656
45. Rangel-Moreno J, Carragher DM, de la Luz Garcia-Hernandez M, Hwang JY, Kusser K, Hartson L, et al. The development of inducible bronchus-associated lymphoid tissue depends on IL-17. *Nat Immunol* (2011) 12(7):639–46. doi:10.1038/ni.2053
46. Peters A, Pitcher LA, Sullivan JM, Mitsdoerffer M, Acton SE, Franz B, et al. Th17 cells induce ectopic lymphoid follicles in central nervous system tissue inflammation. *Immunity* (2011) 35(6):986–96. doi:10.1016/j.immuni.2011.10.015
47. Roos AB, Sandén C, Mori M, Bjermer L, Stampfli MR, Erjefält JS. IL-17A is elevated in end-stage chronic obstructive pulmonary disease and contributes to cigarette smoke-induced lymphoid neogenesis. *Am J Respir Crit Care Med* (2015) 191(11):1232–41. doi:10.1164/rccm.201410-1861OC
48. Deteix C, Attuil-Audenis V, Duthey A, Patey N, McGregor B, Dubois V, et al. Intragraft Th17 infiltrate promotes lymphoid neogenesis and hastens clinical chronic rejection. *J Immunol* (2010) 184(9):5344–51. doi:10.4049/jimmunol.0902999
49. Cañete JD, Celis R, Yeremenko N, Sanmartí R, van Duivenvoorde L, Ramírez J, et al. Ectopic lymphoid neogenesis is strongly associated with activation of the IL-23 pathway in rheumatoid synovitis. *Arthritis Res Ther* (2015) 17:173. doi:10.1186/s13075-015-0688-0
50. Barone F, Nayar S, Campos J, Cloake T, Withers DR, Toellner KM, et al. IL-22 regulates lymphoid chemokine production and assembly of tertiary lymphoid organs. *Proc Natl Acad Sci U S A* (2015) 112(35):11024–9. doi:10.1073/pnas.1503315112
51. Jones GW, Bombardieri M, Greenhill CJ, McLeod L, Nerviani A, Rocher-Ros V, et al. Interleukin-27 inhibits ectopic lymphoid-like structure development in early inflammatory arthritis. *J Exp Med* (2015) 212(11):1793–802. doi:10.1084/jem.20132307
52. Fridman WH, Pagès F, Sautès-Fridman C, Galon J. The immune contexture in human tumours: impact on clinical outcome. *Nat Rev Cancer* (2012) 12(4):298–306. doi:10.1038/nrc3245
53. Becht E, Giraldo NA, Germain C, de Reyniès A, Laurent-Puig P, Zucman-Rossi J, et al. Immune contexture, immunoscore, and malignant cell molecular subgroups for prognostic and theranostic classifications of cancers. *Adv Immunol* (2016) 130:95–190. doi:10.1016/bs.ai.2015.12.002
54. Kocks JR, Davalos-Misslitz AC, Hintzen G, Ohl L, Förster R. Regulatory T cells interfere with the development of bronchus-associated lymphoid tissue. *J Exp Med* (2007) 204(4):723–34. doi:10.1084/jem.20061424
55. Gobert M, Treilleux I, Bendriss-Vermare N, Bachelot T, Goddard-Leon S, Arfi V, et al. Regulatory T cells recruited through CCL22/CCR4 are selectively activated in lymphoid infiltrates surrounding primary breast tumors and lead to an adverse clinical outcome. *Cancer Res* (2009) 69(5):2000–9. doi:10.1158/0008-5472.CAN-08-2360
56. Hindley JP, Jones E, Smart K, Bridgeman H, Lauder SN, Ondondo B, et al. T-cell trafficking facilitated by high endothelial venules is required for tumor control after regulatory T-cell depletion. *Cancer Res* (2012) 72(21):5473–82. doi:10.1158/0008-5472.CAN-12-1912
57. Foo SY, Zhang V, Lalwani A, Lynch JP, Zhuang A, Lam CE, et al. Regulatory T cells prevent inducible BALT formation by dampening neutrophilic inflammation. *J Immunol* (2015) 194(9):4567–76. doi:10.4049/jimmunol.1400909
58. Joshi NS, Akama-Garren EH, Lu Y, Lee DY, Chang GP, Li A, et al. Regulatory T cells in tumor-associated tertiary lymphoid structures suppress anti-tumor T cell responses. *Immunity* (2015) 43(3):579–90. doi:10.1016/j.immuni.2015.08.006
59. Mebius, Reina E. Organogenesis of lymphoid tissues. *Nat Rev Immunol* (2003) 3(4):292–303. doi:10.1038/nri1054
60. Dejardin E, Droin NM, Delhase M, Haas E, Cao Y, Makris C, et al. The lymphotoxin-beta receptor induces different patterns of gene expression via two NF-kappaB pathways. *Immunity* (2002) 17(4):525–35. doi:10.1016/S1074-7613(02)00423-5
61. Meier D, Bornmann C, Chappaz S, Schmutz S, Otten LA, Ceredig R, et al. Ectopic lymphoid-organ development occurs through interleukin 7-mediated enhanced survival of lymphoid-tissue-inducer cells. *Immunity* (2007) 26(5):643–54. doi:10.1016/j.immuni.2007.04.009
62. Seo YB, Im SJ, Namkoong H, Kim SW, Choi YW, Kang MC, et al. Crucial roles of interleukin-7 in the development of T follicular helper cells and in the induction of humoral immunity. *J Virol* (2014) 88(16):8998–9009. doi:10.1128/JVI.00534-14
63. Lee LF, Logronio K, Tu GH, Zhai W, Ni I, Mei L, et al. Anti-IL-7 Receptor-α reverses established type 1 diabetes in non-obese diabetic mice by modulating effector T-cell function. *Proc Natl Acad Sci U S A* (2012) 109(31):12674–9. doi:10.1073/pnas.1203795109
64. Vicari AP, Ait-Yahia S, Chemin K, Mueller A, Zlotnik A, Caux C. Antitumor effects of the mouse chemokine 6Ckine/SLC through angiostatic and immunological mechanisms. *J Immunol* (2000) 165(4):1992–2000. doi:10.4049/jimmunol.165.4.1992
65. Nomura T, Hasegawa H, Kohno M, Sasaki M, Fujita S. Enhancement of anti-tumor immunity by tumor cells transfected with the secondary lymphoid tissue chemokine EBI-1-ligand chemokine and stromal cell-derived factor-1alpha chemokine genes. *Int J Cancer* (2001) 91(5):597–606. doi:10.1002/1097-0215(200002)9999:9999<::AID-IJC1107>3.0.CO;2-J
66. Yang SC, Batra RK, Hillinger S, Reckamp KL, Strieter RM, Dubinett SM, et al. Intrapulmonary administration of CCL21 gene-modified dendritic cells reduces tumor burden in spontaneous murine bronchoalveolar cell carcinoma. *Cancer Res* (2006) 66(6):3205–13. doi:10.1158/0008-5472.CAN-05-3619
67. Kuchen S, Robbins R, Sims GP, Sheng C, Phillips TM, Lipsky PE, et al. Essential role of IL-21 in B cell activation, expansion, and plasma cell generation during CD4 + T cell-B cell collaboration. *J Immunol* (2007) 179(9):5886–96. doi:10.4049/jimmunol.179.9.5886
68. Attridge K, Wang CJ, Wardzinski L, Kenefeck R, Chamberlain JL, Manzotti C, et al. IL-21 inhibits T cell IL-2 production and impairs treg homeostasis. *Blood* (2012) 119(20):4656–64. doi:10.1182/blood-2011-10-388546
69. Maldonado L, Teague JE, Morrow MP, Jotova I, Wu TC, Wang C, et al. Intramuscular therapeutic vaccination targeting HPV16 induces T cell responses that localize in mucosal lesions. *Sci Transl Med* (2014) 6(221):221ra13. doi:10.1126/scitranslmed.3007323
70. Lutz ER, Wu AA, Bigelow E, Sharma R, Mo G, Soares K, et al. Immunotherapy converts non-immunogenic pancreatic tumors into immunogenic foci of immune regulation. *Cancer Immunol Res* (2014) 2(7):616–31. doi:10.1158/2326-6066.CIR-14-0027

13

Ectopic Tertiary Lymphoid Tissue in Inflammatory Bowel Disease: Protective or Provocateur?

Eóin N. McNamee[1] and Jesús Rivera-Nieves[2]*

[1] *Mucosal Inflammation Program, Department of Anesthesiology, School of Medicine, University of Colorado – Anschutz Medical Campus, Aurora, CO, USA,* [2] *Division of Gastroenterology, Inflammatory Bowel Disease Center, San Diego VAMC, University of California San Diego, La Jolla, CA, USA*

Correspondence:
Eóin N. McNamee
eoin.mcnamee@ucdenver.edu

Organized lymphoid tissues like the thymus first appeared in jawed vertebrates around 500 million years ago and have evolved to equip the host with a network of specialized sites, strategically located to orchestrate strict immune-surveillance and efficient immune responses autonomously. The gut-associated lymphoid tissues maintain a mostly tolerant environment to dampen our responses to daily dietary and microbial products in the intestine. However, when this homeostasis is perturbed by chronic inflammation, the intestine is able to develop florid organized tertiary lymphoid tissues (TLT), which heralds the onset of regional immune dysregulation. While TLT are a pathologic hallmark of Crohn's disease (CD), their role in the overall process remains largely enigmatic. A critical question remains; are intestinal TLT generated by the immune infiltrated intestine to modulate immune responses and rebuild tolerance to the microbiota or are they playing a more sinister role by generating dysregulated responses that perpetuate disease? Herein, we discuss the main theories of intestinal TLT neogenesis and focus on the most recent findings that open new perspectives to their role in inflammatory bowel disease.

Keywords: tertiary lymphoid tissue, ectopic lymphoid follicle, Crohn's disease, inflammatory bowel disease

> Quis custodiet ipsos custodes
> "Who will guard the guardians?" from Juvenal (Satire VI, lines 347–8).

Intrinsic to the gastrointestinal tract, gut-associated lymphoid tissue (GALT) are the sentinels of the enteric immune system and guard the host from an ever-present microbial and antigenic assault. Cryptopatches (CP), isolated lymphoid follicles (ILF), Peyer patches (PP), and the chains of mesenteric lymph nodes (MLN) respond to microbial and immune signals, allowing for rapid remodeling during infection and disease. However, during periods where chronic inflammation persists in the setting of failed immunoregulation, such as in inflammatory bowel diseases (IBD), a dysfunctional lymphatic system and the development of ectopic tertiary lymphoid tissue (TLT) develop as a consistent pathological hallmark. Understanding the function of TLT and the myriad of cellular events leading to their development is becoming an area of intense clinical interest, as their

---

Abbreviations: AID, activation-induced deaminase; BALT, bronchus associated lymphoid tissue; CD, Crohn's disease; FDC, follicular dendritic cell; GALT, gut-associated lymphoid tissue; GC, germinal center; HEV, high endothelial venule; IBD, inflammatory bowel disease; ILC, innate lymphoid cell; ILF, isolated lymphoid follicle, SLO, secondary lymph node; LP, lamina propria; LTβR, lymphotoxin beta receptor; LTi, lymphoid tissue inducer cells; MLN, mesenteric lymph node; MMP, matrix metalloprotease; NOD1, nucleotide-binding oligomerization domain containing 1; RORγ, ROR-related orphan receptor gamma; SFB, segmented filamentous bacterium; Tfh, follicular helper T cells; TLT, tertiary lymphoid tissue; UC, ulcerative colitis.

role in pathophysiology remains enigmatic. A critical question remains unanswered; do TLT develop to protect the vulnerable, immune-compromised intestine or do they play a more sinister role in driving autoimmune processes and perpetuate disease?

GUT-ASSOCIATED LYMPHOID TISSUE: *GATEKEEPERS IN HOST DEFENSE*

The GALT is the largest collection of lymphoid tissues in the body, consisting of both organized lymphoid tissues (MLN and PP) and more diffusely scattered lymphocytes in the intestinal lamina propria (LP) and intraepithelial space. With the immunologic maturation of the intestine after birth, aggregates of organized leukocyte populations form CP and ILF and collectively with PP and MLN are a crucial interface between the host and commensal bacteria.

Prenatal GALT Neogenesis

During lymph node development in embryogenesis, a novel subset of $CD4^+$ $CD3^-$ cells, was identified to play a crucial initiating role (1). Now termed lymphoid tissue inducer (LTi) cells, these hematopoietic progenitors signal to mesenchymal cell subsets (stromal organizer cells) within the developing lymph node Anlagen [reviewed in Ref. (2)]. Initial signaling *via* stromal-derived LTβR with its ligand, lymphotoxin-$\alpha_1\beta_2$ ($LT\alpha_1\beta_2$) on LTi's, drives a cascade of chemokine and stromal markers, which recruit and organize immune cells into the developing lymphoid tissue (2). LTi are now identified as members of the innate lymphoid cells (ILC) [specifically type 3 ILC (ILC3)], which express the transcription factors, helix–loop–helix protein inhibitor of DNA binding 2 (ID2) and RAR-related orphan receptor gamma$^+$ ($ROR\gamma t^+$), in addition to the cytokines IL-22 and IL-17a.

Lymphoid tissue inducer cells (ILC3) play a particularly crucial role in development of GALT *in utero* [Reviewed in Ref. (3–5)]. For example, MLN develops at embryonic day E11.5, following colonization of the anlagen with $LT\alpha_1\beta_2^+$ LTi's and activation of lymphotoxin-β receptor-expressing (LTβR) stromal organizer cells (6, 7). The importance of this interaction is evident from early murine studies where mice deficient for both RORγt and LTβR lack MLN (4, 8). Interestingly, while distinct regulatory cytokine/chemokine circuits (such as IL-7, LTβ, CXCL13/CXCR5) control MLN function and organization, their absence does not interfere with MLN development (9–12). Of interest, recent work has demonstrated that while $LT\beta R^{-/-}$ mice fail to develop secondary lymph nodes (SLO), in the setting of excessive TNF production during intestinal inflammation, TNF-α (transgenic over-expression in $TNF^{\Delta ARE/+}$ mice) over-rides the canonical requirement for LTi cells and drives a lymphoid neogenesis program, including the induction of homeostatic chemokines (13). Thus, subtle differences may still remain between homeostasis and chronic inflammation for the ontogeny and regulation of MLN formation.

Peyer patches, which are scattered along the anti-mesenteric border of the small intestine, drain to the mesenteric lymphatic system *via* efferent lymphatic vessels and directly sample antigen from the gut lumen *via*, specialized microfold cells (M cells) (14, 15). The development of PP in the fetal intestine takes place later than MLN (E11.5) between E.15.5 and E18.5 and is also critically dependent on LTβR signaling and $CD11c^+$ dendritic cells (DC) (16, 17). This is most evident by the observation that mice deficient in LTα and LTβ, and as such for their membrane ligand $LT\alpha_1\beta_2$, lack mature PP (8, 9). Critically, LTβR ligation signals *via* the alternative NFκB pathway to induce CXCL13 and recruit LTi and $CXCR5^+$ B cells for PP maturation (6, 18). In addition, while TNF is not required for MLN ontogeny *in utero*, TNF and TNFRI (and signaling *via* classical NFκB pathway) are required for PP development (19, 20).

Postnatal GALT Neogenesis – Integrating Environmental and Commensal Stimuli

Aside from the developmental program of GALT organogenesis, the mammalian intestine adapts and responds to their postnatal colonization by enteric flora with the induction of CP and ILFs.

Cryptopatches are aggregates of approximately 1000 cells composed of LTi cells and chemokine producing dendritic (DC) and stromal cells found around the crypts of the small intestine (21, 22). In response to commensal bacterial stimuli, CP recruit B cells and CD4 T cells to develop into ILF and play a major regulatory role in the intestine by producing Immunoglobulin A (IgA) (23). ILFs are loosely organized clusters of B cells, DC, and T cells that resemble secondary lymphoid organs (SLO) in their cellular components (24, 25). A series of pioneering studies extended on this observation and demonstrated that CP and ILFs utilize similar pathways to SLO for development, following stimulation by a TNF-Lymphotoxin signaling axis (21–27). Expression of the chemokine receptor CCR6 by B cells is critical for expansion of ILFs. The CCR6 ligand, CCL20 is expressed by the epithelial cells that overlay the B cell follicles and its expression, is regulated by $LT\alpha_1\beta_2$ signaling (28).

Recent work has broadened our understanding for the role of ILFs, and a general consensus is that they act in a tolerogenic manner to control intestinal immune responses by generating both IgA^+ plasma cells and regulatory T cells (26, 29, 30). It is now apparent that intestinal ILF form a feedback loop with commensal bacteria, whereby there is reciprocal crosstalk. As an example, the induction of the NOD1 receptor (nucleotide-binding oligomerization domain containing 1) in intestinal epithelial cells by Gram-negative bacteria induces ILFs from CP precursors (31). Conversely and strikingly, in the absence of ILFs (following LTβR-IgG treatment), there is a 10-fold expansion of bacterial flora (31). It is not surprising then that ILFs have been tasked with building postnatal intestinal immune tolerance, *via* generation of IgA and Th17 responses (32). Of note however is that the chain of molecular events required for ectopic lymphoid tissue development under conditions of chronic inflammation and their role in the pathogenesis of CD are less clear.

INTESTINAL TERTIARY LYMPHOID TISSUE IN INFLAMMATORY BOWEL DISEASE

While SLO is developmentally controlled with fixed anatomic locations, chronic inflammation in peripheral tissues can give rise to the florid development of TLT neogenesis [reviewed in

Ref. (33)]. Unlike SLO, TLT do not possess a capsule and as such are not true organs *per se* but rather a highly organized cluster of immune cells, which develop regional segregation similar to SLO. While intestinal ILF are loosely organized clusters of B cells, T cells, and DCs, TLT are defined by the presence of densely packed and active germinal centers (GCs) often with mature follicular dendritic cell (FDC) networks (34). They are further defined by presenting with CD4$^+$ T cell and DC clusters in addition to a mature fibroblastic stromal network (e.g., VCAM1$^+$). TLT often develop around lymphatic vessels and a hallmark indication of mature TLT is the development of specialized high endothelial venules (HEV) within and around follicles (35, 36). As HEV facilitate recruitment of naive (CD62L$^+$) T cells into the T cell cortex of SLO (37), their presence in TLT has raised the possibility that TLT bypass the need for SLO by recruiting and educating naive T cells aberrantly in inflamed peripheral tissues.

The Inflammatory Bowel Diseases, Crohn's Disease, and Ulcerative Colitis

Inflammatory bowel diseases are a collective of chronic intestinal pathologies predominantly represented by Crohn's disease (CD) and ulcerative colitis (UC). There are fundamental differences between the two, being best characterized as immune-mediated rather than autoimmune, as up to date no single autoantibody has been identified. The etiology of IBD remains elusive but involves complex interactions between genetic, environmental, and immunoregulatory factors. Current hypotheses propose that damage to the intestinal mucosa occurs as a result of a dysregulated immune response triggered by microbial antigens (38, 39) that eventually becomes autonomous. The resulting increased leukocytic infiltrate within the intestinal mucosa release a cocktail of enzymes, reactive oxygen species, and cytokines initiating and perpetuating tissue damage and disease. Regarding tissue distribution, UC involves strictly the colon, while CD can involve any segment of the GI tract, from the mouth to the anus, but predominantly the immunologically rich terminal ileum in 2/3 of patients. UC is also a continuous superficial disease, involving predominantly the colonic mucosa, while CD is discontinuous and penetrating, involving all layers of the intestine from the mucosa to the serosa.

The prevailing histopathologic hallmarks of CD during its early investigation were occluded lymphatic vessels, lymphocytic lymphangitis, and inflammatory "T_H1" granulomas. Significantly, these cardinal signs of chronic disease were found in or around ectopic tertiary lymphoid follicles in the inflamed LP [(40–43); Reviewed in Ref. (44)]. Indeed, the presentation of TLT in patient biopsies appears to be a predominant feature of CD [in a recent study, TLT were present in 22 out of 24 patients assessed by immunohistochemistry (45)]. In addition, the presence of TLT at the base of aphthous ulcers is also the earliest endoscopically evident lesion in CD and their appearance heralds recurrent disease within the neoterminal ileum after ilectomy (46–48). In light of these findings, the functional relevance of intestinal TLT and their impact on the etiology and pathogenesis of CD has remained enigmatic, with limited empirical evidence as to their role.

A critical question that remains unanswered is the origin of TLT and whether they are generated *de novo* within the chronically inflamed intestine or predetermined. While the components of mature intestinal TLT include CD4$^+$ T cell clusters, follicular DC, HEV networks, and mature fibroblastic stroma clusters (VCAM1$^+$ ICAM1$^+$) (34), it is unclear whether they arise *de novo*, specifically during chronic inflammation. This question is also at the root of our understanding the functional role of TLT during chronic intestinal disease. While homeostatic ILFs represent a source of IgA to maintain tolerance to commensal bacteria, the transformation of ILF into mature TLT [as has been suggested (23)] could indicate a final detrimental step in the development of intestinal immune dysregulation and the loss of immune-tolerance. The anatomic location of both ILF and TLT within the normal and inflamed intestine may also shed light on their respective functions. While ILFs contain a dome of epithelia containing M cells, TLT are often present at sites of epithelial barrier loss (aphthous ulcers in CD) and around occluded lymphatic vessels in the LP (44, 45). In addition, as CD presents with transmural inflammatory infiltrates, TLT follicles may also be present in the deeper layers of the intestine including the muscle and surrounding mesenteric adipose tissue (e.g., "creeping fat" that encases inflamed intestine in a subset of patients with CD).

Elegant recent work has demonstrated that on a background of failed anti-microbial immunity ($ROR\gamma t^{-/-}$ mice; lacking ILC3 and T_H17 responses) combined with a loss of epithelial barrier function (DSS-colitis), mice develop an aggressive colitis in addition to florid TLT neogenesis (49). Antibiotic treatment reversed this pathology and TLT development confirming its dependence on a commensal microbial insult. However, it is worth noting that the phenotype of TLT that were generated in $ROR\gamma t^{-/-}$ mice contributed to systemic pathology, produced high levels of AID (to facilitate class-switch recombination), and were strikingly attenuated following intravenous immunoglobulin (IVIG) treatment (49). Our work and others has further demonstrated that in the $TNF^{\Delta ARE/+}$ mouse model of Crohn's-like ileitis [$TNF^{\Delta ARE/+}$; a transgenic mouse line with a 69-bp deletion of the 3′UTR for TNF, allowing for overexpression of TNF mRNA (50)], TLT develop during chronic disease and correspond with both a loss of immune tolerance and a prominent dysbiosis of commensal microflora (34, 51, 52). Thus, the presence of TLT during chronic intestinal inflammation clearly heralds a failure of organ-specific immune regulation and the establishment of dysregulated immunity. As such, distinct intestinal TLT may develop based upon the inflammatory environments [tolerogenic CP-ILF induction from commensal bacteria versus inflammation-induced TLT (CP independent); as has been previously postulated (5)].

POSSIBLE CLASSICAL AND NON-CLASSICAL CUES FOR INTESTINAL B CELL FOLLICLE DEVELOPMENT

A vast literature has demonstrated that the molecular cues and cellular machinery required for secondary lymph node development are also utilized for the generation of ectopic TLT during chronic inflammation. For example, Lymphotoxin-β receptor signaling on LTi cells ($LT\alpha_1\beta_2^+$ LTi and $LT\beta R^+$ stromal cells) remains a cardinal requirement for both the generation and organization of SLO. This was elegantly demonstrated by the lack of secondary lymph nodes in the LTα, LTβ, and LTβR-deficient mice (6, 9). In addition, antibody blockade of LTβR signaling *in vivo* dissociates ectopic TLT structures in a multitude of settings using preclinical mouse models of inflammatory diseases (49, 53–55).

However, there is also an ever-increasing body of work identifying novel immune pathways that can by-pass the classical sequence for tertiary lymphangiogenesis (depicted in **Figure 1**). While iILC subsets (to which lymphoid tissue inducer (LTi) cells belong to) are critical for mucosal immunity and for the development of lymph node Anlagen, some reports have identified LTi-redundant mechanisms for TLT development (13, 56, 57). This includes the development of small intestinal TLT driven by TNF-overproduction in the absence of LTi signals (13). TNF production from M_1-like macrophage also confers an LTi phenotype in stromal cells to generate TLT, independent of LTβR signaling (58). Conversely, in the absence of ILC3 and Th17 anti-microbial responses (*RORγt*$^{-/-}$) or *LTα*$^{-/-}$, mice develop florid TLT development during colonic inflammatory insults (49, 59). Thus, the cardinal role of the ILC3–Th17 axis in TLT function, during chronic intestinal inflammation and in the heterogeneous and anatomically distinct subsets of IBD, warrants further investigation (**Table 1**).

Innate and Adaptive Sources of IL-22

IL-22 is a member of the IL-10 cytokine family that is predominantly expressed by Th17, γδT cells, and ILC3 and plays a critical role in anti-microbial defense at mucosal surfaces (60, 61). Recent work has demonstrated a role for IL-22 in the control of both TLT development and function (62). In a viral-induced model of Sjögrens syndrome, delivery of adenovirus into the salivary glands induced development of TLT that was dependent on IL-22 production, initially from NK1.1⁺ and γδT cells, with expression during chronic disease predominated by classical αβT cells. The authors demonstrate that IL-22 maintained CXCL13

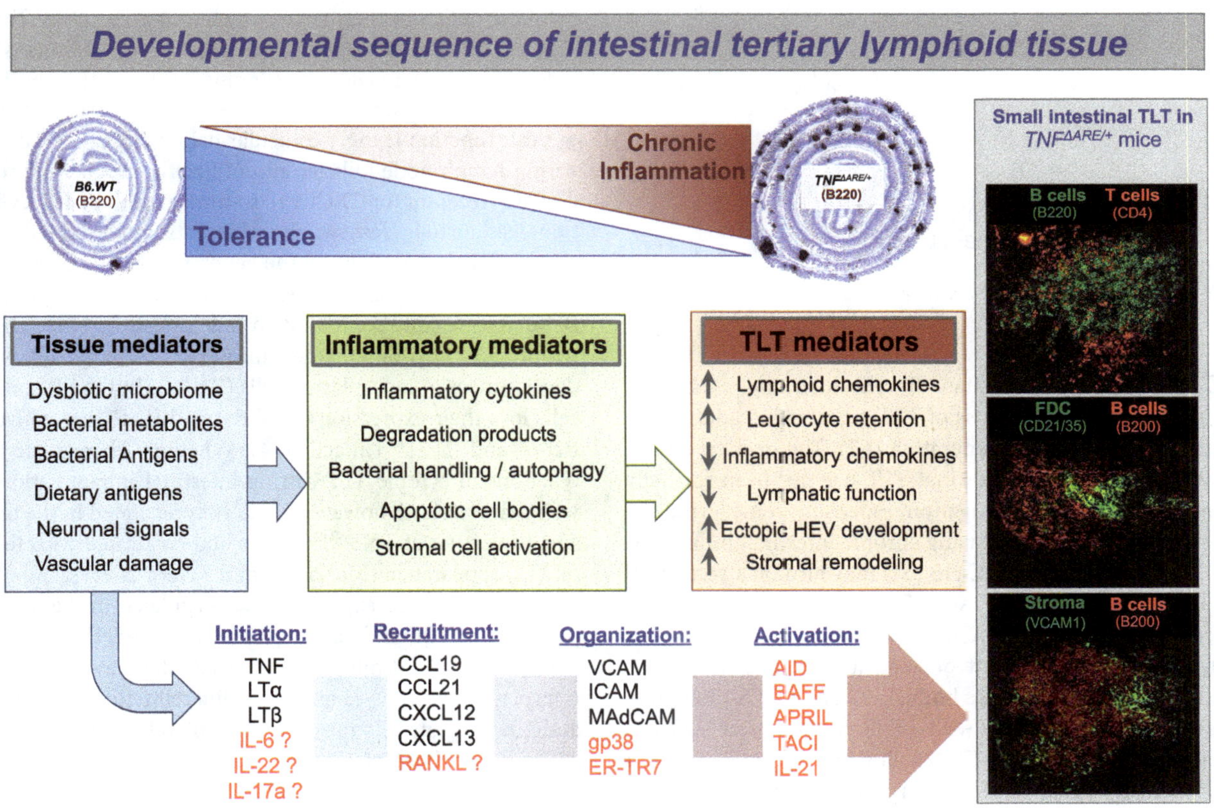

FIGURE 1 | Propose developmental sequence of intestinal tertiary lymphoid tissue. Presented here is a proposed sequence of small intestinal tertiary lymphoid tissue neogenesis in the setting of inflammatory bowel disease. On a background of failed immunoregulation and loss of intestinal tolerance, the florid development of ectopic tertiary lymphoid tissue follicles is a cardinal sign of both Crohn's disease and TNF-transgenic mice with ileitis (TNF$^{\Delta ARE/+}$). The plasticity of these ectopic lymphoid follicles is demonstrated by the observation that they resolve, for example, after removal of bacterial stimuli by antibiotic treatment or following anti-inflammatory interventions (34, 119). As the etiology of Crohn's disease is unknown and proposed to be a result of uncontrolled immune activation to intestinal bacteria in genetically susceptible individuals, we have proposed plausible options from the myriad of potential initiating and organizing signals. TLT development is sure to follow a loss of tissue integrity, chronic activation of inflammatory mediators, and stabilization of maturation events to maintain complex TLT architecture. BAFF, B cell activating factor; APRIL, a proliferation inducing ligand; TACI, TNFR homolog transmembrane activator and Ca^{2+} modulator and CAML interactor [APRIL and BAFF receptor]; ER-TR7, anti-reticular fibroblasts and reticular fibroblast marker; gp38, podoplanin; RANKL, receptor activator of nuclear factor kappa-B ligand/TNFSF11.

TABLE 1 | Incidence of tertiary lymphoid tissue development in human and mouse intestine.

Condition/model	Location	Lymphoid component(s)	Reference
Human			
Helicobacter Pylori	Stomach	B/T cells, HEV, CXCL13	(120, 121)
Crohn's disease	Ileum/ Colon	B/T cells, lymphoid follicular inflammation	(44–46, 122)
Ilectomy (Crohn's disease)	Terminal ileum	Aphthous ulcers, ulcers >8mm, fibrotic strictures rare	(48)
Colorectal carcinoma	Colon	B/T cells, FDC, CXCL13, CCL19, CCL21	(123, 124)
Mice			
Disease model			
Autoimmune gastritis	Stomach	B/T cells, CXCL13, FDC, autoantibodies	(125, 126)
Helicobacter Pylori	Stomach	B/T cells, FDC, GC, CXCR5, CXCL13	(127–129)
TNF-transgenic (*TNF*$^{\Delta ARE}$)	Ileum	B/T cells, FDC, GC CCL19, CCL21, CXCL13	(13, 34)
Prion disease ($LT\alpha^{-/-}/LT\beta^{-/-}$)	Small intestine	B cells, FDC, CR1/CR2	(130)
DSS-colitis ($ROR\gamma t^{-/-}$)	Colon	B/T cells, Th1, autoantibodies, LTBR-dependent	(49)
DSS-colitis ($LT\alpha^{-/-}$)	Colon	B/T cells, CD8	(59)
Anti-LTβR *in utero*	Small intestine	B/T cells, GC, IgA, Th17	(25, 32, 59)
Genetic model			
$CCR7^{-/-}$	Stomach	B/T cells, FDC, CCL21, CXCL13	(131)
$AID^{-/-}$	Small intestine	B/T cells, FDC, hyper IgM	(132)
$CnAalpha^{+/-}$	Small intestine	B/T cells, CD11b, TFG-β, IFNγ	(133)
$IL\text{-}25^{-/-}$	Small intestine	B cells, CD11b, CD11c	(134)
CXCL13-transgenic	Ileum	LTi, IL-22, LTα, LTβ, CXCL13	(65)

and CXCL12 levels to facilitate B cell clustering. Strikingly, IL-22 blockade resulted in loss of TLT structure in addition to anti-nuclear autoantibody generation (62). The involvement of IL-22 in the function of intestinal TLT has not been formally assessed, but warrants investigation, especially considering the major role played by IL-22 during chronic intestinal inflammation (63, 64). The IL-22–CXCL13 axis may also be a reciprocal one, as over-expression of CXCL13 in the intestine facilitates the recruitment of IL-22⁺ ILCs, B cell clustering, and the generation of ILFs, independent of aberrant inflammation (65). A governing signal that drives both IL-22 and CXCL13 expression is integrated by LTβR, with LTβR initiating an ILC-DC cross talk *via* IL-23 to induce IL-22 following intestinal infection with *Citrobacter rodentium* (66). Surprisingly however, recombinant IL-22 administration can restore TLT formation in the colon of LTβR-deficient mice, suggesting that IL-22 can directly and independently impact TLT organization during intestinal infection (67).

ILC- and Th17-Derived IL-17a

Other members of the Th17 family, most notably IL-17a, have been implicated in the development of bronchus associated lymphoid tissues (BALT) during lung infections and in a mouse model of Multiple sclerosis (EAE) (68–70). Following infection with *P. aeruginosa*, mice develop extensive BALT formation, which is dependent on IL-17a-driven CXCL12 from the lung stroma (69). In a second study, Rangel-Moreno and colleagues demonstrated that neonatal mice developed BALT following repeated administration of bacterial lipopolysaccharide (LPS), initiated by IL-17-induced CXCL13. Of note, the generation of CXCL13 was also independent of LTβR in this study (68). As the small intestine is the physiologic site for Th17 generation (71, 72), targeted interruption of this cytokine family may reveal a critical role in intestinal TLT function. In line with this, one recent study has demonstrated that segmented filamentous bacteria (SFB) stimulated the postnatal development of ILF and TLT, which substituted for PP as inductive sites for intestinal IgA and SFB-specific T helper 17 (Th17) cell responses (32). How this integrates with chronic intestinal inflammation and the impact of SFB-induced IgA and Th17 from PP and ILF structures during intestinal disease remain to be clarified.

T Follicular Helper Cells and IL-21

Upon antigen stimulation, naive $CD4^+$ helper T cells differentiate into effector subsets with distinctive functions based on the cytokine milieu of their environment (e.g., Th1, Th2, Th17, and T_{reg}). A critical function of helper $CD4^+$ T cells subsets is to provide stimulatory signals to developing B cells for the generation of appropriate antibody responses. The cardinal $CD4^+$ T cell to carry out this function is the T follicular helper cell (Tfh). Tfh localize within lymph node follicles and utilize the chemokine receptor, CXCR5 (receptor for CXCL13) to stimulate and instruct GC reactions leading to Ig class switch and somatic mutation. Tfh perform much of their functions by the generation of the cytokines IL-6 and IL-21 and under the instruction of the transcription factor Bcl-6. An elegant recent study has demonstrated that Th17 cells within PP trans-differentiate into IL-21⁺ Tfh to aid with the development of IgA^+ plasma cells (73, 74). In the PP, some T_H17 cells lose their expression of RORγt and IL-17 and convert into Bcl-6⁺ and IL-21⁺ Tfh cells (74). Whether Tfh regulate the GC reactions in ectopic TLT during intestinal inflammation is not well characterized; however, IL-21 is upregulated in the inflamed small intestine of $TNF^{\Delta ARE/+}$ mice and correlated with the onset of TLT appearance (McNamee and Rivera-Nieves, unpublished observation). IL-21 expression is upregulated in the intestine of patients with IBD and downregulated in anti-TNF responsive CD patients (75, 76). While most current studies have focused on the interplay between IL-21 and Th17 differentiation (77), how IL-21 and Tfh integrate into the organization and function of intestinal TLT have not been assessed.

Regulatory T Cells

Foxp3⁺ $CD4^+$ regulatory T cells (T_{reg}) have a unique ability to repress chronic inflammation and are critical for the generation and maintenance of intestinal tolerance and prevention of autoimmunity (78–81). They mediate their suppressive effects by intimately controlling DC activation and by repressing effector T cell proliferation (79, 80, 82). Of note, failed immunoregulation and loss of T_{reg} function is a hallmark of both human IBD and preclinical models (83–85). The first study to demonstrate a link between TLT development and T_{reg} function utilized *CCR7*$^{-/-}$ mice. CCR7 expression is generally high on CD4$^+$ Foxp3$^+$ T_{reg}'s and CD103$^+$ regulatory DC. *CCR7*$^{-/-}$ mice have a global loss of these two cell types and inability to control overt inflammation (51). Strikingly, neonatal *CCR7*$^{-/-}$ mice developed BALT without the addition of an extrinsic inflammatory stimulus (86, 87). Importantly, the authors inhibited ectopic BALT follicle development with the adoptive transfer of functional T_{reg} from wild-type mice (87). Thus, the inability of T_{reg} to control chronic intestinal inflammation may facilitate the development and function of TLT during IBD (83–85); however, this has yet to be formally investigated experimentally.

Follicular Dendritic Cells

In the setting of either IBD or in preclinical models that present with TLT, it has not yet been delineated if lymphoid chemokines from stromal "organizer" cells precede the development of intestinal TLT, or if their activation is dependent on the influx of TNF$^+$ and $LT\alpha_1\beta_2^+$ leukocytes. This question is of clinical interest as current biologic interventions in IBD are predominantly aimed at depleting lymphocytes, and their affects on stromal compartment in maintaining chronic tissue inflammation are poorly understood. One such cell subset that is critical for active SLO and mature TLT organization, yet understudied, is the FDC. FDC are highly specialized stromal cells, derived from pericytes, arising within active SLO GCs and chronically inflamed tissues to organize TLT (88, 89). FDC form a reticular scaffold for B cells to generate and maintain GC reactions. They possess a unique recycling mechanism to protect captured antigen from degradation and retain it for long-term presentation to B cells with antibody complexes or on complement receptors CR1 and CR2(90). In addition, FDC express CXCL13 and BAFF, which are essential for the recruitment and survival of CXCR5$^+$ B cells in GC follicles (91). TLTs require chronic antigenic stimulation for their maintenance and the tonic supply of lymphoid chemokines to conserve their structure. FDCs can perform both of these functions (*via* CR1/CR2 and CXCL13), and their appearance within intestinal TLT heralds the onset of chronic disease and lack of tolerance; however, their source and function during IBD is unknown and warrants investigation. An intriguing question remains whether intestinal FDC can maintain tonic IgA or IgG production from their neighboring B cells.

INTESTINAL TLT IN IBD AND EXTRAINTESTINAL DISEASE

Are Intestinal B Cells Contributing to Immune Dysregulation *via* Generation of Autoreactive or Microflora-Reactive Antibodies?

The classical definition of IBDs (and in particular CD) is that they are "immune-mediated" conditions, triggered by a dysregulated host immune response to commensal microbiome in genetically susceptible individuals and perpetuated by an autonomous or independent dysregulated immune response, which might then become independent of bacterial stimuli. While auto-reactive effector CD4$^+$ helper T cell subsets drive a dysregulated immune pathology in CD, neither CD nor UC fall into the category of being classical "autoimmune" conditions, as a pathologic autoantibody has not been identified. However, there is a clear precedent for dysregulated B cells responses in IBD subsets and serological evidence for autoantibodies being generated (92). For example, anti-neutrophil antibodies (ANCA and p-ANCA) are present in patients with UC (60–80%) and to a lesser extent, CD (5–25%) (93–95). Increased concentrations IgG and IgA antibodies to *Saccharomyces cerevisiae* (ASCAs) (brewer's yeast) are found in 60–70% of patients with CD (96), while IgG antibodies against the *Escherichia coli* outer membrane porin (OmpC) is identified in 55% of CD patients (97). IgG antibodies to the flagellin CBir1 is associated with small-bowel, internal-penetrating, and fibrostenotic disease, and defines a subgroup of CD patients not previously recognized by other serologic responses (92, 98).

Of note, there is now evidence that the magnitude of immune response to different microbial antigens (ASCA and OmpC) in patients with CD is associated with the severity of the disease course (fibrostenosis, internal perforating disease, and the need for small-bowel surgery) (99). Thus, a loss of immune tolerance and generation of autoreactive B cell responses are clear clinical features of CD. Whether this process takes place within the intestinal (and TLT follicles) or is a peripheral response (e.g., spleen and bone marrow) is yet to be determined.

Are Intestinal TLT a Mucosal Source for the Generation of Extraintestinal Disease during IBD?

A clinical hallmark of IBD is the development of extraintestinal manifestations during its disease course. These include inflammation of the joints, skin, eyes, and hepatobiliary tract, which are the most usually affected sites (100). An interesting observation is that TLT are a predominant feature of CD pathologies, and patients with CD are more likely than UC patients to have immune-mediated (arthritis, eye, skin, and liver) extraintestinal manifestations: 20.1% CD versus 10.4% UC, with arthropathy significantly more common in CD (12.9%) (100). Of note, altered intestinal bacterial diversity and dissemination of specific species have been postulated as a mucosal origin for arthritis (101–104). In addition, in a TNF-transgenic model of small intestinal CD and polyarthritis (TNF$^{\Delta ARE}$), the temporal onset of arthritis correlates with microbial dysbiosis and the development of intestinal TLT (34, 50, 52). Thus there is precedent that intestinal TLT may aberrantly develop antibodies on a background of failed immunoregulation and thus integrate into a mechanism of systemic immune dysregulation.

WHAT ARE THE ANTIGENIC STIMULI DRIVING THE DEVELOPMENT OF INTESTINAL B CELL FOLLICLES IN TLT?

There are several mechanisms that may underlie the increased numbers of ectopic B-cell follicles in the intestine of patients with IBD. This may be the result of non-specific polyclonal proliferation of B-cells, responding to the local production of B-cell activating factors such as cytokines (IL-6, IL-21, LTβ, and TNFα) in the inflamed gut. Alternatively and more likely, follicular B-cells within intestinal TLT may indicate a specific humoral immune reaction. There remains limited data on the (oligo) clonality of B cells from IBD patients during active disease or in preclinical models to address this. In addition, it is presently unclear against which antigen(s) are intestinal B-cells proliferating. Presumably both microbial and auto-antigens [including degradation products from extracellular matrix (ECM)] should be considered in the setting of TLT during intestinal immune dysregulation (see **Figure 1**).

Intestinal Dysbiosis and Chronic Bacterial Infection

The increase in lymphocytes in the intestine during IBD and their organization into ectopic B cell lymphoid follicles are consistent with an orchestrated adaptive immune response, which is believed to develop in relation to chronic microbial colonization. Several observations favor this hypothesis, including a temporal correlation between the development of small intestinal TLT and a marked dysbiosis of the commensal microbiome (34, 52, 59) (see **Figure 1**). Alterations of the commensal flora are now considered a feature of human IBD, and our understanding of the profound effects that has on intestinal immune homeostasis is rudimentary [reviewed in Ref. (105)]. Patients with IBD respond favorably to antibiotics and fecal diversion, and have greater antibody titers against indigenous bacteria than unaffected individuals (105, 106). Inflammatory lesions are more pronounced in areas of the intestine that contain the greatest number of bacteria. The data in animal models provide further evidence for the involvement of gut bacteria in IBD. Pre-treatment with antibiotics has been shown to alleviate intestinal inflammation in several animal models (107).

Extracellular Matrix Products and Molecular Mimicry

A specific immune response against self-antigens present in intestinal tissue could also be the initiating trigger for ectopic TLT generation. In the intestine of patients with IBD, there is a chronic inflammatory response present with the active recruitment of inflammatory cells and concomitant tissue damage. A resulting immune response can then be directed against intestinal matrix proteins, which can be recognized as neo-antigens. The ECM, composed of proteoglycans (including hyaluronan), collagens, elastin, and non-collagenous glycoproteins in turn both regulates and adapts to this inflammatory milieu. In fact, accumulation of ECM products has been shown to activate and recruit immune cells like T cells and monocytes during IBD (108). Proteolytic degradation of ECM components is a pathognomonic feature of a multitude of inflammatory and degenerative diseases [reviewed in Ref. (109)] and is mainly under the control of specific disintegrins and metalloproteinases (110). In addition, products of infectious agents, e.g., heat shock proteins and enzymes responsible for citrullination, have been shown in several models to induce immune reactivity. For example, several citrullinated autoantigens can be identified in tests for anti-citrullinated peptide antibodies (ACPA; Anti-cyclic Citrullinated Peptide; Anti-CCP), keratin, fibrinogen, fibronectin (FN), collagen, and vimentin from patients with arthritis (111, 112). It is plausible that infiltrating B cells, attracted by the TLT chemokine gradients, are educated against "self" proteins/immune complexes and start producing antibodies against the ECM degradation products. This has been demonstrated in both the joints of patients wit arthritis and in the lungs of patients with emphysema (both sites for TLT development) (112–114).

SUMMARY

It has been estimated that the intestine-associated GALT constitute approximately 50% of our immune cells and both the prenatally defined MLN and PP along with the postnatal induced CP and ILF maintain a remarkably tolerant environment. A staggering reality of IBDs is that the control of the collective regional immune system fails with dire consequences for the host. The florid appearance of TLT within the chronically inflamed intestine may indicate an attempt to support the failed immunoregulatory pathways and restore control of dysregulated inflammation. There remains a dearth of knowledge on the biological role played by TLT utilizing chronic models of IBD in addition to limited human data. Understanding how TLT integrate into the pathophysiology of IBD remains a critical question in our understanding of intestinal immunity.

FUTURE DIRECTIONS AND KNOWLEDGE GAPS

Since its discovery in 1932, the earliest histopathologic features of CD have included the extensive TLT formation within the inflamed mucosa. However, over 80 years later, our understanding of the role(s) of intestinal TLT in CD remains elusive and a crucial need for empirical evidence as to their function remains. The most pertinent question remains as to whether TLT are driving dysregulated immune pathology (e.g., autoantibodies or naive T cell education) or whether they trigger exuberant immune responses at sites of bacterial invasion or neo-antigen exposure (e.g., generation of IgA). Recent work has started to investigate similar questions in the setting of mesenteric fat-associated tertiary lymphoid follicles and has elegantly demonstrated for the first time somatic hypermutation and IgG generation *in situ* within TLT (115). Surprisingly, an exhaustive cellular profile of TLTs in human CD tissues has not been performed. As such, basic questions as to the cellular make up and as such, immune profile of TLT during active inflammation in CD is limited (e.g., do they produce IgA or IgG?). In addition, how TLT respond to current therapeutic interventions during CD is limited, and hampered by the inability to assess their presence or response to treatments *via* endoscopic or histologic means (e.g., with limited tissue from pinch biopsies).

A therapeutic gap also remains for the site-directed targeting of TLT structures while sparing lymph node physiology and the ability to rapidly respond to infections (e.g., either to selectively induce intestinal ILF to increase IgA and antimicrobial defense or to deplete ectopic TLT in situations where they generate autoantibodies and aberrantly activate naive T cells). For example, while a plethora of studies have utilized Lymphotoxin-β receptor blockade to disaggregate mature TLTs, few report on the subsequent impact on disease pathology. In addition, while LTβR inhibition will inhibit clustering of TLT in almost all preclinical models of disease, it has profound effects on lymph node and splenic architecture, e.g., loss of marginal zone macrophage and B cells (116), disruption of GCs, HEV repression (117), and altered DC ratios (118). While these experiments serve as proof-of-principle studies, the site-directed delivery of therapeutics that target TLT function may prove a more viable modality for the treatment of chronic inflammatory diseases, with limited effects on systemic anti-microbial immunity.

An improved understanding of TLT development and function will shed light on critical questions pertaining to intestinal immunity and host defense, and future detailed investigations into the functional role of TLT in intestinal immune dysregulation are sure to expand our understanding of the pathogenesis of CD.

AUTHOR CONTRIBUTIONS

EM and JR-N decided on the emphasis and outlined the article. EM wrote the main body of the piece. JR-N edited the piece.

FUNDING

EN is supported by grants from the Crohn's and Colitis foundation of America (#2570174, #162444). JR-N is supported by grants from the National Institutes of Health (DK108670) and BLRD VA Merit Review award (1I01BX001051).

REFERENCES

1. Mebius RE, Rennert P, Weissman IL. Developing lymph nodes collect CD4+CD3- LTbeta+ cells that can differentiate to APC, NK cells, and follicular cells but not T or B cells. *Immunity* (1997) 7:493–504. doi:10.1016/S1074-7613(00)80371-4
2. van de Pavert SA, Mebius RE. New insights into the development of lymphoid tissues. *Nat Rev Immunol* (2010) 10:664–74. doi:10.1038/nri2832
3. Mebius RE. Organogenesis of lymphoid tissues. *Nat Rev Immunol* (2003) 3:292–303. doi:10.1038/nri1054
4. Eberl G, Marmon S, Sunshine MJ, Rennert PD, Choi Y, Littman DR. An essential function for the nuclear receptor RORgamma(t) in the generation of fetal lymphoid tissue inducer cells. *Nat Immunol* (2004) 5:64–73. doi:10.1038/ni1022
5. Eberl G, Lochner M. The development of intestinal lymphoid tissues at the interface of self and microbiota. *Mucosal Immunol* (2009) 2:478–85. doi:10.1038/mi.2009.114
6. Rennert PD, James D, Mackay F, Browning JL, Hochman PS. Lymph node genesis is induced by signaling through the lymphotoxin beta receptor. *Immunity* (1998) 9:71–9. doi:10.1016/S1074-7613(00)80589-0
7. Mebius RE, Streeter PR, Michie S, Butcher EC, Weissman IL. A developmental switch in lymphocyte homing receptor and endothelial vascular addressin expression regulates lymphocyte homing and permits CD4+ CD3- cells to colonize lymph nodes. *Proc Natl Acad Sci U S A* (1996) 93:11019–24. doi:10.1073/pnas.93.20.11019
8. De Togni P, Goellner J, Ruddle NH, Streeter PR, Fick A, Mariathasan S, et al. Abnormal development of peripheral lymphoid organs in mice deficient in lymphotoxin. *Science* (1994) 264:703–7. doi:10.1126/science.8171322
9. Koni PA, Sacca R, Lawton P, Browning JL, Ruddle NH, Flavell RA. Distinct roles in lymphoid organogenesis for lymphotoxins alpha and beta revealed in lymphotoxin beta-deficient mice. *Immunity* (1997) 6:491–500. doi:10.1016/S1074-7613(00)80292-7
10. Ansel KM, Ngo VN, Hyman PL, Luther SA, Forster R, Sedgwick JD, et al. A chemokine-driven positive feedback loop organizes lymphoid follicles. *Nature* (2000) 406:309–14. doi:10.1038/35018581
11. Forster R, Mattis AE, Kremmer E, Wolf E, Brem G, Lipp M. A putative chemokine receptor, BLR1, directs B cell migration to defined lymphoid organs and specific anatomic compartments of the spleen. *Cell* (1996) 87:1037–47. doi:10.1016/S0092-8674(00)81798-5
12. Cao X, Shores EW, Hu-Li J, Anver MR, Kelsall BL, Russell SM, et al. Defective lymphoid development in mice lacking expression of the common cytokine receptor gamma chain. *Immunity* (1995) 2:223–38. doi:10.1016/1074-7613(95)90047-0
13. Furtado GC, Pacer ME, Bongers G, Benezech C, He Z, Chen L, et al. TNFalpha-dependent development of lymphoid tissue in the absence of RORgammat(+) lymphoid tissue inducer cells. *Mucosal Immunol* (2014) 7:602–14. doi:10.1038/mi.2013.79
14. Schuurman HJ, Kuper CF, Vos JG. Histopathology of the immune system as a tool to assess immunotoxicity. *Toxicology* (1994) 86:187–212. doi:10.1016/0300-483X(94)90004-3
15. Gebert A, Rothkotter HJ, Pabst R. M cells in Peyer's patches of the intestine. *Int Rev Cytol* (1996) 167:91–159. doi:10.1016/S0074-7696(08)61346-7
16. Adachi S, Yoshida H, Kataoka H, Nishikawa S. Three distinctive steps in Peyer's patch formation of murine embryo. *Int Immunol* (1997) 9:507–14. doi:10.1093/intimm/9.4.507
17. Veiga-Fernandes H, Coles MC, Foster KE, Patel A, Williams A, Natarajan D, et al. Tyrosine kinase receptor RET is a key regulator of Peyer's patch organogenesis. *Nature* (2007) 446:547–51. doi:10.1038/nature05597
18. Dejardin E, Droin NM, Delhase M, Haas E, Cao Y, Makris C, et al. The lymphotoxin-beta receptor induces different patterns of gene expression via two NF-kappaB pathways. *Immunity* (2002) 17:525–35. doi:10.1016/S1074-7613(02)00423-5
19. Machleidt T, Kramer B, Adam D, Neumann B, Schutze S, Wiegmann K, et al. Function of the p55 tumor necrosis factor receptor "death domain" mediated by phosphatidylcholine-specific phospholipase C. *J Exp Med* (1996) 184:725–33. doi:10.1084/jem.184.2.725
20. Neumann B, Luz A, Pfeffer K, Holzmann B. Defective Peyer's patch organogenesis in mice lacking the 55-kD receptor for tumor necrosis factor. *J Exp Med* (1996) 184:259–64. doi:10.1084/jem.184.1.259
21. Kanamori Y, Ishimaru K, Nanno M, Maki K, Ikuta K, Nariuchi H, et al. Identification of novel lymphoid tissues in murine intestinal mucosa where clusters of c-kit+ IL-7R+ Thy1+ lympho-hemopoietic progenitors develop. *J Exp Med* (1996) 184:1449–59. doi:10.1084/jem.184.4.1449
22. Pabst O, Herbrand H, Friedrichsen M, Velaga S, Dorsch M, Berhardt G, et al. Adaptation of solitary intestinal lymphoid tissue in response to microbiota and chemokine receptor CCR7 signaling. *J Immunol* (2006) 177:6824–32. doi:10.4049/jimmunol.177.10.6824
23. Lorenz RG, Newberry RD. Isolated lymphoid follicles can function as sites for induction of mucosal immune responses. *Ann N Y Acad Sci* (2004) 1029:44–57. doi:10.1196/annals.1309.006
24. Hamada H, Hiroi T, Nishiyama Y, Takahashi H, Masunaga Y, Hachimura S, et al. Identification of multiple isolated lymphoid follicles on the antimesenteric wall of the mouse small intestine. *J Immunol* (2002) 168:57–64. doi:10.4049/jimmunol.168.1.57
25. Lorenz RG, Chaplin DD, McDonald KG, McDonough JS, Newberry RD. Isolated lymphoid follicle formation is inducible and dependent upon lymphotoxin-sufficient B lymphocytes, lymphotoxin beta receptor, and TNF receptor I function. *J Immunol* (2003) 170:5475–82. doi:10.4049/jimmunol.170.11.5475
26. Pearson C, Uhlig HH, Powrie F. Lymphoid microenvironments and innate lymphoid cells in the gut. *Trends Immunol* (2012) 33:289–96. doi:10.1016/j.it.2012.04.004
27. Taylor RT, Lugering A, Newell KA, Williams IR. Intestinal cryptopatch formation in mice requires lymphotoxin alpha and the lymphotoxin beta receptor. *J Immunol* (2004) 173:7183–9. doi:10.4049/jimmunol.173.12.7183

28. McDonald KG, McDonough JS, Wang C, Kucharzik T, Williams IR, Newberry RD. CC chemokine receptor 6 expression by B lymphocytes is essential for the development of isolated lymphoid follicles. *Am J Pathol* (2007) 170:1229–40. doi:10.2353/ajpath.2007.060817
29. Tsuji M, Suzuki K, Kitamura H, Maruya M, Kinoshita K, Ivanov II, et al. Requirement for lymphoid tissue-inducer cells in isolated follicle formation and T cell-independent immunoglobulin A generation in the gut. *Immunity* (2008) 29:261–71. doi:10.1016/j.immuni.2008.05.014
30. Wang C, McDonald KG, McDonough JS, Newberry RD. Murine isolated lymphoid follicles contain follicular B lymphocytes with a mucosal phenotype. *Am J Physiol Gastrointest Liver Physiol* (2006) 291:G595–604. doi:10.1152/ajpgi.00525.2005
31. Bouskra D, Brezillon C, Berard M, Werts C, Varona R, Boneca IG, et al. Lymphoid tissue genesis induced by commensals through NOD1 regulates intestinal homeostasis. *Nature* (2008) 456:507–10. doi:10.1038/nature07450
32. Lecuyer E, Rakotobe S, Lengline-Garnier H, Lebreton C, Picard M, Juste C, et al. Segmented filamentous bacterium uses secondary and tertiary lymphoid tissues to induce gut IgA and specific T helper 17 cell responses. *Immunity* (2014) 40:608–20. doi:10.1016/j.immuni.2014.03.009
33. Drayton DL, Liao S, Mounzer RH, Ruddle NH. Lymphoid organ development: from ontogeny to neogenesis. *Nat Immunol* (2006) 7:344–53. doi:10.1038/ni1330
34. McNamee EN, Masterson JC, Jedlicka P, Collins CB, Williams IR, Rivera-Nieves J. Ectopic lymphoid tissue alters the chemokine gradient, increases lymphocyte retention and exacerbates murine ileitis. *Gut* (2013) 62:53–62. doi:10.1136/gutjnl-2011-301272
35. Kratz A, Campos-Neto A, Hanson MS, Ruddle NH. Chronic inflammation caused by lymphotoxin is lymphoid neogenesis. *J Exp Med* (1996) 183:1461–72. doi:10.1084/jem.183.4.1461
36. Drayton DL, Ying X, Lee J, Lesslauer W, Ruddle NH. Ectopic LT alpha beta directs lymphoid organ neogenesis with concomitant expression of peripheral node addressin and a HEV-restricted sulfotransferase. *J Exp Med* (2003) 197:1153–63. doi:10.1084/jem.20021761
37. Bistrup A, Tsay D, Shenoy P, Singer MS, Bangia N, Luther SA, et al. Detection of a sulfotransferase (HEC-GlcNAc6ST) in high endothelial venules of lymph nodes and in high endothelial venule-like vessels within ectopic lymphoid aggregates: relationship to the MECA-79 epitope. *Am J Pathol* (2004) 164:1635–44. doi:10.1016/S0002-9440(10)63722-4
38. Fiocchi C. Inflammatory bowel disease: etiology and pathogenesis. *Gastroenterology* (1998) 115:182–205. doi:10.1016/S0016-5085(98)70381-6
39. Nagler-Anderson C. Man the barrier! Strategic defences in the intestinal mucosa. *Nat Rev Immunol* (2001) 1:59–67. doi:10.1038/35095573
40. Von Der Weid PY, Rehal S. Lymphatic pump function in the inflamed gut. *Ann N Y Acad Sci* (2010) 1207(Suppl 1):E69–74. doi:10.1111/j.1749-6632.2010.05715.x
41. Rahier JF, De Beauce S, Dubuquoy L, Erdual E, Colombel JF, Jouret-Mourin A, et al. Increased lymphatic vessel density and lymphangiogenesis in inflammatory bowel disease. *Aliment Pharmacol Ther* (2011) 34:533–43. doi:10.1111/j.1365-2036.2011.04759.x
42. D'Alessio S, Tacconi C, Fiocchi C, Danese S. Advances in therapeutic interventions targeting the vascular and lymphatic endothelium in inflammatory bowel disease. *Curr Opin Gastroenterol* (2013) 29:608–13. doi:10.1097/MOG.0b013e328365d37c
43. von der Weid PY, Rehal S, Ferraz JG. Role of the lymphatic system in the pathogenesis of Crohn's disease. *Curr Opin Gastroenterol* (2011) 27:335–41. doi:10.1097/MOG.0b013e3283476e8f
44. Van Kruiningen HJ, Colombel JF. The forgotten role of lymphangitis in Crohn's disease. *Gut* (2008) 57:1–4. doi:10.1136/gut.2007.123166
45. Sura R, Colombel JF, Van Kruiningen HJ. Lymphatics, tertiary lymphoid organs and the granulomas of Crohn's disease: an immunohistochemical study. *Aliment Pharmacol Ther* (2011) 33:930–9. doi:10.1111/j.1365-2036.2011.04605.x
46. Fujimura Y, Kamoi R, Iida M. Pathogenesis of aphthoid ulcers in Crohn's disease: correlative findings by magnifying colonoscopy, electron microscopy, and immunohistochemistry. *Gut* (1996) 38:724–32. doi:10.1136/gut.38.5.724
47. Rutgeerts P, Geboes K, Vantrappen G, Kerremans R, Coenegrachts JL, Coremans G. Natural history of recurrent Crohn's disease at the ileocolonic anastomosis after curative surgery. *Gut* (1984) 25:665–72. doi:10.1136/gut.25.6.665
48. Olaison G, Smedh K, Sjodahl R. Natural course of Crohn's disease after ileocolic resection: endoscopically visualised ileal ulcers preceding symptoms. *Gut* (1992) 33:331–5. doi:10.1136/gut.33.3.331
49. Lochner M, Ohnmacht C, Presley L, Bruhns P, Si-Tahar M, Sawa S, et al. Microbiota-induced tertiary lymphoid tissues aggravate inflammatory disease in the absence of RORgamma t and LTi cells. *J Exp Med* (2011) 208:125–34. doi:10.1084/jem.20100052
50. Kontoyiannis D, Pasparakis M, Pizarro TT, Cominelli F, Kollias G. Impaired on/off regulation of TNF biosynthesis in mice lacking TNF AU-rich elements: implications for joint and gut-associated immunopathologies. *Immunity* (1999) 10:387–98. doi:10.1016/S1074-7613(00)80038-2
51. McNamee EN, Masterson JC, Veny M, Collins CB, Jedlicka P, Byrne FR, et al. Chemokine receptor CCR7 regulates the intestinal TH1/TH17/Treg balance during Crohn's-like murine ileitis. *J Leukoc Biol* (2015) 97:1011–22. doi:10.1189/jlb.3HI0614-303R
52. Schaubeck M, Clavel T, Calasan J, Lagkouvardos I, Haange SB, Jehmlich N, et al. Dysbiotic gut microbiota causes transmissible Crohn's disease-like ileitis independent of failure in antimicrobial defence. *Gut* (2016) 65:225–37. doi:10.1136/gutjnl-2015-309333
53. Gatumu MK, Skarstein K, Papandile A, Browning JL, Fava RA, Bolstad AI. Blockade of lymphotoxin-beta receptor signaling reduces aspects of Sjogren's syndrome in salivary glands of non-obese diabetic mice. *Arthritis Res Ther* (2009) 11:R24. doi:10.1186/ar2617
54. Fava RA, Kennedy SM, Wood SG, Bolstad AI, Bienkowska J, Papandile A, et al. Lymphotoxin-beta receptor blockade reduces CXCL13 in lacrimal glands and improves corneal integrity in the NOD model of Sjogren's syndrome. *Arthritis Res Ther* (2011) 13:R182. doi:10.1186/ar3507
55. Luther SA, Lopez T, Bai W, Hanahan D, Cyster JG. BLC expression in pancreatic islets causes B cell recruitment and lymphotoxin-dependent lymphoid neogenesis. *Immunity* (2000) 12:471–81. doi:10.1016/S1074-7613(00)80199-5
56. Marinkovic T, Garin A, Yokota Y, Fu YX, Ruddle NH, Furtado GC, et al. Interaction of mature CD3+CD4+ T cells with dendritic cells triggers the development of tertiary lymphoid structures in the thyroid. *J Clin Invest* (2006) 116:2622–32. doi:10.1172/JCI28993
57. Grabner R, Lotzer K, Dopping S, Hildner M, Radke D, Beer M, et al. Lymphotoxin beta receptor signaling promotes tertiary lymphoid organogenesis in the aorta adventitia of aged ApoE-/- mice. *J Exp Med* (2009) 206:233–48. doi:10.1084/jem.20080752
58. Guedj K, Khallou-Laschet J, Clement M, Morvan M, Gaston AT, Fornasa G, et al. M1 macrophages act as LTbetaR-independent lymphoid tissue inducer cells during atherosclerosis-related lymphoid neogenesis. *Cardiovasc Res* (2014) 101:434–43. doi:10.1093/cvr/cvt263
59. Spahn TW, Herbst H, Rennert PD, Lugering N, Maaser C, Kraft M, et al. Induction of colitis in mice deficient of Peyer's patches and mesenteric lymph nodes is associated with increased disease severity and formation of colonic lymphoid patches. *Am J Pathol* (2002) 161:2273–82. doi:10.1016/S0002-9440(10)64503-8
60. Takatori H, Kanno Y, Watford WT, Tato CM, Weiss G, Ivanov II, et al. Lymphoid tissue inducer-like cells are an innate source of IL-17 and IL-22. *J Exp Med* (2009) 206:35–41. doi:10.1084/jem.20072713
61. Wolk K, Kunz S, Witte E, Friedrich M, Asadullah K, Sabat R. IL-22 increases the innate immunity of tissues. *Immunity* (2004) 21:241–54. doi:10.1016/j.immuni.2004.07.007
62. Barone F, Nayar S, Campos J, Cloake T, Withers DR, Toellner KM, et al. IL-22 regulates lymphoid chemokine production and assembly of tertiary lymphoid organs. *Proc Natl Acad Sci U S A* (2015) 112:11024–9. doi:10.1073/pnas.1503315112
63. Sugimoto K, Ogawa A, Mizoguchi E, Shimomura Y, Andoh A, Bhan AK, et al. IL-22 ameliorates intestinal inflammation in a mouse model of ulcerative colitis. *J Clin Invest* (2008) 118:534–44. doi:10.1172/JCI33194
64. Pickert G, Neufert C, Leppkes M, Zheng Y, Wittkopf N, Warntjen M, et al. STAT3 links IL-22 signaling in intestinal epithelial cells to mucosal wound healing. *J Exp Med* (2009) 206:1465–72. doi:10.1084/jem.20082683
65. Marchesi F, Martin AP, Thirunarayanan N, Devany E, Mayer L, Grisotto MG, et al. CXCL13 expression in the gut promotes accumulation of IL-22-producing

lymphoid tissue-inducer cells, and formation of isolated lymphoid follicles. *Mucosal Immunol* (2009) 2:486–94. doi:10.1038/mi.2009.113
66. Tumanov AV, Koroleva EP, Guo X, Wang Y, Kruglov A, Nedospasov S, et al. Lymphotoxin controls the IL-22 protection pathway in gut innate lymphoid cells during mucosal pathogen challenge. *Cell Host Microbe* (2011) 10:44–53. doi:10.1016/j.chom.2011.06.002
67. Ota N, Wong K, Valdez PA, Zheng Y, Crellin NK, Diehl L, et al. IL-22 bridges the lymphotoxin pathway with the maintenance of colonic lymphoid structures during infection with *Citrobacter rodentium*. *Nat Immunol* (2011) 12:941–8. doi:10.1038/ni.2089
68. Rangel-Moreno J, Carragher DM, de la Luz Garcia-Hernandez M, Hwang JY, Kusser K, Hartson L, et al. The development of inducible bronchus-associated lymphoid tissue depends on IL-17. *Nat Immunol* (2011) 12: 639–46. doi:10.1038/ni.2053
69. Fleige H, Ravens S, Moschovakis GL, Bolter J, Willenzon S, Sutter G, et al. IL-17-induced CXCL12 recruits B cells and induces follicle formation in BALT in the absence of differentiated FDCs. *J Exp Med* (2014) 211:643–51. doi:10.1084/jem.20131737
70. Peters A, Pitcher LA, Sullivan JM, Mitsdoerffer M, Acton SE, Franz B, et al. Th17 cells induce ectopic lymphoid follicles in central nervous system tissue inflammation. *Immunity* (2011) 35:986–96. doi:10.1016/j.immuni.2011.10.015
71. Esplugues E, Huber S, Gagliani N, Hauser AE, Town T, Wan YY, et al. Control of TH17 cells occurs in the small intestine. *Nature* (2011) 475:514–8. doi:10.1038/nature10228
72. Geem D, Medina-Contreras O, McBride M, Newberry RD, Koni PA, Denning TL. Specific microbiota-induced intestinal Th17 differentiation requires MHC class II but not GALT and mesenteric lymph nodes. *J Immunol* (2014) 193:431–8. doi:10.4049/jimmunol.1303167
73. Milpied PJ, McHeyzer-Williams MG. High-affinity IgA needs TH17 cell functional plasticity. *Nat Immunol* (2013) 14:313–5. doi:10.1038/ni.2567
74. Hirota K, Turner JE, Villa M, Duarte JH, Demengeot J, Steinmetz OM, et al. Plasticity of Th17 cells in Peyer's patches is responsible for the induction of T cell-dependent IgA responses. *Nat Immunol* (2013) 14:372–9. doi:10.1038/ni.2552
75. Yamamoto-Furusho JK, Miranda-Perez E, Fonseca-Camarillo G, Sanchez-Munoz F, Barreto-Zuniga R, Dominguez-Lopez A. Interleukin 21 expression is increased in rectal biopsies from patients with ulcerative colitis. *Inflamm Bowel Dis* (2010) 16:1090. doi:10.1002/ibd.21135
76. Liu C, Xia X, Wu W, Wu R, Tang M, Chen T, et al. Anti-tumour necrosis factor therapy enhances mucosal healing through down-regulation of interleukin-21 expression and T helper type 17 cell infiltration in Crohn's disease. *Clin Exp Immunol* (2013) 173:102–11. doi:10.1111/cei.12084
77. Yang L, Anderson DE, Baecher-Allan C, Hastings WD, Bettelli E, Oukka M, et al. IL-21 and TGF-beta are required for differentiation of human T(H)17 cells. *Nature* (2008) 454:350–2. doi:10.1038/nature07021
78. Sakaguchi S, Sakaguchi N, Asano M, Itoh M, Toda M. Immunologic self-tolerance maintained by activated T cells expressing IL-2 receptor alpha-chains (CD25). Breakdown of a single mechanism of self-tolerance causes various autoimmune diseases. *J Immunol* (1995) 155:1151–64.
79. Thornton AM, Shevach EM. CD4+CD25+ immunoregulatory T cells suppress polyclonal T cell activation in vitro by inhibiting interleukin 2 production. *J Exp Med* (1998) 188:287–96. doi:10.1084/jem.188.2.287
80. Nakamura K, Kitani A, Strober W. Cell contact-dependent immunosuppression by CD4(+)CD25(+) regulatory T cells is mediated by cell surface-bound transforming growth factor beta. *J Exp Med* (2001) 194:629–44. doi:10.1084/jem.194.5.629
81. Villablanca EJ, De Calisto J, Torregrosa Paredes P, Cassani B, Nguyen DD, Gabrielsson S, et al. beta7 integrins are required to give rise to intestinal mononuclear phagocytes with tolerogenic potential. *Gut* (2014) 63:1431–40. doi:10.1136/gutjnl-2013-305386
82. Serra P, Amrani A, Yamanouchi J, Han B, Thiessen S, Utsugi T, et al. CD40 ligation releases immature dendritic cells from the control of regulatory CD4+CD25+ T cells. *Immunity* (2003) 19:877–89. doi:10.1016/S1074-7613(03)00327-3
83. Collins CB, Aherne CM, McNamee EN, Lebsack MD, Eltzschig H, Jedlicka P, et al. Flt3 ligand expands CD103(+) dendritic cells and FoxP3(+) T regulatory cells, and attenuates Crohn's-like murine ileitis. *Gut* (2012) 61:1154–62. doi:10.1136/gutjnl-2011-300820
84. Collins CB, Aherne CM, Kominsky D, McNamee EN, Lebsack MD, Eltzschig H, et al. Retinoic acid attenuates ileitis by restoring the balance between T-helper 17 and T regulatory cells. *Gastroenterology* (2011) 141:1821–31. doi:10.1053/j.gastro.2011.05.049
85. Wermers JD, McNamee EN, Wurbel MA, Jedlicka P, Rivera-Nieves J. The chemokine receptor CCR9 is required for the T-cell-mediated regulation of chronic ileitis in mice. *Gastroenterology* (2011) 140(1526–35):e3. doi:10.1053/j.gastro.2011.01.044
86. Ueha S, Yoneyama H, Hontsu S, Kurachi M, Kitabatake M, Abe J, et al. CCR7 mediates the migration of Foxp3+ regulatory T cells to the paracortical areas of peripheral lymph nodes through high endothelial venules. *J Leukoc Biol* (2007) 82:1230–8. doi:10.1189/jlb.0906574
87. Kocks JR, Davalos-Misslitz AC, Hintzen G, Ohl L, Forster R. Regulatory T cells interfere with the development of bronchus-associated lymphoid tissue. *J Exp Med* (2007) 204:723–34 doi:10.1084/jem.20061424
88. Aguzzi A, Kranich J, Krautler NJ. Follicular dendritic cells: origin, phenotype, and function in health and disease. *Trends Immunol* (2014) 35:105–13. doi:10.1016/j.it.2013.11.001
89. Krautler NJ, Kana V, Kranich J, Tian Y, Perera D, Lemm D, et al. Follicular dendritic cells emerge from ubiquitous perivascular precursors. *Cell* (2012) 150:194–206. doi:10.1016/j.cell.2012.05.032
90. Heesters BA, Chatterjee P, Kim YA, Gonzalez SF, Kuligowski MP, Kirchhausen T, et al. Endocytosis and recycling of immune complexes by follicular dendritic cells enhances B cell antigen binding and activation. *Immunity* (2013) 38:1164–75. doi:10.1016/j.immuni.2013.02.023
91. Allen CD, Cyster JG. Follicular dendritic cell networks of primary follicles and germinal centers: phenotype and function. *Semin Immunol* (2008) 20:14–25. doi:10.1016/j.smim.2007.12.001
92. Bossuyt X. Serologic markers in inflammatory bowel disease. *Clin Chem* (2006) 52:171–81. doi:10.1373/clinchem.2005.058560
93. Terjung B, Worman HJ, Herzog V, Sauerbruch T, Spengler U. Differentiation of antineutrophil nuclear antibodies in inflammatory bowel and autoimmune liver diseases from antineutrophil cytoplasmic antibodies (p-ANCA) using immunofluorescence microscopy. *Clin Exp Immunol* (2001) 126:37–46. doi:10.1046/j.1365-2249.2001.01649.x
94. Saxon A, Shanahan F, Landers C, Ganz T, Targan S. A distinct subset of antineutrophil cytoplasmic antibodies is associated with inflammatory bowel disease. *J Allergy Clin Immunol* (1990) 86:202–10. doi:10.1016/S0091-6749(05)80067-3
95. Rump JA, Scholmerich J, Gross V, Roth M, Helfesrieder R, Rautmann A, et al. A new type of perinuclear anti-neutrophil cytoplasmic antibody (p-ANCA) in active ulcerative colitis but not in Crohn's disease. *Immunobiology* (1990) 181:406–13. doi:10.1016/S0171-2985(11)80509-7
96. Main J, McKenzie H, Yeaman GR, Kerr MA, Robson D, Pennington CR, et al. Antibody to *Saccharomyces cerevisiae* (bakers' yeast) in Crohn's disease. *BMJ* (1988) 297:1105–6. doi:10.1136/bmj.297.6656.1105
97. Cohavy O, Bruckner D, Gordon LK, Misra R, Wei B, Eggena ME, et al. Colonic bacteria express an ulcerative colitis pANCA-related protein epitope. *Infect Immun* (2000) 68:1542–8. doi:10.1128/IAI.68.3.1542-1548.2000
98. Targan SR, Landers CJ, Yang H, Lodes MJ, Cong Y, Papadakis KA, et al. Antibodies to CBir1 flagellin define a unique response that is associated independently with complicated Crohn's disease. *Gastroenterology* (2005) 128:2020–8. doi:10.1053/j.gastro.2005.03.046
99. Mow WS, Vasiliauskas EA, Lin YC, Fleshner PR, Papadakis KA, Taylor KD, et al. Association of antibody responses to microbial antigens and complications of small bowel Crohn's disease. *Gastroenterology* (2004) 126:414–24. doi:10.1053/j.gastro.2003.11.015
100. Isene R, Bernklev T, Høie O, Munkholm P, Tsianos E, Stockbrugger R, et al. Extraintestinal manifestations in Crohn's disease and ulcerative colitis: results from a prospective, population-based European inception cohort. *Scand J Gastroenterol* (2015) 50:300–5. doi:10.3109/00365521.2014.991752
101. Scher JU, Sczesnak A, Longman RS, Segata N, Ubeda C, Bielski C, et al. Expansion of intestinal *Prevotella copri* correlates with enhanced susceptibility to arthritis. *Elife* (2013) 2:e01202. doi:10.7554/eLife.01202
102. Aoki S, Yoshikawa K, Yokoyama T, Nonogaki T, Iwasaki S, Mitsui T, et al. Role of enteric bacteria in the pathogenesis of rheumatoid arthritis: evidence for antibodies to enterobacterial common antigens in rheumatoid sera and synovial fluids. *Ann Rheum Dis* (1996) 55:363–9. doi:10.1136/ard.55.6.363

103. Vaahtovuo J, Munukka E, Korkeamaki M, Luukkainen R, Toivanen P. Fecal microbiota in early rheumatoid arthritis. *J Rheumatol* (2008) 35:1500–5.
104. Kuhn KA, Pedraza I, Demoruelle MK. Mucosal immune responses to microbiota in the development of autoimmune disease. *Rheum Dis Clin North Am* (2014) 40:711–25. doi:10.1016/j.rdc.2014.07.013
105. Round JL, Mazmanian SK. The gut microbiota shapes intestinal immune responses during health and disease. *Nat Rev Immunol* (2009) 9:313–23. doi:10.1038/nri2515
106. Elson CO. Commensal bacteria as targets in Crohn's disease. *Gastroenterology* (2000) 119:254–7. doi:10.1053/gast.2000.9159
107. Sartor RB. The influence of normal microbial flora on the development of chronic mucosal inflammation. *Res Immunol* (1997) 148:567–76. doi:10.1016/S0923-2494(98)80151-X
108. de La Motte CA, Hascall VC, Calabro A, Yen-Lieberman B, Strong SA. Mononuclear leukocytes preferentially bind via CD44 to hyaluronan on human intestinal mucosal smooth muscle cells after virus infection or treatment with poly(I.C). *J Biol Chem* (1999) 274:30747–55. doi:10.1074/jbc.274.43.30747
109. Jarvelainen H, Sainio A, Koulu M, Wight TN, Penttinen R. Extracellular matrix molecules: potential targets in pharmacotherapy. *Pharmacol Rev* (2009) 61:198–223. doi:10.1124/pr.109.001289
110. Visse R, Nagase H. Matrix metalloproteinases and tissue inhibitors of metalloproteinases: structure, function, and biochemistry. *Circ Res* (2003) 92:827–39. doi:10.1161/01.RES.0000070112.80711.3D
111. van der Woude D, Rantapaa-Dahlqvist S, Ioan-Facsinay A, Onnekink C, Schwarte CM, Verpoort KN, et al. Epitope spreading of the anti-citrullinated protein antibody response occurs before disease onset and is associated with the disease course of early arthritis. *Ann Rheum Dis* (2010) 69:1554–61. doi:10.1136/ard.2009.124537
112. Kuhn KA, Kulik L, Tomooka B, Braschler KJ, Arend WP, Robinson WH, et al. Antibodies against citrullinated proteins enhance tissue injury in experimental autoimmune arthritis. *J Clin Invest* (2006) 116:961–73. doi:10.1172/JCI25422
113. Buckley CD, Barone F, Nayar S, Benezech C, Caamano J. Stromal cells in chronic inflammation and tertiary lymphoid organ formation. *Annu Rev Immunol* (2015) 33:715–45. doi:10.1146/annurev-immunol-032713-120252
114. Lee SH, Goswami S, Grudo A, Song LZ, Bandi V, Goodnight-White S, et al. Antielastin autoimmunity in tobacco smoking-induced emphysema. *Nat Med* (2007) 13:567–9. doi:10.1038/nm1583
115. Benezech C, Luu NT, Walker JA, Kruglov AA, Loo Y, Nakamura K, et al. Inflammation-induced formation of fat-associated lymphoid clusters. *Nat Immunol* (2015) 16:819–28. doi:10.1038/ni.3215
116. Chiang EY, Kolumam GA, Yu X, Francesco M, Ivelja S, Peng I, et al. Targeted depletion of lymphotoxin-alpha-expressing TH1 and TH17 cells inhibits autoimmune disease. *Nat Med* (2009) 15:766–73. doi:10.1038/nm.1984
117. Browning JL, Allaire N, Ngam-Ek A, Notidis E, Hunt J, Perrin S, et al. Lymphotoxin-beta receptor signaling is required for the homeostatic control of HEV differentiation and function. *Immunity* (2005) 23:539–50. doi:10.1016/j.immuni.2005.10.002
118. De Trez C, Schneider K, Potter K, Droin N, Fulton J, Norris PS, et al. The inhibitory HVEM-BTLA pathway counter regulates lymphotoxin receptor signaling to achieve homeostasis of dendritic cells. *J Immunol* (2008) 180:238–48. doi:10.4049/jimmunol.180.1.238
119. Roulis M, Bongers G, Armaka M, Salviano T, He Z, Singh A, et al. Host and microbiota interactions are critical for development of murine Crohn's-like ileitis. *Mucosal Immunol* (2016) 9:787–97. doi:10.1038/mi.2015.102
120. Kobayashi M, Mitoma J, Nakamura N, Katsuyama T, Nakayama J, Fukuda M. Induction of peripheral lymph node addressin in human gastric mucosa infected by *Helicobacter pylori*. *Proc Natl Acad Sci U S A* (2004) 101:17807–12. doi:10.1073/pnas.0407503101
121. Mazzucchelli L, Blaser A, Kappeler A, Schärli P, Laissue JA, Baggiolini M, et al. BCA-1 is highly expressed in *Helicobacter pylori*-induced mucosa-associated lymphoid tissue and gastric lymphoma. *J Clin Invest* (1999) 104:R49–54. doi:10.1172/JCI7830
122. Kaiserling E. Newly-formed lymph nodes in the submucosa in chronic inflammatory bowel disease. *Lymphology* (2001) 34:22–9.
123. Coppola D, Nebozhyn M, Khalil F, Dai H, Yeatman T, Loboda A, et al. Unique ectopic lymph node-like structures present in human primary colorectal carcinoma are identified by immune gene array profiling. *Am J Pathol* (2011) 179:37–45. doi:10.1016/j.ajpath.2011.03.007
124. Bergomas F, Grizzi F, Doni A, Pesce S, Laghi L, Allavena P, et al. Tertiary intratumor lymphoid tissue in colo-rectal cancer. *Cancers (Basel)* (2011) 4:1–10. doi:10.3390/cancers4010001
125. Katakai T, Hara T, Sugai M, Gonda H, Shimizu A. Th1-biased tertiary lymphoid tissue supported by CXC chemokine ligand 13-producing stromal network in chronic lesions of autoimmune gastritis. *J Immunol* (2003) 171:4359–68. doi:10.4049/jimmunol.171.8.4359
126. Katakai T, Nomura T, Gonda H, Sugai M, Agata Y, Nishio A, et al. Spontaneous large-scale lymphoid neogenesis and balanced autoimmunity versus tolerance in the stomach of H+/K+-ATPase-reactive TCR transgenic mouse. *J Immunol* (2006) 177:7858–67. doi:10.4049/jimmunol.177.11.7858
127. Winter S, Loddenkemper C, Aebischer A, Räbel K, Hoffmann K, Meyer TF, et al. The chemokine receptor CXCR5 is pivotal for ectopic mucosa-associated lymphoid tissue neogenesis in chronic *Helicobacter pylori*-induced inflammation. *J Mol Med (Berl)* (2010) 88:1169–80. doi:10.1007/s00109-010-0658-6
128. Shomer NH, Fox JG, Juedes AE, Ruddle NH. *Helicobacter*-induced chronic active lymphoid aggregates have characteristics of tertiary lymphoid tissue. *Infect Immun* (2003) 71:3572–7. doi:10.1128/IAI.71.6.3572-3577.2003
129. Yamamoto K, Nishiumi S, Yang L, Klimatcheva E, Pandina T, Takahashi S, et al. Anti-CXCL13 antibody can inhibit the formation of gastric lymphoid follicles induced by *Helicobacter* infection. *Mucosal Immunol* (2014) 7:1244–54. doi:10.1038/mi.2014.14
130. Glaysher BR, Mabbott NA. Role of the GALT in scrapie agent neuroinvasion from the intestine. *J Immunol* (2007) 178:3757–66. doi:10.4049/jimmunol.178.6.3757
131. Höpken UE, Wengner AM, Loddenkemper C, Stein H, Heimesaat MM, Rehm A, et al. CCR7 deficiency causes ectopic lymphoid neogenesis and disturbed mucosal tissue integrity. *Blood* (2007) 109:886–95. doi:10.1182/blood-2006-03-013532
132. Fagarasan S, Muramatsu M, Suzuki K, Nagaoka H, Hiai H, Honjo T. Critical roles of activation-induced cytidine deaminase in the homeostasis of gut flora. *Science* (2002) 298:1424–7. doi:10.1126/science.1077336
133. Kelly FM, Reddy RN, Roberts BR, Gangappa S, Williams IR, Gooch JL. TGF-beta upregulation drives tertiary lymphoid organ formation and kidney dysfunction in calcineurin A-alpha heterozygous mice. *Am J Physiol Renal Physiol* (2009) 296:F512–20. doi:10.1152/ajprenal.90629.2008
134. Halle S, Bumann D, Herbrand H, Willer Y, Dähne S, Förster R, et al. Solitary intestinal lymphoid tissue provides a productive port of entry for *Salmonella enterica* serovar Typhimurium. *Infect Immun* (2007) 75:1577–85. doi:10.1128/IAI.01392-06

14

Inducible Bronchus-Associated Lymphoid Tissue: Taming Inflammation in the Lung

Ji Young Hwang, Troy D. Randall and Aaron Silva-Sanchez*

Division of Clinical Immunology and Rheumatology, Department of Medicine, University of Alabama at Birmingham, Birmingham, AL, USA

***Correspondence:**
Troy D. Randall
randallt@uab.edu

Following pulmonary inflammation, leukocytes that infiltrate the lung often assemble into structures known as inducible Bronchus-Associated Lymphoid Tissue (iBALT). Like conventional lymphoid organs, areas of iBALT have segregated B and T cell areas, specialized stromal cells, high endothelial venules, and lymphatic vessels. After inflammation is resolved, iBALT is maintained for months, independently of inflammation. Once iBALT is formed, it participates in immune responses to pulmonary antigens, including those that are unrelated to the iBALT-initiating antigen, and often alters the clinical course of disease. However, the mechanisms that govern immune responses in iBALT and determine how iBALT impacts local and systemic immunity are poorly understood. Here, we review our current understanding of iBALT formation and discuss how iBALT participates in pulmonary immunity.

Keywords: inducible bronchus-associated lymphoid tissue, tertiary lymphoid organ, ectopic lymphoid organ, lymphoid neogenesis, germinal center

INTRODUCTION

The evolutionary emergence of lymphocytes with diversified antigen receptors allows the immune system to recognize and respond to a myriad of unknown antigens. However, despite the enormous number of B cells and T cells in the naive compartment, the frequency of B cells or T cells with any particular specificity is miniscule, necessitating efficient mechanisms to acquire and present antigens to the responding lymphocytes (1). Moreover, B and T cells of the same specificity must find one another and interact in a cognate way in order to differentiate into effector cells (2). In order to accomplish these goals, the immune system has evolved a system of secondary lymphoid organs (3).

Secondary lymphoid organs, such as spleen, lymph nodes, Peyer's patches, and other mucosa-associated lymphoid tissues, recruit naive B and T cells from the blood and sample antigens from local non-lymphoid organs and mucosal surfaces, thereby allowing naive lymphocytes to efficiently peruse antigens from all the tissues of an entire organism without having to migrate through those tissues themselves (4). Moreover, secondary lymphoid organs are highly organized and contain architectural domains that facilitate sequential cellular interactions between antigen-presenting cells and lymphocytes and efficiently promote B and T cell activation, selection, and differentiation (1) – ultimately increasing the efficiency of the immune response.

Mammals, birds, and bony fish have easily recognizable secondary lymphoid organs and tissues with some of the characteristics of secondary lymphoid organs are observed in the gut lamina propria of cartilaginous fish, such as sharks (5). In fact, the appearance of cell clusters containing two types of adaptive immune cells can be traced back to pharynx of the lamprey (6), a jawless vertebrate and one of the oldest organisms to have an adaptive immune system (7). Thus, most vertebrates have evolved some type of tissue that is specialized to promote interactions between various cells of the adaptive immune system. Other authors have recently reviewed the evolutionary aspects of lymphoid organs (5); therefore, in this review, we will focus only on the developmental and functional aspects of lymphoid tissues in the lung.

Most secondary lymphoid organs in mice and humans develop embryonically in the absence of microbial stimulation or foreign antigens (8). However, the structure and function of some secondary lymphoid organs, particularly those at mucosal surfaces, is dramatically altered upon exposure to environmental antigens and commensal organisms (9). For example, Peyer's patches in the small intestine dramatically increase in size and complexity following commensal colonization (10, 11). Similarly, Nasal-Associated Lymphoid Tissue in rodents does not completely develop until after birth and this process is accelerated by microbial exposure (12). Strikingly, the appendix of rabbits is both a primary and secondary lymphoid tissue that is functionally dependent on microbial colonization (13). More importantly, however, some lymphoid tissues, known as tertiary lymphoid tissues, develop *only* after environmental exposure to microbes, pathogens, or inflammatory stimuli. Tertiary lymphoid tissues form in a wide variety of organs, including pancreas (14), thyroid (15), thymus (16), salivary gland (17, 18), brain (19), liver (20), kidney (21), and others (22), but in this review, we will focus on tertiary lymphoid tissue that forms in the lung, known as inducible Bronchus-Associated Lymphoid Tissue or iBALT.

Although the lungs of mice and humans normally lack organized lymphoid tissue, areas of iBALT form in the lungs following some types of infection or inflammation (23, 24) (**Table 1**). iBALT is a classic example of a tertiary lymphoid tissue, since it does not develop in a pre-programed way and its occurrence, size, and number in the lung depends on the type and duration of antigenic exposure (25, 26). Areas of iBALT are observed in the lungs of mammals (27–31) and birds (32–34) and are likely found in all air-breathing vertebrates. However, iBALT is most well characterized in the lungs of rodents and humans. Here we will summarize below the results of studies from these species.

GENERAL FEATURES OF iBALT

As the name indicates, iBALT does not occur at random sites in the lungs, but develops in close proximity to the basal side of the bronchial epithelium (35), often in the perivascular space of pulmonary blood vessels (36, 37). The leukocytes comprising iBALT are arranged in two zones, the B cell follicle and the T cell zone (37), in a way that resembles the organization of conventional secondary lymphoid organs. The B cell follicles of iBALT contain tight clusters of IgD^{+} follicular B cells grouped around a network of stromal cells, known as follicular dendritic

TABLE 1 | Association of iBALT with infectious and inflammatory diseases of the lung.

Disease	Important finding	Reference
COPD	SERPINEE2 prevents iBALT formation, inhibits thrombin	(119)
	CXCL13 expression associated with iBALT	(190)
	iBALT associated with COPD stage	(192)
	iBALT associated with uptake of pulmonary antigens	(198)
	Increase in dendritic cells in iBALT of COPD patients	(199)
	CCL20-driven accumulation of dendritic cells in iBALT	(200)
	Increased B follicles in COPD patients	(201)
	iBALT found in smokers and asthmatics	(210)
	CCR7 involved in iBALT formation after cigarette smoke	(195)
Particulate exposure	Exposure to diesel exhaust particles promotes iBALT	(88)
	Cigarette smoke-induced iBALT	(89)
	iBALT associated with response to silica	(226)
Pulmonary arterial hypertension	Formation of iBALT in patients with PAH	(92)
	Association of IL-17 in the formation of iBALT in PAH	(93)
Hypersensitivity pneumonitis	iBALT associated with hypersensitivity pneumonitis	(189)
	iBALT areas found in hypersensitivity pneumonitis	(209)
Rheumatoid lung disease	iBALT found in patients with rheumatoid lung disease	(208)
Sjogren syndrome	IL-22 promotes CXCL13 expression and iBALT formation	(18)
Allograft rejection	iBALT formation associated with lung transplant rejection	(218)
	iBALT formation associated with lung transplant tolerance	(222)
Allergy/asthma	Pulmonary challenge of rats with antigens	(35)
	Pulmonary challenge of rats with HRP	(62)
	Pulmonary challenge with OVA leads to IgE in iBALT	(90)
	IL-5 overexpression and eosinophils lead to iBALT	(129)
	iBALT is sufficient for immunity to allergens	(176)
	Local IgE production in iBALT in aspergillosis	(211)
	Poor association of iBALT with asthma in non-smokers	(212)
Viral infection	iBALT independently promotes immunity to influenza	(23)
	iBALT in mink infected with Aleutian disease virus	(28)
	CXCL13, CCL19, and CCL21 are important for iBALT function	(56)
	iBALT formation after infection with modified vaccinia ankara	(65)
	iBALT accelerates immunity to pneumovirus	(82)
	Infection of mice with murine cytomegalovirus	(85)
	Dendritic cell – dependence of iBALT	(121)
	Immunologic memory maintained in iBALT	(180)
	iBALT-mediated immunity to SARS, influenza	(181)
	Acceleration of CD4 responses by iBALT	(67)
Bacterial infection	iBALT in humans with bacterial infections	(29)
	iBALT in goats with *Pasteurella haemolytica*	(31)

(Continued)

TABLE 1 | Continued

Disease	Important finding	Reference
	Lymphatics around iBALT after *Mycoplasma pulmonis* infection	(64)
	Infection of pigs with *Actinobacillus pleuropneumoniae*	(25)
	Pulmonary exposure to LPS leads to IL-17-dependent iBALT	(78)
	iBALT in pigs exposed to hemolytic *streptococcus*	(81)
	Formation of iBALT in human fetuses with amnionitis	(83)
	Mycobacterium tuberculosis induces iBALT in mice	(87)
	IL-17-dependent iBALT formation *Pseudomonas aruginosa*	(94)
	IL-17-dependent CXCL13 after *M. tuberculosis*	(100)
	IL-23 maintains iBALT and granulomas in *M tuberculosis*	(98)
	iBALT is sufficient for immunity to *M tuberculosis*	(175)
	iBALT is sufficient for immunity to *M tuberculosis*	(177)
	Pulmonary vaccination to *F. tulerensis* promotes iBALT	(182)
	Lymphoid chemokines maintain iBALT in *tuberculosis*	(185)
	iBALT recruits CXCR5 + T cells in *tuberculosis*	(186)
	Human tuberculosis granulomas resemble iBALT	(187)
	Vaccination elicits iBALT and protects from tuberculosis	(188)
Lung cancer	iBALT associated with good prognosis in lung cancer	(224)
	iBALT associated with ILC3 cells in lung cancer	(225)
Spontaneous iBALT	IL-6 overexpression leads to iBALT	(130)
	Oncostatin M overexpression leads to iBALT	(131)
	Poor Treg function in CCR7$^{-/-}$ mice leads to iBALT	(127)
Lung fibrosis	Reduced bleomycin-induced fibrosis in lungs with iBALT	(227)
	Reduced bleomycin-induced fibrosis in lungs with iBALT	(228)

cells (FDCs), that express CD21, CXCL13, and lymphotoxin (LT) β receptor (LTβR) (38–41) (**Figure 1B**). B cell follicles in reactive iBALT areas may contain large germinal centers (23), in which B cells are rapidly dividing in response to antigen. These germinal centers will also contain activated CD4 T cells, known as T follicular helper (Tfh) cells (42, 43) (**Figure 1A**). The T cell zone of iBALT surrounds the B cell follicles and contains CD4 and CD8 T cells as well as conventional dendritic cells (DCs) (24, 44) (**Figure 1A**).

The compartmentalization of B and T cell areas in iBALT requires specialized fibroblastic cells, usually referred to as stromal cells. Stromal cells in the B cell follicle are primarily FDCs, which express CXCL13, a chemokine that attracts CXCL13-expressing cells like B cells and Tfh cells (42, 45, 46). Stromal cells are also observed in the T cell zones of iBALT and are likely similar to the fibroblastic reticular cells (FRCs) found in the T zones of conventional secondary lymphoid organs (47, 48). These cells express chemokines like CCL19 and CCL21 (49–51), which attract naive T cells and activated DCs (45, 52, 53). T zone stromal cells also produce IL-7 (54, 55), a cytokine important for the survival of naive lymphocytes.

In addition to the stromal cells that support the B and T cell areas, iBALT often features high endothelial venules (HEVs) (56), which are specialized blood vessels that express homing and adhesion molecules as well as chemokines that together recruit lymphocytes from the blood (57). HEVs in iBALT are located just outside the B cell follicle in the T cell zone (56). Although one might assume that iBALT is a mucosal lymphoid tissue based on its location in the lung, the HEVs of iBALT express peripheral lymph node addressin (PNAd) like the HEVs of peripheral lymph nodes (56), but do not express mucosal addressin cell adhesion molecule (MAdCAM), which is prominently expressed by mesenteric lymph nodes and Peyer's patches in the intestine (58). HEVs in iBALT also express (or display) CCL21 (56), which is likely important for the recruitment of naive lymphocytes from the blood.

Given that iBALT is located underneath the bronchial epithelium, one might assume that it acquires antigens directly from the lumen of the airways *via* epithelial M cells. Although antigen-transporting M cells have been reported in the iBALT of some species (35, 59, 60), they are not consistently observed and many areas of iBALT do not have the classic structure of a mucosal lymphoid tissue, with a dome epithelium overlaying the B cell follicle (61). It is not clear at this time whether this inconsistency in the structure of iBALT is due to differences in species, the way in which iBALT is formed or the duration/magnitude of antigen exposure (62).

Despite the lack of obvious M cells in many iBALT areas, there are also lymphatic vessels that surround the B cell follicle and likely facilitate the uptake of antigens. In the normal lung, lymphatics originate from two distinct locations, one set of lymphatics originate from the parenchyma and follows the pulmonary veins toward the draining lymph node, and the other set originates around the connective tissue between the airways and veins, and follows the airways toward the draining lymph node (63). New data show that additional lymphatic vessels are generated during lung inflammation surrounding the iBALT areas, apparently by sprouting from the existing lymphatic network (64). Given the placement of iBALT in the perivascular space next to large airways, we expect that afferent lymphatics drain from the distal portions of the lung toward iBALT. The best evidence for this model is the ability of iBALT to collect labeled DCs and particulates (23, 64, 65).

Lymph nodes have both afferent and efferent lymphatics, whereas most mucosal lymphoid tissues have only efferent lymphatics that connect to downstream lymph nodes and ultimately to the blood. We assume that many of the lymphatics associated with iBALT are efferent lymphatics that allow cells within iBALT to re-enter the circulation. In fact, we expect that iBALT follows the conventional model of lymphoid recirculation in which naive B and T cells enter iBALT from the blood through PNAd-expressing HEVs and then exit iBALT *via* efferent lymphatic vessels (66). Efferent lymphatic vessels would also allow activated effector and memory lymphocytes to exit iBALT and re-enter the circulation. Although the ability of efferent lymphatics to collect cells primed in iBALT and

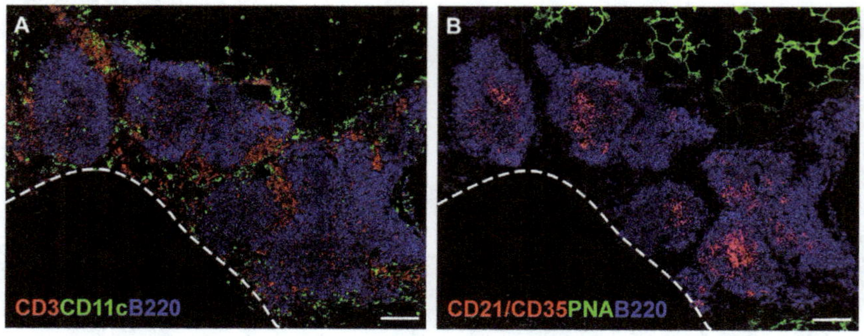

FIGURE 1 | The structure of iBALT. C57BL/6 mice were intranasally administered LPS on days 3, 5, 7, 9, and 11 after birth, and lungs were obtained 6 weeks after the last LPS administration. **(A)** Frozen sections were probed with anti-CD3 (red), anti-CD11c (green), and anti-B220 (Blue), and images were acquired on a Nikon Eclipse Ti microscope using the 20× objective. The dashed line indicates the position of a blood vessel. Scale bar indicates 200 μm. **(B)** Frozen sections were probed with anti-CD21/35 (red), peanut agglutinin (PNA - green), and anti-B220 (blue), and images were acquired on a Nikon Eclipse Ti microscope using the 20× objective. Scale bar indicates 200 μm.

drain them to the downstream mediastinal lymph node has not been directly demonstrated, recent data show that the presence of iBALT promotes more rapid responses in the draining LN (67), suggesting that iBALT is connected to downstream lymph nodes and can alter the trafficking of antigen-bearing DCs and primed lymphocytes. Importantly, new data show that lymphatic endothelial cells in iBALT areas are more than just highways for leukocyte trafficking. In addition to producing the chemoattractant, CCL21, lymphatic endothelial cells also produce IL-7 and contribute to the maintenance of memory T cells (68). Thus, the lymphatic vessels surrounding iBALT likely have multiple functions.

iBALT DEVELOPMENT

Secondary lymphoid organs, such as lymph nodes and Peyer's patches, form independently of antigenic or inflammatory stimuli in a highly ordered process that occurs during embryogenesis at very specific times (8) and reviewed in Ref. (69). Once that developmental window is passed, lymph nodes are no longer able to develop, even if all the necessary cells and molecules are present (8). In contrast, the development of iBALT requires an inflammatory or infectious stimulus in most species (25, 26, 70–73), including rats (74–77), mice (78), goats (79), chicken (33), and humans (29, 73, 80), and its development can be initiated throughout life. In contrast, pigs are reported to form iBALT in the lungs during fetal development (81). However, it is unclear whether this observation reflects a species or developmental difference.

Although the formation of iBALT is not restricted to a developmental window during embryogenesis, it seems to form more easily in the neonatal period just after birth (78, 82). For example, iBALT is found in the lungs of healthy adult humans at a relatively low frequency (83) but is found with increasing frequencies in the lungs of children and infants (29, 73, 83). The incidence of iBALT increases dramatically in all age groups following infection (70, 72, 73) but is highest in the lungs of infected children and infants and, most strikingly, is a prominent feature in 100% of late-term fetuses miscarried as a result of amnionitis (29), which results from an *in utero* pulmonary infection.

In part, the increased frequency of iBALT in the lungs of neonates and infants might reflect the initial exposure of a naive individual to stimuli such as pulmonary pathogens, microbial products, and allergens (25). However, the neonatal immune system also seems to favor the development of iBALT and other tertiary lymphoid tissues in mice living in controlled environments (78, 82, 84). For example, the injection of cell suspensions from dissociated lymph nodes into the skin of neonatal mice leads to the formation of highly organized lymphoid tissues (84), whereas the injection of the same cells into adults does not (84). Similarly, the repeated intranasal administration of the microbial product, LPS, to neonatal C57BL/6 mice induces iBALT formation, whereas repeated intranasal administration of LPS to weanling or adult C57BL/6 mice does not (78, 82). In another example, pulmonary infection of neonatal mice with cytomegalovirus (CMV) promotes the formation of Nodular Inflammatory Foci (NIF), whereas the pulmonary infection of adult mice with CMV does not (85, 86). NIFs are similar to iBALT in that they seem to support adaptive immune responses in the lung, but NIFs lack a B cell follicle and contain mostly a mix of CD8 T cells and DCs (85). At this point, it is unclear whether BALT and NIF formation are products of two different types of immune responses or whether CMV diverts the immune response leading to NIF formation as a byproduct and preventing BALT formation.

Interestingly, the preferential ability of neonates to form tertiary lymphoid tissues is less striking in BALB/c mice, as the pulmonary administration of LPS on a single day is sufficient to trigger iBALT formation in both neonatal and adult BALB/c mice (82). Moreover, other investigators have observed iBALT formation in adult mice following a variety of pulmonary challenges, including infections (87), particulates (88, 89), and allergens (90). Thus, the ability to trigger iBALT formation (or NIF formation) at particular stages of development likely reflects the inflammatory environment at the time of challenge and the type and duration of the challenge.

Given that the structure of iBALT is similar to that of conventional secondary lymphoid organs, it is not too surprising that the cytokines and chemokines (as well as their receptors) that are important for the development of secondary lymphoid organs are also important for the development of iBALT. For example, CXCL13 and its receptor, CXCR5 are required for the formation and maintenance of B cell follicles in both secondary lymphoid organs (45) and in iBALT (56). Similarly, the ligands for CCR7, CCL19, and CCL21 are important for the organization of the T cell zone and for the recruitment of lymphocytes from the blood through HEVs in both conventional lymphoid organs (45) and iBALT (56). Moreover, under steady state conditions, the expression of CXCL13, CCL19, and CCL21 is controlled by LT signaling through its receptors, LTβR and TNFR1 in both lymph nodes (91) and iBALT (78). However, during iBALT development, the expression of CXCL13 and CCL19 is controlled by IL-17 and possibly other inflammatory cytokines – independently of LT (78). Although IL-17 promotes the expression of CXCL13, CCL19, and other inflammatory chemokines during iBALT development, once iBALT is formed and inflammation is resolved, the expression of CXCL13 and CCL19 is maintained by LT signaling, independently of IL-17 (78). Thus, LT and IL-17 act at different times during iBALT development (**Figure 2**).

IL-17 is also important for iBALT formation in patients with pulmonary arterial hypertension (92, 93). As might be expected, the expression of lymphoid chemokines, CXCL13, CCL19, and CCL21 in the iBALT areas of these patients correlated with the frequency of RORγt-expressing T cells, presumably Th17 cells (92). Similarly, the pulmonary administration of heat-killed *Pseudomonas aeruginosa* (HK-Pa) to mice promotes iBALT formation in an IL-17-dependent fashion (94). Interestingly, in HK-Pa-treated mice, IL-17 mediates the aggregation of B cells by

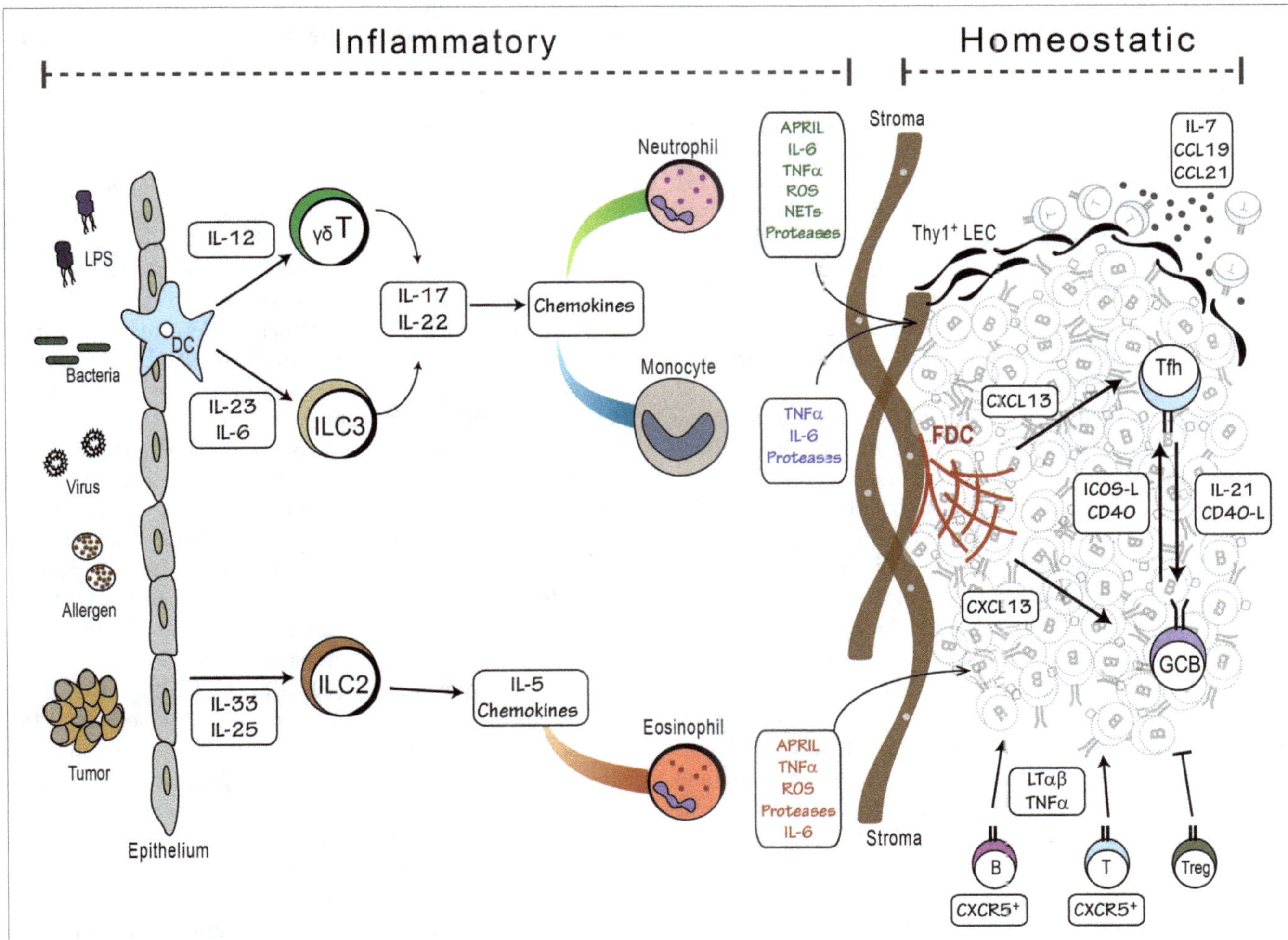

FIGURE 2 | Model of iBALT development. The development of iBALT can be initiated by a wide variety of stimuli, including microbial products, bacteria, viruses, allergens, tumors, and particulates (left side), which trigger the activation and cytokine production from epithelial cells and dendritic cells. Innate cells, such as ILCs and $\gamma\delta$T cells, become activated and produce cytokines and chemokines that attract inflammatory cells like neutrophils, monocytes, and eosinophils. Granulocytes produce cytokines that promote B cell activation as well as proteases and reactive oxygen that activate stromal cell precursors. These activities would all occur during an inflammatory process. Once mature B and T cells are recruited to the lung, they reinforce the differentiation of stromal cells into mature FDCs and FRCs that respectively support the B and T cell areas of iBALT. Once inflammation is resolved, the lymphocytes, dendritic cells, and stromal cells can maintain the iBALT structure using homeostatic mechanisms – lymphotoxin and chemokines – for months.

CXCL12, rather than CXCL13 (94). However, IL-17 is not always required for the formation of iBALT. For example, pulmonary infection of IL-17-deficient mice with Modified Vaccinia virus Ankara (MVA) promotes the formation of a classic iBALT structure (94). Despite the absence of IL-17, lymphoid chemokines, such as CXCL13 are still expressed, possibly as a result of reduced Treg activity (95) or complement-mediated neutrophil recruitment (96) as will be discussed later in this review. Thus, there are multiple ways to recruit lymphocytes to the lung and organize them into iBALT-type structures. Nevertheless, IL-17 seems to be an important cytokine in the development of ectopic lymphoid tissues in multiple locations (19, 97).

IL-22 is also important for iBALT formation (18, 98). Although IL-22 is most well known to act on epithelial cells in the lung and gut to trigger anti-microbial defenses and promote epithelial repair (99), the IL-22 receptor is also expressed on stromal cells in the B cell follicle of iBALT (18). In addition, the LPS-induced development of iBALT is impaired in the absence of IL-22 (18). Moreover, the lymphoid domains of tuberculosis granulomas, which resemble iBALT, are also disrupted in the absence of IL-22 – the FDC network is smaller, the B cell follicle is smaller and CXCL13 expression is reduced (98, 100). IL-22 is also important for the formation of other ectopic follicles, as the overexpression of IL-22 in the salivary gland strongly promotes the formation of ectopic follicles in that tissue (18). Interestingly, the IL-22 receptor is also expressed by stromal cells and FDCs in other locations, particularly following inflammation (101). However, IL-22 is not required for lymph node development or for the differentiation of stromal cells in lymph nodes (69). Thus, the requirement for IL-22 also distinguishes the development of iBALT from the development of conventional lymphoid tissues.

Another important difference in the development of lymph nodes and iBALT is the requirement for lymphoid tissue inducer (LTi) cells. LTi cells are a subset of innate lymphoid cells (ILCs) that are dependent on the transcription factors, RORγt and Id2, and express cytokines like TNF, LT, IL-22, and IL-17 (102, 103). LTi cells express CXCR5 and CCR7 and, during embryogenesis, home to developing lymph nodes (104), where they express LTα and LTβ and, through the actions of the LTβR and TNFR1, promote the differentiation of local mesenchymal cells into mature fibroblastic stromal cells that form the scaffold of secondary lymphoid organs (38, 105–109). Importantly, LTi cells are essential for the development of lymph nodes, as mice lacking RORγt or Id2 completely lack lymph nodes and Peyer's patches (102, 110, 111). Given that LTi cells express IL-17, IL-22, and LT, one might expect that these cells would also be required for iBALT formation. However, mice lacking RORγt and Id2 (and therefore lacking LTi cells) generate fully formed iBALT structures in the lungs (78). Thus, LTi cells are not required (although they may be involved) in the development of iBALT (**Figure 2**).

The differential requirement for LTi cells in the development of iBALT and lymph nodes probably reflects the difference in when these tissues are formed. Conventional lymph nodes form during embryogenesis in the absence of antigen or inflammation in an environment that lacks mature B and T cells (8). In contrast, iBALT forms after birth following exposure to antigenic and inflammatory stimuli that trigger the activation of mature lymphocytes. Given that the neonatal lung has mature T cells, such as γδT cells and Tfh cells that express TNF, IL-17, IL-22, and LT (78); these cells may functionally replace LTi cells for promoting iBALT development in postnatal mice.

Although IL-17 promotes the expression of CXCL13 and CXCL12, which in turn recruit B cells and Tfh cells, this process may not entirely explain the role of IL-17 in iBALT formation. For example, IL-17 is most well known for promoting the expression of CXCL9, CXCL10, and CXCL11 (112, 113) as well as cytokines, like G-CSF, that strongly attract inflammatory cells like neutrophils. These chemokines and cytokines are also dramatically upregulated in an IL-17-dependent manner following pulmonary LPS exposure in neonates (78). In fact, large numbers of neutrophils are recruited to the lungs of LPS-exposed neonates and are required for iBALT formation (82). Neutrophils are important for the production of APRIL and IL-21, which maintain B cell activation and survival and thereby help to promote iBALT formation (82). Interestingly, neonates are prone to granulocytosis (114, 115), which may help to explain why the formation of iBALT occurs more easily in this age group.

Other studies also support the role of neurophils in the formatin of iBALT. For example, mice doubly deficient for the genes encoding the NQO1 and NQO2 proteins, two neutrophil-expressed enzymes that limit ROS generation, spontaneously develop iBALT (116). NQO1$^{-/-}$NQO2$^{-/-}$mice have increased numbers of granulocytes in the peripheral blood and, in the lungs, have areas of iBALT with elevated numbers of neutrophils (116). However, it is not clear from these studies whether the elevated production of reactive oxygen directly promotes iBALT or whether the elevated numbers of neutrophils in the lung perform some other function that promotes iBALT formation.

Neutrophils may also play a role in the spontaneous formation of iBALT in Serpine2-deficient (SE2$^{-/-}$) mice. Serpine2 is a protease inhibitor that inhibits proteases like thrombin, trypsin, urokinase plasminogen activator (uPA), and plasmin, but not elastase (117, 118). These mice spontaneously develop iBALT in their lungs as early as 8 weeks after birth (119). The formation of iBALT in SE2$^{-/-}$ mice is associated with the excessive expression of both inflammatory (CXCL9, CXCL10, and CXCL11) and homeostatic (CXCL12, CXCL19, and CCL19) chemokines as well as heightened thrombin activity (119). Importantly, the pulmonary administration of thrombin to the lungs of WT mice promotes an NFkB-dependent increase in chemokine expression from epithelial cells. Thrombin also activates protease-activated receptors (PARs) on neutrophils and endothelial cells and promotes neutrophil chemotaxis (120), suggesting that neutrophils may play a role in this process. Given the role of proteases in COPD, a lung disease in which iBALT may contribute to pathology, it is likely that protease-mediated processes will be an important contributing pathway in iBALT formation.

CD11c-expressing DCs are also important for the formation and the maintenance of iBALT. For example, mice depleted of CD11c-expressing cells rapidly lose existing areas of iBALT (94, 121) and the depletion of CD11c-expressing cells following the pulmonary administration of LPS to neonates prevents iBALT formation (78). Conversely, the pulmonary administration of bone marrow-derived DCs (BMDCs) promotes the formation of iBALT structures (121). CD11c-expressing DCs may promote iBALT formation/maintenance directly by providing LT (121) or indirectly by supporting the activation of T cells and B cells. In addition, depending on how they are activated, DCs are potent sources of IL-23, which acts on ILC3 cells (122, 123), γδT cells (124), and even CD4 T cells (125) to promote their production of IL-17. One caveat to the interpretation of these studies is that alveolar macrophages also express CD11c and will be deleted in CD11c-DTR mice. Moreover, BMDCs are actually a mix of true DCs and macrophages (126). Thus, macrophages may play an important, although poorly understood, role in the development and maintenance of iBALT.

Regulatory T cells (Tregs) limit local immune responses and, not surprisingly, can restrain the formation of iBALT. For example, CCR7-deficient mice spontaneously form iBALT (127), in part, because CCR7-deficient Tregs are poorly recruited to the lymph node, which prevents them from inhibiting effector T cell responses. This process can be mimicked by the blockade of CD62L-dependent lymph node homing (127). However, the interpretation of these studies is complicated. Does poor T cell homing to the lymph node lead to increased homing to the lung, regardless of whether Tregs are working properly? Does depletion of Tregs or impairment of their activity promote autoimmunity and therefore local pulmonary inflammation and the development of iBALT? There is also a connection between Tregs and neutrophils, as the selective depletion of FoxP3$^+$ Tregs in neonatal mice increases the number of neutrophils and promotes iBALT formation (82), whereas the targeted depletion of neutrophils significantly reduces the number and size of iBALT areas following intranasal LPS administration. Thus, Tregs play an inhibitory role in iBALT development consistent with their immunosuppressive activities.

Although the mechanisms that recruit leukocytes to the lung are clearly important in the formation of iBALT, the resolution of pulmonary inflammation will also likely play a role. In other words, if leukocytes are recruited to a site faster than they can be cleared, then they will build up over time and, upon reaching a critical mass, may spontaneously assemble into a lymphoid tissue like iBALT (128). In support of this idea, the treatment of mice with the S1P1R agonist, FTY720, also promotes iBALT development, possibly by retaining cells in the lungs (127). One mechanism for clearing cells from the lung is drainage *via* lymphatic vessels (64), which are concentrated surrounding iBALT areas (64). In fact, infection of mice with *Mycoplasma pulmonis* induces large areas of iBALT and increases the number and volume of intrapulmonary lymphatics (64). The increase in lymphatics is mediated by signaling through VEGF-R2 and VEGF-R3. However, the simultaneous blockade of both receptors does not impede iBALT development (64). These data suggest that differentiation of lung lymphatics and VEGF play a marginal role in the development of iBALT; however, the newly generated lymphatics surrounding iBALT areas are likely to be important in regulating pulmonary inflammation and edema in response to subsequent respiratory infections.

Although the development of iBALT following exposure to microbes or microbial products provides information about normal physiological processes, these types of experiments are complicated to interpret due to the wide array of pathways that may be triggered by infection. To avoid this problem, some investigators have used the reductionist approach of overexpressing individual cytokines in the lung. In three separate reports, all of them using an adenovirus expression system, the forced overexpression of IL-5 (129), human IL-6/IL16R (130), or the IL-6 family member, oncostatin M (OSM) (131) in mouse lungs successfully generated iBALT structures. Interestingly, these pro-inflammatory cytokines have the potential to activate B cells (129, 131–133), which we know are important for the production of LT and the differentiation of lung stromal cells into FDCs. However, the overexpression of OSM and IL-5 also promoted the accumulation of eosinophils in the lungs. Thus, the local activation of eosinophils may functionally replace the role of neutrophils in these circumstances and provide cytokines, reactive oxygen, or proteases that facilitate the formation of iBALT.

TOWARD A MODEL OF iBALT DEVELOPMENT

The formation of iBALT depends on pulmonary infection or inflammation, and it seems that a wide variety of stimuli, including bacteria, viruses, microbial products, allergens, and even tumors, are capable of triggering this process (**Figure 2**). In most cases, repetitive exposures (LPS, allergens), infectious agents (viruses, bacteria), or long-lasting stimuli (particulates) are required, suggesting that a transient inflammatory response is generally not sufficient to promote iBALT formation. Given the diverse nature of the stimuli capable of inducing iBALT formation; it is difficult to find a single pathway that is common to all. However, the recruitment of granulocytes (neutrophils or eosinophils) does seem to be a prominent feature of most models. Importantly, both neutrophils and eosinophils produce a variety of cytokines that help FDC differentiation (TNFα, LTβ), B cell activation (APRIL, IL-6), and promote the recruitment of more neutrophils (IL-23, G-CSF) or eosinophils (eotaxin, IL-5) (134, 135). They also make proteases and reactive oxygen that likely trigger receptors or cause damage in a way that promotes the accumulation of activated lymphocytes (136–138). These processes seem to be particularly active in neonates, perhaps because neonates are prone to heightened neutrophilia (114, 139), have a relatively high frequency of IL-17-producing γδ-T cells (140) or ILCs (103), and a relatively low frequency of Tregs (141–143).

Additional neutrophil functions may also be important for iBALT formation or function. For example, during acute inflammation, neutrophils die *via* Fas-mediated apoptosis (144), and are subsequently cleared by macrophages (145). However, neutrophils may also die in a way that leads to the production of neutrophil extracellular traps (NETs) – a process called NETosis (146). Exposure of neutrophils to reactive-oxygen species as well as activation by LPS, IFNγ, or CXCL8 can favor NETosis over apoptosis (147), and lead to an increase in IL-23 and IL-17 (148), which would favor iBALT formation. A hallmark characteristic of NETs is that neutrophil granule contents (histones, antimicrobial peptides, neutrophil elastase, and cytokines) remain attached to the expulsed DNA (147). Moreover, NET production is associated with lung fibroblast differentiation (149), as well as the processing and bioactivation of IL-33 by elastase (150), which triggers IL-17F production by bronchial epithelial cells (151). Once produced, IL-17 may become trapped on the NETs (149) and further increase the neutrophil recruitment to the lungs and the differentiation/activation of lung stroma, again leading to iBALT formation (**Figure 2**). This idea is consistent with data showing that NETs contribute to the control of pulmonary infection with *Streptococcus suis* in pigs and promote iBALT formation (152, 153).

Although iBALT development is triggered by inflammation, it can be maintained for months in the absence of inflammation by homeostatic mechanisms (78, 154). These mechanisms are the same as those that maintain the structure of conventional lymphoid tissues (**Figure 1**). For example, once B cell follicles are formed, B cells constitutively produce LT and TNF (41), which helps maintain the FDC network, HEVs, and lymphatic vessels (41). In turn, the stromal cells of the B and T cell zones make homeostatic cytokines, like IL-7 (54), and homeostatic chemokines, like CXCL12, CXCL13, CCL19, CCL20, and CCL21 (91), all of which act to recruit lymphocytes, direct their homing to the proper architectural domains, promote their survival and maintain the expression of LT and TNF, which support the stromal cells (91). Thus, once they are established, lymphocytes and stromal cells reinforce each other's survival and differentiation in the absence of inflammatory cytokines or chemokines. Of course, in many chronic inflammatory conditions in the lung, both the inflammatory and homeostatic mechanisms operate simultaneously, which likely leads to continuous iBALT expansion and pathological outcomes.

Many of these same mechanisms are involved in the formation of tertiary lymphoid tissues in a variety of organs other than the lung. For example, tertiary lymphoid organs form in the brains of patients with multiple sclerosis (155, 156). The local expression of homeostatic chemokines, such as CXCL13, CCL19, and CCL21, correlates with the formation of these tissues (157) and soluble LTβR can suppress their formation and ameliorate the symptoms of EAE (156). Moreover, Th17 cells are involved in the pathogenesis of EAE and multiple sclerosis (158), and IL-17 is involved in lymphoid neogenesis by promoting the expression of lymphoid chemokines (19) and for the differentiation of local stromal cells (159). Thus, some of the same inflammatory and homeostatic pathways are involved in the formation of ectopic lymphoid tissues in the lungs and the brain.

Transgenic models also reveal similarities and differences between target organs in the formation of tertiary lymphoid tissues. For example, the pancreas develops tertiary lymphoid tissues, particularly in the context of diabetes (14, 160). CXCL13 is required for the organization of B cell follicles in the pancreas (161, 162), whereas chemokines like CCL21 and CCL19 are involved in recruiting B and T cells to the site and cytokines like IL-7 are important for their survival (49, 163, 164). Again, the LT and TNF signaling pathways are important for the maintenance of chemokine expression and the differentiation of stromal cells (164, 165), but their contribution to inflammation and diabetes is different (166). Interestingly, mice that express a CCL21 transgene in the pancreas develop well-defined ectopic lymphoid tissues, whereas mice expressing CCL21 in the skin do not (167). Thus, although there are clear commonalities in the pathways that promote ectopic lymphoid tissues in different organs, some striking differences that can probably be attributed to the different types of cells present in each target organ.

Exposure to a particular inflammatory stimulus will also likely dictate what pathways are involved in ectopic lymphoid tissue formation. For example, DCs (15, 168), CCL21 (169), and the LTβR (170) are required for the formation of ectopic follicles in the thyroid without a requirement for Id2-dependent LTi cells (15). However, the over-expression of CXCL13 in the gut promotes the formation of isolated lymphoid follicles *via* the recruitment of IL-22-expressing ILC3 cells (171). IL-17 is also involved in the formation of ectopic follicles in the gut (172), suggesting that Th17 responses to commensal organisms are likely driving the formation of tertiary lymphoid tissues in this location. Thus, the local inflammatory milieu and resident cell types likely dictate organ-specific pathways that promote the formation of tertiary lymphoid tissues in each non-lymphoid organ.

ROLE OF iBALT IN PULMONARY IMMUNE RESPONSES TO INFECTION

Given that iBALT structurally resembles conventional secondary lymphoid organs, one might assume that it performs similar functions, i.e., promoting encounters between naive lymphocytes that are recruited from the blood and antigen-presenting cells that have migrated from the lumen of the airways. However, this hypothesis is difficult to demonstrate experimentally. We and others have used LT-deficient mice, which lack conventional secondary lymphoid organs (173), to show that immune responses to a variety of antigens can be initiated directly in the lung (23, 174, 175). For example, LT-deficient mice generate nearly normal primary B and T cell responses to a pulmonary infection with influenza virus (23, 174). Similarly, LT-deficient mice are capable of generating primary immune responses following pulmonary exposure to allergens (176) and *Mycobacterium tuberculosis* (175, 177). Thus, conventional secondary lymphoid organs are not necessary for generating immune responses to the pulmonary antigens and pathogens that have been tested.

Despite their ability to generate primary immune responses, LT-deficient mice are not entirely immunocompetent. In particular, the DCs in LT-deficient mice have defects in survival and migration (178), in part due to poor expression of homeostatic chemokines. As a result, LT-deficient mice succumb to lower doses of influenza and fare worse than their normal counterparts, even though they do make primary immune responses. The generation of bone marrow chimeras (in which WT bone marrow is transferred into LT-deficient mice) circumvents the problems associated with LT deficiency, but does not restore lymph nodes or Peyer's patches. Thus, upon the removal of the spleen, these mice lack all conventional secondary lymphoid organs and are known as Spleen, Lymph node and Peyer's patch-deficient (SLP) mice. Importantly, SLP mice generate primary immune responses to influenza without any delay (23). Immune responses in SLP mice are initiated in the lung, in well-organized areas of iBALT. Moreover, germinal center responses are observed in the lungs of SLP mice and germinal enters can be observed in the B cell follicles of iBALT (69, 155, 179). In addition, influenza-specific memory T cells are generated and maintained in SLP mice, as are long-lived antibody-secreting cells (180). Most surprisingly, influenza-infected SLP mice fare better than WT mice, even in the absence of conventional secondary lymphoid organs (23). This result is likely due to slightly reduced T cell responses in SLP mice, which leads to reduced production of inflammatory cytokines, like TNF and IL-6, both of which contribute to weight loss and morbidity. Thus, iBALT areas in the lung are capable of generating primary immune responses, maintaining memory cells, and reducing morbidity and mortality associated with pulmonary infections.

Once iBALT is formed, it is maintained in the lungs for months, often in the absence of the original stimulus that triggered its formation (78). Moreover, once iBALT is formed, it acts like any other lymphoid organ and can recruit naive B and T cells and support their activation in response to antigens that are unrelated to the antigens that triggered iBALT formation. For instance, iBALT generated in response to *Mycobacterium tuberculosis* infection can recruit naive OVA-specific CD4 T cells and support their activation upon subsequent pulmonary exposure to OVA, without contributions from conventional secondary lymphoid organs (175, 177). Moreover, the transfer of DCs loaded with OVA peptide to mice in which iBALT was induced following pulmonary infection with MVA primes naive OVA-specific CD8 T cells in the lung (23, 65). Together, these data suggest that the specificity of naive T cell priming can be different from the antigenic stimulation that initially induced iBALT.

The presence of iBALT in normal mice also has dramatic consequences on the resulting immune response and clinical outcomes. For example, mice that have iBALT induced by pulmonary instillation of protein nanoparticles clear virus more rapidly and lose less weight following influenza infection (67, 181). In these mice, the kinetics of influenza-specific $CD4^+$ T cells in the lymph node parallels that in the lung, suggesting that they are being primed in both locations simultaneously (67). The presence of iBALT also provides a beneficial effect with SARS-coronavirus and pneumovirus, which are cleared more rapidly in mice with iBALT by an accelerated antibody response (181). Similarly, mice that have iBALT induced as a result of neonatal LPS exposure lose less weight and clear pneumovirus faster than mice without iBALT (82). Importantly, the CD4 T cell response to pneumovirus is accelerated in mice with iBALT (82) suggesting that the presence of iBALT in the lung leads to faster, more efficient pulmonary immune responses that promote rapid viral clearance and reduce morbidity after infection. Thus, iBALT is beneficial in the context of respiratory virus infection.

The presence of iBALT is also protective in the context of bacterial infections. For example, intranasal vaccination with LPS and recombinant porin B from *Francisella tulerensis* induces highly organized iBALT structures (182) and confers improved survival and more efficient bacterial control upon challenge with the *Francisella tulerensis* vaccine strain (182). Similarly, iBALT induced with nanoparticles confers protection against subsequent challenge with *Coxiella burnetii* (181).

In addition to its role in resolving acute bacterial infections in the lung, iBALT also helps control chronic pulmonary infection with *Mycobacteria tuberculosis* (MTB). A hallmark of MTB infection is the formation of granulomas, clusters of lymphocytes that surround MTB-infected macrophages and contain infection (183). Granulomas exhibit many of the features of iBALT and B cell follicles containing germinal centers, and FDCs are often observed in MTB granulomas in mice (87, 184–186), humans (187), and monkeys (186, 188). Monkeys with latent MTB infection maintain large, well-organized areas of iBALT surrounding granulomas (186), whereas monkeys with active disease have fewer and less organized areas of iBALT. Thus, the maintenance of good iBALT structures seems to be important for the control of MTB. In fact, the activity of iBALT is sufficient to prime MTB-specific IFNγ-producing CD4 T cells and control infection, without contributions from conventional secondary lymphoid organs (175).

In fact, chronic pulmonary infection with MTB progressively leads to iBALT development, with progressive increases in the expression of both CCL19 and CXCL13 (87, 185). Importantly, the loss of these chemokines in $CXCL13^{-/-}$ mice or *plt/plt* mice (lacking both CCL19 and CCL21) leads to disrupted iBALT architecture and delayed granuloma formation (185). CXCL13 seems to be most important for generating proper granulomas and for recruiting CXCR5-expressing T cells to the lungs (185), whereas granuloma formation is relatively normal in *plt/plt* mice, but the Th1 response is delayed (185). Consistent with the poor immune response in these mice, the titers of MTB are higher in the lungs of both $CXCL13^{-/-}$ mice and in *plt/plt* mice and are even higher in the lungs of $CXCL13^{-/-}$ x *plt/plt* mice.

Given that CXCL13 expression depends on IL-17 during pulmonary inflammatory conditions it is not surprising that IL-17 is important in immunity to MTB following vaccination (184). In fact, intranasal vaccination of mice with MTB in combination with type II heat labile enterotoxin, elicits MTB-specific Th17 cells (100). Upon subsequent challenge with MTB, the memory Th17 cells elicit pulmonary expression of CXCL13, which recruits CXCR5-expressing T cells to the granuloma (100, 186). Consequently, MTB-specific Th1 cells activate macrophages and control infection.

Although iBALT seems consistently beneficial in the context of experimental models of infection, children and young adults with chronic or recurrent pneumonia develop iBALT areas in their lungs that are associated with bronchiolar damage (189), indicating that iBALT may contribute to bronchial pathology. Moreover, it is described in rabbits that collagens in the deeper layers of the bronchial wall are disrupted when iBALT is present (75), again supporting an association in pathologic context. However, the actual function of iBALT in these cases is difficult to assess.

iBALT IN CHRONIC PULMONARY DISEASES

Patients with chronic pulmonary diseases often develop areas of iBALT. For example, patients with Chronic Obstructive Pulmonary Disease (COPD) develop areas of iBALT adjacent to their small airways (190). In fact, the Global Initiative for Chronic Obstructive Lung Disease (GOLD) has classified COPD patients into five-stages based on airflow limitation (191), and there is a strong correlation between the patients in GOLD stages 3 and 4 (severe and very severe) with the percentage of iBALT follicles in the airway and lymphocyte infiltration, compared to GOLD stages 1 and 2 (mild and moderate) patients (192). These studies also show a positive correlation between CXCL13 expression and lymphoid follicle density (192), suggesting that B cells accumulate in iBALT-like areas *via* a CXCL13-dependent mechanism. Interestingly, B cells in the iBALT areas of COPD patients may be capable of making their own CXCL13 (190). However, inflammatory chemokine receptors, such as CXCR3, are also found on B cells of COPD patients (193), suggesting a role of both inflammatory and homeostatic recruitment of B cells. As suggested in other studies, LT is also important for the formation of iBALT in the context of COPD (194, 195). Cytokines like BAFF are also important for the activation or survival of B cells in COPD lungs (196). B cells not only make antibodies but also activate macrophages in the context of COPD (197), which contributes to disease pathology. Similarly, Langerin-expressing DCs are found surrounding iBALT areas in COPD patients (198, 199) and their numbers positively correlate with the severity of COPD (199, 200). Consistent with these observations, mouse models of chronic cigarette smoke-induced COPD also identify iBALT areas in the lungs (89), and the numbers of iBALT areas are greater in mice exposed for longer periods.

Given that iBALT is associated with the most severe forms of COPD (192, 201), one could argue that iBALT contributes to pathology and is detrimental for the host. Conversely, one could argue that the elevated inflammation and lung damage in patients with more severe COPD promote iBALT formation. Consistent with this idea, patients with COPD often have elevated expression of thrombin in their airways (202, 203), which is associated with pulmonary inflammation and damage (204, 205). Interestingly, mice lacking the Serine Protease Inhibitor, SERPINE2, spontaneously develop chronic pulmonary inflammation and form iBALT-like structures in their lungs (119). Thus, pathways of damage and inflammation in chronic lung disease may promote iBALT. Finally, patients with COPD often develop bacterial infections in their lung, which exacerbates disease (206). Thus, iBALT may form as a consequence of infection and, based on studies in mice, may actually be providing a benefit to the patient, despite the severity of disease.

The development of iBALT is also associated with another chronic lung condition, hypersensitivity pneumonitis. Hypersensitivity pneumonitis is caused by a chronic exposure to environmental organic dusts or molds, resulting in immune-driven inflammation (207). Often referred to as "farmer's lung" hypersensitivity pneumonitis is typically the result of repeated exposure to a particular pulmonary antigen, such as moldy hay. Thus, iBALT structures in the lungs of hypersensitivity pneumonitis patients are often very reactive and contain enormous germinal centers (208, 209).

Given the dramatic enlargement of iBALT areas in an antigen-driven disease like hypersensitivity pneumonitis, one might expect that patients with allergen-driven asthma would also develop extensive areas of iBALT. In fact, the appearance of iBALT-like structures (isolated aggregations of lymphoid cells or IALC) is observed in asthmatic patients and is greater in number and size compared to those in non-asthmatics (210). In addition, the appearance of iBALT-like areas in asthmatics correlates with airway wall thickening and increases in eosinophil infiltration. Furthermore, the progressive organization of iBALT positively correlates with the severity of asthma symptoms, suggesting that iBALT may be responding to external antigens and exacerbating pulmonary pathology. Similarly, patients with allergic bronchopulmonary aspergillosis also develop iBALT areas, some of which have allergen-specific IgE-expressing B cells in the germinal centers (211), again suggesting an involvement of iBALT in pathology. These observations can be mimicked in mice by sensitization and pulmonary challenge with OVA, which promotes the differentiation of OVA-specific, IgE-secreting plasma cells in iBALT structures in the lungs and increases airway hyperresponsiveness (90). However, the presence of iBALT does not always correlate with the development or progression of allergy or asthma, as a study of cross-country skiers finds iBALT at a similar frequency in normal and asthmatic individuals (independent of smoking status) and does not correlate iBALT with either respiratory allergy or airway hyperresponsiveness (212). Thus, the causal relationship between iBALT and pulmonary allergies or asthma remains enigmatic.

Well-developed iBALT is also commonly found in patients with pulmonary complications of rheumatoid arthritis (RA) (208). These structures are highly reactive, with polarized germinal centers that nearly fill the B cell follicles. Plasma cells secreting antibodies specific for citrullinated proteins are found surrounding the iBALT areas. Given that antibodies against citrullinated proteins are highly specific for RA (213) and are known to be pathologic (214), these data suggest that iBALT areas are contributing to autoimmune disease. Similar structures are observed in a subset of patients with pulmonary manifestations of Sjogren's syndrome (SS) (208). SS is also an autoimmune disease that is characterized with an autoantibody production (215). Interestingly, the lungs of both RA and SS patients with pulmonary disease have extraordinary increases in the expression of the chemokines, CXCL13 and CXCL12 (216), which likely contribute to the recruitment of lymphocytes and the formation of iBALT areas in the lung, comparable to what is observed in the salivary glands of SS patients (217). Again, these data suggest that iBALT contributes to the local production of autoantibodies and correlates with local pathology.

Immune responses against transplanted organs are similar to autoimmune responses in that alloantigens, like autoantigens, persist forever – sometimes promoting the development of ectopic lymphoid tissues like iBALT (218). For instance, iBALT is observed around small airways in a rat model of orthotopic lung transplantation (219) and, given the local immune reactivity, is thought to contribute to the rejection of the transplanted lungs. Similarly transplanted hearts and kidneys also develop ectopic lymphoid tissues that are associated with the production of antibodies directed against donor MHC-I molecules (220). Interestingly, treatment of heart allograft recipients with LTβR–Ig fusion protein abolished the formation of tertiary lymphoid tissues, attenuated the autoantibody response, and prevented graft rejection (221), suggesting again that local lymphoid tissues play a role in local immune reactivity. However, the long-term acceptance of lung allografts is also associated with the formation of iBALT (222). In this case, the acceptance of the graft is dependent on the accumulation of $Foxp3^+$ Tregs that accumulate in iBALT areas. Thus, the formation of iBALT can promote tolerance (222) as well as immune reactivity and understanding how it might perform these functions will be important for future studies to determine.

Local immune reactivity and the formation of ectopic lymphoid tissues are also important for immunity against tumors (223). For example, some patients with non-small-cell lung cancer (NSCLC) develop lymphocyte clusters, called tumor-induced BALT (Ti-BALT) (224), which are associated with more favorable clinical outcomes. Presumably, DCs within Ti-BALT present tumor-associated antigens to T cells and enhance the efficiency of the immune response. In addition, ILC3 that express natural cytotoxicity receptors (NCRs) accumulate in Ti-BALT, and their frequency positively correlates with Ti-BALT formation and negatively correlates with tumor growth (225). Thus, in this context, the presence of iBALT is associated with productive immunity rather than tolerance.

HOW DOES BALT DO IT?

There is little doubt that iBALT promotes productive immunity to a wide variety of infectious agents. It also correlates with inflammatory lung diseases, immunity against lung tumors, and transplant rejection. These data might suggest that the presence of iBALT leads to bigger and faster immune responses, which would be "good" for immunity against infection and "bad" for autoimmunity and chronic inflammation. However, there are clear instances in which iBALT correlates with tolerance against allografts and may even reduce inflammation associated with inflammatory diseases like asthma. Thus, the function(s) of iBALT are much more complex than initially thought.

How might iBALT accelerate immune responses and simultaneously suppress inflammatory responses? One possible mechanism involves the formation of additional lymphatic vessels around the iBALT follicles (64, 208), which by efficiently gathering pulmonary DCs, might accelerate immune responses and concentrate the local inflammatory response in the areas of iBALT – away from the remainder of the lung parenchyma. One can envision this process as sequestering antigens, pathogens, and cells in iBALT areas in order to control inflammation and pathology and also to efficiently eliminate or contain pathogens, like MTB. In fact, static imaging shows that inhaled antigens and particulates, such as diesel exhaust (88) or silica (226) accumulate in iBALT areas, effectively sequestering them and potentially reducing their ability to trigger inflammation.

A similar mechanism may be acting in $CCR7^{-/-}$ mice, which spontaneously develop iBALT in the context of rheumatoid lung disease (127, 195), but are simultaneously protected from developing bleomycin-induced pulmonary fibrosis (227). In addition, mice that develop iBALT as a consequence of autoimmunity are also protected from bleomycin-induced fibrosis (228). One possible explanation for these results is that following bleomycin administration, the iBALT areas rapidly sequester the drug or efficiently drain it out of the lung *via* lymphatics, thereby reducing its ability to trigger a fibrotic response.

One can extend this idea to antigens and allergens that are taken up by phagocytic cells in the lung. The areas of iBALT may efficiently collect antigen-bearing DCs or macrophages *via* lymphatics or other mechanisms, promoting their concentration in areas devoted to T and B cell priming, and simultaneously depleting them from the rest of the lung. In fact, plasmacytoid DCs (pDCs) in patients with asthma and in patients with mild moderate COPD are found concentrated in iBALT areas of the lung (229) where they may promote the local differentiation of Tregs (230, 231). In addition, lymphatic vessels in iBALT provide a survival niche for memory CD4 T cells by providing IL-7. Interestingly, lymphatic endothelial cells also produce cytokines like IL-33 as well as chemokines like CCL21 (68), all of which may contribute to trafficking, activation, and survival of lymphocytes. These possibilities highlight the potential regulatory function of iBALT in the context of inflammatory diseases.

CONCLUDING REMARKS

The delicate mucosal surface of the lung is constantly exposed to pathogens and environmental antigens, but in most cases manages to generate immune responses that are sufficient to clear pathogens without causing undue damage. The presence of iBALT clearly plays a role in this process by modulating local immune responses in a way that accelerates immunity to pathogens and, in some cases, ameliorating chronic inflammation. One might argue that iBALT achieves both these effects by sequestering antigens and cells in small areas of lymphoid tissue in the lung. However, the factors that control the activity of iBALT are unclear and will undoubtedly be the focus of future studies. Once we understand the pathways that control the development and function of iBALT, we may be able to target therapies that promote or inhibit these activities, depending on the context.

AUTHOR CONTRIBUTIONS

All authors listed, have made substantial, direct and intellectual contribution to the work, and approved it for publication.

FUNDING

This work was supported by grants, HL69409, AI100127, AI097357, and AR48311 from the National Institutes of Health.

REFERENCES

1. Goodnow CC. Chance encounters and organized rendezvous. *Immunol Rev* (1997) 156:5–10. doi:10.1111/j.1600-065X.1997.tb00954.x
2. MacLennan IC, Gulbranson-Judge A, Toellner KM, Casamayor-Palleja M, Chan E, Sze DM, et al. The changing preference of T and B cells for partners as T-dependent antibody responses develop. *Immunol Rev* (1997) 156:53–66. doi:10.1111/j.1600-065X.1997.tb00958.x
3. Danilova N. The evolution of adaptive immunity. *Adv Exp Med Biol* (2012) 738:218–35. doi:10.1007/978-1-4614-1680-7_13
4. Girard JP, Moussion C, Forster R. HEVs, lymphatics and homeostatic immune cell trafficking in lymph nodes. *Nat Rev Immunol* (2012) 12:762–73. doi:10.1038/nri3298
5. Boehm T, Hess I, Swann JB. Evolution of lymphoid tissues. *Trends Immunol* (2012) 33:315–21. doi:10.1016/j.it.2012.02.005
6. Amemiya CT, Saha NR, Zapata A. Evolution and development of immunological structures in the lamprey. *Curr Opin Immunol* (2007) 19:535–41. doi:10.1016/j.coi.2007.08.003
7. Rast JP, Buckley KM. Lamprey immunity is far from primitive. *Proc Natl Acad Sci U S A* (2013) 110:5746–7. doi:10.1073/pnas.1303541110
8. Rennert PD, Browning JL, Mebius R, Mackay F, Hochman PS. Surface lymphotoxin alpha/beta complex is required for the development of peripheral lymphoid organs. *J Exp Med* (1996) 184:1999–2006. doi:10.1084/jem.184.5.1999
9. Randall TD, Mebius RE. The development and function of mucosal lymphoid tissues: a balancing act with micro-organisms. *Mucosal Immunol* (2014) 7:455–66. doi:10.1038/mi.2014.11
10. Hashi H, Yoshida H, Honda K, Fraser S, Kubo H, Awane M, et al. Compartmentalization of Peyer's patch anlagen before lymphocyte entry. *J Immunol* (2001) 166:3702–9. doi:10.4049/jimmunol.166.6.3702
11. Nishikawa S, Nishikawa S, Honda K, Hashi H, Yoshida H. Peyer's patch organogenesis as a programmed inflammation: a hypothetical model. *Cytokine Growth Factor Rev* (1998) 9:213–20. doi:10.1016/S1359-6101(98)00014-8
12. Krege J, Seth S, Hardtke S, Davalos-Misslitz AC, Forster R. Antigen-dependent rescue of nose-associated lymphoid tissue (NALT) development independent of LTbetaR and CXCR5 signaling. *Eur J Immunol* (2009) 39:2765–78. doi:10.1002/eji.200939422
13. Pospisil R, Mage RG. Rabbit appendix: a site of development and selection of the B cell repertoire. *Curr Top Microbiol Immunol* (1998) 229:59–70.
14. Kendall PL, Yu G, Woodward EJ, Thomas JW. Tertiary lymphoid structures in the pancreas promote selection of B lymphocytes in autoimmune diabetes. *J Immunol* (2007) 178:5643–51. doi:10.4049/jimmunol.178.9.5643
15. Marinkovic T, Garin A, Yokota Y, Fu YX, Ruddle NH, Furtado GC, et al. Interaction of mature CD3+CD4+ T cells with dendritic cells triggers the development of tertiary lymphoid structures in the thyroid. *J Clin Invest* (2006) 116:2622–32. doi:10.1172/JCI28993
16. Weiss JM, Cufi P, Le Panse R, Berrih-Aknin S. The thymus in autoimmune myasthenia gravis: paradigm for a tertiary lymphoid organ. *Rev Neurol* (2013) 169:640–9. doi:10.1016/j.neurol.2013.02.005
17. Astorri E, Scrivo R, Bombardieri M, Picarelli G, Pecorella I, Porzia A, et al. CX3CL1 and CX3CR1 expression in tertiary lymphoid structures in salivary gland infiltrates: fractalkine contribution to lymphoid neogenesis in Sjogren's syndrome. *Rheumatology* (2014) 53:611–20. doi:10.1093/rheumatology/ket401
18. Barone F, Nayar S, Campos J, Cloake T, Withers DR, Toellner KM, et al. IL-22 regulates lymphoid chemokine production and assembly of tertiary lymphoid organs. *Proc Natl Acad Sci U S A* (2015) 112:11024–9. doi:10.1073/pnas.1503315112
19. Peters A, Pitcher LA, Sullivan JM, Mitsdoerffer M, Acton SE, Franz B, et al. Th17 cells induce ectopic lymphoid follicles in central nervous system tissue inflammation. *Immunity* (2011) 35:986–96. doi:10.1016/j.immuni.2011.10.015
20. Shomer NH, Fox JG, Juedes AE, Ruddle NH. Helicobacter-induced chronic active lymphoid aggregates have characteristics of tertiary lymphoid tissue. *Infect Immun* (2003) 71:3572–7. doi:10.1128/IAI.71.6.3572-3577.2003
21. Pei G, Zeng R, Han M, Liao P, Zhou X, Li Y, et al. Renal interstitial infiltration and tertiary lymphoid organ neogenesis in IgA nephropathy. *Clin J Am Soc Nephrol* (2014) 9:255–64. doi:10.2215/CJN.01150113
22. Ruddle NH. Lymphatic vessels and tertiary lymphoid organs. *J Clin Invest* (2014) 124:953–9. doi:10.1172/JCI71611
23. Moyron-Quiroz JE, Rangel-Moreno J, Kusser K, Hartson L, Sprague F, Goodrich S, et al. Role of inducible bronchus associated lymphoid tissue (iBALT) in respiratory immunity. *Nat Med* (2004) 10:927–34. doi:10.1038/nm1091
24. Randall TD. Bronchus-associated lymphoid tissue (BALT) structure and function. *Adv Immunol* (2010) 107:187–241. doi:10.1016/B978-0-12-381300-8.00007-1
25. Delventhal S, Hensel A, Petzoldt K, Pabst R. Effects of microbial stimulation on the number, size and activity of bronchus-associated lymphoid tissue (BALT) structures in the pig. *Int J Exp Pathol* (1992) 73:351–7.
26. Tschernig T, Pabst R. Bronchus-associated lymphoid tissue (BALT) is not present in the normal adult lung but in different diseases. *Pathobiology* (2000) 68:1–8. doi:10.1159/000028109
27. Gregson RL, Davey MJ, Prentice DE. Bronchus-associated lymphoid tissue (BALT) in the laboratory-bred and wild rat, *Rattus norvegicus*. *Lab Anim* (1979) 13:239–43. doi:10.1258/002367779780937735
28. Jericho KW. Intrapulmonary lymphoid tissue in mink infected with Aleutian disease virus. *Res Vet Sci* (1982) 32:206–12.
29. Gould SJ, Isaacson PG. Bronchus-associated lymphoid tissue (BALT) in human fetal and infant lung. *J Pathol* (1993) 169:229–34. doi:10.1002/path.1711690209
30. Pabst R, Binns RM. The immune system of the respiratory tract in pigs. *Vet Immunol Immunopathol* (1994) 43:151–6. doi:10.1016/0165-2427(94)90131-7
31. Effendy AW, Zamri-Saad M, Maswati MA, Ismail MS, Jamil SM. Stimulation of the bronchus-associated lymphoid tissue of goats and its effect on in vitro colonization by *Pasteurella haemolytica*. *Vet Res Commun* (1998) 22:147–53. doi:10.1023/A:1006064703662
32. Fagerland JA, Arp LH. Structure and development of bronchus-associated lymphoid tissue in conventionally reared broiler chickens. *Avian Dis* (1993) 37:10–8. doi:10.2307/1591451
33. Jeurissen SH, Janse EM, Koch G, De Boer GF. Postnatal development of mucosa-associated lymphoid tissues in chickens. *Cell Tissue Res* (1989) 258:119–24. doi:10.1007/BF00223151
34. Smialek M, Tykalowski B, Stenzel T, Koncicki A. Local immunity of the respiratory mucosal system in chickens and turkeys. *Pol J Vet Sci* (2011) 14:291–7.
35. Gregson RL, Davey MJ, Prentice DE. The response of rat bronchus-associated lymphoid tissue to local antigenic challenge. *Br J Exp Pathol* (1979) 60:471–82.
36. Kawamata N, Xu B, Nishijima H, Aoyama K, Kusumoto M, Takeuchi T, et al. Expression of endothelia and lymphocyte adhesion molecules in bronchus-associated lymphoid tissue (BALT) in adult human lung. *Respir Res* (2009) 10:97. doi:10.1186/1465-9921-10-97
37. Woodland DL, Randall TD. Anatomical features of anti-viral immunity in the respiratory tract. *Semin Immunol* (2004) 16:163–70. doi:10.1016/j.smim.2004.02.003
38. Matsumoto M, Fu YX, Molina H, Chaplin DD. Lymphotoxin-alpha-deficient and TNF receptor-I-deficient mice define developmental and functional characteristics of germinal centers. *Immunol Rev* (1997) 156:137–44. doi:10.1111/j.1600-065X.1997.tb00965.x
39. Endres R, Alimzhanov MB, Plitz T, Futterer A, Kosco-Vilbois MH, Nedospasov SA, et al. Mature follicular dendritic cell networks depend on expression of lymphotoxin beta receptor by radioresistant stromal cells and of lymphotoxin beta and tumor necrosis factor by B cells. *J Exp Med* (1999) 189:159–68. doi:10.1084/jem.189.1.159
40. Futterer A, Mink K, Luz A, Kosco-Vilbois MH, Pfeffer K. The lymphotoxin beta receptor controls organogenesis and affinity maturation in peripheral lymphoid tissues. *Immunity* (1998) 9:59–70. doi:10.1016/S1074-7613(00)80588-9
41. Gonzalez M, Mackay F, Browning JL, Kosco-Vilbois MH, Noelle RJ. The sequential role of lymphotoxin and B cells in the development of splenic follicles. *J Exp Med* (1998) 187:997–1007. doi:10.1084/jem.187.7.997
42. Vinuesa CG, Linterman MA, Goodnow CC, Randall KL. T cells and follicular dendritic cells in germinal center B-cell formation and selection. *Immunol Rev* (2010) 237:72–89. doi:10.1111/j.1600-065X.2010.00937.x
43. Vinuesa CG, Linterman MA, Yu D, MacLennan IC. Follicular helper T cells. *Annu Rev Immunol* (2016) 34:335–68. doi:10.1146/annurev-immunol-041015-055605

44. Pabst R, Tschernig T. Lymphocytes in the lung: an often neglected cell. Numbers, characterization and compartmentalization. *Anat Embryol (Berl)* (1995) 192:293–9. doi:10.1007/BF00710098
45. Muller G, Hopken UE, Lipp M. The impact of CCR7 and CXCR5 on lymphoid organ development and systemic immunity. *Immunol Rev* (2003) 195:117–35. doi:10.1034/j.1600-065X.2003.00073.x
46. Gunn MD, Ngo VN, Ansel KM, Ekland EH, Cyster JG, Williams LT. A B-cell-homing chemokine made in lymphoid follicles activates Burkitt's lymphoma receptor-1. *Nature* (1998) 391:799–803. doi:10.1038/35876
47. Chai Q, Onder L, Scandella E, Gil-Cruz C, Perez-Shibayama C, Cupovic J, et al. Maturation of lymph node fibroblastic reticular cells from myofibroblastic precursors is critical for antiviral immunity. *Immunity* (2013) 38:1013–24. doi:10.1016/j.immuni.2013.03.012
48. Cremasco V, Woodruff MC, Onder L, Cupovic J, Nieves-Bonilla JM, Schildberg FA, et al. B cell homeostasis and follicle confines are governed by fibroblastic reticular cells. *Nat Immunol* (2014) 15:973–81. doi:10.1038/ni.2965
49. Luther SA, Bidgol A, Hargreaves DC, Schmidt A, Xu Y, Paniyadi J, et al. Differing activities of homeostatic chemokines CCL19, CCL21, and CXCL12 in lymphocyte and dendritic cell recruitment and lymphoid neogenesis. *J Immunol* (2002) 169:424–33. doi:10.4049/jimmunol.169.1.424
50. Mori S, Nakano H, Aritomi K, Wang CR, Gunn MD, Kakiuchi T. Mice lacking expression of the chemokines CCL21-ser and CCL19 (plt mice) demonstrate delayed but enhanced T cell immune responses. *J Exp Med* (2001) 193:207–18. doi:10.1084/jem.193.2.207
51. Vassileva G, Soto H, Zlotnik A, Nakano H, Kakiuchi T, Hedrick JA, et al. The reduced expression of 6Ckine in the plt mouse results from the deletion of one of two 6Ckine genes. *J Exp Med* (1999) 190:1183–8. doi:10.1084/jem.190.8.1183
52. Jang MH, Sougawa N, Tanaka T, Hirata T, Hiroi T, Tohya K, et al. CCR7 is critically important for migration of dendritic cells in intestinal lamina propria to mesenteric lymph nodes. *J Immunol* (2006) 176:803–10. doi:10.4049/jimmunol.176.2.803
53. Forster R, Schubel A, Breitfeld D, Kremmer E, Renner-Muller I, Wolf E, et al. CCR7 coordinates the primary immune response by establishing functional microenvironments in secondary lymphoid organs. *Cell* (1999) 99:23–33. doi:10.1016/S0092-8674(00)80059-8
54. Onder L, Narang P, Scandella E, Chai Q, Iolyeva M, Hoorweg K, et al. IL-7-producing stromal cells are critical for lymph node remodeling. *Blood* (2012) 120:4675–83. doi:10.1182/blood-2012-03-416859
55. Link A, Vogt TK, Favre S, Britschgi MR, Acha-Orbea H, Hinz B, et al. Fibroblastic reticular cells in lymph nodes regulate the homeostasis of naive T cells. *Nat Immunol* (2007) 8:1255–65. doi:10.1038/ni1513
56. Rangel-Moreno J, Moyron-Quiroz JE, Hartson L, Kusser K, Randall TD. Pulmonary expression of CXC chemokine ligand 13, CC chemokine ligand 19, and CC chemokine ligand 21 is essential for local immunity to influenza. *Proc Natl Acad Sci U S A* (2007) 104:10577–82. doi:10.1073/pnas.0700591104
57. Miyasaka M, Tanaka T. Lymphocyte trafficking across high endothelial venules: dogmas and enigmas. *Nat Rev Immunol* (2004) 4:360–70. doi:10.1038/nri1354
58. Gorfu G, Rivera-Nieves J, Ley K. Role of beta7 integrins in intestinal lymphocyte homing and retention. *Curr Mol Med* (2009) 9:836–50. doi:10.2174/156652409789105525
59. Sminia T, van der Brugge-Gamelkoorn GJ, Jeurissen SH. Structure and function of bronchus-associated lymphoid tissue (BALT). *Crit Rev Immunol* (1989) 9:119–50.
60. Tango M, Suzuki E, Gejyo F, Ushiki T. The presence of specialized epithelial cells on the bronchus-associated lymphoid tissue (BALT) in the mouse. *Arch Histol Cytol* (2000) 63:81–9. doi:10.1679/aohc.63.81
61. Mowat AM, Viney JL. The anatomical basis of intestinal immunity. *Immunol Rev* (1997) 156:145–66. doi:10.1111/j.1600-065X.1997.tb00966.x
62. van der Brugge-Gamelkoorn GJ, van de Ende M, Sminia T. Changes occurring in the epithelium covering the bronchus-associated lymphoid tissue of rats after intratracheal challenge with horseradish peroxidase. *Cell Tissue Res* (1986) 245:439–44. doi:10.1007/BF00213952
63. Kretschmer S, Dethlefsen I, Hagner-Benes S, Marsh LM, Garn H, Konig P. Visualization of intrapulmonary lymph vessels in healthy and inflamed murine lung using CD90/Thy-1 as a marker. *PLoS One* (2013) 8:e55201. doi:10.1371/journal.pone.0055201
64. Baluk P, Adams A, Phillips K, Feng J, Hong YK, Brown MB, et al. Preferential lymphatic growth in bronchus-associated lymphoid tissue in sustained lung inflammation. *Am J Pathol* (2014) 184:1577–92. doi:10.1016/j.ajpath.2014.01.021
65. Halle S, Dujardin HC, Bakocevic N, Fleige H, Danzer H, Willenzon S, et al. Induced bronchus-associated lymphoid tissue serves as a general priming site for T cells and is maintained by dendritic cells. *J Exp Med* (2009) 206:2593–601. doi:10.1084/jem.20091472
66. Picker LJ. Mechanisms of lymphocyte homing. *Curr Opin Immunol* (1992) 4:277–86. doi:10.1016/0952-7915(92)90077-R
67. Richert LE, Harmsen AL, Rynda-Apple A, Wiley JA, Servid AE, Douglas T, et al. Inducible bronchus-associated lymphoid tissue (iBALT) synergizes with local lymph nodes during antiviral CD4+ T cell responses. *Lymphat Res Biol* (2013) 11:196–202. doi:10.1089/lrb.2013.0015
68. Shinoda K, Hirahara K, Iinuma T, Ichikawa T, Suzuki AS, Sugaya K, et al. Thy1+IL-7+ lymphatic endothelial cells in iBALT provide a survival niche for memory T-helper cells in allergic airway inflammation. *Proc Natl Acad Sci U S A* (2016) 113:E2842–51. doi:10.1073/pnas.1512600113
69. Randall TD, Carragher DM, Rangel-Moreno J. Development of secondary lymphoid organs. *Annu Rev Immunol* (2008) 26:627–50. doi:10.1146/annurev.immunol.26.021607.090257
70. Delventhal S, Brandis A, Ostertag H, Pabst R. Low incidence of bronchus-associated lymphoid tissue (BALT) in chronically inflamed human lungs. *Virchows Arch B Cell Pathol Incl Mol Pathol* (1992) 62:271–4. doi:10.1007/BF02899692
71. Hiller AS, Tschernig T, Kleemann WJ, Pabst R. Bronchus-associated lymphoid tissue (BALT) and larynx-associated lymphoid tissue (LALT) are found at different frequencies in children, adolescents and adults. *Scand J Immunol* (1998) 47:159–62. doi:10.1046/j.1365-3083.1998.00276.x
72. Pabst R, Gehrke I. Is the bronchus-associated lymphoid tissue (BALT) an integral structure of the lung in normal mammals, including humans? *Am J Respir Cell Mol Biol* (1990) 3:131–5. doi:10.1165/ajrcmb/3.2.131
73. Tschernig T, Kleemann WJ, Pabst R. Bronchus-associated lymphoid tissue (BALT) in the lungs of children who had died from sudden infant death syndrome and other causes. *Thorax* (1995) 50:658–60. doi:10.1136/thx.50.6.658
74. Bienenstock J. Bronchus-associated lymphoid tissue. *Int Arch Allergy Appl Immunol* (1985) 76(Suppl 1):62–9. doi:10.1159/000233736
75. Bienenstock J, Johnston N, Perey DY. Bronchial lymphoid tissue. I. Morphologic characteristics. *Lab Invest* (1973) 28:686–92.
76. Simecka JW, Davis JK, Cassell GH. Distribution of Ia antigens and T lymphocyte subpopulations in rat lungs. *Immunology* (1986) 57:93–8.
77. Gregson RL, Davey MJ, Prentice DE. Postnatal development of bronchus-associated lymphoid tissue (BALT) in the rat, *Rattus norvegicus*. *Lab Anim* (1979) 13:231–8. doi:10.1258/002367779780937870
78. Rangel-Moreno J, Carragher DM, de la Luz Garcia-Hernandez M, Hwang JY, Kusser K, Hartson L, et al. The development of inducible bronchus-associated lymphoid tissue depends on IL-17. *Nat Immunol* (2011) 12:639–46. doi:10.1038/ni.2053
79. Barman NN, Bhattacharyya R, Upadhyaya TN, Baishya G. Development of bronchus-associated lymphoid tissue in goats. *Lung* (1996) 174:127–31. doi:10.1007/BF00177706
80. Holt PG. Development of bronchus associated lymphoid tissue (BALT) in human lung disease: a normal host defence mechanism awaiting therapeutic exploitation? *Thorax* (1993) 48:1097–8. doi:10.1136/thx.48.11.1097
81. Jericho KW, Derbyshire JB, Jones JE. Intrapulmonary lymphoid tissue of pigs exposed to aerosols of haemolytic streptococcus group L and porcine adenovirus. *J Comp Pathol* (1971) 81:1–11. doi:10.1016/0021-9975(71)90049-1
82. Foo SY, Zhang V, Lalwani A, Lynch JP, Zhuang A, Lam CE, et al. Regulatory T cells prevent inducible BALT formation by dampening neutrophilic inflammation. *J Immunol* (2015) 194:4567–76. doi:10.4049/jimmunol.1400909
83. Ersch J, Tschernig T, Stallmach T. Frequency and potential cause of bronchus-associated lymphoid tissue in fetal lungs. *Pediatr Allergy Immunol* (2005) 16:295–8. doi:10.1111/j.1399-3038.2005.00269.x
84. Cupedo T, Jansen W, Kraal G, Mebius RE. Induction of secondary and tertiary lymphoid structures in the skin. *Immunity* (2004) 21:655–67. doi:10.1016/j.immuni.2004.09.006

85. Stahl FR, Heller K, Halle S, Keyser KA, Busche A, Marquardt A, et al. Nodular inflammatory foci are sites of T cell priming and control of murine cytomegalovirus infection in the neonatal lung. *PLoS Pathog* (2013) 9:e1003828. doi:10.1371/journal.ppat.1003828
86. Stahl FR, Keyser KA, Heller K, Bischoff Y, Halle S, Wagner K, et al. Mck2-dependent infection of alveolar macrophages promotes replication of MCMV in nodular inflammatory foci of the neonatal lung. *Mucosal Immunol* (2015) 8:57–67. doi:10.1038/mi.2014.42
87. Kahnert A, Hopken UE, Stein M, Bandermann S, Lipp M, Kaufmann SH. *Mycobacterium tuberculosis* triggers formation of lymphoid structure in murine lungs. *J Infect Dis* (2007) 195:46–54. doi:10.1086/508894
88. Hiramatsu K, Azuma A, Kudoh S, Desaki M, Takizawa H, Sugawara I. Inhalation of diesel exhaust for three months affects major cytokine expression and induces bronchus-associated lymphoid tissue formation in murine lungs. *Exp Lung Res* (2003) 29:607–22. doi:10.1080/01902140390240140
89. van der Strate BW, Postma DS, Brandsma CA, Melgert BN, Luinge MA, Geerlings M, et al. Cigarette smoke-induced emphysema: a role for the B cell? *Am J Respir Crit Care Med* (2006) 173:751–8. doi:10.1164/rccm.200504-594OC
90. Chvatchko Y, Kosco-Vilbois MH, Herren S, Lefort J, Bonnefoy JY. Germinal center formation and local immunoglobulin E (IgE) production in the lung after an airway antigenic challenge. *J Exp Med* (1996) 184:2353–60. doi:10.1084/jem.184.6.2353
91. Ngo VN, Korner H, Gunn MD, Schmidt KN, Riminton DS, Cooper MD, et al. Lymphotoxin alpha/beta and tumor necrosis factor are required for stromal cell expression of homing chemokines in B and T cell areas of the spleen. *J Exp Med* (1999) 189:403–12. doi:10.1084/jem.189.2.403
92. Perros F, Dorfmuller P, Montani D, Hammad H, Waelput W, Girerd B, et al. Pulmonary lymphoid neogenesis in idiopathic pulmonary arterial hypertension. *Am J Respir Crit Care Med* (2012) 185:311–21. doi:10.1164/rccm.201105-0927OC
93. Hautefort A, Girerd B, Montani D, Cohen-Kaminsky S, Price L, Lambrecht BN, et al. T-helper 17 cell polarization in pulmonary arterial hypertension. *Chest* (2015) 147:1610–20. doi:10.1378/chest.14-1678
94. Fleige H, Ravens S, Moschovakis GL, Bolter J, Willenzon S, Sutter G, et al. IL-17-induced CXCL12 recruits B cells and induces follicle formation in BALT in the absence of differentiated FDCs. *J Exp Med* (2014) 211:643–51. doi:10.1084/jem.20131737
95. Fletcher HA, Pathan AA, Berthoud TK, Dunachie SJ, Whelan KT, Alder NC, et al. Boosting BCG vaccination with MVA85A down-regulates the immunoregulatory cytokine TGF-beta1. *Vaccine* (2008) 26:5269–75. doi:10.1016/j.vaccine.2008.07.040
96. Price PJ, Banki Z, Scheideler A, Stoiber H, Verschoor A, Sutter G, et al. Complement component C5 recruits neutrophils in the absence of C3 during respiratory infection with modified vaccinia virus Ankara. *J Immunol* (2015) 194:1164–8. doi:10.4049/jimmunol.1301410
97. Grogan JL, Ouyang W. A role for Th17 cells in the regulation of tertiary lymphoid follicles. *Eur J Immunol* (2012) 42:2255–62. doi:10.1002/eji.201242656
98. Khader SA, Guglani L, Rangel-Moreno J, Gopal R, Junecko BA, Fountain JJ, et al. IL-23 is required for long-term control of *Mycobacterium tuberculosis* and B cell follicle formation in the infected lung. *J Immunol* (2011) 187:5402–7. doi:10.4049/jimmunol.1101377
99. Eidenschenk C, Rutz S, Liesenfeld O, Ouyang W. Role of IL-22 in microbial host defense. *Curr Top Microbiol Immunol* (2014) 380:213–36. doi:10.1007/978-3-662-43492-5_10
100. Gopal R, Rangel-Moreno J, Slight S, Lin Y, Nawar HF, Fallert Junecko BA, et al. Interleukin-17-dependent CXCL13 mediates mucosal vaccine-induced immunity against tuberculosis. *Mucosal Immunol* (2013) 6:972–84. doi:10.1038/mi.2012.135
101. Corneth OB, Reijmers RM, Mus AM, Asmawidjaja PS, van Hamburg JP, Papazian N, et al. Loss of IL-22 inhibits autoantibody formation in collagen-induced arthritis in mice. *Eur J Immunol* (2016) 46(6):1404–14. doi:10.1002/eji.201546241
102. Eberl G, Littman DR. The role of the nuclear hormone receptor RORgammat in the development of lymph nodes and Peyer's patches. *Immunol Rev* (2003) 195:81–90. doi:10.1034/j.1600-065X.2003.00074.x
103. Cupedo T, Kraal G, Mebius RE. The role of CD45+CD4+CD3- cells in lymphoid organ development. *Immunol Rev* (2002) 189:41–50. doi:10.1034/j.1600-065X.2002.18905.x
104. van de Pavert SA, Olivier BJ, Goverse G, Vondenhoff MF, Greuter M, Beke P, et al. Chemokine CXCL13 is essential for lymph node initiation and is induced by retinoic acid and neuronal stimulation. *Nat Immunol* (2009) 10:1193–9. doi:10.1038/ni.1789
105. Matsumoto M, Mariathasan S, Nahm MH, Baranyay F, Peschon JJ, Chaplin DD. Role of lymphotoxin and the type I TNF receptor in the formation of germinal centers. *Science* (1996) 271:1289–91. doi:10.1126/science.271.5253.1289
106. Ngo VN, Cornall RJ, Cyster JG. Splenic T zone development is B cell dependent. *J Exp Med* (2001) 194:1649–60. doi:10.1084/jem.194.11.1649
107. Dubey LK, Lebon L, Mosconi I, Yang CY, Scandella E, Ludewig B, et al. Lymphotoxin-dependent B cell-FRC crosstalk promotes De Novo Follicle formation and antibody production following intestinal helminth infection. *Cell Rep* (2016) 15:1527–41. doi:10.1016/j.celrep.2016.04.023
108. Fletcher AL, Acton SE, Knoblich K. Lymph node fibroblastic reticular cells in health and disease. *Nat Rev Immunol* (2015) 15:350–61. doi:10.1038/nri3846
109. Lu TT, Browning JL. Role of the lymphotoxin/LIGHT system in the development and maintenance of reticular networks and vasculature in lymphoid tissues. *Front Immunol* (2014) 5:47. doi:10.3389/fimmu.2014.00047
110. Nagatake T, Fukuyama S, Kim DY, Goda K, Igarashi O, Sato S, et al. Id2-, RORgammat-, and LTbetaR-independent initiation of lymphoid organogenesis in ocular immunity. *J Exp Med* (2009) 206:2351–64. doi:10.1084/jem.20091436
111. Yokota Y, Mansouri A, Mori S, Sugawara S, Adachi S, Nishikawa S, et al. Development of peripheral lymphoid organs and natural killer cells depends on the helix-loop-helix inhibitor Id2. *Nature* (1999) 397:702–6. doi:10.1038/17812
112. McAleer JP, Kolls JK. Directing traffic: IL-17 and IL-22 coordinate pulmonary immune defense. *Immunol Rev* (2014) 260:129–44. doi:10.1111/imr.12183
113. Schwarzenberger P, La Russa V, Miller A, Ye P, Huang W, Zieske A, et al. IL-17 stimulates granulopoiesis in mice: use of an alternate, novel gene therapy-derived method for in vivo evaluation of cytokines. *J Immunol* (1998) 161:6383–9.
114. Manroe BL, Weinberg AG, Rosenfeld CR, Browne R. The neonatal blood count in health and disease. I. Reference values for neutrophilic cells. *J Pediatr* (1979) 95:89–98. doi:10.1016/S0022-3476(79)80096-7
115. Weinberg AG, Rosenfeld CR, Manroe BL, Browne R. Neonatal blood cell count in health and disease. II. Values for lymphocytes, monocytes, and eosinophils. *J Pediatr* (1985) 106:462–6. doi:10.1016/S0022-3476(85)80681-8
116. Das A, Kole L, Wang L, Barrios R, Moorthy B, Jaiswal AK. BALT development and augmentation of hyperoxic lung injury in mice deficient in NQO1 and NQO2. *Free Radic Biol Med* (2006) 40:1843–56. doi:10.1016/j.freeradbiomed.2006.01.025
117. Bouton MC, Boulaftali Y, Richard B, Arocas V, Michel JB, Jandrot-Perrus M. Emerging role of serpinE2/protease nexin-1 in hemostasis and vascular biology. *Blood* (2012) 119:2452–7. doi:10.1182/blood-2011-10-387464
118. Baker JB, Low DA, Simmer RL, Cunningham DD. Protease-nexin: a cellular component that links thrombin and plasminogen activator and mediates their binding to cells. *Cell* (1980) 21:37–45. doi:10.1016/0092-8674(80)90112-9
119. Solleti SK, Srisuma S, Bhattacharya S, Rangel-Moreno J, Bijli KM, Randall TD, et al. Serpine2 deficiency results in lung lymphocyte accumulation and bronchus-associated lymphoid tissue formation. *FASEB J* (2016). doi:10.1096/fj.201500159R
120. Bizios R, Lai L, Fenton JW II, Malik AB. Thrombin-induced chemotaxis and aggregation of neutrophils. *J Cell Physiol* (1986) 128:485–90. doi:10.1002/jcp.1041280318
121. GeurtsvanKessel CH, Willart MA, Bergen IM, van Rijt LS, Muskens F, Elewaut D, et al. Dendritic cells are crucial for maintenance of tertiary lymphoid structures in the lung of influenza virus-infected mice. *J Exp Med* (2009) 206:2339–49. doi:10.1084/jem.20090410
122. Geremia A, Arancibia-Carcamo CV, Fleming MP, Rust N, Singh B, Mortensen NJ, et al. IL-23-responsive innate lymphoid cells are increased in inflammatory bowel disease. *J Exp Med* (2011) 208:1127–33. doi:10.1084/jem.20101712
123. Buonocore S, Ahern PP, Uhlig HH, Ivanov II, Littman DR, Maloy KJ, et al. Innate lymphoid cells drive interleukin-23-dependent innate intestinal pathology. *Nature* (2010) 464:1371–5. doi:10.1038/nature08949
124. Sutton CE, Lalor SJ, Sweeney CM, Brereton CF, Lavelle EC, Mills KH. Interleukin-1 and IL-23 induce innate IL-17 production from gammadelta

T cells, amplifying Th17 responses and autoimmunity. *Immunity* (2009) 31:331–41. doi:10.1016/j.immuni.2009.08.001

125. Langrish CL, Chen Y, Blumenschein WM, Mattson J, Basham B, Sedgwick JD, et al. IL-23 drives a pathogenic T cell population that induces autoimmune inflammation. *J Exp Med* (2005) 201:233–40. doi:10.1084/jem.20041257
126. Helft J, Bottcher J, Chakravarty P, Zelenay S, Huotari J, Schraml BU, et al. GM-CSF mouse bone marrow cultures comprise a heterogeneous population of CD11c(+)MHCII(+) macrophages and dendritic cells. *Immunity* (2015) 42:1197–211. doi:10.1016/j.immuni.2015.05.018
127. Kocks JR, Davalos-Misslitz AC, Hintzen G, Ohl L, Forster R. Regulatory T cells interfere with the development of bronchus-associated lymphoid tissue. *J Exp Med* (2007) 204:723–34. doi:10.1084/jem.20061424
128. Thaunat O, Kerjaschki D, Nicoletti A. Is defective lymphatic drainage a trigger for lymphoid neogenesis? *Trends Immunol* (2006) 27:441–5. doi:10.1016/j.it.2006.08.003
129. Lee JJ, McGarry MP, Farmer SC, Denzler KL, Larson KA, Carrigan PE, et al. Interleukin-5 expression in the lung epithelium of transgenic mice leads to pulmonary changes pathognomonic of asthma. *J Exp Med* (1997) 185:2143–56. doi:10.1084/jem.185.12.2143
130. Goya S, Matsuoka H, Mori M, Morishita H, Kida H, Kobashi Y, et al. Sustained interleukin-6 signalling leads to the development of lymphoid organ-like structures in the lung. *J Pathol* (2003) 200:82–7. doi:10.1002/path.1321
131. Botelho FM, Rangel-Moreno J, Fritz D, Randall TD, Xing Z, Richards CD. Pulmonary expression of oncostatin M (OSM) promotes inducible BALT formation independently of IL-6, despite a role for IL-6 in OSM-driven pulmonary inflammation. *J Immunol* (2013) 191:1453–64. doi:10.4049/jimmunol.1203318
132. Mizoguchi C, Uehara S, Akira S, Takatsu K. IL-5 induces IgG1 isotype switch recombination in mouse CD38-activated sIgD-positive B lymphocytes. *J Immunol* (1999) 162:2812–9.
133. Kishimoto T. IL-6: from its discovery to clinical applications. *Int Immunol* (2010) 22:347–52. doi:10.1093/intimm/dxq030
134. Ravin KA, Loy M. The eosinophil in infection. *Clin Rev Allergy Immunol* (2015) 50(2):214–27. doi:10.1007/s12016-015-8525-4
135. Tecchio C, Micheletti A, Cassatella MA. Neutrophil-derived cytokines: facts beyond expression. *Front Immunol* (2014) 5:508. doi:10.3389/fimmu.2014.00508
136. Koga H, Miyahara N, Fuchimoto Y, Ikeda G, Waseda K, Ono K, et al. Inhibition of neutrophil elastase attenuates airway hyperresponsiveness and inflammation in a mouse model of secondary allergen challenge: neutrophil elastase inhibition attenuates allergic airway responses. *Respir Res* (2013) 14:8. doi:10.1186/1465-9921-14-8
137. Meyer-Hoffert U, Wiedow O. Neutrophil serine proteases: mediators of innate immune responses. *Curr Opin Hematol* (2011) 18:19–24. doi:10.1097/MOH.0b013e32834115d1
138. Felton JM, Lucas CD, Rossi AG, Dransfield I. Eosinophils in the lung – modulating apoptosis and efferocytosis in airway inflammation. *Front Immunol* (2014) 5:302. doi:10.3389/fimmu.2014.00302
139. Barak Y, Blachar Y, Levin S. Neonatal neutrophilia: possible role of a humoral granulopoietic factor. *Pediatr Res* (1980) 14:1026–8. doi:10.1203/00006450-198009000-00002
140. Hayes SM, Sirr A, Jacob S, Sim GK, Augustin A. Role of IL-7 in the shaping of the pulmonary gamma delta T cell repertoire. *J Immunol* (1996) 156:2723–9.
141. McGrath-Morrow SA, Lee S, Gibbs K, Lopez A, Collaco JM, Neptune E, et al. Immune response to intrapharyngeal LPS in neonatal and juvenile mice. *Am J Respir Cell Mol Biol* (2015) 52:323–31. doi:10.1165/rcmb.2014-0100OC
142. Miethke AG, Saxena V, Shivakumar P, Sabla GE, Simmons J, Chougnet CA. Post-natal paucity of regulatory T cells and control of NK cell activation in experimental biliary atresia. *J Hepatol* (2010) 52:718–26. doi:10.1016/j.jhep.2009.12.027
143. Torow N, Yu K, Hassani K, Freitag J, Schulz O, Basic M, et al. Active suppression of intestinal CD4(+)TCRalphabeta(+) T-lymphocyte maturation during the postnatal period. *Nat Commun* (2015) 6:7725. doi:10.1038/ncomms8725
144. Liles WC, Kiener PA, Ledbetter JA, Aruffo A, Klebanoff SJ. Differential expression of Fas (CD95) and Fas ligand on normal human phagocytes: implications for the regulation of apoptosis in neutrophils. *J Exp Med* (1996) 184:429–40. doi:10.1084/jem.184.2.429
145. Borges VM, Vandivier RW, McPhillips KA, Kench JA, Morimoto K, Groshong SD, et al. TNFalpha inhibits apoptotic cell clearance in the lung, exacerbating acute inflammation. *Am J Physiol Lung Cell Mol Physiol* (2009) 297:L586–95. doi:10.1152/ajplung.90569.2008
146. Remijsen Q, Kuijpers TW, Wirawan E, Lippens S, Vandenabeele P, Vanden Berghe T. Dying for a cause: NETosis, mechanisms behind an antimicrobial cell death modality. *Cell Death Differ* (2011) 18:581–8. doi:10.1038/cdd.2011.1
147. Almyroudis NG, Grimm MJ, Davidson BA, Rohm M, Urban CF, Segal BH. NETosis and NADPH oxidase: at the intersection of host defense, inflammation, and injury. *Front Immunol* (2013) 4:45. doi:10.3389/fimmu.2013.00045
148. Stark MA, Huo Y, Burcin TL, Morris MA, Olson TS, Ley K. Phagocytosis of apoptotic neutrophils regulates granulopoiesis via IL-23 and IL-17. *Immunity* (2005) 22:285–94. doi:10.1016/j.immuni.2005.01.011
149. Chrysanthopoulou A, Mitroulis I, Apostolidou E, Arelaki S, Mikroulis D, Konstantinidis T, et al. Neutrophil extracellular traps promote differentiation and function of fibroblasts. *J Pathol* (2014) 233:294–307. doi:10.1002/path.4359
150. Lefrancais E, Roga S, Gautier V, Gonzalez-de-Peredo A, Monsarrat B, Girard JP, et al. IL-33 is processed into mature bioactive forms by neutrophil elastase and cathepsin G. *Proc Natl Acad Sci U S A* (2012) 109:1673–8. doi:10.1073/pnas.1115884109
151. Fujita J, Kawaguchi M, Kokubu F, Ohara G, Ota K, Huang SK, et al. Interleukin-33 induces interleukin-17F in bronchial epithelial cells. *Allergy* (2012) 67:744–50. doi:10.1111/j.1398-9995.2012.02825.x
152. Soerensen CM, Holmskov U, Aalbaek B, Boye M, Heegaard PM, Nielsen OL. Pulmonary infections in swine induce altered porcine surfactant protein D expression and localization to dendritic cells in bronchial-associated lymphoid tissue. *Immunology* (2005) 115:526–35. doi:10.1111/j.1365-2567.2005.02189.x
153. Zhao J, Lin L, Fu L, Han L, Zhang A. Neutrophils extracellular Taps play an important role in clearance of *Streptococcus suis* in vivo. *Microbiol Immunol* (2016) 60(4):228–33. doi:10.1111/1348-0421.12367
154. Morissette MC, Jobse BN, Thayaparan D, Nikota JK, Shen P, Labiris NR, et al. Persistence of pulmonary tertiary lymphoid tissues and anti-nuclear antibodies following cessation of cigarette smoke exposure. *Respir Res* (2014) 15:49. doi:10.1186/1465-9921-15-49
155. Aloisi F, Pujol-Borrell R. Lymphoid neogenesis in chronic inflammatory diseases. *Nat Rev Immunol* (2006) 6:205–17. doi:10.1038/nri1786
156. Columba-Cabezas S, Griguoli M, Rosicarelli B, Magliozzi R, Ria F, Serafini B, et al. Suppression of established experimental autoimmune encephalomyelitis and formation of meningeal lymphoid follicles by lymphotoxin beta receptor-Ig fusion protein. *J Neuroimmunol* (2006) 179:76–86. doi:10.1016/j.jneuroim.2006.06.015
157. Aloisi F, Columba-Cabezas S, Franciotta D, Rosicarelli B, Magliozzi R, Reynolds R, et al. Lymphoid chemokines in chronic neuroinflammation. *J Neuroimmunol* (2008) 198:106–12. doi:10.1016/j.jneuroim.2008.04.025
158. Gaublomme JT, Yosef N, Lee Y, Gertner RS, Yang LV, Wu C, et al. Single-cell genomics unveils critical regulators of Th17 cell pathogenicity. *Cell* (2015) 163:1400–12. doi:10.1016/j.cell.2015.11.009
159. Pikor NB, Astarita JL, Summers-Deluca L, Galicia G, Qu J, Ward LA, et al. Integration of Th17- and lymphotoxin-derived signals initiates meningeal-resident stromal cell remodeling to propagate neuroinflammation. *Immunity* (2015) 43:1160–73. doi:10.1016/j.immuni.2015.11.010
160. Astorri E, Bombardieri M, Gabba S, Peakman M, Pozzilli P, Pitzalis C. Evolution of ectopic lymphoid neogenesis and in situ autoantibody production in autoimmune nonobese diabetic mice: cellular and molecular characterization of tertiary lymphoid structures in pancreatic islets. *J Immunol* (2010) 185:3359–68. doi:10.4049/jimmunol.1001836
161. Henry RA, Kendall PL. CXCL13 blockade disrupts B lymphocyte organization in tertiary lymphoid structures without altering B cell receptor bias or preventing diabetes in nonobese diabetic mice. *J Immunol* (2010) 185:1460–5. doi:10.4049/jimmunol.0903710
162. Luther SA, Lopez T, Bai W, Hanahan D, Cyster JG. BLC expression in pancreatic islets causes B cell recruitment and lymphotoxin-dependent lymphoid neogenesis. *Immunity* (2000) 12:471–81. doi:10.1016/S1074-7613(00)80199-5
163. Fan L, Reilly CR, Luo Y, Dorf ME, Lo D. Cutting edge: ectopic expression of the chemokine TCA4/SLC is sufficient to trigger lymphoid neogenesis. *J Immunol* (2000) 164:3955–9. doi:10.4049/jimmunol.164.8.3955

164. Luther SA, Ansel KM, Cyster JG. Overlapping roles of CXCL13, interleukin 7 receptor alpha, and CCR7 ligands in lymph node development. *J Exp Med* (2003) 197:1191–8. doi:10.1084/jem.20021294
165. Kratz A, Campos-Neto A, Hanson MS, Ruddle NH. Chronic inflammation caused by lymphotoxin is lymphoid neogenesis. *J Exp Med* (1996) 183:1461–72. doi:10.1084/jem.183.4.1461
166. Picarella DE, Kratz A, Li CB, Ruddle NH, Flavell RA. Transgenic tumor necrosis factor (TNF)-alpha production in pancreatic islets leads to insulitis, not diabetes. Distinct patterns of inflammation in TNF-alpha and TNF-beta transgenic mice. *J Immunol* (1993) 150:4136–50.
167. Chen SC, Vassileva G, Kinsley D, Holzmann S, Manfra D, Wiekowski MT, et al. Ectopic expression of the murine chemokines CCL21a and CCL21b induces the formation of lymph node-like structures in pancreas, but not skin, of transgenic mice. *J Immunol* (2002) 168:1001–8. doi:10.4049/jimmunol.168.3.1001
168. Muniz LR, Pacer ME, Lira SA, Furtado GC. A critical role for dendritic cells in the formation of lymphatic vessels within tertiary lymphoid structures. *J Immunol* (2011) 187:828–34. doi:10.4049/jimmunol.1004233
169. Martin AP, Coronel EC, Sano G, Chen SC, Vassileva G, Canasto-Chibuque C, et al. A novel model for lymphocytic infiltration of the thyroid gland generated by transgenic expression of the CC chemokine CCL21. *J Immunol* (2004) 173:4791–8. doi:10.4049/jimmunol.173.8.4791
170. Furtado GC, Marinkovic T, Martin AP, Garin A, Hoch B, Hubner W, et al. Lymphotoxin beta receptor signaling is required for inflammatory lymphangiogenesis in the thyroid. *Proc Natl Acad Sci U S A* (2007) 104:5026–31. doi:10.1073/pnas.0606697104
171. Marchesi F, Martin AP, Thirunarayanan N, Devany E, Mayer L, Grisotto MG, et al. CXCL13 expression in the gut promotes accumulation of IL-22-producing lymphoid tissue-inducer cells, and formation of isolated lymphoid follicles. *Mucosal Immunol* (2009) 2:486–94. doi:10.1038/mi.2009.113
172. Pearson C, Uhlig HH, Powrie F. Lymphoid microenvironments and innate lymphoid cells in the gut. *Trends Immunol* (2012) 33:289–96. doi:10.1016/j.it.2012.04.004
173. De Togni P, Goellner J, Ruddle NH, Streeter PR, Fick A, Mariathasan S, et al. Abnormal development of peripheral lymphoid organs in mice deficient in lymphotoxin. *Science* (1994) 264:703–7. doi:10.1126/science.8171322
174. Lund FE, Partida-Sanchez S, Lee BO, Kusser KL, Hartson L, Hogan RJ, et al. Lymphotoxin-alpha-deficient mice make delayed, but effective, T and B cell responses to influenza. *J Immunol* (2002) 169:5236–43. doi:10.4049/jimmunol.169.9.5236
175. Day TA, Koch M, Nouailles G, Jacobsen M, Kosmiadi GA, Miekley D, et al. Secondary lymphoid organs are dispensable for the development of T-cell-mediated immunity during tuberculosis. *Eur J Immunol* (2010) 40:1663–73. doi:10.1002/eji.201040299
176. Constant SL, Brogdon JL, Piggott DA, Herrick CA, Visintin I, Ruddle NH, et al. Resident lung antigen-presenting cells have the capacity to promote Th2 T cell differentiation in situ. *J Clin Invest* (2002) 110:1441–8. doi:10.1172/JCI0216109
177. Kashino SS, Vallerskog T, Martens G, Troudt J, Keyser A, Taylor J, et al. Initiation of acquired immunity in the lungs of mice lacking lymph nodes after infection with aerosolized *Mycobacterium tuberculosis*. *Am J Pathol* (2010) 176:198–204. doi:10.2353/ajpath.2010.090446
178. Kabashima K, Banks TA, Ansel KM, Lu TT, Ware CF, Cyster JG. Intrinsic lymphotoxin-beta receptor requirement for homeostasis of lymphoid tissue dendritic cells. *Immunity* (2005) 22:439–50. doi:10.1016/j.immuni.2005.02.007
179. Mebius RE. Organogenesis of lymphoid tissues. *Nat Rev Immunol* (2003) 3:292–303. doi:10.1038/nri1054
180. Moyron-Quiroz JE, Rangel-Moreno J, Hartson L, Kusser K, Tighe MP, Klonowski KD, et al. Persistence and responsiveness of immunologic memory in the absence of secondary lymphoid organs. *Immunity* (2006) 25:643–54. doi:10.1016/j.immuni.2006.08.022
181. Wiley JA, Richert LE, Swain SD, Harmsen A, Barnard DL, Randall TD, et al. Inducible bronchus-associated lymphoid tissue elicited by a protein cage nanoparticle enhances protection in mice against diverse respiratory viruses. *PLoS One* (2009) 4:e7142. doi:10.1371/journal.pone.0007142
182. Chiavolini D, Rangel-Moreno J, Berg G, Christian K, Oliveira-Nascimento L, Weir S, et al. Bronchus-associated lymphoid tissue (BALT) and survival in a vaccine mouse model of tularemia. *PLoS One* (2010) 5:e11156. doi:10.1371/journal.pone.0011156
183. Ramakrishnan L. Revisiting the role of the granuloma in tuberculosis. *Nat Rev Immunol* (2012) 12:352–66. doi:10.1038/nri3211
184. Khader SA, Bell GK, Pearl JE, Fountain JJ, Rangel-Moreno J, Cilley GE, et al. IL-23 and IL-17 in the establishment of protective pulmonary CD4+ T cell responses after vaccination and during *Mycobacterium tuberculosis* challenge. *Nat Immunol* (2007) 8:369–77. doi:10.1038/ni1449
185. Khader SA, Rangel-Moreno J, Fountain JJ, Martino CA, Reiley WW, Pearl JE, et al. In a murine tuberculosis model, the absence of homeostatic chemokines delays granuloma formation and protective immunity. *J Immunol* (2009) 183:8004–14. doi:10.4049/jimmunol.0901937
186. Slight SR, Rangel-Moreno J, Gopal R, Lin Y, Fallert Junecko BA, Mehra S, et al. CXCR5(+) T helper cells mediate protective immunity against tuberculosis. *J Clin Invest* (2013) 123:712–26. doi: 10.1172/JCI65728
187. Ulrichs T, Kosmiadi GA, Trusov V, Jorg S, Pradl L, Titukhina M, et al. Human tuberculous granulomas induce peripheral lymphoid follicle-like structures to orchestrate local host defence in the lung. *J Pathol* (2004) 204:217–28. doi:10.1002/path.1628
188. Kaushal D, Foreman TW, Gautam US, Alvarez X, Adekambi T, Rangel-Moreno J, et al. Mucosal vaccination with attenuated *Mycobacterium tuberculosis* induces strong central memory responses and protects against tuberculosis. *Nat Commun* (2015) 6:8533. doi:10.1038/ncomms9533
189. Meuwissen HJ, Hussain M. Bronchus-associated lymphoid tissue in human lung: correlation of hyperplasia with chronic pulmonary disease. *Clin Immunol Immunopathol* (1982) 23:548–61. doi:10.1016/0090-1229(82)90139-8
190. Litsiou E, Semitekolou M, Galani IE, Morianos I, Tsoutsa A, Kara P, et al. CXCL13 production in B cells via Toll-like receptor/lymphotoxin receptor signaling is involved in lymphoid neogenesis in chronic obstructive pulmonary disease. *Am J Respir Crit Care Med* (2013) 187:1194–202. doi:10.1164/rccm.201208-1543OC
191. Pauwels RA, Rabe KF. Burden and clinical features of chronic obstructive pulmonary disease (COPD). *Lancet* (2004) 364:613–20. doi:10.1016/S0140-6736(04)16855-4
192. Hogg JC, Chu F, Utokaparch S, Woods R, Elliott WM, Buzatu L, et al. The nature of small-airway obstruction in chronic obstructive pulmonary disease. *N Engl J Med* (2004) 350:2645–53. doi:10.1056/NEJMoa032158
193. Kelsen SG, Aksoy MO, Georgy M, Hershman R, Ji R, Li X, et al. Lymphoid follicle cells in chronic obstructive pulmonary disease overexpress the chemokine receptor CXCR3. *Am J Respir Crit Care Med* (2009) 179:799–805. doi:10.1164/rccm.200807-1089OC
194. Demoor T, Bracke KR, Maes T, Vandooren B, Elewaut D, Pilette C, et al. Role of lymphotoxin-alpha in cigarette smoke-induced inflammation and lymphoid neogenesis. *Eur Respir J* (2009) 34:405–16. doi:10.1183/09031936.00101408
195. Demoor T, Bracke KR, Vermaelen KY, Dupont L, Joos GF, Brusselle GG. CCR7 modulates pulmonary and lymph node inflammatory responses in cigarette smoke-exposed mice. *J Immunol* (2009) 183:8186–94. doi:10.4049/jimmunol.0902015
196. Polverino F, Cosio BG, Pons J, Laucho-Contreras M, Tejera P, Iglesias A, et al. B cell-activating factor. An orchestrator of lymphoid follicles in severe chronic obstructive pulmonary disease. *Am J Respir Crit Care Med* (2015) 192:695–705. doi:10.1164/rccm.201501-0107OC
197. John-Schuster G, Gunter S, Hager K, Conlon TM, Eickelberg O, Yildirim AO. Inflammaging increases susceptibility to cigarette smoke-induced COPD. *Oncotarget* (2015) 7:30068–30083. doi:10.18632/oncotarget.4027
198. Mori M, Andersson CK, Svedberg KA, Glader P, Bergqvist A, Shikhagaie M, et al. Appearance of remodelled and dendritic cell-rich alveolar-lymphoid interfaces provides a structural basis for increased alveolar antigen uptake in chronic obstructive pulmonary disease. *Thorax* (2013) 68:521–31. doi:10.1136/thoraxjnl-2012-202879
199. Van Pottelberge GR, Bracke KR, Demedts IK, De Rijck K, Reinartz SM, van Drunen CM, et al. Selective accumulation of langerhans-type dendritic cells in small airways of patients with COPD. *Respir Res* (2010) 11:35. doi:10.1186/1465-9921-11-35
200. Demedts IK, Bracke KR, Van Pottelberge G, Testelmans D, Verleden GM, Vermassen FE, et al. Accumulation of dendritic cells and increased CCL20 levels in the airways of patients with chronic obstructive pulmonary disease. *Am J Respir Crit Care Med* (2007) 175:998–1005. doi:10.1164/rccm.200608-1113OC

201. Gosman MM, Willemse BW, Jansen DF, Lapperre TS, van Schadewijk A, Hiemstra PS, et al. Increased number of B-cells in bronchial biopsies in COPD. *Eur Respir J* (2006) 27:60–4. doi:10.1183/09031936.06.00007005
202. Jankowski M, Undas A, Kaczmarek P, Butenas S. Activated factor XI and tissue factor in chronic obstructive pulmonary disease: links with inflammation and thrombin generation. *Thromb Res* (2011) 127:242–6. doi:10.1016/j.thromres.2010.11.005
203. Ashitani J, Mukae H, Arimura Y, Matsukura S. Elevated plasma procoagulant and fibrinolytic markers in patients with chronic obstructive pulmonary disease. *Intern Med* (2002) 41:181–5. doi:10.2169/internalmedicine.41.181
204. Leonard A, Marando C, Rahman A, Fazal F. Thrombin selectively engages LIM kinase 1 and slingshot-1L phosphatase to regulate NF-kappaB activation and endothelial cell inflammation. *Am J Physiol Lung Cell Mol Physiol* (2013) 305:L651–64. doi:10.1152/ajplung.00071.2013
205. Lin CH, Yu MC, Chiang CC, Bien MY, Chien MH, Chen BC. Thrombin-induced NF-kappaB activation and IL-8/CXCL8 release is mediated by c-Src-dependent Shc, Raf-1, and ERK pathways in lung epithelial cells. *Cell Signal* (2013) 25:1166–75. doi:10.1016/j.cellsig.2013.01.018
206. Sethi S. New developments in the pathogenesis of acute exacerbations of chronic obstructive pulmonary disease. *Curr Opin Infect Dis* (2004) 17:113–9. doi:10.1097/00001432-200404000-00008
207. Bourke SJ, Dalphin JC, Boyd G, McSharry C, Baldwin CI, Calvert JE. Hypersensitivity pneumonitis: current concepts. *Eur Respir J Suppl* (2001) 32:81s–92s.
208. Rangel-Moreno J, Hartson L, Navarro C, Gaxiola M, Selman M, Randall TD. Inducible bronchus-associated lymphoid tissue (iBALT) in patients with pulmonary complications of rheumatoid arthritis. *J Clin Invest* (2006) 116:3183–94. doi:10.1172/JCI28756
209. Suda T, Chida K, Hayakawa H, Imokawa S, Iwata M, Nakamura H, et al. Development of bronchus-associated lymphoid tissue in chronic hypersensitivity pneumonitis. *Chest* (1999) 115:357–63. doi:10.1378/chest.115.2.357
210. Elliot JG, Jensen CM, Mutavdzic S, Lamb JP, Carroll NG, James AL. Aggregations of lymphoid cells in the airways of nonsmokers, smokers, and subjects with asthma. *Am J Respir Crit Care Med* (2004) 169:712–8. doi:10.1164/rccm.200308-1167OC
211. Slavin RG, Gleich GJ, Hutcheson PS, Kephart GM, Knutsen AP, Tsai CC. Localization of IgE to lung germinal lymphoid follicles in a patient with allergic bronchopulmonary aspergillosis. *J Allergy Clin Immunol* (1992) 90:1006–8. doi:10.1016/0091-6749(92)90479-L
212. Sue-Chu M, Karjalainen EM, Altraja A, Laitinen A, Laitinen LA, Naess AB, et al. Lymphoid aggregates in endobronchial biopsies from young elite cross-country skiers. *Am J Respir Crit Care Med* (1998) 158:597–601. doi:10.1164/ajrccm.158.2.9711012
213. Niewold TB, Harrison MJ, Paget SA. Anti-CCP antibody testing as a diagnostic and prognostic tool in rheumatoid arthritis. *QJM* (2007) 100:193–201. doi:10.1093/qjmed/hcm015
214. Schellekens GA, de Jong BA, van den Hoogen FH, van de Putte LB, van Venrooij WJ. Citrulline is an essential constituent of antigenic determinants recognized by rheumatoid arthritis-specific autoantibodies. *J Clin Invest* (1998) 101:273–81. doi:10.1172/JCI1316
215. Horsfall AC, Rose LM, Maini RN. Autoantibody synthesis in salivary glands of Sjogren's syndrome patients. *J Autoimmun* (1989) 2:559–68. doi:10.1016/0896-8411(89)90189-3
216. Bleul CC, Fuhlbrigge RC, Casasnovas JM, Aiuti A, Springer TA. A highly efficacious lymphocyte chemoattractant, stromal cell-derived factor 1 (SDF-1). *J Exp Med* (1996) 184:1101–9. doi:10.1084/jem.184.3.1101
217. Amft N, Curnow SJ, Scheel-Toellner D, Devadas A, Oates J, Crocker J, et al. Ectopic expression of the B cell-attracting chemokine BCA-1 (CXCL13) on endothelial cells and within lymphoid follicles contributes to the establishment of germinal center-like structures in Sjogren's syndrome. *Arthritis Rheum* (2001) 44:2633–41. doi:10.1002/1529-0131(200111)44:11<2633::AID-ART443>3.0.CO;2-9
218. Sato M, Hirayama S, Hwang DM, Lara-Guerra H, Wagnetz D, Waddell TK, et al. The role of intrapulmonary de novo lymphoid tissue in obliterative bronchiolitis after lung transplantation. *J Immunol* (2009) 182:7307–16. doi:10.4049/jimmunol.0803606
219. van Panhuys N, Perret R, Prout M, Ronchese F, Le Gros G. Effector lymphoid tissue and its crucial role in protective immunity. *Trends Immunol* (2005) 26:242–7. doi:10.1016/j.it.2005.03.005
220. Thaunat O, Field AC, Dai J, Louedec L, Patey N, Bloch MF, et al. Lymphoid neogenesis in chronic rejection: evidence for a local humoral alloimmune response. *Proc Natl Acad Sci U S A* (2005) 102:14723–8. doi:10.1073/pnas.0507223102
221. Motallebzadeh R, Rehakova S, Conlon TM, Win TS, Callaghan CJ, Goddard M, et al. Blocking lymphotoxin signaling abrogates the development of ectopic lymphoid tissue within cardiac allografts and inhibits effector antibody responses. *FASEB J* (2012) 26:51–62. doi:10.1096/fj.11-186973
222. Li W, Bribriesco AC, Nava RG, Brescia AA, Ibricevic A, Spahn JH, et al. Lung transplant acceptance is facilitated by early events in the graft and is associated with lymphoid neogenesis. *Mucosal Immunol* (2012) 5:544–54. doi:10.1038/mi.2012.30
223. Randall TD, Kern JA. Tertiary lymphoid structures target the antitumor immune response to lung cancer. *Am J Respir Crit Care Med* (2014) 189:767–9. doi:10.1164/rccm.201402-0317ED
224. Dieu-Nosjean MC, Antoine M, Danel C, Heudes D, Wislez M, Poulot V, et al. Long-term survival for patients with non-small-cell lung cancer with intratumoral lymphoid structures. *J Clin Oncol* (2008) 26:4410–7. doi:10.1200/JCO.2007.15.0284
225. Carrega P, Loiacono F, Di Carlo E, Scaramuccia A, Mora M, Conte R, et al. NCR(+) ILC3 concentrate in human lung cancer and associate with intratumoral lymphoid structures. *Nat Commun* (2015) 6:8280. doi:10.1038/ncomms9280
226. Davis GS, Pfeiffer LM, Hemenway DR. Expansion of interferon-gamma-producing lung lymphocytes in mouse silicosis. *Am J Respir Cell Mol Biol* (1999) 20:813–24. doi:10.1165/ajrcmb.20.4.3407
227. Trujillo G, Hartigan AJ, Hogaboam CM. T regulatory cells and attenuated bleomycin-induced fibrosis in lungs of CCR7-/- mice. *Fibrogenesis Tissue Repair* (2010) 3:18. doi:10.1186/1755-1536-3-18
228. Shilling RA, Williams JW, Perera J, Berry E, Wu Q, Cummings OW, et al. Autoreactive T and B cells induce the development of bronchus-associated lymphoid tissue in the lung. *Am J Respir Cell Mol Biol* (2013) 48:406–14. doi:10.1165/rcmb.2012-0065OC
229. Van Pottelberge GR, Bracke KR, Van den Broeck S, Reinartz SM, van Drunen CM, Wouters EF, et al. Plasmacytoid dendritic cells in pulmonary lymphoid follicles of patients with COPD. *Eur Respir J* (2010) 36:781–91. doi:10.1183/09031936.00140409
230. Gilliet M, Liu YJ. Generation of human CD8 T regulatory cells by CD40 ligand-activated plasmacytoid dendritic cells. *J Exp Med* (2002) 195:695–704. doi:10.1084/jem.20011603
231. Puccetti P, Fallarino F. Generation of T cell regulatory activity by plasmacytoid dendritic cells and tryptophan catabolism. *Blood Cells Mol Dis* (2008) 40:101–5. doi:10.1016/j.bcmd.2007.06.026

15

Development and Function of Secondary and Tertiary Lymphoid Organs in the Small Intestine and the Colon

Manuela Buettner[1] *and Matthias Lochner*[2*]

[1] *Central Animal Facility, Institute of Laboratory Animal Science, Hannover Medical School, Hannover, Germany,* [2] *Institute of Infection Immunology, TWINCORE, Centre for Experimental and Clinical Infection Research, a joint venture between the Medical School Hannover (MHH) and the Helmholtz Centre for Infection Research (HZI), Hannover, Germany*

Correspondence:
Matthias Lochner
matthias.lochner@twincore.de

The immune system of the gut has evolved a number of specific lymphoid structures that contribute to homeostasis in the face of microbial colonization and food-derived antigenic challenge. These lymphoid organs encompass Peyer's patches (PP) in the small intestine and their colonic counterparts that develop in a programed fashion before birth. In addition, the gut harbors a network of lymphoid tissues that is commonly designated as solitary intestinal lymphoid tissues (SILT). In contrast to PP, SILT develop strictly after birth and consist of a dynamic continuum of structures ranging from small cryptopatches (CP) to large, mature isolated lymphoid follicles (ILF). Although the development of PP and SILT follow similar principles, such as an early clustering of lymphoid tissue inducer (LTi) cells and the requirement for lymphotoxin beta (LTβ) receptor-mediated signaling, the formation of CP and their further maturation into ILF is associated with additional intrinsic and environmental signals. Moreover, recent data also indicate that specific differences exist in the regulation of ILF formation between the small intestine and the colon. Importantly, intestinal inflammation in both mice and humans is associated with a strong expansion of the lymphoid network in the gut. Recent experiments in mice suggest that these structures, although they resemble large, mature ILF in appearance, may represent *de novo*-induced tertiary lymphoid organs (TLO). While, so far, it is not clear whether intestinal TLO contribute to the exacerbation of inflammatory pathology, it has been shown that ILF provide the critical microenvironment necessary for the induction of an effective host response upon infection with enteric bacterial pathogens. Regarding the importance of ILF for intestinal immunity, interfering with the development and maturation of these lymphoid tissues may offer novel means for manipulating the immune response during intestinal infection or inflammation.

Keywords: isolated lymphoid follicles, cryptopatch, lymphoid tissue inducer cells, tertiary lymphoid organs, small intestine, large intestine

---

Abbreviations: CP, cryptopatches; ILC, innate lymphoid cells; ILF, isolated lymphoid follicles; LTi, lymphoid tissue inducer; LTo, lymphoid tissue organizer; PP, Peyer's patches; SILT, solitary intestinal lymphoid tissues; SLO, secondary lymphoid organs; TLO, tertiary lymphoid organs.

INTRODUCTION

Lymphatic organs were described very early in history. The first description of the spleen was made in Egypt 3000 years B.C., and the mesenteric lymph node was mentioned by Herophilus in 335–280 B.C. (1, 2). The thymus was characterized in the fifteenth century, but the immunological function of these organs was recognized not until the twentieth century (2, 3). The thymus and bone marrow are referred to as primary lymphatic organs and represent the places in the body where T and B lymphocytes development and selection takes place. Secondary lymphatic organs (SLO), such as the spleen and lymph nodes (LN), develop at predetermined locations during embryonic development and provide the microenvironment that is required for lymphocyte activation and differentiation into regulatory or effector cells. The strategic positioning of SLO allows optimal sampling of self- and non-self-derived antigens that reach the SLO *via* the bloodstream (spleen) or the afferent lymphatics, which also transport antigen-presenting cells from tissues toward the SLO. In addition to the programed development of SLO, it is now well appreciated that structured lymphoid organs can also develop after birth in response to an ongoing immune reaction. These organized lymphoid aggregates resemble SLO and are designated as tertiary lymphoid organs (TLO) or ectopic lymphoid tissues. Formation of TLO has been observed in almost every tissue of the body under inflammatory conditions associated with autoimmunity, infection, or cancer [summarized in Pitzalis et al. (4)].

The mucosal surfaces of the body represent a major entry site for non-self antigens. It is, thus, not surprising that these barrier sites are surveyed by specific SLO that can be differentiated according to their location as nasal-associated lymphoid tissues (NALT), bronchus-associated lymphoid tissues (BALT), or gut-associated lymphoid tissues (GALT). It is, in particular, the intestine that has evolved a range of unique lymphoid organs, reflecting the extraordinary challenge for the intestinal immune system of maintaining tolerance to food antigens and the complex commensal microbiota, while at the same time preserving tissue integrity and the ability to fight harmful pathogens. In this review, we will focus on the different types of intestinal lymphoid organs, their development, and function in intestinal inflammation and infection. We will, furthermore, point out similarities and specific differences regarding the development and maturation of lymphoid tissues between the small intestine and the colon. A special focus will be set on isolated lymphoid follicles (ILF), which show features of TLO such as the postnatal development and the requirement for additional activating signals to promote their formation.

PROGRAMED SLO DEVELOPMENT IN THE GUT

The principal molecular mechanisms that govern the development of SLO have been extensively characterized during the past two decades (5, 6), and various cell types and factors were identified to be crucial for their development. In the gut, a chain of several LN embedded in the mesenteric membranes drain antigens from the intestine. Despite their common location, the mesenteric (m)LN that drain the small intestine and colon in mice can be separated anatomically and by distinct specificities in their immunological functions (7). The development of mLN follows the general molecular processes described for LN formation, which we will first summarize here, before pointing out major similarities and differences to the development of another major SLO in the gut, the Peyer's patches (PP).

Similar to all other LN, mLN formation starts during embryogenesis *in utero* and proceeds until the development is completely finished after birth. The mLN are the first LN to develop in the mouse, probably starting already around embryonic day (E) 9–12.5 (8). Nerve fibers were identified as potential producers of retinaldehyde dehydrogenase 2 (RALDH2) (5, 9), an enzyme that converts retinal into retinoic acid (RA). RA induces the production of the chemokine CXCL13 by mesenchymal cells in the LN primordium (also designated as LN anlagen). The origin of these mesenchymal cells is not completely clear, but adipocyte progenitor cells were shown to differentiate into LN stromal cells *via* lymphotoxin beta receptor (LTβR) signaling and upregulation of CXCL13 (10). At E13, mesenchymal cells surround endothelial cells (EC), which express EC markers such as podoplanin (also known as gp38), intercellular adhesion molecule (ICAM)-1, and Lyve1$^+$ and produce CCL21 (5, 11). CXCL13 and CCL21 together attract a population of CD3$^-$ CD4$^{+/-}$ CD45$^+$ lymphoid tissue inducer (LTi) cells into the developing LN primordium (5, 11). LTi cells differentiate from fetal liver cells and have been characterized as IL-7Rα$^+$, RA receptor-related orphan receptor (ROR)γt$^+$, CXCR5$^+$, CD117$^+$, and RANKL$^+$ (12). It has become clear that LTi cells belong to a group of lymphoid cells that is now commonly designated as innate lymphoid cells (ILC) (13). LTi cells resemble group 3 ILC, due to the shared requirement for RORγt expression for their generation and function. Yet, LTi cells may form an independent ILC subset, since they were shown to develop from a specific LTi precursor aside from all other ILC subsets (14, 15). Importantly, LTi cells also express lymphotoxin (LT) $\alpha_1\beta_2$ on their surface, which binds to LTβR on gp38$^+$ stromal lymphoid tissue organizer (LTo) cells (11). Notably, stromal LTo cells express markers found on mesenchymal cells such as platelet-derived growth factor receptor (PDGFR) α (11), indicating that these cells originate from the mesenchymal cells present in the LN anlagen. The binding of LT$\alpha_1\beta_2$ and LTβR is essential for LN development, as deficiency for LTα, LTβ, or LTβR results in the absence of LN (8, 16, 17). Therefore, the initial clustering of LTi cells and their interaction with stromal LTo cells marks an important step in LN development. Activated LTo cells start to express high levels of ICAM-1, VCAM-1, and MAdCAM-1 (11), which paves the way for further recruitment and retention of hematopoietic cells into the developing LN. IL-7 and RANKL (also known as TRANCE) produced by LTi and LTo cells were both found to be inducers of LT$\alpha_1\beta_2$. Likewise, LT$\alpha_1\beta_2$ signaling to LTβR leads to the production of IL-7 and RANKL, resulting in a positive feedback loop, and the accumulation of more LTi cells to the LN primordium (18). Loss of IL-7 or RANKL was shown to result in abnormal LN microarchitecture or even complete absence of LN due to altered LTi cell migration or high endothelial venule (HEV) formation, respectively (18, 19).

The connection of HEV and lymphatic vessels to the LN mediated by LTo cells *via* VEGF-C production enables lymphocytes to colonize the LN and to migrate to their distinct B- and T-cell zones (20). LTo cells eventually differentiate into LN stromal cell subsets such as fibroblastic reticular cells (FRC) and follicular dendritic cells (FDC).

PEYER'S PATCHES DEVELOPMENT

The development of PP starts on E12.5–15.5 (21, 22). Similar to LN development, LTi cells play a pivotal role in the formation of PP, as in the absence of LTi cells in RORγt- or ID2-deficient mice PP fail to develop (23, 24). Recruitment of LTi cells to the PP primordium depends on the chemokine CXCL13 and its receptor CXCR5. However, whereas PP were described to be absent or strongly reduced in CXCL13- or CXCR5-deficient animals (25, 26), mLN were still present, even in mice with a combined deficiency in CXCR5 and CCR7, the receptor for CCL19/CCL21 (26–28). The expression of the adhesion molecule β1 integrin on LTi cells directs them to VCAM1$^+$ stromal LTo cells (29), and IL-7/RANKL expression by LTo cells leads to an upregulated expression of $LT\alpha_1\beta_2$ by LTi cells (30). In contrast to LN development, however, both IL-7 and RANKL seem not to be pivotal for the development of PP, as PP primordia were detectable in IL-7$^{-/-}$ mice at E18 (31) and small PP develop in RANKL$^{-/-}$ mice (32). More important in the formation of PP seems to be the IL-7Rα or receptor tyrosine kinase Kit expression on LTi cells (19, 21, 31). The formation of PP primordia in IL-7Rα$^{-/-}$ mice is disturbed and not detectable, and a defect Kit/Kit ligand axis resulted in a reduced PP development (19, 21). Importantly, the first cell population unique for PP formation and responsible for the clustering of LTi cells in the intestine is of hematopoietic origin. These cells were detected to be CD45$^+$, IL7Rα$^-$ CD4$^+$, CD3$^-$ CD11c$^+$ and showed similarities to dendritic cells (DC) from the adult spleen (22). These CD11c$^+$ cells express two molecules known to be pivotal in PP formation: LTβ and the receptor tyrosine kinase RET. Deficiency for one of these molecules resulted in complete loss of PP development. Furthermore, RET signaling was observed to be dependent on different RET ligands (Artn and Nrtn) expressed on VCAM1$^+$ stromal cells. However, the loss of one of these ligands only resulted in a reduced number of PP. Thus, although similar molecules and signaling pathways govern both the formation of PP and LN, there are specific differences in the relative requirement for specific cell types and factors during their development.

SPECIAL LYMPHOID ORGANS OF THE SMALL INTESTINE – THE CP/ILF NETWORK

In addition to the PP, the small intestine harbors a large number of organized lymphoid structures that are commonly designated as solitary intestinal lymphoid tissues (SILT). In contrast to PP and all other secondary lymphoid organs, SILT development in the small intestine of mice is initiated during the early postnatal phase and starts with the accumulation of RORγt$^+$ IL-7Rα$^+$ LTi cells into small clusters named cryptopatches (CP), according to their anatomical location at the bottom of intestinal crypts (33, 34). While in the first days after birth lymphocytes in the intestine are almost exclusively found in the nascent PP (35), CP start to recruit lymphocytes during the following weeks and develop into ILF. Around 100–200 ILF can be found in the small intestine of a mouse, that contain variable numbers of cells and can reach the size of a single PP follicle (36). Large, mature ILF contain mainly B cells as well as a number of interspersed LTi cells and few CD4$^+$ T cells, which do, however, not segregate into a confined T cell zone (34, 36). ILF and their CP precursors also contain CD11c$^+$ CD11b$^-$ DC, which play an important role for the development and structural maintenance of ILFs (37). Most of the B cells within ILF are conventional B-2 B cells, of which around 10% represent IgA$^+$ plasma cells (36). Accordingly, mature ILF have been shown to contain germinal centers and serve as inductive sites for antigen-specific IgA responses (38). In addition, ILF have been proposed to be a major site for T cell-independent B cell class switch to IgA (39). Similar to PP, the epithelium adjacent to mature ILF shows the characteristics of a follicle-associated epithelium containing M cells that allow for direct uptake of antigens from the intestinal lumen (36, 40). An overview on the structure and cellularity of the different lymphoid organs of the small intestine is given in **Figure 1**.

The development of ILF follows similar molecular principles that have been described for the development of PP, such as the interaction of $LT\alpha_1\beta_2$ expressed by LTi cells with the LTβR on VCAM-1$^+$ stromal LTo cells as a critical requirement for the development of CP (40, 41). Transition from CP into ILF in the small intestine depends on the secretion of the B cell recruiting chemokine CXCL13 by stromal cells and CD11c$^+$ DC within CP/ILF (37). Consequently, either the deficiency for CXCL13 or its receptor CXCR5 results in the absence of ILF, whereas the numbers of CP is not affected (37, 42). It should be emphasized here that the development of CP, although initiated after birth, proceeds in the absence of any exogenous inflammatory stimuli. Furthermore, the formation of small intestinal SILT strictly depends on LTi cells, as evidenced by the absence of these structures in RORγt-deficient mice, which lack all LTi cells in the intestine (34, 39). Taking this into account, it is, thus, reasonable to consider ILF as true SLO. Unlike the development of all other SLO, however, the formation of ILF is not completely "programed," and still requires additional input from environmental factors.

Evidence for the requirement of specific dietary products for the development of SILT stems from studies showing that mice deficient for the Aryl hydrocarbon receptor (Ahr) show an almost complete lack of CP/ILF in their small intestines, while the formation of PP or LN was not affected (43, 44). Natural ligands for the Ahr include polyphenols and glucosinolates that can be found in Brassicaceae plants (such as broccoli or cauliflower). Feeding mice with a synthetic diet devoid of any plant-derived products resulted in the absence of CP and ILF at 4 weeks after birth, a phenotype that could be completely restored by the addition of the Ahr ligand indole-3-carbinol to the diet (43). Importantly, tissue-specific deletion of Ahr in RORγt$^+$ ILC was sufficient to impair the development of CP, further demonstrating the importance of these cells for CP/ILF induction. Although the exact molecular mechanisms remain elusive, it is likely that Ahr does not regulate the function, but rather the pool size of RORγt$^+$ ILC

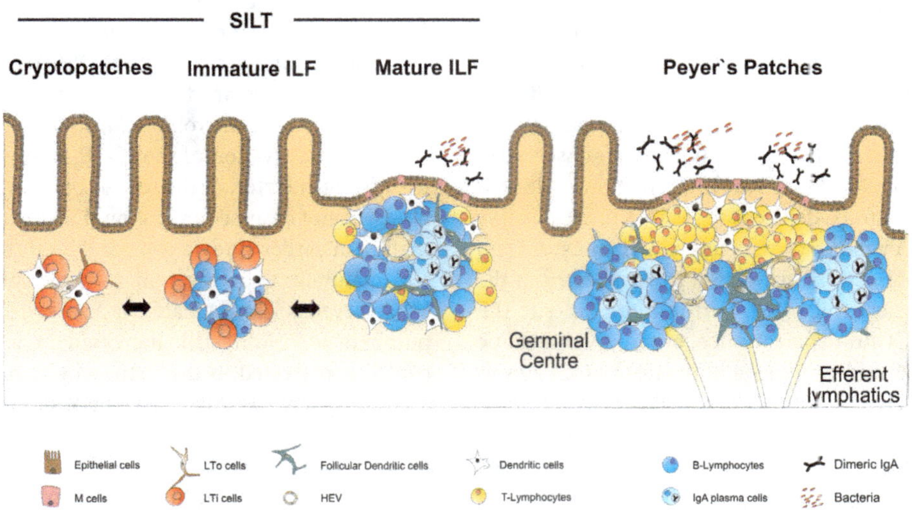

FIGURE 1 | Overview on the anatomy and structure of CP, ILF, and PP in the small intestine. SILT consists of a dynamic continuum of structures ranging from small cryptopatches (CP) to large mature isolated lymphoid follicles (ILF). CP start to develop into immature ILF by recruiting B cells. Mature ILF contain one big B cell follicle and develop germinal centers, vascular structures, and a follicle-associated epithelium. PP represent the most structured lymphoid organs in the intestine, containing several B cell follicles and distinct T and B cell areas.

after birth, since ILC-specific loss of Ahr was shown to interfere with the postnatal expansion/survival of these cells (43, 44). Vitamin A, a dietary component, was also recently found to be required for normal numbers of RORγt$^+$ ILC and ILF formation (45). Although the different stages of the SILT (CP, immature and mature ILF) were present in mice fed with a vitamin A-deficient diet, their total numbers were reduced in the middle and distal part of the intestine. It is likely that the development of fewer SILT in these mice is a consequence of the reduced numbers of RORγt$^+$ ILC upon vitamin A deficiency.

Besides this unexpected role of dietary products in the initial steps of ILF formation, it is less surprising that the intestinal microbiota also plays a role in the regulation of SILT development. In this regard, it has been observed that the small intestine of germ-free mice contain normal numbers of CP and some small immature ILF which harbor only few B cells, whereas the transition into mature ILF depends on the presence of a bacterial microbiota (33, 46, 47). A range of receptors and adaptor molecules involved in the recognition of bacteria-derived molecular patterns, including toll-like receptors (TLR) 2/4, myeloid differentiation primary response gene (MyD) 88, and nucleotide-binding oligomerization domain-containing protein (NOD) 2, were shown to contribute to the maturation of small intestinal ILF (47). In the same study, a more specific role in the early transition of CP into immature ILF was proposed for NOD1, which recognizes peptidoglycans (PGN) derived from Gram-negative bacteria. NOD1, which is expressed in small intestinal epithelial cells, induces upon recognition of PGN the secretion of factors, such as CCL20 or β-defensin 3 (mBD3). Both factors are ligands for CCR6, which is expressed by B cells and LTi cells. Thus, activation of NOD1 may regulate the formation of ILF by activating LTi cells and by supporting the CCR6-dependent recruitment of B cells to CP (48). Supporting this hypothesis, mice deficient either for CCR6 or mBD3 fail to develop ILF, and a similar phenotype could be observed in mice treated with a CCL20 neutralizing antibody (47).

LYMPHOID ORGANS OF THE COLON – SIMILARITIES AND DIFFERENCES TO SMALL INTESTINE

Interestingly, most of the factors and molecular mechanisms that govern the development of PP and SILT have been analyzed in the small intestine, while the formation of the respective lymphoid tissues in the colon has not been comprehensively studied until recently. Similar to the small intestine, also the colon of mice harbors distinct lymphoid tissues. Colonic patches represent the equivalents of PP in the small intestine. They are usually composed of two or more large B cell follicles with separate T cell areas and contain CD35$^+$ FDCs as well as vessels with HEV. As in the small intestine, also SILT exists, which resemble in its appearance its small intestinal counterpart, ranging from small CP-like structures to mature colonic ILF containing one big B cell follicle with CD35$^+$ FDC, but no defined T cell area (49, 50). As for PP, the development of colonic patches starts *in utero* with clustering of RORγt-expressing LTi cells and their interaction with VCAM-1$^+$ stromal cells. Although the initial clustering of LTi cells at colonic patch primordium seems to be independent of LTα$_1$β$_2$–LTβR interaction, the further development into colonic patches strictly requires activation of this pathway as well as the sustained expression of CXCL13 (49). SILT development in the colon starts after birth with the clustering of LTi cells into CP-like structures surrounded by CD11c$^+$ cells, and the successful formation of these structures depends again on signaling *via* the LTβR pathway. Despite these important similarities, it is getting increasingly clear that also striking differences exist between the processes of lymphoid tissue formation in the small intestine and the colon (summarized in **Figure 2**). CXCL13 for example, while required for the formation of colonic patches and the recruitment of B cells into small intestinal CP, seems to be dispensable for colonic SILT formation, as numerous colonic ILF were observed in CXCL13-deficient mice (49). Likewise, ILF formation is blocked in the small intestine of mice deficient for RANKL, presumably due to a role for this cytokine in inducing CXCL13 expression in stromal cells. In contrast, ILF formation is not affected in the colon of RANKL-deficient mice (51). Furthermore, colonic ILF develop normally in CCR6-deficient mice, even though colonic LTi cells express CCR6, and expression of the ligand CCL20 was shown to be decreased in the colon of LTα-deficient mice, which fail to develop colonic lymphoid tissues (49). This indicates that in contrast to the small intestine, SILT formation in the colon is less dependent on the CCR6–CCL20 axis. Most striking, however, is the notion that microbiota-derived signals seem to be much less important for the formation of mature colonic ILF as compared to the small intestine. Two recent studies showed that in germ-free mice the formation of the whole spectrum of SILT in the colon is not significantly impaired (49, 50). Yet, MyD88 signaling was found to be necessary for full colonic ILF maturation, even in the absence of the microbiota (49). Whether MyD88 signaling is induced by activation of the IL-1R family, which also signal *via* the MyD88 adaptor, or the release of endogenous TLR ligands is, however, not clear so far. It should be mentioned in that respect, that in an earlier study a role for TLR2/4 was shown for colonic ILF maturation, however in a microbiota-dependent manner (47). Nevertheless, Donaldson and colleagues even found the numbers of colonic ILF increased in germ-free mice, which could be corrected in their study by transferring these mice to a conventional housing (50). Interestingly, intestinal colonization of germ-free mice with microbiota was accompanied by upregulation of colonic IL-25 expression. IL-25 is produced upon microbial colonization by the intestinal epithelium, and it has been demonstrated that commensal microbiota-induced IL-25 production dampens the activity of RORγt⁺ ILC and reduces

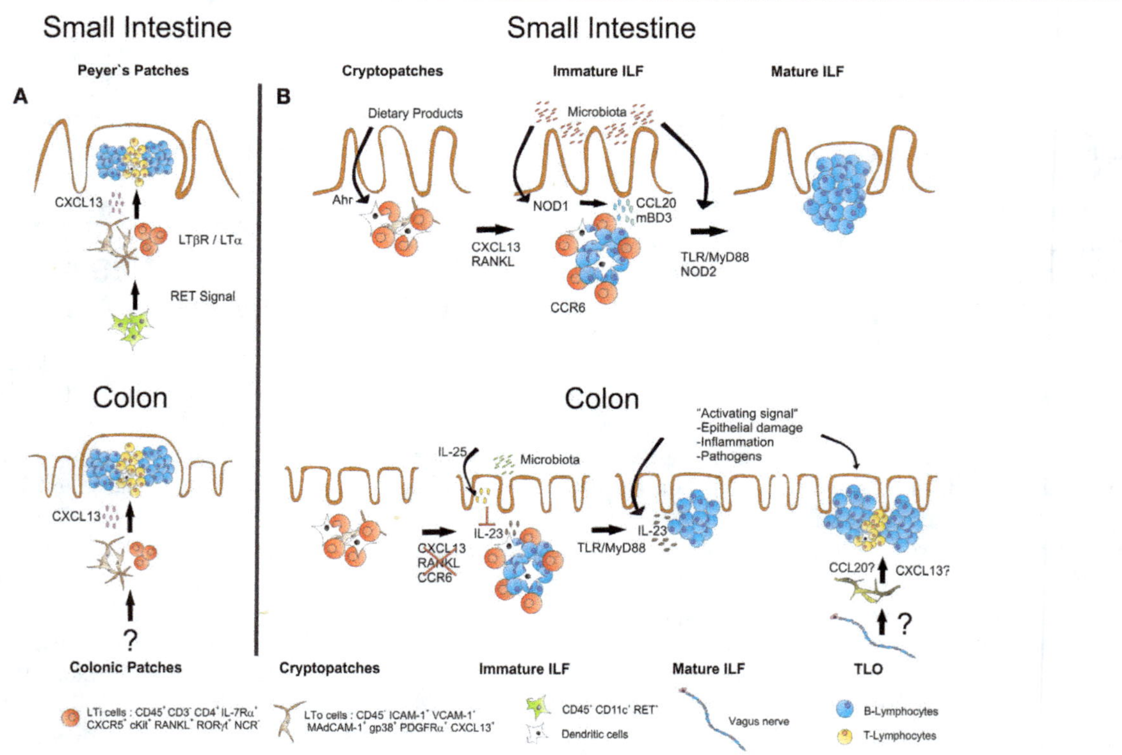

FIGURE 2 | Similarities and differences in the development of small intestinal and colonic lymphoid tissues. (A) Development of both PP and colonic patches starts before birth with the clustering of $LT\alpha_1\beta_2$-expressing IL-7Rα⁺RORγt⁺ LTi cells together with LTo cells. LTi cell clustering and further development of both PP and colonic patches requires expression of CXCL13 and is dependent on LT-signaling. Whether the initial clustering of LTi cells in the colon depends on RET-expressing IL7Rα⁻CD11c⁺ cells, as it has been described for PP development, is not known. **(B)** ILF formation in both small intestine and colon starts after birth with the clustering of IL-7Rα⁺RORγt⁺ LTi cells in CP. Maintenance and further development of these structures into ILF requires LT signaling in both small intestine and the colon. In the small intestine, also signaling *via* the Ahr and the expression of CXCL13, RANKL and CCR6 is required, and the commensal microbiota induce ILF formation and maturation *via* activation of signaling pathways that include NOD1, NOD2, TLRs, and MyD88. In the colon, ILF formation does not seem to critically depend on CXCL13, RANKL, and CCR6. There, the presence of commensal microbiota rather inhibits ILF maturation, probably by inducing IL-25 production from the epithelium, which in turn diminishes the secretion of IL-23, a cytokine that specifically promotes ILF maturation in the colon. Signals associated with intestinal inflammation or infection with enteric pathogens also induce ILF formation and maturation. Intestinal inflammation or infection may also result in the induction of TLO that form independently of LTi cells. TLO may be discriminated from ILF by structural differences such as the presence of T cell areas. A role for the intestinal nervous system for TLO induction in intestinal inflammation has been suggested.

IL-23 expression in the intestine (52, 53). Indeed, colonic ILF development was increased in IL-25-deficient mice (50). This was associated with enhanced expression of IL-23, suggesting that IL-25 may influence colonic ILF maturation by negatively regulating IL-23 production. The authors could confirm this hypothesis by showing that IL-23p19-deficient mice displayed a colon-specific decrease in ILF numbers, and identified colonic (but not small intestinal) CD11c+ cells within ILF as a source for IL-23 production. Thus, the commensal microbiota may still be important for regulating the status of the colonic SILT, however, by a process different from the small intestine, involving IL-23 as an important (and colon-specific) factor for ILF development.

ILF IN INTESTINAL INFLAMMATION

Despite the findings that ILF formation in the small intestine and the colon is initiated after birth and requires additional environmental factors, these structures may still be considered as SLO, since their development depends on the programed initial clustering of LTi cells into CP. In contrast, TLO can form as a consequence of an inflammatory process and are independent of the programed clustering of LTi cells. As the intestinal SILT already represents a flexible system of "inducible" SLO, the question remains whether true TLO do also develop in this organ during inflammation. Evidence that TLO induction, indeed, occurs in the intestine comes from studies using RORγt-deficient mice, which lack all RORγt-dependent ILC and, therefore, all programed peripheral lymphoid tissues, including LN, PP, and colonic patches. In these mice, numerous ILF-like B cell follicles containing germinal centers develop spontaneously in the colon, demonstrating that formation of TLO is possible in the intestine in the absence of LTi cells (54). It is likely that the spontaneous formation of such colonic TLO is compensating for the lack of other intestinal lymphoid tissues or critical components of the intestinal immune system (55). In fact, an increase in colonic ILF has also been observed in mice after the development of mLN, and PP was inhibited by the *in utero* blockage of LTβR and TNFRp55 or in mice that are deficient for the Ahr (43, 56). In RORγt-deficient mice, the development of colonic TLO was still dependent on LTβR signaling, and it was shown that B cells were the critical source of $LT\alpha_1\beta_2$ in the absence of LTi cells (54). The induction of TLO in RORγt-deficient mice was strictly dependent on the microbiota and strongly enhanced upon induction of intestinal inflammation with dextran sodium sulfate (DSS). Interestingly, there was an intriguing correlation between the presence of TLO in the colon of RORγt-deficient mice and the severity of the colonic inflammation. The pathology could be reverted to levels seen in wild-type control mice by blocking the development of TLO using a LTβR–Ig fusion protein, suggesting that the TLO in this model indeed contribute to the severity of colitis. This finding complements data from other studies suggesting that increased formation of mucosal lymphoid tissues is associated with an exacerbation of intestinal pathology. In TNFΔARE mice, which serve as a TNFα-dependent model of Crohn's Ileitis, induction of TLO within the chronically inflamed terminal ileum was observed (57). Aberrant production of CCL19 and CCL21 by these structures enhanced the density of infiltrating effector memory T cells and augmented their retention in the inflamed intestine, contributing to the perpetuation of ileitis. Also, the B cell follicles that develop in the colon of Ahr-deficient mice have been associated with intestinal pathology, such as the formation of anal prolapse, colonic hyperplasia, and increased inflammation upon intestinal infection (43, 58). There is ample evidence also from other studies in mice and in men that intestinal inflammation is associated with enhanced formation of structured lymphoid tissues (59–66) (summarized in **Table 1**). Yet, the contribution of these lymphoid organs to the perpetuation or exacerbation of the inflammatory pathology was, in the cases where it was tested, less evident.

Of note, the question whether the lymphoid organs that form in intestinal inflammatory diseases also represent *de novo*-induced TLO instead of ILF that develop as SLO within the SILT network is, as of now, not completely clear. In this regard, the group of Reina Mebius recently reported the *de novo* formation of lymphoid tissues in the colon of mice treated with DSS (66). Although these structures showed all hallmarks of mature ILF in terms of the presence of B cell follicles, DC, FDC, and a vascular network, they also presented a distinct T cell area. It is likely that these lymphoid structures indeed represent *de novo*-formed TLO, since they were not observed in non-treated control mice. Thus, despite the lack of a marker allowing to definitely discriminate ILF from TLO, it may be possible to distinguish inflammation-induced TLO from ILF by structural differences, such as the presence of defined T cell areas. Interestingly, the same study also suggested a specific role for the nervous system in colonic TLO formation. It was shown that disrupting the

TABLE 1 | Formation of lymphoid follicles in intestinal inflammation.

Species	Phenotype	Reference
$Ahr^{-/-}$ mice	Spontaneous lymphoid follicle formation in colon, anal prolapse, and increased intestinal inflammation upon infection	Fernandez-Salguero et al. (58) and Kiss et al. (43)
$ROR\gamma t^{-/-}$ mice	Spontaneous lymphoid follicle formation in colon, increased follicle numbers and enhanced pathology during DSS colitis. Blocking of lymphoid follicle formation reduced pathology	Lochner et al. (54)
TNFΔARE mice	Lymphoid follicle induction in terminal ileum during spontaneous ileitis	McNamee et al. (57)
WT mice	Lymphoid follicle induction in the colon upon DSS colitis	Olivier et al. (66)
CD40L/B tg mice	Lymphoid follicle formation in small intestine and colon during spontaneous colitis	Kawamura et al. (65)
LN/PP-deficient mice	Formation of lymphoid follicles during DSS colitis, no correlation with disease severity	Spahn et al. (64)
Human	*De novo* formation of lymphoid follicle in UC and CD	Kaiserling (62)
Human	Description of lymphoid aggregates in UC lesions	Carlsen et al. (63)
Human	Description of lymphoid aggregates in CD lesions	Makiyama et al. (59), Surawicz and Belic (60), and Fujimura et al. (61)

UC, ulcerative colitis; CD, Crohn's disease.

innervation of the proximal colon by the vagus nerve prevented the induction of TLO upon DSS treatment, as a consequence of insufficient upregulation of CXCL13 and CCL20 expression by colonic stromal cells.

ILF IN INTESTINAL INFECTION

Under steady-state conditions, SILT functions mainly as a dynamic expandable system that contributes to the regulation of the intestinal commensal microbiota by the induction of IgA [reviewed in Ref. (38)]. It has been shown that ILF, as well as other gut lymphoid organs, harbor in their interior populations of specific commensal bacteria, such as *Alcaligenes* spp., *Achromobacter* spp., and others (67, 68). These lymphoid tissue-resident commensals could stimulate local ILC3 and T cell responses and induce the secretion of IL-10, which limited proinflammatory responses in the steady-state and protected mice during DSS-induced colitis (69). Besides their role in establishing mutualism between the host and the commensal microbiota, ILF may, however, also participate in the immune response against specific intestinal pathogens. In that respect, it has been shown that in mice lacking LNs and PP, but not ILF, *Salmonella typhimurium*-specific IgA responses could be induced upon oral infection with this pathogen (70). *Candidatus arthromicus* [also known as segmented filamentous bacteria (SFB)] has been described as a bacterial strain with marked immunostimulatory properties, although it does not cause overt immunopathology (71). SFB colonizes mainly the terminal ileum of mice, where it can directly attach to the epithelium and induce the maturation of several intestinal immune functions, including IgA production and Th17 induction (72, 73). In mice containing a normal set of lymphoid organs, PP represent a major site for SFB-induced IgA production (74). However, when mice were made devoid of LN, PP, as well as CP-derived ILF by LTβR–Ig treatment, SFB induced the formation of small intestinal TLO capable of initiating an IgA response to SFB. Interestingly, IgA-induction against a non-adherent and non-virulent strain of *Escherichia coli* occurred in PP, but was completely abolished in mice lacking PP. Overall, these data suggest that specific bacteria with immunostimulatory or pathogenic properties can stimulate the formation of ILF, which can substitute for PP as inductive sites for intestinal IgA. Interestingly, pathogen-induced formation of lymphoid follicles has also been observed in the mucosal tissue of the stomach. Although the stomach generally lacks organized or diffused lymphoid tissues, infection with *Helicobacter pylori* can induce the development of gastric lymphoid follicles in mice, presumably in an LTi cell-dependent manner (75). Of note, also intestinal parasites, such as the nematode *Trichuris muris* can induce the formation of ILFs in the colon of infected mice (76).

Evidence for a functional role of ILFs in host protection against intestinal infection comes from studies using the bacterium *Citrobacter rodentium*, a non-invasive Gram-negative mouse enteric pathogen that forms attaching and effacing (A/E) lesions in the intestinal epithelium, modeling the infection process of the human pathogens, enterohemorrhagic *E. coli* (EHEC) and enteropathogenic *E. coli* (EPEC) (77). During the early phase of infection, RORγt$^+$ ILC3 produces large amounts of IL-22 (78–80), which has a major protective role, e.g., by inducing the expression of antimicrobial proteins, such as RegIIIβ and RegIIIγ, by intestinal epithelial cells (81). Mice that lack ILC3 are highly susceptible to intestinal infection with *C. rodentium* (78, 80), largely recapitulating the phenotype of IL-22-deficient mice (82). Importantly, the LTβR-pathway also plays an essential role for the defense against this pathogen, since LTβR-deficient mice were found to be highly susceptible to *C. rodentium* and to succumb rapidly upon infection (83, 84). It turned out that RORγt$^+$ ILC were the critical cell type for the activation of LTβR-signaling *via* their surface expression of LT$\alpha_1\beta_2$ (84–86). It was furthermore demonstrated that the LT pathway was required for the subsequent induction of IL-22 production by ILC. Intriguingly, IL-22$^+$ ILC closely interacted with DCs in colonic ILF, and it was shown that LTβR-expression by CD11c$^+$ DC is a prerequisite for IL-22 induction in ILC (86). The data provided by the study of Tumanov and colleagues suggest that ILF, indeed, provide the necessary microenvironment for the close interaction between RORγt$^+$ ILC and DC. The LT$\alpha_1\beta_2$–LTβR-mediated interaction results in IL-23 secretion by the DC, which in turn activates IL-22 production from the ILC. Importantly, both disruption of the LTβR pathway and IL-22 deficiency interfered with the induction of ILF and impaired their structural integrity (85). However, the surprising role of IL-22 for ILF formation was only observed after infection with *C. rodentium*, but not during the steady state. Together, these findings indicate that ILF not only provide the critical environment for the induction of an effective immune response toward intestinal infection but also demonstrate an important role for RORγt$^+$ ILC-derived IL-22 for the induction and maintenance of ILF under infectious conditions in the gut. Notably, a critical role of IL-22 has also been reported recently in a model of adenovirus-induced development of TLO in the salivary glands of mice (87). In the absence of IL-22, the recruitment of B cells into the developing TLO structures was significantly impaired, resulting in a strong reduction of autoantibody formation. It was shown that IL-22 production was necessary for the upregulation of CXCL12 and CXCL13 from epithelial and stromal cells within TLO, and therapeutic blocking of IL-22 inhibited the expression of both chemokines and the correct assembly of TLO. Although ILC were identified as IL-22 producers, the majority of cells expressing this cytokine at the early phase were γδ T cells and αβ T cells at the later stage. These findings together, thus, suggest important regulatory role for IL-22 in the formation of lymphoid organs under inflammatory or infectious conditions at mucosal sites.

CONCLUDING REMARKS

In contrast to most other lymphoid tissues of the body, the formation of ILF in the gut is initiated after birth and unfolds upon the reception of environmental signals associated with the uptake of food-derived compounds and microbial colonization. Despite these differences, ILF can be considered as SLO, since their development strictly requires the LTi-dependent formation of CP. This distinguishes ILF from TLO, which can be induced also in the absence of LTi cells and in response to an inflammatory trigger. Recent experiments in mice suggest that inflammation not only leads to an expansion of the existing SILT network but also to the induction of TLO in the gut. Although it is not clear so far, to what extent TLO contribute to the inflammatory process and pathology in intestinal inflammation, disrupting TLO formation may represent a strategy for the treatment of chronic inflammatory disorders. Regarding its prominent role in lymphoid neogenesis, targeting the LTβR pathway may prove effective in blocking TLO development during inflammation. However, the human phase II studies that analyzed therapeutics targeting the lymphotoxin pathway showed only very limited effects in improving the symptoms of primary Sjögren's syndrome or rheumatoid arthritis (88, 89). Another promising approach to interfere with TLO development is the blockade or neutralization of CXCL13 in order to prevent B cell recruitment into lymphoid structures. In this regard, antibody-mediated neutralization of CXCL13 in a mouse model for Sjögren's syndrome resulted in improved disease phenotype and reduced lymphoid follicles in the submandibular glands (90). CXCL13 neutralization had also a beneficial effect in mouse models for rheumatoid arthritis and multiple sclerosis (91), although the effect on TLO formation was not determined in this study. Blocking CXCL13 in the NOD-mouse model for diabetes disrupted the organization of TLO in the pancreas of the mice, however, without affecting disease severity (92). These findings indicate that the effect of anti-CXCL13 treatment may be influenced by the specific characteristics of the inflammatory model. In that respect, it will be interesting to see whether blocking of CXCL13 also impacts on gut inflammation and TLO development in the intestine.

Besides the well-known factors that are required for the development of ILF, there are also cytokines like IL-22 entering the stage that may have a specific function in ILF biology. Also, IL-23, besides its established proinflammatory role within the T_H17–IL-23 axis (93), seems to influence ILF formation specifically in the colon, and has been associated with TLO formation in rheumatoid arthritis (94). Also, IL-17, which together with IL-22 is produced by neonatal RORγt$^+$ LTi cells as well as by RORγt-expressing T cell subsets, has been implicated in TLO formation in the lung (95) and in a model of experimental allergic encephalomyelitis (96). Nevertheless, the significance of these cytokines for the development and structural maintenance of organized lymphoid tissues may strongly depend on the inflammatory context and the target organ. While, so far, no role for IL-17 in ILF formation has been reported, its requirement for TLO formation in the lung also depends strongly on the model used (97).

Increasing our knowledge on the similarities, but in particular also the differences, in the mechanisms that govern postnatal development of lymphoid tissues such as ILF in the small intestine and the colon may offer novel strategies for immunomodulation. It should also be taken into account that targeting cytokines, e.g. within the T_H17–IL-23 axis, for the treatment of inflammatory disorders may in addition to the direct anti-inflammatory effects also critically influence the formation and function of lymphoid tissues.

AUTHOR CONTRIBUTIONS

MB and ML contributed equally to designing and writing of the review.

ACKNOWLEDGMENTS

We thank Peyman Ghorbani for critical reading of the manuscript. ML is supported by grants from the Deutsche Forschungsgemeinschaft (DFG) grant No. LO1415/7-1. MB is supported by a grant from the DFG grant No. BO1866/3-1.

REFERENCES

1. Chikly B. Who discovered the lymphatic system. *Lymphology* (1997) 30:186–93.
2. Boehm T, Bleul CC. The evolutionary history of lymphoid organs. *Nat Immunol* (2007) 8:131–5. doi:10.1038/ni1435
3. Miller JF. Immunological function of the thymus. *Lancet* (1961) 2:748–9. doi:10.1016/S0140-6736(61)90693-6
4. Pitzalis C, Jones GW, Bombardieri M, Jones SA. Ectopic lymphoid-like structures in infection, cancer and autoimmunity. *Nat Rev Immunol* (2014) 14:447–62. doi:10.1038/nri3700
5. van de Pavert SA, Olivier BJ, Goverse G, Vondenhoff MF, Greuter M, Beke P, et al. Chemokine CXCL13 is essential for lymph node initiation and is induced by retinoic acid and neuronal stimulation. *Nat Immunol* (2009) 10:1193–9. doi:10.1038/ni.1789
6. Burger NB, Stuurman KE, Kok E, Konijn T, Schooneman D, Niederreither K, et al. Involvement of neurons and retinoic acid in lymphatic development: new insights in increased nuchal translucency. *Prenat Diagn* (2014) 34:1312–9. doi:10.1002/pd.4473
7. Houston SA, Cerovic V, Thomson C, Brewer J, Mowat AM, Milling S. The lymph nodes draining the small intestine and colon are anatomically separate and immunologically distinct. *Mucosal Immunol* (2016) 9:468–78. doi:10.1038/mi.2015.77
8. Rennert PD, James D, Mackay F, Browning JL, Hochman PS. Lymph node genesis is induced by signaling through the lymphotoxin beta receptor. *Immunity* (1998) 9:71–9. doi:10.1016/S1074-7613(00)80589-0
9. Buckley CD, Barone F, Nayar S, Benezech C, Caamano J. Stromal cells in chronic inflammation and tertiary lymphoid organ formation. *Annu Rev Immunol* (2015) 33:715–45. doi:10.1146/annurev-immunol-032713-120252
10. Benezech C, Mader E, Desanti G, Khan M, Nakamura K, White A, et al. Lymphotoxin-beta receptor signaling through NF-kappaB2-RelB pathway reprograms adipocyte precursors as lymph node stromal cells. *Immunity* (2012) 37:721–34. doi:10.1016/j.immuni.2012.06.010
11. Benezech C, White A, Mader E, Serre K, Parnell S, Pfeffer K, et al. Ontogeny of stromal organizer cells during lymph node development. *J Immunol* (2010) 184:4521–30. doi:10.4049/jimmunol.0903113
12. van de Pavert SA, Mebius RE. New insights into the development of lymphoid tissues. *Nat Rev Immunol* (2010) 10:664–74. doi:10.1038/nri2832
13. Spits H, Artis D, Colonna M, Diefenbach A, Di Santo JP, Eberl G, et al. Innate lymphoid cells – a proposal for uniform nomenclature. *Nat Rev Immunol* (2013) 13:145–9. doi:10.1038/nri3365
14. Constantinides MG, Mcdonald BD, Verhoef PA, Bendelac A. A committed precursor to innate lymphoid cells. *Nature* (2014) 508:397–401. doi:10.1038/nature13047
15. Ishizuka IE, Chea S, Gudjonson H, Constantinides MG, Dinner AR, Bendelac A, et al. Single-cell analysis defines the divergence between the innate lymphoid cell lineage and lymphoid tissue-inducer cell lineage. *Nat Immunol* (2016) 17:269–76. doi:10.1038/ni.3344
16. Mariathasan S, Matsumoto M, Baranyay F, Nahm MH, Kanagawa O, Chaplin DD. Absence of lymph nodes in lymphotoxin-alpha(LT alpha)-deficient mice is due to abnormal organ development, not defective lymphocyte migration. *J Inflamm* (1995) 45:72–8.
17. Alimzhanov MB, Kuprash DV, Kosco-Vilbois MH, Luz A, Turetskaya RL, Tarakhovsky A, et al. Abnormal development of secondary lymphoid tissues in lymphotoxin beta-deficient mice. *Proc Natl Acad Sci U S A* (1997) 94:9302–7. doi:10.1073/pnas.94.17.9302
18. Sugiyama M, Nakato G, Jinnohara T, Akiba H, Okumura K, Ohno H, et al. Expression pattern changes and function of RANKL during mouse lymph

node microarchitecture development. *Int Immunol* (2012) 24:369–78. doi:10.1093/intimm/dxs002
19. Chappaz S, Gartner C, Rodewald HR, Finke D. Kit ligand and Il7 differentially regulate Peyer's patch and lymph node development. *J Immunol* (2010) 185:3514–9. doi:10.4049/jimmunol.1000665
20. Vondenhoff MF, Greuter M, Goverse G, Elewaut D, Dewint P, Ware CF, et al. LTbetaR signaling induces cytokine expression and up-regulates lymphangiogenic factors in lymph node anlagen. *J Immunol* (2009) 182:5439–45. doi:10.4049/jimmunol.0801165
21. Adachi S, Yoshida H, Honda K, Maki K, Saijo K, Ikuta K, et al. Essential role of IL-7 receptor alpha in the formation of Peyer's patch anlage. *Int Immunol* (1998) 10:1–6. doi:10.1093/intimm/10.1.1
22. Veiga-Fernandes H, Coles MC, Foster KE, Patel A, Williams A, Natarajan D, et al. Tyrosine kinase receptor RET is a key regulator of Peyer's patch organogenesis. *Nature* (2007) 446:547–51. doi:10.1038/nature05597
23. Eberl G, Marmon S, Sunshine MJ, Rennert PD, Choi Y, Littman DR. An essential function for the nuclear receptor RORgamma(t) in the generation of fetal lymphoid tissue inducer cells. *Nat Immunol* (2004) 5:64–73. doi:10.1038/ni1022
24. Boos MD, Yokota Y, Eberl G, Kee BL. Mature natural killer cell and lymphoid tissue-inducing cell development requires Id2-mediated suppression of E protein activity. *J Exp Med* (2007) 204:1119–30. doi:10.1084/jem.20061959
25. Forster R, Mattis AE, Kremmer E, Wolf E, Brem G, Lipp M. A putative chemokine receptor, BLR1, directs B cell migration to defined lymphoid organs and specific anatomic compartments of the spleen. *Cell* (1996) 87:1037–47. doi:10.1016/S0092-8674(00)81798-5
26. Ansel KM, Ngo VN, Hyman PL, Luther SA, Forster R, Sedgwick JD, et al. A chemokine-driven positive feedback loop organizes lymphoid follicles. *Nature* (2000) 406:309–14. doi:10.1038/35018581
27. Luther SA, Ansel KM, Cyster JG. Overlapping roles of CXCL13, interleukin 7 receptor alpha, and CCR7 ligands in lymph node development. *J Exp Med* (2003) 197:1191–8. doi:10.1084/jem.20021294
28. Ohl L, Henning G, Krautwald S, Lipp M, Hardtke S, Bernhardt G, et al. Cooperating mechanisms of CXCR5 and CCR7 in development and organization of secondary lymphoid organs. *J Exp Med* (2003) 197:1199–204. doi:10.1084/jem.20030169
29. Finke D, Acha-Orbea H, Mattis A, Lipp M, Kraehenbuhl J. CD4+CD3- cells induce Peyer's patch development: role of alpha4beta1 integrin activation by CXCR5. *Immunity* (2002) 17:363–73. doi:10.1016/S1074-7613(02)00395-3
30. Yoshida H, Naito A, Inoue J, Satoh M, Santee-Cooper SM, Ware CF, et al. Different cytokines induce surface lymphotoxin-alphabeta on IL-7 receptor-alpha cells that differentially engender lymph nodes and Peyer's patches. *Immunity* (2002) 17:823–33. doi:10.1016/S1074-7613(02)00479-X
31. Nishikawa S, Honda K, Vieira P, Yoshida H. Organogenesis of peripheral lymphoid organs. *Immunol Rev* (2003) 195:72–80. doi:10.1034/j.1600-065X.2003.00063.x
32. Kong YY, Yoshida H, Sarosi I, Tan HL, Timms E, Capparelli C, et al. OPGL is a key regulator of osteoclastogenesis, lymphocyte development and lymph-node organogenesis. *Nature* (1999) 397:315–23. doi:10.1038/16852
33. Kanamori Y, Ishimaru K, Nanno M, Maki K, Ikuta K, Nariuchi H, et al. Identification of novel lymphoid tissues in murine intestinal mucosa where clusters of c-kit+ IL-7R+ Thy1+ lympho-hemopoietic progenitors develop. *J Exp Med* (1996) 184:1449–59. doi:10.1084/jem.184.4.1449
34. Eberl G, Littman DR. Thymic origin of intestinal alphabeta T cells revealed by fate mapping of RORgammat+ cells. *Science* (2004) 305:248–51. doi:10.1126/science.1096472
35. Torow N, Yu K, Hassani K, Freitag J, Schulz O, Basic M, et al. Active suppression of intestinal CD4(+)TCRalphabeta(+) T-lymphocyte maturation during the postnatal period. *Nat Commun* (2015) 6:7725. doi:10.1038/ncomms8725
36. Hamada H, Hiroi T, Nishiyama Y, Takahashi H, Masunaga Y, Hachimura S, et al. Identification of multiple isolated lymphoid follicles on the antimesenteric wall of the mouse small intestine. *J Immunol* (2002) 168:57–64. doi:10.4049/jimmunol.168.1.57
37. McDonald KG, Mcdonough JS, Dieckgraefe BK, Newberry RD. Dendritic cells produce CXCL13 and participate in the development of murine small intestine lymphoid tissues. *Am J Pathol* (2010) 176:2367–77. doi:10.2353/ajpath.2010.090723
38. Knoop KA, Newberry RD. Isolated lymphoid follicles are dynamic reservoirs for the induction of intestinal IgA. *Front Immunol* (2012) 3:84. doi:10.3389/fimmu.2012.00084
39. Tsuji M, Suzuki K, Kitamura H, Maruya M, Kinoshita K, Ivanov II, et al. Requirement for lymphoid tissue-inducer cells in isolated follicle formation and T cell-independent immunoglobulin A generation in the gut. *Immunity* (2008) 29:261–71. doi:10.1016/j.immuni.2008.05.014
40. Lorenz RG, Chaplin DD, Mcdonald KG, Mcdonough JS, Newberry RD. Isolated lymphoid follicle formation is inducible and dependent upon lymphotoxin-sufficient B lymphocytes, lymphotoxin beta receptor, and TNF receptor I function. *J Immunol* (2003) 170:5475–82. doi:10.4049/jimmunol.170.11.5475
41. Taylor RT, Lugering A, Newell KA, Williams IR. Intestinal cryptopatch formation in mice requires lymphotoxin alpha and the lymphotoxin beta receptor. *J Immunol* (2004) 173:7183–9. doi:10.4049/jimmunol.173.12.7183
42. Velaga S, Herbrand H, Friedrichsen M, Jiong T, Dorsch M, Hoffmann MW, et al. Chemokine receptor CXCR5 supports solitary intestinal lymphoid tissue formation, B cell homing, and induction of intestinal IgA responses. *J Immunol* (2009) 182:2610–9. doi:10.4049/jimmunol.0801141
43. Kiss EA, Vonarbourg C, Kopfmann S, Hobeika E, Finke D, Esser C, et al. Natural aryl hydrocarbon receptor ligands control organogenesis of intestinal lymphoid follicles. *Science* (2011) 334:1561–5. doi:10.1126/science.1214914
44. Lee JS, Cella M, Mcdonald KG, Garlanda C, Kennedy GD, Nukaya M, et al. AHR drives the development of gut ILC22 cells and postnatal lymphoid tissues via pathways dependent on and independent of Notch. *Nat Immunol* (2012) 13:144–51. doi:10.1038/ni.2187
45. Goverse G, Labao-Almeida C, Ferreira M, Molenaar R, Wahlen S, Konijn T, et al. Vitamin A controls the presence of RORgamma+ innate lymphoid cells and lymphoid tissue in the small intestine. *J Immunol* (2016) 196:5148–55. doi:10.4049/jimmunol.1501106
46. Pabst O, Herbrand H, Friedrichsen M, Velaga S, Dorsch M, Berhardt G, et al. Adaptation of solitary intestinal lymphoid tissue in response to microbiota and chemokine receptor CCR7 signaling. *J Immunol* (2006) 177:6824–32. doi:10.4049/jimmunol.177.10.6824
47. Bouskra D, Brezillon C, Berard M, Werts C, Varona R, Boneca IG, et al. Lymphoid tissue genesis induced by commensals through NOD1 regulates intestinal homeostasis. *Nature* (2008) 456:507–10. doi:10.1038/nature07450
48. McDonald KG, Mcdonough JS, Wang C, Kucharzik T, Williams IR, Newberry RD. CC chemokine receptor 6 expression by B lymphocytes is essential for the development of isolated lymphoid follicles. *Am J Pathol* (2007) 170:1229–40. doi:10.2353/ajpath.2007.060817
49. Baptista AP, Olivier BJ, Goverse G, Greuter M, Knippenberg M, Kusser K, et al. Colonic patch and colonic SILT development are independent and differentially regulated events. *Mucosal Immunol* (2013) 6:511–21. doi:10.1038/mi.2012.90
50. Donaldson DS, Bradford BM, Artis D, Mabbott NA. Reciprocal regulation of lymphoid tissue development in the large intestine by IL-25 and IL-23. *Mucosal Immunol* (2015) 8:582–95. doi:10.1038/mi.2014.90
51. Knoop KA, Butler BR, Kumar N, Newberry RD, Williams IR. Distinct developmental requirements for isolated lymphoid follicle formation in the small and large intestine: RANKL is essential only in the small intestine. *Am J Pathol* (2011) 179:1861–71. doi:10.1016/j.ajpath.2011.06.004
52. Zaph C, Du Y, Saenz SA, Nair MG, Perrigoue JG, Taylor BC, et al. Commensal-dependent expression of IL-25 regulates the IL-23-IL-17 axis in the intestine. *J Exp Med* (2008) 205:2191–8. doi:10.1084/jem.20080720
53. Sawa S, Lochner M, Satoh-Takayama N, Dulauroy S, Berard M, Kleinschek M, et al. RORgammat+ innate lymphoid cells regulate intestinal homeostasis by integrating negative signals from the symbiotic microbiota. *Nat Immunol* (2011) 12:320–6. doi:10.1038/ni.2002
54. Lochner M, Ohnmacht C, Presley L, Bruhns P, Si-Tahar M, Sawa S, et al. Microbiota-induced tertiary lymphoid tissues aggravate inflammatory disease in the absence of RORgamma t and LTi cells. *J Exp Med* (2011) 208:125–34. doi:10.1084/jem.20100052
55. Ohnmacht C, Marques R, Presley L, Sawa S, Lochner M, Eberl G. Intestinal microbiota, evolution of the immune system and the bad reputation of pro-inflammatory immunity. *Cell Microbiol* (2011) 13:653–9. doi:10.1111/j.1462-5822.2011.01577.x

56. Kweon MN, Yamamoto M, Rennert PD, Park EJ, Lee AY, Chang SY, et al. Prenatal blockage of lymphotoxin beta receptor and TNF receptor p55 signaling cascade resulted in the acceleration of tissue genesis for isolated lymphoid follicles in the large intestine. *J Immunol* (2005) 174:4365–72. doi:10.4049/jimmunol.174.7.4365
57. McNamee EN, Masterson JC, Jedlicka P, Collins CB, Williams IR, Rivera-Nieves J. Ectopic lymphoid tissue alters the chemokine gradient, increases lymphocyte retention and exacerbates murine ileitis. *Gut* (2013) 62:53–62. doi:10.1136/gutjnl-2011-301272
58. Fernandez-Salguero PM, Ward JM, Sundberg JP, Gonzalez FJ. Lesions of aryl-hydrocarbon receptor-deficient mice. *Vet Pathol* (1997) 34:605–14. doi:10.1177/030098589703400609
59. Makiyama K, Bennett MK, Jewell DP. Endoscopic appearances of the rectal mucosa of patients with Crohn's disease visualised with a magnifying colonoscope. *Gut* (1984) 25:337–40. doi:10.1136/gut.25.4.337
60. Surawicz CM, Belic L. Rectal biopsy helps to distinguish acute self-limited colitis from idiopathic inflammatory bowel disease. *Gastroenterology* (1984) 86:104–13.
61. Fujimura Y, Kamoi R, Iida M. Pathogenesis of aphthoid ulcers in Crohn's disease: correlative findings by magnifying colonoscopy, electron microscopy, and immunohistochemistry. *Gut* (1996) 38:724–32. doi:10.1136/gut.38.5.724
62. Kaiserling E. Newly-formed lymph nodes in the submucosa in chronic inflammatory bowel disease. *Lymphology* (2001) 34:22–9.
63. Carlsen HS, Baekkevold ES, Johansen FE, Haraldsen G, Brandtzaeg P. B cell attracting chemokine 1 (CXCL13) and its receptor CXCR5 are expressed in normal and aberrant gut associated lymphoid tissue. *Gut* (2002) 51:364–71. doi:10.1136/gut.51.3.364
64. Spahn TW, Herbst H, Rennert PD, Lugering N, Maaser C, Kraft M, et al. Induction of colitis in mice deficient of Peyer's patches and mesenteric lymph nodes is associated with increased disease severity and formation of colonic lymphoid patches. *Am J Pathol* (2002) 161:2273–82. doi:10.1016/S0002-9440(10)64503-8
65. Kawamura T, Kanai T, Dohi T, Uraushihara K, Totsuka T, Iiyama R, et al. Ectopic CD40 ligand expression on B cells triggers intestinal inflammation. *J Immunol* (2004) 172:6388–97. doi:10.4049/jimmunol.172.10.6388
66. Olivier B, Cailotto C, Van Der Vliet J, Knippenberg M, Greuter MJ, Hilbers F, et al. Vagal innervation is required for the formation of tertiary lymphoid tissue in colitis. *Eur J Immunol* (2016). doi:10.1002/eji.201646370
67. Obata T, Goto Y, Kunisawa J, Sato S, Sakamoto M, Setoyama H, et al. Indigenous opportunistic bacteria inhabit mammalian gut-associated lymphoid tissues and share a mucosal antibody-mediated symbiosis. *Proc Natl Acad Sci U S A* (2010) 107:7419–24. doi:10.1073/pnas.1001061107
68. Sonnenberg GF, Monticelli LA, Alenghat T, Fung TC, Hutnick NA, Kunisawa J, et al. Innate lymphoid cells promote anatomical containment of lymphoid-resident commensal bacteria. *Science* (2012) 336:1321–5. doi:10.1126/science.1222551
69. Fung TC, Bessman NJ, Hepworth MR, Kumar N, Shibata N, Kobuley D, et al. Lymphoid-tissue-resident commensal bacteria promote members of the IL-10 cytokine family to establish mutualism. *Immunity* (2016) 44:634–46. doi:10.1016/j.immuni.2016.02.019
70. Lorenz RG, Newberry RD. Isolated lymphoid follicles can function as sites for induction of mucosal immune responses. *Ann N Y Acad Sci* (2004) 1029:44–57. doi:10.1196/annals.1309.006
71. Schnupf P, Gaboriau-Routhiau V, Cerf-Bensussan N. Host interactions with segmented filamentous bacteria: an unusual trade-off that drives the post-natal maturation of the gut immune system. *Semin Immunol* (2013) 25:342–51. doi:10.1016/j.smim.2013.09.001
72. Gaboriau-Routhiau V, Rakotobe S, Lecuyer E, Mulder I, Lan A, Bridonneau C, et al. The key role of segmented filamentous bacteria in the coordinated maturation of gut helper T cell responses. *Immunity* (2009) 31:677–89. doi:10.1016/j.immuni.2009.08.020
73. Ivanov II, Atarashi K, Manel N, Brodie EL, Shima T, Karaoz U, et al. Induction of intestinal Th17 cells by segmented filamentous bacteria. *Cell* (2009) 139:485–98. doi:10.1016/j.cell.2009.09.033
74. Lecuyer E, Rakotobe S, Lengline-Garnier H, Lebreton C, Picard M, Juste C, et al. Segmented filamentous bacterium uses secondary and tertiary lymphoid tissues to induce gut IgA and specific T helper 17 cell responses. *Immunity* (2014) 40:608–20. doi:10.1016/j.immuni.2014.03.009
75. Shiu J, Piazuelo MB, Ding H, Czinn SJ, Drakes ML, Banerjee A, et al. Gastric LTi cells promote lymphoid follicle formation but are limited by IRAK-M and do not alter microbial growth. *Mucosal Immunol* (2015) 8:1047–59. doi:10.1038/mi.2014.132
76. Little MC, Bell LV, Cliffe LJ, Else KJ. The characterization of intraepithelial lymphocytes, lamina propria leukocytes, and isolated lymphoid follicles in the large intestine of mice infected with the intestinal nematode parasite *Trichuris muris*. *J Immunol* (2005) 175:6713–22. doi:10.4049/jimmunol.175.10.6713
77. Mundy R, Macdonald TT, Dougan G, Frankel G, Wiles S. *Citrobacter rodentium* of mice and man. *Cell Microbiol* (2005) 7:1697–706. doi:10.1111/j.1462-5822.2005.00625.x
78. Satoh-Takayama N, Vosshenrich CA, Lesjean-Pottier S, Sawa S, Lochner M, Rattis F, et al. Microbial flora drives interleukin 22 production in intestinal NKp46+ cells that provide innate mucosal immune defense. *Immunity* (2008) 29:958–70. doi:10.1016/j.immuni.2008.11.001
79. Cella M, Fuchs A, Vermi W, Facchetti F, Otero K, Lennerz JK, et al. A human natural killer cell subset provides an innate source of IL-22 for mucosal immunity. *Nature* (2009) 457:722–5. doi:10.1038/nature07537
80. Sonnenberg GF, Monticelli LA, Elloso MM, Fouser LA, Artis D. CD4(+) lymphoid tissue-inducer cells promote innate immunity in the gut. *Immunity* (2011) 34:122–34. doi:10.1016/j.immuni.2010.12.009
81. Liang SC, Tan XY, Luxenberg DP, Karim R, Dunussi-Joannopoulos K, Collins M, et al. Interleukin (IL)-22 and IL-17 are coexpressed by Th17 cells and cooperatively enhance expression of antimicrobial peptides. *J Exp Med* (2006) 203:2271–9. doi:10.1084/jem.20061308
82. Zheng Y, Valdez PA, Danilenko DM, Hu Y, Sa SM, Gong Q, et al. Interleukin-22 mediates early host defense against attaching and effacing bacterial pathogens. *Nat Med* (2008) 14:282–9. doi:10.1038/nm1720
83. Spahn TW, Maaser C, Eckmann L, Heidemann J, Lugering A, Newberry R, et al. The lymphotoxin-beta receptor is critical for control of murine *Citrobacter rodentium*-induced colitis. *Gastroenterology* (2004) 127:1463–73. doi:10.1053/j.gastro.2004.08.022
84. Wang Y, Koroleva EP, Kruglov AA, Kuprash DV, Nedospasov SA, Fu YX, et al. Lymphotoxin beta receptor signaling in intestinal epithelial cells orchestrates innate immune responses against mucosal bacterial infection. *Immunity* (2010) 32:403–13. doi:10.1016/j.immuni.2010.02.011
85. Ota N, Wong K, Valdez PA, Zheng Y, Crellin NK, Diehl L, et al. IL-22 bridges the lymphotoxin pathway with the maintenance of colonic lymphoid structures during infection with *Citrobacter rodentium*. *Nat Immunol* (2011) 12:941–8. doi:10.1038/ni.2089
86. Tumanov AV, Koroleva EP, Guo X, Wang Y, Kruglov A, Nedospasov S, et al. Lymphotoxin controls the IL-22 protection pathway in gut innate lymphoid cells during mucosal pathogen challenge. *Cell Host Microbe* (2011) 10:44–53. doi:10.1016/j.chom.2011.06.002
87. Barone F, Nayar S, Campos J, Cloake T, Withers DR, Toellner KM, et al. IL-22 regulates lymphoid chemokine production and assembly of tertiary lymphoid organs. *Proc Natl Acad Sci U S A* (2015) 112:11024–9. doi:10.1073/pnas.1503315112
88. Kennedy WP, Simon JA, Offutt C, Horn P, Herman A, Townsend MJ, et al. Efficacy and safety of pateclizumab (anti-lymphotoxin-alpha) compared to adalimumab in rheumatoid arthritis: a head-to-head phase 2 randomized controlled study (The ALTARA Study). *Arthritis Res Ther* (2014) 16:467. doi:10.1186/s13075-014-0467-3
89. St.Clair EW, Baer AN, Noaiseh G, Parke A, Coca A, Utset T, et al. The clinical efficacy and safety of baminercept, a lymphotoxin-beta receptor fusion protein, in primary Sjögren's syndrome: results from a randomized, double-blind, placebo-controlled phase II trial. *Arthritis Rheumatol* (2015) 67(Suppl 10). Available at: http://acrabstracts.org/abstract/the-clinical-efficacy-and-safety-of-baminercept-a-lymphotoxin-beta-receptor-fusion-protein-in-primary-sjogrens-syndrome-results-from-a-randomized-double-blind-placebo-controlled-phase-ii-trial/
90. Kramer JM, Klimatcheva E, Rothstein TL. CXCL13 is elevated in Sjogren's syndrome in mice and humans and is implicated in disease pathogenesis. *J Leukoc Biol* (2013) 94:1079–89. doi:10.1189/jlb.0113036
91. Klimatcheva E, Pandina T, Reilly C, Torno S, Bussler H, Scrivens M, et al. CXCL13 antibody for the treatment of autoimmune disorders. *BMC Immunol* (2015) 16:6. doi:10.1186/s12865-015-0068-1

92. Henry RA, Kendall PL. CXCL13 blockade disrupts B lymphocyte organization in tertiary lymphoid structures without altering B cell receptor bias or preventing diabetes in nonobese diabetic mice. *J Immunol* (2010) 185:1460–5. doi:10.4049/jimmunol.0903710
93. Gaffen SL, Jain R, Garg AV, Cua DJ. The IL-23-IL-17 immune axis: from mechanisms to therapeutic testing. *Nat Rev Immunol* (2014) 14:585–600. doi:10.1038/nri3707
94. Canete JD, Celis R, Yeremenko N, Sanmarti R, Van Duivenvoorde L, Ramirez J, et al. Ectopic lymphoid neogenesis is strongly associated with activation of the IL-23 pathway in rheumatoid synovitis. *Arthritis Res Ther* (2015) 17:173. doi:10.1186/s13075-015-0688-0
95. Rangel-Moreno J, Carragher DM, de la Luz Garcia-Hernandez M, Hwang JY, Kusser K, Hartson L, et al. The development of inducible bronchus-associated lymphoid tissue depends on IL-17. *Nat Immunol* (2011) 12: 639–46. doi:10.1038/ni.2053
96. Peters A, Pitcher LA, Sullivan JM, Mitsdoerffer M, Acton SE, Franz B, et al. Th17 cells induce ectopic lymphoid follicles in central nervous system tissue inflammation. *Immunity* (2011) 35:986–96. doi:10.1016/j.immuni.2011.10.015
97. Fleige H, Ravens S, Moschovakis GL, Bolter J, Willenzon S, Sutter G, et al. IL-17-induced CXCL12 recruits B cells and induces follicle formation in BALT in the absence of differentiated FDCs. *J Exp Med* (2014) 211:643–51. doi:10.1084/jem.20131737

16

Tertiary Lymphoid Organs in Cancer Tissues

Nobuyoshi Hiraoka[1,2,3], Yoshinori Ino[2,3] and Rie Yamazaki-Itoh[2]*

[1] Division of Pathology and Clinical Laboratories, National Cancer Center Hospital, Tokyo, Japan, [2] Division of Molecular Pathology, National Cancer Center Research Institute, Tokyo, Japan, [3] Division of Analytical Pathology, National Cancer Center Research Institute, Tokyo, Japan

***Correspondence:**
Nobuyoshi Hiraoka
nhiraoka@ncc.go.jp

Tertiary lymphoid organs (TLOs) are induced postnatally in non-lymphoid tissues such as those affected by chronic infections, autoimmune diseases, and chronic allograft rejection, and also in cancer tissues. TLOs are thought to provide important lymphocytic functional environments for both cellular and humoral immunity, similar to lymph nodes or Peyer's patches. TLOs have a structure similar to that of lymph nodes or Peyer's patches, including T cell zones, B cell follicles, and high endothelial venules (HEV) without encapsulation. Here, we review recent advances in our knowledge of TLOs in human solid cancers, including their location, structure, methods of evaluation, and clinicopathological impact. We also discuss the formation and/or maintenance of TLOs in cancer tissues in association with the tumor immune microenvironment, cancer invasion, and the tissue structure of the cancer stroma.

Keywords: tertiary lymphoid organs, cancer, tumor immunology, tissue structure, tumor microenvironment

INTRODUCTION

Cancer tissue is composed of cancer cells and a stroma (alternatively referred to as the cancer microenvironment or tumor microenvironment), and cancer cells themselves, the cancer stroma, and their interaction can determine the biological behavior of the cancer (1). The cancer stroma is composed of vessels, fibroblasts, immune cells, and an extracellular matrix, making cancer tissue analogous to a form of organ. The host immune system is one of the leading players in the tumor microenvironment (1), and plays a critical role in tumor surveillance (2–4). The host antitumor immune reaction differs according to tumor type, tumor developmental stage, and the tissue from which the tumor develops. For example, colon cancers with many gene mutations such as those with microsatellite instability (MSI) tend to be immunogenic with a higher number of tumor-infiltrating lymphocytes (TILs) (5, 6), and many respond to immunotherapy with immune checkpoint inhibitors, although many patients with colon cancer do not achieve the same degree of effect with any given immunotherapy due to non-immunogenicity of the tumor (7).

Tumor-infiltrating immune cells often represent the host immune reaction. The presence of high numbers of TILs has been found to be a major predictor of favorable clinical outcome in many types of solid cancer, such as colorectal, lung, ovarian, and pancreatic cancers (8, 9). Cells of myeloid lineage, such as macrophages, granulocytes, and mast cells, also infiltrate tumor tissues, especially macrophages, which are usually the most abundant cells infiltrating tumor tissues, and these myeloid cells exert many biological effects in cancer (10–16). These tumor-infiltrating myeloid cells have also been shown to be prognostically significant (9, 12). The tumor immune microenvironment shows a drastic change during the natural history of tumor development and progression, i.e., from an immune reaction to immune tolerance during the progression of multi-step carcinogenesis (17–19). Meanwhile, inflammatory responses affect tumor development at different stages, including initiation, promotion, malignant conversion, invasion, and metastasis (20). Tumor-infiltrating immune cells engage in extensive and dynamic cross-talk with cancer cells, and some of the molecular events that mediate this dialog have been revealed (20). Accumulated evidence suggests that even the same types or subsets of tumor-infiltrating immune cells sometimes have different and opposite effects on patient outcome (8, 21).

The central mechanism involved in cellular immune reactions begins when immature dendritic cells (DCs) take up foreign antigens and then migrate to regional lymph nodes to present the antigens to T cells. The cognate T cells then proliferate and begin to remove the foreign antigens. The B cell-mediated immune response is mainly humoral, and occurs in peripheral lymphoid organs such as lymph nodes or the spleen. Thus, lymph nodes, Peyer's patches, and the spleen act as a lymphocytic functional environment for both cellular and humoral immunity, and these lymphoid organs are referred to as secondary lymphoid organs (SLOs) or tissues, in contrast to the primary lymphoid organs (PLOs) – the thymus and bone marrow – where lymphocytes are produced and educated. These PLOs and SLOs develop during embryogenesis and early life. Postnatal lymphoid organs with a morphology similar to SLOs are induced to form in non-lymphoid tissues such as those associated with chronic inflammation, chronic allograft rejection, or cancer, and these are known as tertiary lymphoid organs (TLOs) or structures (alternatively, ectopic lymphoid structures). TLOs are generally induced in areas of extensive local activation of cellular and humoral immune responses. TLOs are thought to play roles in immune responses that are similar to those of SLOs (22–26). One type of TLO, bronchus-associated lymphoid tissue (BALT), can independently initiate local B- and T-cell responses (24) and serves as a reservoir of memory B and T cells (23). Mice with BALT are strikingly more resistant to pulmonary infection with a variety of infectious agents than mice without BALT (24, 26). Dieu-Nosjean et al. have observed TLO components in lung cancers that are very similar (but not identical) to those of SLOs, being active in cellular and humoral immune responses (27, 28). In comparison to SLOs, TLOs are located very much closer to, or within, lesions and have similar immune function. Therefore, TLOs act as a front line base or bridgehead on the "immune battlefield."

DEFINITION, LOCATION, AND STRUCTURE OF TLOs

Tertiary lymphoid organs can develop in various kinds of inflamed and non-lymphoid tissues including those associated with chronic infections, autoimmune diseases, chronic allograft rejection, and several solid cancers (29–34). TLOs are organized lymphoid structures similar to SLOs, characterized by B-cell follicles, T-cell zones, and specialized vessels known as high endothelial venules (HEVs), although TLOs are not encapsulated and supplied by afferent lymphatics.

Lymphocytic infiltration, lymphocyte trafficking, and lymphocyte homing are accurately regulated by several types of chemotactic factors and adhesion molecules expressed or demonstrated on endothelial cells or along the pathways of lymphocytic movement (35–37). The lymphocyte trafficking system allows appropriate subset of lymphocytes with appropriate activity deploy to appropriate sites, areas, or tissues with appropriate timing. Effector or effector memory lymphocytes infiltrate into inflamed tissues, although large numbers of lymphocytes, particularly naive and central memory lymphocytes, accumulate in TLOs by homing through the HEVs from the blood by a multi-step mechanism that involves L-selectin-, chemokine-, and integrin-mediated lymphocyte-endothelial cell interaction (35, 36, 38). HEVs specifically express L-selectin ligands, including peripheral node addressin (PNAd), which are sulfated sialyl Lewis X molecules whose carbohydrate structures and biological function have been clarified by our group and others (37, 39–44). Chemokines CCL19 and CCL21 are necessary for the recruitment and disposition of T cells and DCs within lymphoid tissue, and chemokine CXCL13 functions in the recruitment and disposition of B cells. These chemokines are also involved in lymphoid neogenesis (29–34).

Location of TLOs in Cancer Tissues

Tumor-associated TLOs can be located peritumorally or intratumorally (**Figure 1**). The majority of TLOs in cancer tissues develop in peritumoral areas, and are characterized as TLOs at the invasive front (or invasive margin), forming a wall around the cancer tissue. Peritumoral TLOs are positioned just outside the cancer tissue or in the periphery of the cancer (within the cancer-invasive area). Intratumoral TLOs are much rarer than peritumoral TLOs in common types of cancer, but the frequency of intratumoral TLOs varies depending on the tissue of cancer origin and the tumor type. If intratumoral TLOs are relatively abundant in a tumor type that usually shows only a low frequency of them, this suggests that the tumor is a limited or rather specialized case.

Structures of TLOs

Tertiary lymphoid organs have a structure similar to that of lymph nodes or Peyer's patches. In addition to the histology, the constituent cells of TLOs and the molecules they express are quite similar to those in SLOs, as would be expected (46–48). T-zone T cells are $CD62L^+$ and mainly central memory $CD4^+$ T cells or naive T cells that accumulate *via* HEVs from the blood stream. The T cell area also contains immature and $CD208^+$ mature DCs. The density of HEVs is strongly correlated with the density of $CD3^+$ T cells, $CD8^+$ T cells, $CD20^+$ B cells, and $CD208^+$ mature DCs (49). The B-cell follicle is composed of a mantle of naive B cells, surrounding a germinal center (GC) composed of highly proliferating B cells and a network of $CD21^+$ follicular DCs. Development of the GC structure represents an active immune reaction, and the density of GCs in lung and breast cancers has been significantly correlated with patient outcome (48, 50, 51). In addition to lymphoid chemokines (CCL19, CCL21, CXCL13) and adhesion molecules (ICAM-2, ICAM-3, VCAM-1, MAdCAM-1), CCL17, CCL22, and IL16 are found in TLOs (48, 50–52). One interesting feature in lung cancer is that no $NKp46^+$ NK cells are detected in TLOs (47), thus allowing

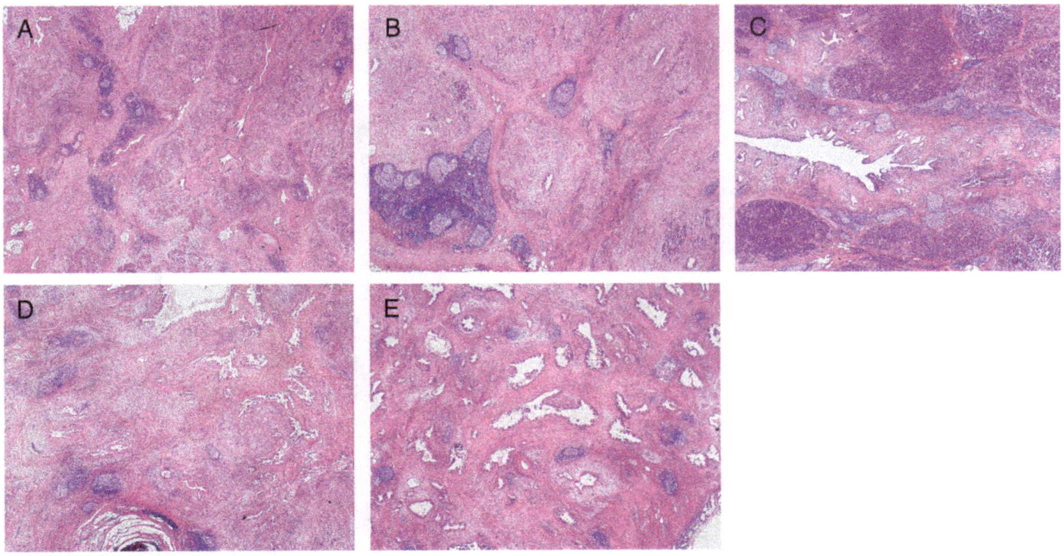

FIGURE 1 | Histological features of TLOs (45) in chronic pancreatitis (A), IgG4-related lymphoplasmacytic sclerosing pancreatitis (autoimmune pancreatitis) (B,C), and pancreatic ductal adenocarcinoma (PDAC) (D,E). TLOs are distributed evenly in inflamed tissues **(A,B)** and sometimes concentrated near the target structure (around ducts) **(C)**. In contrast, cancer tissue is surrounded by peritumoral TLOs **(D)** and a rare pancreatic cancer case has intratumoral TLOs **(D)**. Common PDAC has a paucity of vessels and lacks intratumoral TLOs, although limited cases do have intratumoral TLOs that are richer in tumor-infiltrating lymphocytes and retain relatively intact vascular networks consisting of arterioles, venules, and capillaries without cancer invasion.

them to be distinguished from SLOs. NK cells and DCs are co-localized in lymph nodes, and their interaction enhances NK cell proliferation, IFN-γ secretion, and cytotoxic function, as well as promoting DC maturation (47).

CLINICOPATHOLOGICAL IMPACT OF TLOs IN HUMAN CANCERS

The presence of TLOs in cancer tissues has been reported to be a favorable prognostic indicator (**Table 1**) (45, 48, 50–68), although some studies have concluded that this is not always the case (55, 60), or may only apply to exceptional cancers such as renal cell carcinoma (61).

Evaluation of TLOs

It is important to detect the presence of TLOs in both tumors and the tissues surrounding them. However, there is still no consensus regarding the best method for evaluation of TLOs as different approaches may be needed according to the types of cancer or the tissues from which they develop. Recent studies have detected TLOs using a combination of histological and immunohistochemical methods according to whether the TLOs have B-cell follicles, T-cell zones, and HEVs detected by immune-labeling for $CD20^+$ cells, $CD3^+$ cells, and $PNAd^+$ vessels, respectively (**Figure 2**). This offers a basic approach that can evaluate the clinicopathological and biological characteristics of TLOs from a neutral viewpoint. Other methods have adopted a morphological approach, or the use of specific markers such as lymphoid aggregates with $CD208^+$ mature DCs, or the expression profiles of chemokine genes. These are good biomarkers for detection of TLOs with active immune reactions in lung, breast (48, 59), or colon cancers that are significantly correlated with a better patient outcome (57). One potential problem is that these markers are not always specific, for example the detection of $CD208^+$ cells in cancer tissue as representative of the presence of TLOs can be applied to only limited types of cancer where all the $CD208^+$ cells are mature DCs located within TLOs. Lung cancer is a good example of this, although in renal cell carcinoma $CD208^+$ cells are present in non-TLO stroma (61).

Recently, the International TIL Working Group (2014) has informally recommended a method for evaluating TLOs in breast cancer within the existing method for evaluation of TILs (69). In breast cancer, it has been pointed out that TLOs are typically localized in the area surrounding the tumor, and may be localized in normal tissue directly adjacent to the tumor. However, only a limited population of breast cancers has apparent intratumoral TLOs. TILs are counted within the borders of the invasive tumor and exclude TLOs. Lee et al. have evaluated TLOs using this recommended method and observed that TLOs were present mainly around carcinoma *in situ* (CIS) and in adjacent terminal duct lobular units (63, 64).

Frequency of TLOs

The frequency of TLOs varies, and tends to be dependent upon where the TLOs are located and the types of cancer (**Table 1**). At least one peritumoral TLO has been found in more than 90% of cases of colorectal, pancreatic, and breast cancer, while intratumoral TLOs have been observed in only about 15% of colorectal and pancreatic cancers. About 20–40% of skin and oral mucosal cancers have TLOs, where the surfaces of background tissues are covered by squamous cell epithelium.

TABLE 1 | Summary of TLOs in human cancers.

Cancer types	Evaluation	Numbers of case	Location of TLOs	Frequency of TLOs (presence)	Prognostication	Significant association			Reference
						Clinicopathological variables	TIL, TAM	Others	
Breast cancer	IHC (PNAd$^+$ HEV)	146 (Stage I–III)	Mixed (peritumoral and intratumoral)	ND	Favorable (OS, DFS)	No association (tumor size, grade, nodal metastasis, hormone receptor status, adjuvant chemotherapy, CD34$^+$ blood vessel within cancer stroma)	CD3$^+$T, CD8$^+$T, FOXP3$^+$ cells, ratio of FOXP3/CD3[b], CD20$^+$B	[Gene expression] related to Th1 cell orientation, cytotoxic granules, lymphoid chemokines, and T cell homing receptors	(48, 52)
	Histology and IHC with gene expression (Tfh)	794 (Stage I–III, ER$^-$HER2$^-$ 163, HER2$^+$ 120, ER$^+$HER2$^-$ 510)	Mixed (peritumoral and intratumoral)	ND	Favorable (DFS) in all patients, HER2$^+$, or ER$^+$HER2$^-$ patients	ND	Tfh, Th1	[Gene expression] CXCL13	(51)
	Gene expression (Tfh, CXCL13)	996 [preoperative chemotherapy (+)]	Mixed (peritumoral and intratumoral)	ND	Favorable	ND	ND	ND	(51)
	Histology and IHC (CD3$^+$T, CD20$^+$B)	290 (Stage I–III, invasive carcinoma 257, DCIS 33)	Peritumoral	110 (38.6%)	No prognostic	DCIS grade, ER status[b], PR status[b], HER2 status, tumor grade, nodal metastasis, histological TIL	ND	ND	(60)
	Recommended histological criteria (68)	769 (Stage I–III, triple negative breast cancer)	Peritumoral	713 (92.7%: minimal 17.2%, moderate 36.2%, abundant 39.4%)	Favorable (OS[a], DFS[a])	Histological TIL	ND	ND	(64)
	Recommended histological criteria (68)	447 (Stage I to III, HER2$^+$ invasive carcinoma)	Peritumoral	404 (79%: minimal 37.1%, moderate 31.3%, abundant 10.2%)	No prognostic	TIL, ER ALLred score[b], HER2 IHC score, HER2 copy number, DCIS percentage, HLA-A percentage, HLA-ABC percentage	ND	ND	(63)
Colorectal cancer	Gene expression (12 chemokines)	20 (Stage 0–IV$_A$, 10 the highest and 11 the lowest score tumors selected from 326)	Mixed (peritumoral and intratumoral)	ND	Favorable (OS)	No association (sex, tumor grade, tumor site, location, MSI-H/MSS status, tumor stage)	ND	(Gene expression) related to cytotoxicity and DC	(57)
	Histology and IHC	418 (Stage I–IV)	Peritumoral (extra-tumoral)	411 (98.3%)	Favorable (OS)	TNM stage[b], preoperative radiotherapy or chemoradiotherapy[b], deficient mismatch repair enzyme expression	CD3$^+$T, CD8$^+$T, FOXP3$^+$, CD83$^+$ (at invasive front and at stromal); CD3$^+$T, CD8$^+$T (intraepithelial)		(65)
		149 (Stage I–IV)	Peritumoral (extra-tumoral)	147 (98.7%)					(65)
		351 (Stage II 185, stage III 166)	Mixed (peritumoral and intratumoral)	276 (78.6%)	Favorable (DFS) in stage II; no prognostic (DFS) in stage III	PNAd$^+$HEV	CD3$^+$T		(58)
	IHC (PNAd$^+$ HEV)	62 (Duke's A and C)	Peritumoral (extra-tumoral), intratumoral	Peritumoral TLO: 49 (79%); intratumoral TLO: <8 (12.9%)	No prognostic	More advanced disease, no association (MSI status)		ND	(55)

(Continued)

TABLE 1 | Continued

Cancer types	Evaluation	Numbers of case	Location of TLOs	Frequency of TLOs (presence)	Prognostication	Significant association			Reference
						Clinicopathological variables	TIL, TAM	Others	
Lung cancer	IHC (CD208^{+}mature DC)	74 (Stage I to II, ADC 46, SCC 28)	Mixed (peritumoral and intratumoral)	ND	Favorable (OS, DSS, DFS)	No association (sex, smoking history, histology, tumor grade, TNM stage, fibrosis, necrosis, Ki-67 tumor cells)	CD3^{+}T, ratio of CD4/CD8, T-bet^{+}, CD20^{+}B	ND	(46, 50, 59)
	IHC (CD208^{+}mature DC, follicular CD20^{+}B)	122 (Stage III with neoadjuvant chemotherapy)	Mixed (peritumoral and intratumoral)	ND	Favorable (DSS)	ND	ND	An adaptive and specific humoral immune response (+)	(50)
	IHC (CD208^{+}mature DC)	458 (Stage I-IV, ADC 241, SCC 111, others 18, ND 6)						(Gene expression) related to cytotoxicity and Th1	(62)
Germ cell tumor	Histology	6 (Intracranial germinaom 2, seminoma 3, dysgerminoma 1)	Intratumoral TLO	ND	ND	ND	ND	an adaptive and specific humoral immune response (+)	(66)
MALT lymphoma	Histology	20 (salivary gland)	ND	ND	ND	ND	ND	ND	(53)
Skin Merkel cell carcinoma	Histology	21 (Stage I to IV)	Mixed (peritumoral and intratumoral)	8 (38%)	Favorable (DFS)[a], no prognostic (OS)	No association (age, sex, TNM stage, extension status)	Ratio of CD8/ CD4 (at tumor periphery)	ND	(54)
Oral squamous cell carcinoma	Histology and IHC (CD3^{+}T, CD20^{+}B, PNAd^{+}HEV)	80 (Stage I to IV)	Peritumoral predominant	17 (21%)	Favorable (DSS)[a]	No association (age, sex, smoking history, alcohol consumption, tumor site, tumor grade, TNM stage, treatment, HPV status)	ND	ND	(67)
Pancreatic cancer	Histology and IHC (CD3^{+}T, CD20^{+}B, PNAd^{+}HEV)	308 (Stage I to IV)	Intratumoral and peritumoral	Intratumoral TLO 49 (12.9%), peritumoral TLO 308 (100%)	Only intratumoral TLO: favorable (OS, DFS)	Only intratumoral TLO: tumor grade[b], venous invasion[b]	Only intratumoral TLO: CD3^{+}T, CD4^{+}T, CD8^{+}T, ratio of FOXP3/ CD4[b], CD163^{+}M2[b]	Only intratumoral TLO: (gene expression) related to Th1 and Th17	(45)
	Histology and IHC (CD3^{+}T, CD20^{+}B, PNAd^{+}HEV)	226 (Stage I to IV)	Intratumoral and peritumoral	Intratumoral TLO 37 (16.4%), peritumoral TLO 308 (100%)	Only intratumoral TLO: favorable (OS, DFS)	ND			(45)
Renal cell carcinoma	IHC (CD208^{+}mature DC)	135 (Clear cell RCC), 51 ccRCC lung metastasis	Peritumoral?	ND	No prognostic (TLS-DC, OS, DFS), unfavorable (NTLS-DC, peritumoral, OS, DFS)	TLS-DC: PD-1^{+} cells[b], PD-L1, and/or PD-L2^{+} tumor cells[b]	ND	ND	(61)
Cutaneous metastasis of malignant melanoma	Histology and IHC (CD3^{+}T, CD20^{+}B, PNAd^{+}HEV)	29	Mixed (peritumoral and intratumoral)	7 (24% complete TLO), 6 (20% incomplete TLO)	ND	ND	ND	ND	(56)

[a]*By only univariate analysis.*

[b]*Negatively associated.*

ADC, adenocarcinoma; DCIS, ductal carcinoma in situ; DFS, disease-free survival; DSS, disease-specific survival; HPV, human papilloma virus; IHC, immunohistochemistry; MSI-H, microsatellite instability – high; MSS, microsatellite stable; ND, not determined; OS, overall survival; PNAd, peripheral node addressin; SCC, squamous cell carcinoma; TAMs, tumor-associated macrophages; TILs, tumor-infiltrating lymphocytes.

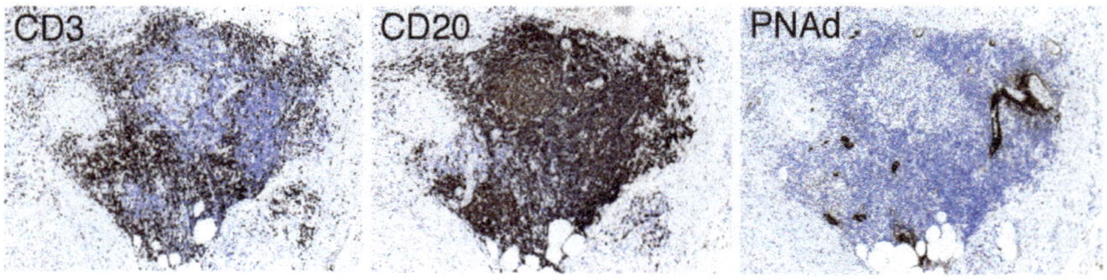

FIGURE 2 | Immunohistochemistry detecting a TLO having B-cell follicles, T-cell zones, and HEVs detected by immune-labeling for CD20⁺ cells, CD3⁺ cells, and PNAd⁺ vessels, respectively (45).

TLOs in oral squamous cell carcinoma are found mainly in the peritumoral stroma within 0.5 mm from the tumor front, in lymphocyte-rich subepithelial areas (67). The density of TLOs in breast cancer shows a marked reduction from DCIS to invasive carcinoma, although other studies have obtained different findings (60).

Prognostic Impact

The presence of TLOs is usually indicative of a favorable prognosis, although a few reports have suggested it may have a rather negative prognostic impact (**Table 1**). Bento et al. reported that the presence of extra-tumoral TLOs in colorectal cancer was significantly associated with more advanced disease (55). Figenschau et al. considered that cases of breast cancer associated with TLOs had a higher tumor grade and a high frequency of lymph nodal metastasis (60). These inconsistent results may explain why no universally accepted method for evaluating TLOs has emerged.

The location of TLOs has not been considered in the majority of previous studies. We have evaluated the clinicopathological impact of both peritumoral and intratumoral TLOs in two different cohorts of patients with pancreatic cancer ($n = 308, 226$). Though the presence and density of peritumoral TLOs were not prognostic, the presence of intratumoral TLOs was an independent prognostic factor. In only five cases (1.6%) that showed a higher density of intratumoral TLOs, four of the patients survived without recurrence at least 7 years after the surgery even though one of them had stage 2A disease, three were stage 2B, and one was stage 4 (45).

Association with Clinicopathologic Variables

The presence of TLOs is basically independent of various clinicopathologic factors in several types of cancer (**Table 1**). Sometimes a few factors may be significantly associated with TLOs, although no definite tendency has yet emerged. The microsatellite instability (MSI) subset of colorectal cancer has been shown to have an immunogenic character with massive TIL, although the relationship between TLOs and MSI is controversial; in colorectal cancers, two studies found no significant association (55, 57) and one study demonstrated a significant association whereby a more marked Crohn's-like lymphoid reaction (extra-tumoral TLOs) was significantly associated with deficient expression of the mismatch repair enzyme (65).

Association with the Immune Microenvironment

The presence and density of TLOs are significantly correlated with immune reaction in many cancers, although there are differences in degree among studies or cancer types (**Table 1**). TILs (TLOs are usually not counted as TILs) are better indicators of the immune microenvironment, as they lie within the tumor that are detected by histological examination, although it is impossible to avoid contamination from lymphocytes infiltrating into tissues surrounding the cancer invasive area or lymphocytes in intratumoral TLOs in assays such as flow cytometry and RT-PCR using cells or tissues prepared on the basis of macroscopic findings.

Tertiary lymphoid organ presence and density are associated with mainly Th1- and cytotoxicity-related cellular immune reactions that commonly occur in cancers of the breast, colorectum, lung, and pancreas (**Table 1**). TLO density is also associated with FOXP3⁺ cells but negatively associated with the FOXP3⁺/CD3⁺T cell ratio or the FOXP3/CD4⁺T cell ratio, and also M2 macrophages in breast and/or pancreatic cancer, being consistent with features mentioned above (45, 48). In the tumor microenvironment associated with TLOs, Th1- and cytotoxicity-related genes are commonly expressed, whereas DC-related genes are expressed in colorectal cancer and Th17-related genes in pancreatic cancer. Th2- and immune inhibition-related genes are not significantly associated with TLOs. The presence and density of TLOs are associated with CD20⁺ B cells. In breast and lung cancers, the size and density, or numbers, of B-cell follicles or GCs are significantly correlated with favorable outcome (50, 51). Furthermore, in lung cancer and germ cell tumors, the presence of B-cell follicles in TLOs shows that the machinery for GC somatic hypermutation and class switch recombination is activated, along with the generation of plasma cells (50, 66). It has been thought that B cells play an important role in antitumor immunity, perhaps by capturing and presenting tumor antigens to T cells or by generating tumor antigen-specific antibodies that target tumor antigens to DCs expressing receptors for antibody constant regions. Germain et al. have stated that the presence of CD208⁺ mature DCs with a high density of B-cell follicles is a strong indicator of outcome in patients with lung cancers (50). Thus, it appears that a high density of TLOs is a good biomarker of a tumor immune microenvironment where active cellular and humoral immune reactions are occurring.

A recent study has also shown that Treg cells actively restrain effector T cells within tumor-associated TLOs. Localized Treg cell depletion in a murine model of lung adenocarcinoma triggers robust effector T cell responses and tumor destruction, suggesting that, in this model, Treg cells in TLOs actively restrain anti-tumor immunity (70). Therefore, in order to enhance the effects of immunotherapy, it is recommended that Treg depletion should be performed.

FORMATION, MAINTENANCE, AND INDUCTION OF TLOs IN CANCER TISSUES

Formation of SLOs and TLOs

The mechanism of SLO formation has been studied actively, and is considered to share a number of features with TLO formation. Details can be found in another review (29–34, 71). Molecular and cellular mechanisms exist for the development of SLOs (29–34, 71). One pathway mainly for organogenesis of lymph nodes is initiated by interaction between $CD3^-CD4^+CD45^+$ lymphoid tissue inducer (LTi) cells and stromal organizer (STo) cells at the lymph node anlagen. These specialized cells are of hematopoietic and mesenchymal lineage, respectively. Retinoic acid, probably derived from nerve fibers, induces the expression of CXCL13 in stromal cells. LTi cells accumulate in response to local expression of CXCL13 to form the first cell clusters. In response to IL-7 and TNFSF11, LTi cells are induced to secrete lymphotoxin (LT) $\alpha_1\beta_2$. Interaction of $LT\alpha_1\beta_2$ expressed on LTi cells with the LTβ receptor (LTβR) expressed on stromal cells allows the latter to differentiate into STo cells, resulting in secretion of the lymphoid chemokines CCL19, CCL21, and CXCL13 to recruit hematopoietic cells and increase the expression of VCAM-1, ICAM-1, and MAdCAM-1 to ensure lymphocyte retention. Chemokines CCL19 and CCL21 interact with their receptor CCR7 to recruit T cells and DCs, and chemokine CXCL13 interacts with the chemokine receptor CXCR5 to recruit B cells. STo cells also secrete VEGF-C, FGF-2, and HGF, which promote development of the lymphatic vasculature and HEVs. STo cells also differentiate into stromal cell lineages including follicular DCs, fibroblastic reticular cells, and marginal reticular cells, which populate lymph nodes and contribute to SLO function. Another pathway operates mainly for Peyer's patch formation. $CD11c^+$ cells engage RET ligand expressed on gut, and RET-dependent signaling leads to expression of $LT\alpha_1\beta_2$ by the $CD11c^+$ cells. Interaction of these $CD11c^+$ cells and $LT\beta R^+$ stromal cells allows the latter to differentiate into STo cells, followed by steps similar to those responsible for formation of lymph nodes. It has been speculated that the mechanism responsible for formation of TLOs is similar to that for SLOs, especially lymph node and mucosal lymphoid tissues, since there are many features of TLOs that are common to the formation of SLOs. Th17, γδT cells expressing IL-17A, or innate lymphoid cell 3 (ILC3) may substitute for LTi cells for development of TLOs (72, 73). These cells share common features with LTi cells, e.g., production of common cytokines such as IL-17A, IL-22, LTβ, TNF, and GM-CSF. T follicular helper (Tfh) cells expressing CXCL13 are also implicated in the regulation of TLOs, representing a key initiator of lymphoid organogenesis that functions upstream of LTβR signaling, promoting B-cell activities, and supporting the generation of high-affinity antibodies at GCs (72, 74, 75). Instead of STo cells, stromal tissue cells such as synovial fibroblasts (e.g., in rheumatoid arthritis) contribute to TLO formation. CXCL13 can be produced by marginal reticular cells, Tfh and follicular DCs, as well as some monocytes/macrophages, a subset of memory T cells, activated B cells, some endothelial cells, stromal cells, or epithelial cells in inflammatory foci. Chemokines, CXCL13, CCL19, CCL21, and CXCL12 are involved in not only the initiation of TLO development, but also maintenance of the highly organized cellular architecture of established SLOs and TLOs.

Formation and Maintenance of TLOs in Cancer Tissues

How do TLOs develop in human cancer tissues? Is the process different from that occurring in chronically inflamed tissue? Currently there is still no complete answer, although it likely involves (1) the state of antitumor immunity (tumor immunogenicity and immune microenvironment) and (2) the state of tissue structures necessary for formation/maintenance of TLOs.

A number of previous studies have indicated that an active immune response is usually present in background tissues with TLOs, both in cancer and chronic inflammation. The structures and contents of TLOs are comparable between these two situations, although cancer-associated TLOs show a high density of Tregs and absence of NK cells. The location of TLOs is another significant point, as mentioned above. In contrast to the evenly distributed TLOs in chronically inflamed tissues, TLOs in the majority of cancers are present in the area surrounding the invasive lesion, i.e., they are peritumoral TLOs. In non-invasive breast cancer (DCIS) (63, 64), it is interesting that non-invasive cancerous ducts or lobules, including peripheral ducts, are surrounded by TLOs, bearing a histological resemblance to a chronic autoimmune reaction. In invasive cancers, almost the entire cancer tissue is surrounded by TLOs, and intratumoral TLOs are rarely present. Etiologically, TLO formation is expected to occur in tissues with active and continuous immune reactions involving active inflammation. This situation is common in tissues surrounding cancer, since the foreign antigens of cancer cells are presented continuously, tissue destruction caused by cancer invasion becomes a trigger of inflammation, and healthy non-cancerous tissue structures (blood vessels, nerve fibers, extracellular matrix, etc.) remain.

Arterioles and venules, which are small-sized arteries and veins, respectively, are associated with TLOs, and nerve fibers are usually found in TLOs in pancreatic cancers and chronic pancreatitis (45). TLOs, which develop in the pancreatic parenchyma in both chronic pancreatitis and pancreatic cancer, are always found in the interlobular spaces, where arterioles, venules, and relatively large nerve fibers are confined (45). It is speculated that these arterioles, venules, and nerve fibers are necessary for formation and/or maintenance of TLOs. The high frequency of arterial or venous invasion by cancer cells reduces the densities of arteries, arterioles, veins, and venules in the pancreatic cancer stroma. Common pancreatic cancers that have a high frequency of venous or arterial invasion lack intratumoral TLOs regardless of whether peritumoral TLOs are present. Conversely, intratumoral TLOs are found in pancreatic cancers with a low frequency of venous or arterial invasion (45).

A high frequency of venous invasion is found in TLOs at the invasive front. It is speculated that peritumoral TLOs in pancreatic cancer are destroyed and dispersed by cancer invasion, mainly venous invasion, and that other TLOs just outside the invasive front are induced to form. These in turn become surrounded by newly invasive cancer tissues, thus becoming new peritumoral TLOs, which are again subjected to invasion and destruction by further cancer invasion. These processes are repeated, resulting in cancer tissue being surrounded by peritumoral TLOs, whereas intratumoral TLOs are absent (**Figure 3**). Peritumoral TLOs can be induced if appropriate immune stimuli are present, since arterioles, venules, and nerve fibers remain intact in the surrounding tissue outside the cancer-invasive area, being consistent with the above hypothesis.

It is noteworthy that pancreatic cancers with intratumoral TLOs show peculiar clinicopathological behavior, with a lower degree of cancer invasiveness, especially to venules, and an active associated immune reaction. In addition, the tumor microenvironment has abundant arterioles and venules without cancer invasion. Furthermore, there are relatively many blood vessels (mainly capillaries) that appear to be morphologically and immunohistochemically intact; there is higher expression of VE-cadherin, which is known to be abundant in quiescent and mature vessels (76, 77), and the density of endothelial cells in the abnormal blood vessels (so-called tumor vessels) is lower, lacking a covering of pericytes positive for α-smooth muscle actin (45). It is suggested that at least partly functional vascular networks are retained, transporting immune cells or other molecules into the cancer tissues, thereby rendering the antitumor immune reaction more effective, although vascular density is exceptionally low within the pancreatic cancer tissue in general (78). Murine vascular studies have shown that vascular normalization in tumors enhances the influx of immune effector cells into the tumor parenchyma and markedly prolongs the survival of tumor-bearing mice (79, 80). Pancreatic cancers with intratumoral TLOs might offer a higher chance of effector immune cells, drugs, or effector molecules coming into contact with cancer cells as a result of immunotherapy, chemotherapy, or molecular targeting therapy.

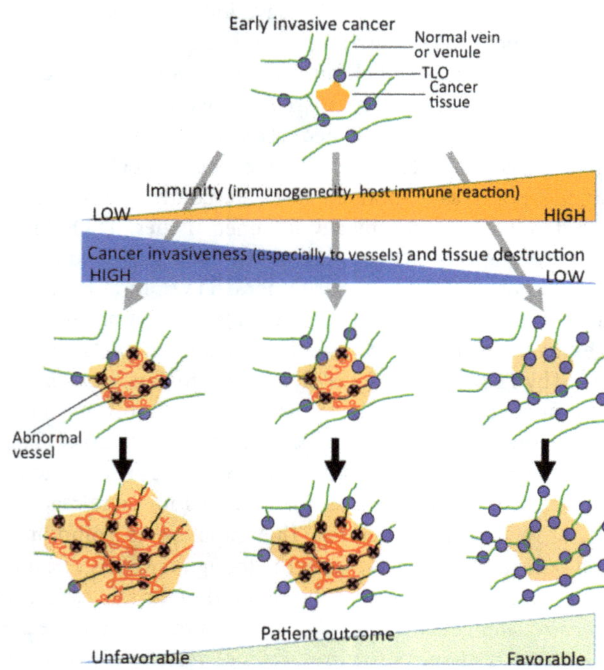

FIGURE 3 | Hypothesis of TLO formation/maintenance in cancer tissue, which likely involves (1) the state of antitumor immunity (tumor immunogenicity and host immune reaction) and (2) cancer invasiveness especially to vessels and tissue destruction that significantly affects the state of tissue structures necessary for formation/maintenance of TLOs. TLOs develop in the locations of venules in association with arterioles, venules, and nerve fibers (45). Cancer tissue that has become remodeled, showing absence of functional vascular networks replaced by abnormal blood vessels after invasion of cancer cells (center and left). Peritumoral TLOs can be induced if appropriate immune stimuli are present. Cancer tissue with intratumoral TLOs (right) shows a lower degree of cancer invasiveness, especially to vessels, and an active associated immune reaction. It retains relatively intact vascular networks, transporting immune cells, or other molecules into the cancer tissues, thereby rendering the antitumor immune reaction more effective. The scheme can apply to various solid cancers, although tendency of TLO development may be modified by tissue- and tumor type-specific properties.

Induction of TLOs after antitumor vaccination has been reported. Two weeks after vaccination with a granulocyte-macrophage colony-stimulating factor (GM-CSF)-secreting pancreatic tumor vaccine (GVAX), intratumoral TLOs with an active cellular and humoral immune response were induced (81). However, it is not clear whether the postvaccination induced TLOs are identical to naturally occurring TLOs, since no comparison of the induced TLOs with naturally occurring TLOs is provided and HEV status is not mentioned in these induced TLOs (81). The induction of TLOs alone did not accurately predict the post-vaccination patient outcome, since TLOs were induced in most vaccinated patients' tumors (85%), although not all tumors from patients with short survival lacked induction of TLOs. Several of the 12 chemokines associated with TLOs in malignant melanoma and colorectal cancer (57, 82) expressed but downregulated in the induced TLOs in patients who have prolonged survival and elevated ratio of effector T cells to Tregs. Meanwhile, TLOs with an active immune reaction were reportedly induced in high-grade cervical intraepithelial neoplasias (CIN2/3) after intramuscular vaccination with HPV16 E6/E7 antigens (83). CIN2/3 can develop cervical squamous cell carcinoma, although no stromal invasion of cancer cells is found. Postvaccination TLOs were induced in the stroma subjacent to residual intraepithelial lesions. The first example is a TLO induced after the pancreatic cancer-associated remodeled tissue, while the second example shows TLOs develop in non-remodeled (but inflammatory) tissue next to the CIN. The second example is similar to the situation at the development of TLOs in persistent active chronic inflammation. It requires further study how TLOs are induced after vaccination more profoundly in the cancer-associated remodeled tissue. Although not all vaccination trials have been able to induce TLOs, these successes might provide clues to the molecular mechanisms occurring in developing TLOs, in addition to development of therapeutic interventions.

HEV Formation and Maintenance

High endothelial venules are specially differentiated vessels that play important roles in the formation of lymphoid organs through accumulation of naive and central memory lymphocytes or other immune cells including DCs by providing an apparatus for extravasation of these cells from the blood stream into lymphoid organs (35–38). For this activity, HEVs specifically express and produce sulfated carbohydrate ligands, L-selectin ligands, and some adhesion molecules such as ICAM-1, VCAM-1, or MAdCAM-1 (36–44). HEV cells do not express lymphoid chemokines (CCL19, CCL21, and CXCL13) but present them at luminal surfaces through binding to scaffold molecules. Thus, HEVs are necessary for active and functional lymphoid organs.

Several studies have revealed that continuous engagement of LTβR on HEVs by $LT\alpha 1\beta 2^+$ cells is critical for the induction and maintenance of HEV gene expression and HEV cell morphology (84, 85). In mice, the major sources of LTα1β2 for HEV regulation in lymphoid tissues are $CD11c^+$ DCs and B cells (86–88). $CD11c^+$ cells and activated B cells contribute to an increase of VEGF production, resulting in proliferation of endothelial cells in lymph nodes. Retention of routes for the recruitment of $CD11c^+$ DCs into TLOs might be necessary in order to maintain the HEV phenotype in TLOs. It is assumed that if these routes are shut down by cancer invasion, HEV function will fail and the cellular content will be reduced, eventually leading to a decline in TLOs. Intratumoral HEVs would be expected to fail easily. In fact, in colorectal cancer, HEVs composed of flattened, atypical endothelial cells without lymphoid aggregates are observed within the tumor, whereas HEVs composed of normal tall columnar to cuboidal-shaped endothelial cells with lymphoid aggregates are found in peritumoral areas (55).

CONCLUDING REMARKS

Reports that have accumulated so far suggest that tumor-associated TLOs in many types of cancers play roles in the initiation and maintenance of active cellular and humoral immune responses against the cancers. Indeed, the presence of TLOs is significantly correlated with a favorable patient outcome and with a tumor immune microenvironment showing responses involving cellular and humoral immunity. The location of TLOs varies according to the type of cancer, and is important for evaluating the pathological significance of TLOs, i.e., whether they develop as a response to the cancer or as a result of secondary inflammatory changes caused by cancer invasion. Although the developmental mechanisms of TLOs are thought to be shared with those of SLO formation, we need to understand them in more detail, particularly the differences between TLOs that develop in non-cancerous tissues and those that develop in tissues remodeled by cancer invasion, and also the factors that trigger TLO development. In order to achieve this, we have to understand the real tumor-associated TLOs more and more with considering relationships of TLOs with cancer cells, and other stromal components including blood vessels, fibroblasts, and extracellular matrix. Unfortunately, any correlation between TLO formation and clinical outcome does not provide much information about the mechanism involved, and therefore both observational studies of human cancer and functional studies using reliable models will be required. It is anticipated that the presence (or higher density) of TLOs may be applicable as not only a prognostic marker but also a biomarker for selection of patients suitable for immunotherapy and/or for monitoring of patients during therapeutic intervention.

AUTHOR CONTRIBUTIONS

Conception and design of the work: NH. Acquisition of data: NH, YI, and RY-I. Writing, review, and/or revision of the manuscript: NH, YI, and RY-I. Final approval of the version: NH, YI, and RY-I. Administrative, technical, or material support: NH, YI, and RY-I. Study supervision: NH.

FUNDING

This work was supported by a Grant-in-Aid for Scientific Research from the Ministry of Education, Culture, Sports, Science and Technology of Japan, a Grant for Japan Agency for Medical Research and Development, and Cancer Research and Development Fund (NH).

REFERENCES

1. Hanahan D, Weinberg RA. Hallmarks of cancer: the next generation. *Cell* (2011) 144:646–74. doi:10.1016/j.cell.2011.02.013
2. Schreiber RD, Old LJ, Smyth MJ. Cancer immunoediting: integrating immunity's roles in cancer suppression and promotion. *Science* (2011) 331:1565–70. doi:10.1126/science.1203486
3. Gajewski TF, Schreiber H, Fu YX. Innate and adaptive immune cells in the tumor microenvironment. *Nat Immunol* (2013) 14:1014–22. doi:10.1038/ni.2703
4. Teng MW, Galon J, Fridman WH, Smyth MJ. From mice to humans: developments in cancer immunoediting. *J Clin Invest* (2015) 125:3338–46. doi:10.1172/JCI80004
5. Gubin MM, Zhang X, Schuster H, Caron E, Ward JP, Noguchi T, et al. Checkpoint blockade cancer immunotherapy targets tumour-specific mutant antigens. *Nature* (2014) 515:577–81. doi:10.1038/nature13988
6. Llosa NJ, Cruise M, Tam A, Wicks EC, Hechenbleikner EM, Taube JM, et al. The vigorous immune microenvironment of microsatellite instable colon cancer is balanced by multiple counter-inhibitory checkpoints. *Cancer Discov* (2015) 5:43–51. doi:10.1158/2159-8290.CD-14-0863
7. Brahmer JR, Tykodi SS, Chow LQ, Hwu WJ, Topalian SL, Hwu P, et al. Safety and activity of anti-PD-L1 antibody in patients with advanced cancer. *N Engl J Med* (2012) 366:2455–65. doi:10.1056/NEJMoa1200694
8. Fridman WH, Pages F, Sautes-Fridman C, Galon J. The immune contexture in human tumours: impact on clinical outcome. *Nat Rev Cancer* (2012) 12:298–306. doi:10.1038/nrc3245
9. Ino Y, Yamazaki-Itoh R, Shimada K, Iwasaki M, Kosuge T, Kanai Y, et al. Immune cell infiltration as an indicator of the immune microenvironment of pancreatic cancer. *Br J Cancer* (2013) 108:914–23. doi:10.1038/bjc.2013.32
10. Gabrilovich DI, Ostrand-Rosenberg S, Bronte V. Coordinated regulation of myeloid cells by tumours. *Nat Rev Immunol* (2012) 12:253–68. doi:10.1038/nri3175
11. Jinushi M, Komohara Y. Tumor-associated macrophages as an emerging target against tumors: creating a new path from bench to bedside. *Biochim Biophys Acta* (2015) 1855:123–30. doi:10.1016/j.bbcan.2015.01.002
12. Komohara Y, Jinushi M, Takeya M. Clinical significance of macrophage heterogeneity in human malignant tumors. *Cancer Sci* (2014) 105:1–8. doi:10.1111/cas.12314

13. Mantovani A, Allavena P, Sica A, Balkwill F. Cancer-related inflammation. *Nature* (2008) 454:436–44. doi:10.1038/nature07205
14. Mantovani A, Sozzani S, Locati M, Allavena P, Sica A. Macrophage polarization: tumor-associated macrophages as a paradigm for polarized M2 mononuclear phagocytes. *Trends Immunol* (2002) 23:549–55. doi:10.1016/S1471-4906(02)02302-5
15. Qian BZ, Pollard JW. Macrophage diversity enhances tumor progression and metastasis. *Cell* (2010) 141:39–51. doi:10.1016/j.cell.2010.03.014
16. Wynn TA, Chawla A, Pollard JW. Macrophage biology in development, homeostasis and disease. *Nature* (2013) 496:445–55. doi:10.1038/nature12034
17. Hiraoka N, Onozato K, Kosuge T, Hirohashi S. Prevalence of FOXP3+ regulatory T cells increases during the progression of pancreatic ductal adenocarcinoma and its premalignant lesions. *Clin Cancer Res* (2006) 12:5423–34. doi:10.1158/1078-0432.CCR-06-0369
18. Hiraoka N, Yamazaki-Itoh R, Ino Y, Mizuguchi Y, Yamada T, Hirohashi S, et al. CXCL17 and ICAM2 are associated with a potential anti-tumor immune response in early intraepithelial stages of human pancreatic carcinogenesis. *Gastroenterology* (2011) 140:310–21. doi:10.1053/j.gastro.2010.10.009
19. Kobayashi N, Hiraoka N, Yamagami W, Ojima H, Kanai Y, Kosuge T, et al. FOXP3+ regulatory T cells affect the development and progression of hepatocarcinogenesis. *Clin Cancer Res* (2007) 13:902–11. doi:10.1158/1078-0432.CCR-06-2363
20. Grivennikov SI, Greten FR, Karin M. Immunity, inflammation, and cancer. *Cell* (2010) 140:883–99. doi:10.1016/j.cell.2010.01.025
21. Remark R, Alifano M, Cremer I, Lupo A, Dieu-Nosjean MC, Riquet M, et al. Characteristics and clinical impacts of the immune environments in colorectal and renal cell carcinoma lung metastases: influence of tumor origin. *Clin Cancer Res* (2013) 19:4079–91. doi:10.1158/1078-0432.CCR-12-3847
22. Geurtsvankessel CH, Willart MA, Bergen IM, Van Rijt LS, Muskens F, Elewaut D, et al. Dendritic cells are crucial for maintenance of tertiary lymphoid structures in the lung of influenza virus-infected mice. *J Exp Med* (2009) 206:2339–49. doi:10.1084/jem.20090410
23. Moyron-Quiroz JE, Rangel-Moreno J, Hartson L, Kusser K, Tighe MP, Klonowski KD, et al. Persistence and responsiveness of immunologic memory in the absence of secondary lymphoid organs. *Immunity* (2006) 25:643–54. doi:10.1016/j.immuni.2006.08.022
24. Moyron-Quiroz JE, Rangel-Moreno J, Kusser K, Hartson L, Sprague F, Goodrich S, et al. Role of inducible bronchus associated lymphoid tissue (iBALT) in respiratory immunity. *Nat Med* (2004) 10:927–34. doi:10.1038/nm1091
25. Schrama D, Voigt H, Eggert AO, Xiang R, Zhou H, Schumacher TN, et al. Immunological tumor destruction in a murine melanoma model by targeted LTalpha independent of secondary lymphoid tissue. *Cancer Immunol Immunother* (2008) 57:85–95. doi:10.1007/s00262-007-0352-x
26. Wiley JA, Richert LE, Swain SD, Harmsen A, Barnard DL, Randall TD, et al. Inducible bronchus-associated lymphoid tissue elicited by a protein cage nanoparticle enhances protection in mice against diverse respiratory viruses. *PLoS One* (2009) 4:e7142. doi:10.1371/journal.pone.0007142
27. Dieu-Nosjean MC, Giraldo NA, Kaplon H, Germain C, Fridman WH, Sautes-Fridman C. Tertiary lymphoid structures, drivers of the anti-tumor responses in human cancers. *Immunol Rev* (2016) 271:260–75. doi:10.1111/imr.12405
28. Dieu-Nosjean MC, Goc J, Giraldo NA, Sautes-Fridman C, Fridman WH. Tertiary lymphoid structures in cancer and beyond. *Trends Immunol* (2014) 35:571–80. doi:10.1016/j.it.2014.09.006
29. Aloisi F, Pujol-Borrell R. Lymphoid neogenesis in chronic inflammatory diseases. *Nat Rev Immunol* (2006) 6:205–17. doi:10.1038/nri1786
30. Carragher DM, Rangel-Moreno J, Randall TD. Ectopic lymphoid tissues and local immunity. *Semin Immunol* (2008) 20:26–42. doi:10.1016/j.smim.2007.12.004
31. Hayasaka H, Taniguchi K, Fukai S, Miyasaka M. Neogenesis and development of the high endothelial venules that mediate lymphocyte trafficking. *Cancer Sci* (2010) 101:2302–8. doi:10.1111/j.1349-7006.2010.01687.x
32. Drayton DL, Liao S, Mounzer RH, Ruddle NH. Lymphoid organ development: from ontogeny to neogenesis. *Nat Immunol* (2006) 7:344–53. doi:10.1038/ni1330
33. Huang HY, Luther SA. Expression and function of interleukin-7 in secondary and tertiary lymphoid organs. *Semin Immunol* (2012) 24:175–89. doi:10.1016/j.smim.2012.02.008
34. Van De Pavert SA, Mebius RE. New insights into the development of lymphoid tissues. *Nat Rev Immunol* (2010) 10:664–74. doi:10.1038/nri2832
35. Von Andrian UH, Mempel TR. Homing and cellular traffic in lymph nodes. *Nat Rev Immunol* (2003) 3:867–78. doi:10.1038/nri1222
36. Girard JP, Moussion C, Forster R. HEVs, lymphatics and homeostatic immune cell trafficking in lymph nodes. *Nat Rev Immunol* (2012) 12:762–73. doi:10.1038/nri3298
37. Rosen SD. Ligands for L-selectin: homing, inflammation, and beyond. *Annu Rev Immunol* (2004) 22:129–56. doi:10.1146/annurev.immunol.21.090501.080131
38. Miyasaka M, Tanaka T. Lymphocyte trafficking across high endothelial venules: dogmas and enigmas. *Nat Rev Immunol* (2004) 4:360–70. doi:10.1038/nri1354
39. Hiraoka N, Petryniak B, Nakayama J, Tsuboi S, Suzuki M, Yeh JC, et al. A novel, high endothelial venule-specific sulfotransferase expresses 6-sulfo sialyl Lewis(x), an L-selectin ligand displayed by CD34. *Immunity* (1999) 11:79–89. doi:10.1016/S1074-7613(00)80083-7
40. Yeh JC, Hiraoka N, Petryniak B, Nakayama J, Ellies LG, Rabuka D, et al. Novel sulfated lymphocyte homing receptors and their control by a Core1 extension beta 1,3-N-acetylglucosaminyltransferase. *Cell* (2001) 105:957–69. doi:10.1016/S0092-8674(01)00394-4
41. Hiraoka N, Kawashima H, Petryniak B, Nakayama J, Mitoma J, Marth JD, et al. Core 2 branching beta1,6-N-acetylglucosaminyltransferase and high endothelial venule-restricted sulfotransferase collaboratively control lymphocyte homing. *J Biol Chem* (2004) 279:3058–67. doi:10.1074/jbc.M311150200
42. Kawashima H, Petryniak B, Hiraoka N, Mitoma J, Huckaby V, Nakayama J, et al. N-acetylglucosamine-6-O-sulfotransferases 1 and 2 cooperatively control lymphocyte homing through L-selectin ligand biosynthesis in high endothelial venules. *Nat Immunol* (2005) 6:1096–104. doi:10.1038/ni1259
43. Mitoma J, Bao X, Petryanik B, Schaerli P, Gauguet JM, Yu SY, et al. Critical functions of N-glycans in L-selectin-mediated lymphocyte homing and recruitment. *Nat Immunol* (2007) 8:409–18. doi:10.1038/ni1442
44. Uchimura K, Gauguet JM, Singer MS, Tsay D, Kannagi R, Muramatsu T, et al. A major class of L-selectin ligands is eliminated in mice deficient in two sulfotransferases expressed in high endothelial venules. *Nat Immunol* (2005) 6:1105–13. doi:10.1038/ni1258
45. Hiraoka N, Ino Y, Yamazaki-Itoh R, Kanai Y, Kosuge T, Shimada K. Intratumoral tertiary lymphoid organ is a favourable prognosticator in patients with pancreatic cancer. *Br J Cancer* (2015) 112:1782–90. doi:10.1038/bjc.2015.145
46. De Chaisemartin L, Goc J, Damotte D, Validire P, Magdeleinat P, Alifano M, et al. Characterization of chemokines and adhesion molecules associated with T cell presence in tertiary lymphoid structures in human lung cancer. *Cancer Res* (2011) 71:6391–9. doi:10.1158/0008-5472.CAN-11-0952
47. Germain C, Gnjatic S, Dieu-Nosjean MC. Tertiary lymphoid structure-associated B cells are key players in anti-tumor immunity. *Front Immunol* (2015) 6:67. doi:10.3389/fimmu.2015.00067
48. Martinet L, Filleron T, Le Guellec S, Rochaix P, Garrido I, Girard JP. High endothelial venule blood vessels for tumor-infiltrating lymphocytes are associated with lymphotoxin beta-producing dendritic cells in human breast cancer. *J Immunol* (2013) 191:2001–8. doi:10.4049/jimmunol.1300872
49. Martinet L, Le Guellec S, Filleron T, Lamant L, Meyer N, Rochaix P, et al. High endothelial venules (HEVs) in human melanoma lesions: major gateways for tumor-infiltrating lymphocytes. *Oncoimmunology* (2012) 1:829–39. doi:10.4161/onci.20492
50. Germain C, Gnjatic S, Tamzalit F, Knockaert S, Remark R, Goc J, et al. Presence of B cells in tertiary lymphoid structures is associated with a protective immunity in patients with lung cancer. *Am J Respir Crit Care Med* (2014) 189:832–44. doi:10.1164/rccm.201309-1611OC
51. Gu-Trantien C, Loi S, Garaud S, Equeter C, Libin M, De Wind A, et al. CD4(+) follicular helper T cell infiltration predicts breast cancer survival. *J Clin Invest* (2013) 123:2873–92. doi:10.1172/JCI67428
52. Martinet L, Garrido I, Filleron T, Le Guellec S, Bellard E, Fournie JJ, et al. Human solid tumors contain high endothelial venules: association with T- and B-lymphocyte infiltration and favorable prognosis in breast cancer. *Cancer Res* (2011) 71:5678–87. doi:10.1158/0008-5472.CAN-11-0431
53. Barone F, Bombardieri M, Rosado MM, Morgan PR, Challacombe SJ, De Vita S, et al. CXCL13, CCL21, and CXCL12 expression in salivary glands of patients with Sjogren's syndrome and MALT lymphoma: association with reactive and malignant areas of lymphoid organization. *J Immunol* (2008) 180:5130–40. doi:10.4049/jimmunol.180.7.5130

54. Behr DS, Peitsch WK, Hametner C, Lasitschka F, Houben R, Schonhaar K, et al. Prognostic value of immune cell infiltration, tertiary lymphoid structures and PD-L1 expression in Merkel cell carcinomas. *Int J Clin Exp Pathol* (2014) 7:7610–21.
55. Bento DC, Jones E, Junaid S, Tull J, Williams GT, Godkin A, et al. High endothelial venules are rare in colorectal cancers but accumulate in extra-tumoral areas with disease progression. *Oncoimmunology* (2015) 4:e974374. doi:10.4161/2162402X.2014.974374
56. Cipponi A, Mercier M, Seremet T, Baurain JF, Theate I, Van Den Oord J, et al. Neogenesis of lymphoid structures and antibody responses occur in human melanoma metastases. *Cancer Res* (2012) 72:3997–4007. doi:10.1158/0008-5472.CAN-12-1377
57. Coppola D, Nebozhyn M, Khalil F, Dai H, Yeatman T, Loboda A, et al. Unique ectopic lymph node-like structures present in human primary colorectal carcinoma are identified by immune gene array profiling. *Am J Pathol* (2011) 179:37–45. doi:10.1016/j.ajpath.2011.03.007
58. Di Caro G, Bergomas F, Grizzi F, Doni A, Bianchi P, Malesci A, et al. Occurrence of tertiary lymphoid tissue is associated with T-cell infiltration and predicts better prognosis in early-stage colorectal cancers. *Clin Cancer Res* (2014) 20:2147–58. doi:10.1158/1078-0432.CCR-13-2590
59. Dieu-Nosjean MC, Antoine M, Danel C, Heudes D, Wislez M, Poulot V, et al. Long-term survival for patients with non-small-cell lung cancer with intratumoral lymphoid structures. *J Clin Oncol* (2008) 26:4410–7. doi:10.1200/JCO.2007.15.0284
60. Figenschau SL, Fismen S, Fenton KA, Fenton C, Mortensen ES. Tertiary lymphoid structures are associated with higher tumor grade in primary operable breast cancer patients. *BMC Cancer* (2015) 15:101. doi:10.1186/s12885-015-1116-1
61. Giraldo NA, Becht E, Pages F, Skliris G, Verkarre V, Vano Y, et al. Orchestration and prognostic significance of immune checkpoints in the microenvironment of primary and metastatic renal cell cancer. *Clin Cancer Res* (2015) 21:3031–40. doi:10.1158/1078-0432.CCR-14-2926
62. Goc J, Germain C, Vo-Bourgais TK, Lupo A, Klein C, Knockaert S, et al. Dendritic cells in tumor-associated tertiary lymphoid structures signal a Th1 cytotoxic immune contexture and license the positive prognostic value of infiltrating CD8+ T cells. *Cancer Res* (2014) 74:705–15. doi:10.1158/0008-5472.CAN-13-1342
63. Lee HJ, Kim JY, Park IA, Song IH, Yu JH, Ahn JH, et al. Prognostic significance of tumor-infiltrating lymphocytes and the tertiary lymphoid structures in HER2-positive breast cancer treated with adjuvant trastuzumab. *Am J Clin Pathol* (2015) 144:278–88. doi:10.1309/AJCPIXUYDVZ0RZ3G
64. Lee HJ, Park IA, Song IH, Shin SJ, Kim JY, Yu JH, et al. Tertiary lymphoid structures: prognostic significance and relationship with tumour-infiltrating lymphocytes in triple-negative breast cancer. *J Clin Pathol* (2016) 69(5):422–30. doi:10.1136/jclinpath-2015-203089
65. Vayrynen JP, Sajanti SA, Klintrup K, Makela J, Herzig KH, Karttunen TJ, et al. Characteristics and significance of colorectal cancer associated lymphoid reaction. *Int J Cancer* (2014) 134:2126–35. doi:10.1002/ijc.28533
66. Willis SN, Mallozzi SS, Rodig SJ, Cronk KM, Mcardel SL, Caron T, et al. The microenvironment of germ cell tumors harbors a prominent antigen-driven humoral response. *J Immunol* (2009) 182:3310–7. doi:10.4049/jimmunol.0803424
67. Wirsing AM, Rikardsen OG, Steigen SE, Uhlin-Hansen L, Hadler-Olsen E. Characterisation and prognostic value of tertiary lymphoid structures in oral squamous cell carcinoma. *BMC Clin Pathol* (2014) 14:38. doi:10.1186/1472-6890-14-38
68. Zhu W, Germain C, Liu Z, Sebastian Y, Devi P, Knockaert S, et al. A high density of tertiary lymphoid structure B cells in lung tumors is associated with increased CD4 T cell receptor repertoire clonality. *Oncoimmunology* (2015) 4:e1051922. doi:10.1080/2162402X.2015.1051922
69. Salgado R, Denkert C, Demaria S, Sirtaine N, Klauschen F, Pruneri G, et al. The evaluation of tumor-infiltrating lymphocytes (TILs) in breast cancer: recommendations by an International TILs Working Group 2014. *Ann Oncol* (2015) 26:259–71. doi:10.1093/annonc/mdu450
70. Joshi NS, Akama-Garren EH, Lu Y, Lee DY, Chang GP, Li A, et al. Regulatory T cells in tumor-associated tertiary lymphoid structures suppress anti-tumor T cell responses. *Immunity* (2015) 43:579–90. doi:10.1016/j.immuni.2015.08.006
71. Mebius RE. Organogenesis of lymphoid tissues. *Nat Rev Immunol* (2003) 3:292–303. doi:10.1038/nri1054
72. Jones GW, Jones SA. Ectopic lymphoid follicles: inducible centres for generating antigen-specific immune responses within tissues. *Immunology* (2016) 147:141–51. doi:10.1111/imm.12554
73. Carrega P, Loiacono F, Di Carlo E, Scaramuccia A, Mora M, Conte R, et al. NCR(+)ILC3 concentrate in human lung cancer and associate with intratumoral lymphoid structures. *Nat Commun* (2015) 6:8280. doi:10.1038/ncomms9280
74. Breitfeld D, Ohl L, Kremmer E, Ellwart J, Sallusto F, Lipp M, et al. Follicular B helper T cells express CXC chemokine receptor 5, localize to B cell follicles, and support immunoglobulin production. *J Exp Med* (2000) 192:1545–52. doi:10.1084/jem.192.11.1545
75. Schaerli P, Willimann K, Lang AB, Lipp M, Loetscher P, Moser B. CXC chemokine receptor 5 expression defines follicular homing T cells with B cell helper function. *J Exp Med* (2000) 192:1553–62. doi:10.1084/jem.192.11.1553
76. Dejana E, Tournier-Lasserve E, Weinstein BM. The control of vascular integrity by endothelial cell junctions: molecular basis and pathological implications. *Dev Cell* (2009) 16:209–21. doi:10.1016/j.devcel.2009.01.004
77. Sawada J, Urakami T, Li F, Urakami A, Zhu W, Fukuda M, et al. Small GTPase R-Ras regulates integrity and functionality of tumor blood vessels. *Cancer Cell* (2012) 22:235–49. doi:10.1016/j.ccr.2012.06.013
78. Olive KP, Jacobetz MA, Davidson CJ, Gopinathan A, Mcintyre D, Honess D, et al. Inhibition of Hedgehog signaling enhances delivery of chemotherapy in a mouse model of pancreatic cancer. *Science* (2009) 324:1457–61. doi:10.1126/science.1171362
79. Carmeliet P, Jain RK. Principles and mechanisms of vessel normalization for cancer and other angiogenic diseases. *Nat Rev Drug Discov* (2011) 10:417–27. doi:10.1038/nrd3455
80. Hamzah J, Jugold M, Kiessling F, Rigby P, Manzur M, Marti HH, et al. Vascular normalization in Rgs5-deficient tumours promotes immune destruction. *Nature* (2008) 453:410–4. doi:10.1038/nature06868
81. Lutz ER, Wu AA, Bigelow E, Sharma R, Mo G, Soares K, et al. Immunotherapy converts nonimmunogenic pancreatic tumors into immunogenic foci of immune regulation. *Cancer Immunol Res* (2014) 2:616–31. doi:10.1158/2326-6066.CIR-14-0027
82. Messina JL, Fenstermacher DA, Eschrich S, Qu X, Berglund AE, Lloyd MC, et al. 12-Chemokine gene signature identifies lymph node-like structures in melanoma: potential for patient selection for immunotherapy? *Sci Rep* (2012) 2:765. doi:10.1038/srep00765
83. Maldonado L, Teague JE, Morrow MP, Jotova I, Wu TC, Wang C, et al. Intramuscular therapeutic vaccination targeting HPV16 induces T cell responses that localize in mucosal lesions. *Sci Transl Med* (2014) 6:221ra13. doi:10.1126/scitranslmed.3007323
84. Browning JL, Allaire N, Ngam-Ek A, Notidis E, Hunt J, Perrin S, et al. Lymphotoxin-beta receptor signaling is required for the homeostatic control of HEV differentiation and function. *Immunity* (2005) 23:539–50. doi:10.1016/j.immuni.2005.10.002
85. Drayton DL, Ying X, Lee J, Lesslauer W, Ruddle NH. Ectopic LT alpha beta directs lymphoid organ neogenesis with concomitant expression of peripheral node addressin and a HEV-restricted sulfotransferase. *J Exp Med* (2003) 197:1153–63. doi:10.1084/jem.20021761
86. Kumar V, Scandella E, Danuser R, Onder L, Nitschke M, Fukui Y, et al. Global lymphoid tissue remodeling during a viral infection is orchestrated by a B cell-lymphotoxin-dependent pathway. *Blood* (2010) 115:4725–33. doi:10.1182/blood-2009-10-250118
87. Liao S, Ruddle NH. Synchrony of high endothelial venules and lymphatic vessels revealed by immunization. *J Immunol* (2006) 177:3369–79. doi:10.4049/jimmunol.177.5.3369
88. Moussion C, Girard JP. Dendritic cells control lymphocyte entry to lymph nodes through high endothelial venules. *Nature* (2011) 479:542–6. doi:10.1038/nature10540

17

Tertiary Lymphoid Organs in Takayasu Arteritis

*Marc Clement[1†], Adrien Galy[2†], Patrick Bruneval[3], Marion Morvan[1], Fabien Hyafil[1,4], Khadija Benali[4], Nicoletta Pasi[5], Lydia Deschamps[6], Quentin Pellenc[7], Thomas Papo[2,8,9], Antonino Nicoletti[1,9] and Karim Sacre[2,8,9]**

[1] INSERM U1148, Université Paris Diderot, PRES Sorbonne Paris Cité, Paris, France, [2] Département de Médecine Interne, Hôpital Bichat, Assistance Publique Hôpitaux de Paris, Université Paris Diderot, PRES Sorbonne Paris Cité, Paris, France, [3] Département de Pathologie, Hôpital Européen Georges Pompidou, Assistance Publique Hôpitaux de Paris, Université Paris Descartes, PRES Sorbonne Paris Cité, Paris, France, [4] Département de Médecine Nucléaire, Hôpital Bichat, Assistance Publique Hôpitaux de Paris, Université Paris Diderot, PRES Sorbonne Paris Cité, Paris, France, [5] Département de Radiologie, Hôpital Bichat, Assistance Publique Hôpitaux de Paris, Université Paris Diderot, PRES Sorbonne Paris Cité, Paris, France, [6] Département de Pathologie, Hôpital Bichat, Assistance Publique Hôpitaux de Paris, Université Paris Diderot, PRES Sorbonne Paris Cité, Paris, France, [7] Département de Chirurgie Vasculaire, Hôpital Bichat, Assistance Publique Hôpitaux de Paris, Université Paris Diderot, PRES Sorbonne Paris Cité, Paris, France, [8] INSERM U1149, Laboratoire d'excellence INFLAMEX, Université Paris Diderot, PRES Sorbonne Paris Cité, Paris, France, [9] Département Hospitalo-Universitaire FIRE (Fibrosis, Inflammation and Remodelling in Renal and Respiratory Diseases), Université Paris Diderot, PRES Sorbonne Paris Cité, Paris, France

***Correspondence:**
Karim Sacre
karim.sacre@aphp.fr

†Marc Clement and Adrien Galy contributed equally to this work.

Objective: The role of B cells in the pathogenesis of Takayasu arteritis (TA) is controversial. We aimed to study the presence of tertiary lymphoid organs (TLOs) in the aortic wall of TA patients.

Methods: Hematoxylin and eosin-stained sections from aorta specimens from patients with TA were screened for TLOs. The presence of B cell aggregates (CD20), follicular dendritic cells (FDCs, CD21), and high endothelial venules (HEVs, PNAd) was investigated by immunohistochemistry. Immune cells from the adventitial layer of one patient were characterized by flow cytometry. Demographic, medical history, laboratory, imaging, treatment, and follow-up data were extracted from medical records.

Results: Aorta specimens from Bentall procedures were available from seven patients (5 females, aged 22–57 years) with TA. Surgical treatment was performed at TA diagnosis (n = 4) or at a median of 108 months (84–156) after TA diagnosis. Disease was active at surgery in four patients according to NIH score. B cell aggregates-TLOs containing HEVs were observed in the adventitia of all but one patient. Of note, ectopic follicles containing CD21$^+$ FDCs were found in all patients (4/4) with increased aortic ^{18}F-fluorodeoxyglucose (FDG) uptake before surgery but were absent in all but one patients (2/3) with no FDG uptake. In addition, flow cytometry analysis confirmed the accumulation of memory/germinal center-like B cells in the adventitial layer and showed the presence of antigen-experienced T follicular helper cells.

Conclusion: Ectopic lymphoid neogenesis displaying functional features can be found in the aortic wall of a subset of patients with active TA. The function of these local B cell clusters on the pathogenesis of TA remains to be elucidated.

Keywords: tertiary lymphoid organs, Takayasu arteritis, B cells, immunopathogenesis

INTRODUCTION

Takayasu arteritis (TA) is a rare primary vasculitis affecting large arteries, especially the aorta, the aortic arch, and its main branches. The etiology of TA is unknown even if it has been proposed that infectious agents play a significant role in the pathogenesis of this disease (1). In addition, while T cells exhibiting a Th1 profile have been implicated in the pathogenesis of TA (1, 2), the role of humoral immunity remains to be elucidated.

Tertiary lymphoid organs (TLOs) are ectopic lymphoid structures that form at sites of chronic inflammation through a process referred as lymphoid neogenesis. TLOs have morphologic features of secondary lymphoid organs including post-capillary high endothelial venules (HEVs) allowing homing of naive cells in the T cell area, an interface between T and B cell zones and germinal center (GC) areas. TLOs have been described in autoimmunity, microbial infection, cancer, chronic allograft rejection, atherosclerosis models, and abdominal aortic aneurysms (3–5). Studies have pinpointed the presence of lymphoid aggregates in the aortic wall of TA patients without distinguishing them from granulomas and have suggested their implication in the physiopathology of TA (6, 7). In addition, pathogenic B cells producing autoantibodies against endothelial cells are found in the blood stream of active TA patients, which suggests that these B cells could be activated within the adventitial layer before recirculating (8). Finally, some TA patients with active disease have a dramatic increase of circulating plasmablasts that are efficiently targeted by depleting anti-CD20 antibodies (9).

We aimed at characterizing the peri-aortic lymphoid aggregates developing in TA patients and at analyzing whether their presence could be associated with the activity of the disease.

MATERIALS AND METHODS

Patients

We conducted a retrospective multicenter study of patients with TA in whom aortic surgery was performed and aortic tissue specimen was available for analysis. All patients fulfilled the American College of Rheumatology and the Sharma-modified Ishikawa criteria for TA (10, 11). Demographic, medical history, laboratory, imaging findings, including ^{18}F-fluoro-deoxyglucose positron emission tomography (FDG-PET), computed tomography angiography (CTA), and/or magnetic resonance imaging (MRI), treatment, and follow-up data were extracted from medical records. The patients' clinical, laboratory, and imaging data, as well as treatments were analyzed at disease onset and at time of surgery. Routine laboratory tests, including C-reactive protein levels, were collected, and disease activity was defined according to the NIH criteria (12). Disease was considered active if NIH score was 2 or more, and inactive otherwise.

Immunohistochemistry on Aortic Samples

Aorta tissues were fixed in 4% PFA, embedded in paraffin, and sectioned at 6 µm. The sections were deparaffinized in toluene, hydrated in ethanol, and incubated in retrieval reagent (R&D Systems) for 20 min. After blocking in 5% BSA, the slides were incubated with purified primary antibody (mouse anti-human CD20, clone L-26; rabbit anti-human CD3, polyclonal, Dako; rat anti-human PNAd, MECA-79, BD Biosciences; rabbit anti-human CD14, clone EPR3653; rabbit anti-human CD21, clone EP3093, Abcam; mouse anti-human CD15, clone HI98, Biolegend) overnight at 4°C. After several washes with PBS, sections were incubated with the appropriate secondary antibody (polyclonal goat anti-rabbit DyLight649; goat anti-mouse rhodamine; goat anti-rat rhodamine; donkey anti-mouse rhodamine, Jackson Immunoresearch) at RT for 30 min and then cover mounted using Prolong Gold Antifade Reagent® (Invitrogen) for microscopy. The resulting fluorescence was detected with a Zeiss Axiovert 200 M microscope equipped with an AxioCam MRm version 3 camera, an ApoTome® system, and AxioVision® image capture software.

Flow Cytometry Analysis

Adventitial layer samples from the aorta were weighed, cut into small pieces (<1 mm), and digested using a previously described protocol (13). After a wash step, the cells were incubated with

TABLE 1 | Patients' baseline characteristics.

Patients	P01	P02	P03	P04	P05	P06	P07
Sex	F	F	M	F	M	F	F
Age	57	26	22	41	42	34	32
Smoker	Yes	Yes	No	No	Yes	No	Yes
Dyslipidemia	Yes	No	No	No	No	Yes	No
Hypertension	Yes	No	Yes	No	Yes	Yes	Yes
Diabetes	No	No	No	Yes	No	No	No
BMI (kg/m^2)	24	24.8	22.8	23	26.6	33.3	21.1
Diagnosis delay (months)	11	3	29	82	96	32	13
Systemic features	Yes	No	No	Yes	Yes	Yes	Yes
Vascular features	No	Yes	Yes	Yes	No	Yes	Yes
C-reactive protein (mg/L)	68	1	4	48	106	11	75
Aortic lesions (type)	IIa (C$^+$P$^-$)	V (C$^+$P$^+$)	V (C$^-$P$^-$)	V (C$^-$P$^-$)	IIb (C$^-$P$^+$)	V (C$^-$P$^-$)	IIb (C$^-$P$^-$)
Disease activity score	3	2	2	4	3	4	4

BMI, body mass index; the type of aortic lesions was defined according to international criteria (14); the disease activity score was assessed according to NIH criteria (12). Systemic features referred to fatigue (n = 4), headache (n = 2), weight loss (n = 1), dizziness (n = 1), arthritis (n = 1), visual disturbance (n = 1), or erythema nodosum (n = 1). Vascular features referred to carotid or subclavian bruit (n = 4), claudication with a diminished or absent pulse (n = 4) and carotidodynia (n = 2).

LIVE/DEAD® Fixable Yellow Dead Cell Stain Kit (Molecular Probes) and stained with the following antibodies: mouse anti-human CD19 brilliant violet 785, clone HIB19 (Biolegend); mouse anti-human CD45 eFluor 605, clone HI30 (eBioscience); mouse anti-human CD3 eFluor 450, clone OKT3 (eBioscience); mouse anti-human CD4 PE-CF594, clone UCHL1 (BD Biosciences); mouse anti-human HLA-DR APC-H7, clone L234; mouse anti-human CD27 brilliant violet 421, clone M-T271; mouse anti-human IgD APC, clone IA6-2; mouse anti-human CD95 FITC, clone DX2 (BD Biosciences); rate anti-human CXCR5 FITC, clone rf8b2 (BD Biosciences); mouse anti-PD-1 PerCP-Cy 5.5, clone EH1 2.1 (BD Biosciences); mouse anti-human CD45RA V450, clone HI100 (BD Biosciences); mouse anti-human Bcl6 PE, clone IG191/A8 (Biolegend). Flow cytometry analysis was performed using an LSR II flow cytometer (BD Biosciences). Data were analyzed with DIVA (BD Biosciences) and FlowJo (TreeStar) software.

Ethical Statement

Our study is a retrospective human non interventional study where subjects were not assigned to treatment; they were assigned to a diagnosis strategy within the current practice; the study involved products with a marketing authorization that are prescribed in the usual manner and used in accordance with authorizations by French agencies; epidemiological methods were used to analyze the data; and information used in the study were collected for clinical care. According to the Public Health French Law (art L 1121-1-1, art L 1121-1-2), written consents and IRB approval are not required for human non interventional studies. Patients were however informed that data collected in medical records might be used for research study in accordance to privacy rule. The study protocol conforms to the ethical guidelines of the 1975 Declaration of Helsinki.

RESULTS

Patients' Characteristics at Disease Onset and Medical Treatment

Aorta specimens were available from 16 patients with TA who underwent surgery between 2009 and 2014. Nine patients were excluded because diagnosis criteria for TA were not met ($n = 7$) or data were missing ($n = 2$). Seven patients (five females and two males) who fulfilled American College of Rheumatology and Ishikawa criteria for TA were studied. The median age at TA diagnosis was 34 years (22–57). Diabetes mellitus and dyslipidemia were present in cases 1 (14.3%) and 2 (28.6%), respectively.

TABLE 2 | Patients' characteristics at surgery.

Patients	P01	P02	P03	P04	P05	P06	P07
General features							
Sex	F	F	M	F	M	F	F
Age at diagnosis (years)	57	26	22	41	42	34	32
Age at surgery (years)	57	33	22	41	51	34	45
C-reactive protein (mg/L)	35	33	4	9	4	11	1
Disease activity score	2	2	2	0	1	3	0
Corticosteroid treatment	No	Yes	No	No	Yes	No	Yes
Immunosuppressive drugs	No	No	No	No	No	No	Yes
Antiplatelet treatment	No	Yes	No	No	Yes	No	Yes
Statin	No	Yes	Yes	Yes	No	Yes	No
Aortic disease							
Wall thickness (mm, CT scan or MRI)	10	NA	7	5	16	5	3.5
Wall contrast enhancement (CT scan or MRI)	NA	NA	No	No	Yes	NA	Yes
PET (SUV max)	4.8	0	1.3	0	5.0	0	7.0
Apparent *in situ* aortic inflammation	Yes	Yes	Yes	No	No	Yes	Yes
Aorta histological findings							
Mononuclear cells infiltrate	M, A	M, A	I, M, A	A	M, A	A	I, M, A
Multinuclear giant cells	M	No	M	No	No	No	M
Sclerosis	A	A	I, M, A	M, A	I, A	I, A	A
Neovascularization	No	M	M	M, A	M, A	No	No
Plasma cell	No	M, A	No	No	M	A	No
Wall thickness	A	A	I	No	I, A	I, A	A
Coexistent atheroma	No	No	No	No	No	Yes	Yes
Vasa vasorum thickening	Yes	No	No	No	No	No	Yes
Interruption of elastic lamina	Yes	Yes	Yes	Yes	Yes	Yes	Yes
Granuloma	M	No	No	No	No	No	M
Tertiary lymphoid organ	A	A	A	No	A	A	A
$CD21^+$ FDCs	++	++	+	−	+	−	++

PET, positron emission tomography; CT, computed tomography; MRI, magnetic resonance imaging; FDCs, follicular dendritic cells; SUV max, maximal standard uptake values; I, intima; M, media; A, adventitia; NA, not available.

The disease activity score was assessed according to NIH criteria (12).

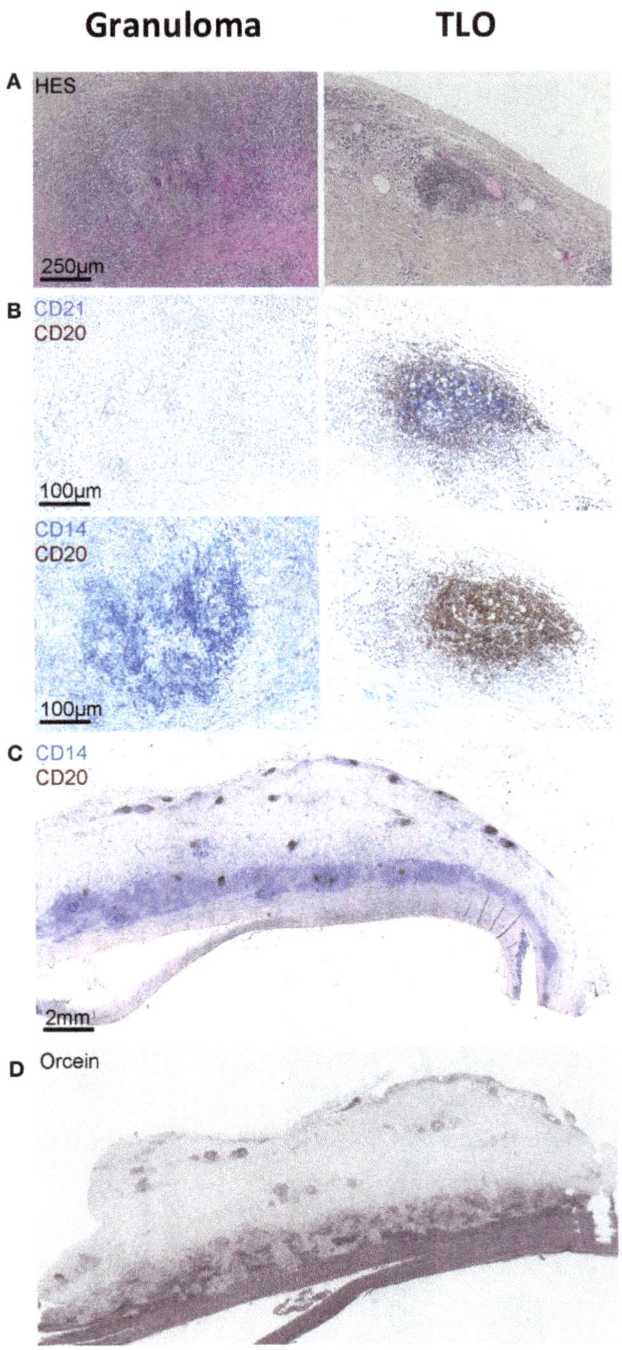

FIGURE 1 | Granulomas versus tertiary lymphoid organs (TLOs) in TA patients. Hematoxylin and eosin staining showing the presence of granuloma [first column **(A)**] in the aortic wall identified as $CD14^{++}CD20^{-}CD21^{-}$ cell aggregates by using a combination of CD21 (blue) CD20 (brown) [first column **(B)**] and CD14 (blue) CD20 (brown) [first column **(B)**] staining. Other cell aggregates also visible on hematoxylin and eosin-stained sections [second column **(A)**] are instead TLOs structures displaying few $CD14^{+}$ cells (blue), many $CD20^{+}$ B cells (brown), and $CD21^{+}$ FDCs (blue) **(B)**. Representative picture **(C)** showing the distribution of granulomas ($CD14^{++}$) in contact with the medial layer and TLOs ($CD20^{++}$) located deeper within the adventitial layer. Orcein staining **(D)** suggests that granulomas are physically implicated in medial destruction, whereas TLOs might develop in response to sustained inflammation in the adventitia.

Tobacco use was reported in four (57.1%) patients. No patients had past history of tuberculosis. The median body mass index was 23.5 kg/m^2 (21.1–33.3). The country of origin was France ($n = 4$), Morocco ($n = 1$), Mali ($n = 1$), and West Congo ($n = 1$).

At disease onset, patients suffered from fatigue ($n = 4$), headache ($n = 2$), carotidodynia ($n = 2$), weight loss ($n = 1$), dizziness ($n = 1$), arthritis ($n = 1$), visual disturbance ($n = 1$), and erythema nodosum ($n = 1$). No patients had fever. One patient was asymptomatic but had asymmetric blood pressure. Hypertension was present at onset ($n = 4$) or occurred ($n = 1$) during the course of the disease. The median delay between the onset of first symptoms and the diagnosis of disease was 29 months (3–96).

Serum C-reactive protein levels were raised in five (71.4%) patients [median 68 mg/L (11–106)]. At TA diagnosis, disease was considered active (NIH score ≥2) in all patients. CT angiography of the aorta was performed at TA diagnosis and showed multiple arterial lesions in all patients. Aorta was involved in all cases (**Table 1**).

All patients received glucocorticoids as first-line treatment. Methotrexate ($n = 3$), infliximab ($n = 2$), azathioprine ($n = 1$), and tocilizumab ($n = 1$) were prescribed during follow-up in four patients.

Patients' Characteristics at Surgery

Surgery was performed at the time of first diagnosis in four patients or during follow-up (84–156 months) in three patients. Disease was active at time of surgery in four patients with a NIH score ranging from 2 to 3, including recent ischemic vascular claudication ($n = 2$), new upper limb bruit ($n = 1$), and/or C-reactive protein >10 mg/L ($n = 3$). Aortic CT angiography displayed an increased circumferential aorta wall thickness (3.5–16 mm, median 7 mm). PET showed an increased FDG uptake in the vascular wall of the thoracic aorta wall in four cases. Three patients, including one with active disease, were still receiving glucocorticoids at time of surgery with a daily dose <10 mg. One patient was under tocilizumab. Antiplatelet treatment and statin were given in cases 3 and 4, respectively (**Table 2**).

Fourteen vascular procedures were done in seven patients (1–3 per patient, mean 1.7). Indications for surgery were aortic regurgitation due to thoracic aneurysm ($n = 7$) and abdominal aorta stenosis with lower limb chronic ischemia ($n = 1$).

Specimens from the thoracic aorta were obtained from Bentall procedures in all cases. At surgery, peri-aortic inflammation was obvious in five patients. Microscopically, prominent fibrosis was observed in intimal ($n = 3$), medial ($n = 2$), and adventitial ($n = 7$) layers, associated with increased intimal ($n = 3$) and adventitial ($n = 5$) thickness. Medial or adventitial inflammation was seen in all cases and involved mononuclear cells ($n = 7$), giant cells ($n = 3$), and plasma wall cells ($n = 3$). The deep portion of the media ($n = 4$) and adventitia ($n = 2$) contained neovessels. Atherosclerotic lesions were detected in two aortic specimens (**Table 2**).

Tertiary Lymphoid Organs in the Aortic Wall

Combination of CD14, CD20, and CD21 staining allowed identification of active TLOs (>90% $CD14^{low}CD20^{+}CD21^{+}$) and

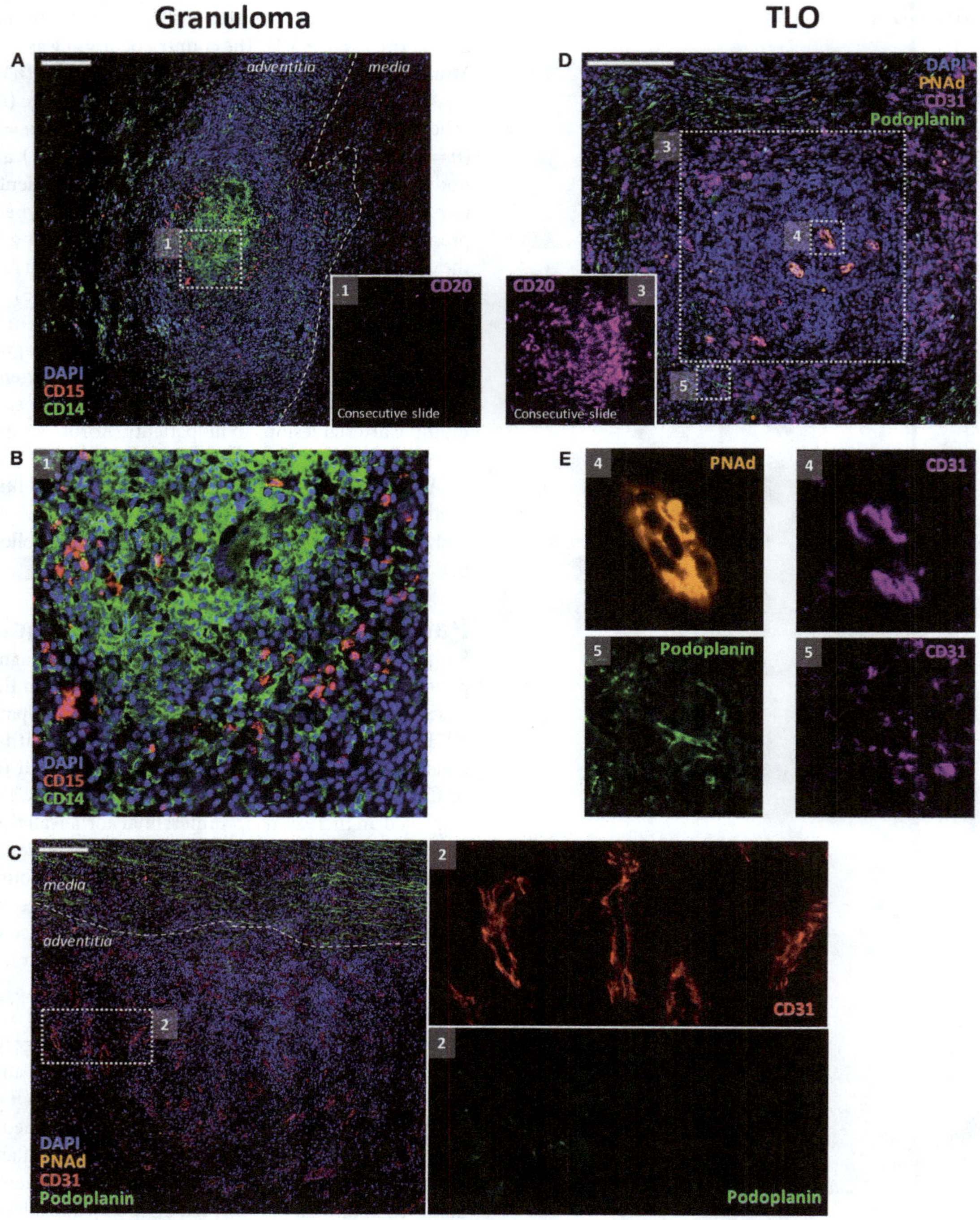

FIGURE 2 | Distinct features of granulomas and TLOs. Granulomas were made of clusters of CD14⁺ cells and of CD15⁺ cells **(A,B)** where very few B cells (inset 1) could be detected. Granulomas were also characterized by an intense angiogenesis [CD31⁺ vessels **(C)** and inset 2]. These adventitial neovessels were PNAd⁻ **(C)**. Few podoplanin + lymphatic vessels were also associated with blood vessels [**(C)** and inset 2]. At variance, CD31⁺ blood vessels with endothelial cells displaying a high endothelial venule phenotype and expressing PNAd [**(E)** and inset 4] were systematically observed within the B cell clusters [**(D)** and inset 3] that are composed of TLOs. A rich network of CD31⁺ Podoplanin⁺ lymphatics was detected around TLOs [**(E)** and inset 5].

granulomas (>90% $CD14^{++}CD20^{-}CD21^{-}$) in the vessel wall. TLOs were observed in the aortic wall in all but one patient. Granulomas were made of macrophages/neutrophils ($CD14^{+}$/$CD15^{+}$) and identified in only two patients. Interestingly, distribution patterns of granulomas and TLOs were distinct: granulomas were in contact with the medial layer, whereas TLOs were located deeper in the adventitial layer (**Figure 1**). Of note, TLOs ($CD20^{+}$ clusters) contained a dense network of

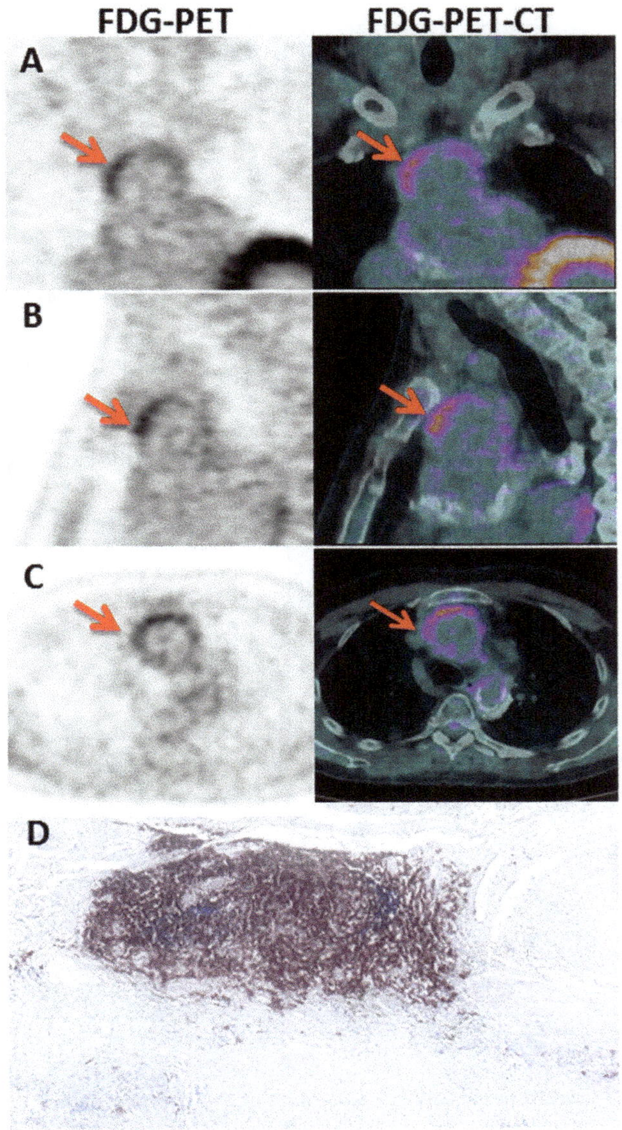

FIGURE 3 | FDG-PET-CT imaging in TA patient. Coronal **(A)**, sagittal **(B)**, and axial **(C)** slices of the thoracic aorta with FDG-PET imaging in P05. Note the presence of a linear, high FDG uptake in the ascending thoracic aorta on PET corresponding to the anterior region of the aortic wall from an aortic aneurysm on corresponding CT images. The left and the right imaging are, respectively, ^{18}FDG PET and fused PET/CT images showing high tracer uptake on the ascending aorta (Red arrows). Hematoxylin and eosin staining **(D)** of CD21$^+$ (blue) CD20$^+$ (brown) TLOs in the adventitial layer of the aortic wall of the same P05 patient.

HEVs (PNAd$^+$) able to recruit naive cells from the periphery. No HEVs were detected within or around CD14$^+$/CD15$^+$ granulomas (**Figure 2**). Of note, the presence of TLOs in the aortic wall was associated with FDG uptake measured by PET-CT scanner (**Figure 3**). Indeed, ectopic follicles containing CD21$^+$ follicular dendritic cells (FDCs) were found in all patients with increased aortic FDG uptake before surgery, but were absent in all but one (2/3) patients with no FDG uptake (**Table 2**).

Memory B Cells and Antigen-Experienced T Follicular Helper Cells in the Aortic Wall

Patient 1 (P01) had a Bentall procedure for aortic regurgitation due to thoracic aortic aneurysm (**Tables 1** and **2**, for clinical details). CTA and FDG-PET revealed active aortic lesions in the ascending aorta and the aortic arch at surgery time.

Flow cytometry analysis of digested fresh tissue samples confirmed the accumulation of live (LIVEDEAD®-negative) B cells (CD45$^+$CD19$^+$HLA-DR$^+$) in the inflammatory adventitial layer of the middle of the aneurysm, as compared to the neck (the portion of the aneurysm that is contiguous with the normal aorta). Local activation of B cells was suspected because most B cells had a memory-like phenotype (CD27$^+$IgD$^-$) and some harbored a GC-like phenotype (CD95$^+$CD24$^-$IgD$^-$CD27^{high}) (**Figure 4**). In addition, flow cytometry analysis of adventitial tissue samples revealed an increase in CD4$^+$ T cells in the core of the aneurysm, most of which had a memory phenotype (CD45RA$^-$). Interestingly, T follicular helper (Tfh) cells (PD1$^+$CXCR5$^+$Bcl6^{high}) were present in the aortic wall as well and were antigen-experienced (CD27$^-$) (**Figure 4**).

DISCUSSION

Takayasu arteritis is a rare form of chronic large vessel vasculitis of unknown origin involving the aorta and its major branches. Over the last decades, T cell-mediated immunity and inflammation have been implicated in the pathogenesis of this disease. Our data show that ectopic lymphoid neogenesis takes place in the aortic wall of patients with active TA and highlight the role of B cells in TA.

Using immunohistochemical examination, mature TLOs were detected in the adventitia of all but one TA aortic specimen. The accumulation of B cells within the adventitia, as well as their organization in TLOs suggests that B cells infiltrate the aortic wall in TA. The structural similarities between TLOs and B cells follicles found in secondary lymphoid organs suggest a local recruitment of naive cells *via* HEV (PNAd$^+$), their activation, as well as the establishment of an immunological humoral memory supported by Tfh cells. We detected by immunostaining both TLOs and granulomas, each displaying distinct cellular composition and occupying different vascular niches. This suggests different functions and involvement in the activity of the disease with TLOs enhancing the destructive properties of granulomas and vice versa.

Analysis of immune adventitial cells revealed a high percentage of memory and antigen-experienced CD4$^+$ T cells and also the presence of cells expressing canonical Tfh cell markers, such as CXCR5, Bcl6, and PD-1. These cells orchestrate B-cell activation, proliferation, and function (15). TLOs development and maintenance in TA may thus depend on the Tfh cell compartment as recently reported in atherosclerosis-prone mice (5). In addition, patients with TA are known to have enhanced interleukine-6 (IL-6) serum levels that parallel disease activity (16) and inhibition of IL-6 by the monoclonal anti-IL-6 receptor antibody tocilizumab is clearly efficient in TA (17). Interestingly, IL-6 is essential for B and Tfh cell differentiation (18) suggesting that immunotherapy against IL-6 could have dampened TLO development in the

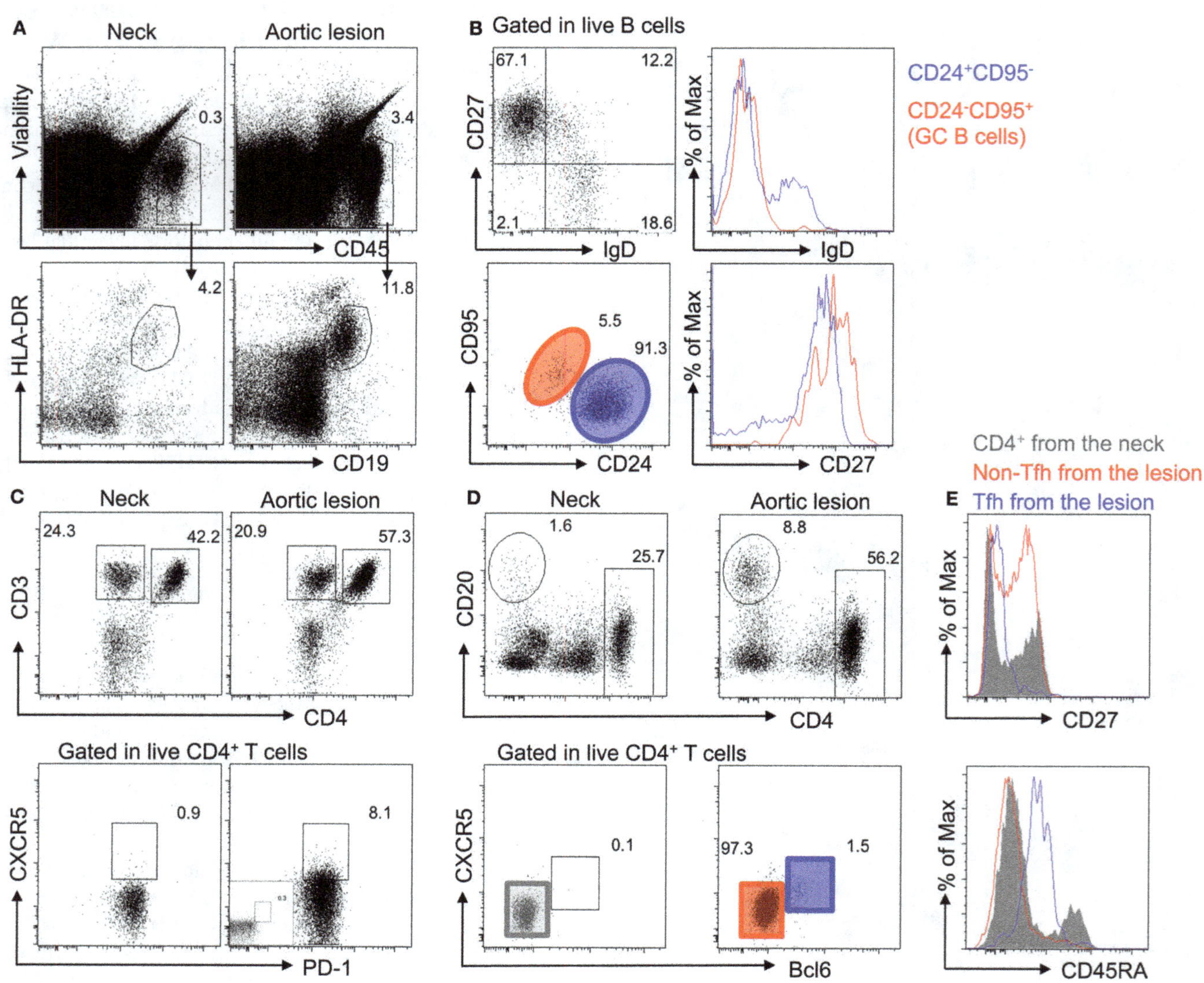

FIGURE 4 | Accumulation of memory B cells, germinal center B cells, and $CD4^+$ T follicular helper cells in the adventitia of TA diseased aortas. **(A)** Accumulation of immune cells ($Viability^-CD45^+$) and B cells ($HLA\text{-}DR^+CD19^+$) analyzed by flow cytometry in the adventitial layer of the core of the aortic lesions of a TA patient (P01) as compared to the neck of the same sample. **(B)** Characterization of B cells in the adventitia of the aortic lesion by flow cytometry shows that most B cells have a memory phenotype ($CD27^+IgD^-$) with some harboring a germinal center phenotype ($CD95^+CD24^-IgD^-CD27^{high}$). **(C)** Flow cytometry analysis of adventitial tissue samples reveals an increase in $CD4^+$ T cells in the aortic lesion (top panel), as well as the presence of $CD4^+$ T cells harboring a Tfh cell phenotype ($PD1^+CXCR5^+$), as compared to aortic tissues sampled in the aneurysmal neck. **(D)** $CXCR5^+CD4^+$ T cells from the adventitia of the core aortic lesion are $Bcl6^{high}$. **(E)** $CD4^+$ T cells from the adventitia of the neck (gray), non-Tfh cells ($CXCR5^-Bcl6^-$; Red), and Tfh cells ($CXCR5^+Bcl6^{high}$; blue) were analyzed for CD27 and CD45RA expression. As compared to $CD4^+$ T cells from the neck, which are a mixture of naive and antigen-experienced ($CD27^-$) and memory cells ($CD45RA^-$), the adventitia of the core of the aortic lesion contains more antigen-experienced and no naive T cells ($CD45RA^+$). Interestingly, Tfh cells in the adventitia are $CD45RA^{int}$ and display an antigen-experienced phenotype ($CD27^-$).

inflamed arteries of TA patients. Thus, our data suggest that the TLOs in TA can support antigen-driven clonal expansion and diversification and contain key elements for driving an immune pathogenic response that could last for decades if long lived plasma cells and memory $CD4^+$ T cells are generated.

Tertiary lymphoid organs can develop in inflamed tissues with a frequency that varies greatly depending on the anatomical sites and diseases. Ectopic lymphoid tissue and lymphoid neogenesis have been observed in infection or immune disorders, including synovia in rheumatoid arthritis (19), salivary glands of patients with Sjogren's syndrome (20), multiple sclerosis, inflammatory bowel diseases, and allografts (4). Although we still do not know what antigenic stimuli trigger their formation, TLOs cannot be considered as simple passive bystander markers of tissue inflammation because they are able to promote auto- or allo-antibody production and activating cellular effectors resulting in organ damage such as chronic inflammatory disorders and allograft rejection (3, 4).

In conclusion, TLOs are detected in the aortic adventitia of TA and comprise Tfh cells, clearly implicating B-cells in active TA. Deciphering whether TLOs are functional and allow the maturation of B cells and the production of antibodies remain to be formally demonstrated. In addition, understanding the respective involvement of local immunological reactions associated with TLO and granuloma formation in the pathogenesis of TA, as well as deciphering the cell types involved and the distinctive factors triggering the formation of each type of leukocyte aggregates, will lead to the development of new therapeutic approaches to treat patients with TA.

AUTHOR CONTRIBUTIONS

KS had full access to all of the data in the study and takes responsibility for the integrity of the data and the accuracy of the data analysis. Study design: MC, AN, and KS. Acquisition of data: MC, AG, PB, MM, FH, KB, NP, LD, QP, TP, AN, and KS. Analysis and interpretation of data: MC, AG, PB, FH, NP, LD, and KS. Manuscript preparation: MC, FH, AN, TP, and KS.

FUNDING

This work was supported by the Institut National de la Santé et de la Recherche Médicale (INSERM), Paris Denis Diderot University, the Région Ile de France (CORDDIM), the Département Hospitalo-Universitaire DHU "FIRE," the Fondation de la Recherche Médicale (FRM), the Fondation de France, and the Agence Nationale de la Recherche (ANR, grant "MI2 ATHLO").

REFERENCES

1. Weyand CM, Goronzy JJ. Immune mechanisms in medium and large-vessel vasculitis. *Nat Rev Rheumatol* (2013) **9**:731–40. doi:10.1038/nrrheum.2013.161
2. Weyand CM, Goronzy JJ. Medium- and large-vessel vasculitis. *N Engl J Med* (2003) **349**:160–9. doi:10.1056/NEJMra022694
3. Drayton DL, Liao S, Mounzer RH, Ruddle NH. Lymphoid organ development: from ontogeny to neogenesis. *Nat Immunol* (2006) **7**:344–53. doi:10.1038/ni1330
4. Aloisi F, Pujol-Borrell R. Lymphoid neogenesis in chronic inflammatory diseases. *Nat Rev Immunol* (2006) **6**:205–17. doi:10.1038/nri1786
5. Clement M, Guedj K, Andreata F, Morvan M, Bey L, Khallou-Laschet J, et al. Control of the T follicular helper-germinal center B-cell axis by CD8(+) regulatory T cells limits atherosclerosis and tertiary lymphoid organ development. *Circulation* (2015) **131**:560–70. doi:10.1161/CIRCULATIONAHA.114.010988
6. Inder SJ, Bobryshev YV, Cherian SM, Wang AY, Lord RS, Masuda K, et al. Immunophenotypic analysis of the aortic wall in Takayasu's arteritis: involvement of lymphocytes, dendritic cells and granulocytes in immuno-inflammatory reactions. *Cardiovasc Surg* (2000) **8**:141–8. doi:10.1016/S0967-2109(99)00100-3
7. Inder SJ, Bobryshev YV, Cherian SM, Lord RS, Masuda K, Yutani C. Accumulation of lymphocytes, dendritic cells, and granulocytes in the aortic wall affected by Takayasu's disease. *Angiology* (2000) **51**:565–79. doi:10.1177/000331970005100705
8. Wang H, Ma J, Wu Q, Luo X, Chen Z, Kou L. Circulating B lymphocytes producing autoantibodies to endothelial cells play a role in the pathogenesis of Takayasu arteritis. *J Vasc Surg* (2011) **53**:174–80. doi:10.1016/j.jvs.2010.06.173
9. Hoyer BF, Mumtaz IM, Loddenkemper K, Bruns A, Sengler C, Hermann KG, et al. Takayasu arteritis is characterised by disturbances of B cell homeostasis and responds to B cell depletion therapy with rituximab. *Ann Rheum Dis* (2012) **71**:75–9. doi:10.1136/ard.2011.153007
10. Arend WP, Michel BA, Bloch DA, Hunder GG, Calabrese LH, Edworthy SM, et al. The American College of Rheumatology 1990 criteria for the classification of Takayasu arteritis. *Arthritis Rheum* (1990) **33**:1129–34. doi:10.1002/art.1780330811
11. Sharma BK, Jain S, Suri S, Numano F. Diagnostic criteria for Takayasu arteritis. *Int J Cardiol* (1996) **54**:S141–7. doi:10.1016/0167-5273(96)02647-2
12. Kerr GS, Hallahan CW, Giordano J, Leavitt RY, Fauci AS, Rottem M, et al. Takayasu arteritis. *Ann Intern Med* (1994) **120**:919–29. doi:10.7326/0003-4819-120-11-199406010-00004
13. Dutertre CA, Clement M, Morvan M, Schäkel K, Castier Y, Alsac JM, et al. Deciphering the stromal and hematopoietic cell network of the adventitia from non-aneurysmal and aneurysmal human aorta. *PLoS One* (2014) **9**:e89983. doi:10.1371/journal.pone.0089983
14. Hata A, Noda M, Moriwaki R, Numano F. Angiographic findings of Takayasu arteritis: new classification. *Int J Cardiol* (1996) **54**:S155–63. doi:10.1016/S0167-5273(96)02813-6
15. Tangye SG, Ma CS, Brink R, Deenick EK. The good, the bad and the ugly - TFH cells in human health and disease. *Nat Rev Immunol* (2013) **13**:412–26. doi:10.1038/nri3447
16. Noris M, Daina E, Gamba S, Bonazzola S, Remuzzi G. Interleukin-6 and RANTES in Takayasu arteritis: a guide for therapeutic decisions? *Circulation* (1999) **100**:55–60. doi:10.1161/01.CIR.100.1.55
17. Mekinian A, Comarmond C, Resche-Rigon M, Mirault T, Kahn JE, Lambert M, et al. Efficacy of biological-targeted treatments in Takayasu arteritis: multicenter, retrospective study of 49 patients. *Circulation* (2015) **132**:1693–700. doi:10.1161/CIRCULATIONAHA.114.014321
18. Choi YS, Eto D, Yang JA, Lao C, Crotty S. Cutting edge: STAT1 is required for IL-6-mediated Bcl6 induction for early follicular helper cell differentiation. *J Immunol* (2013) **190**:3049–53. doi:10.4049/jimmunol.1203032
19. Takemura S, Braun A, Crowson C, Kurtin PJ, Cofield RH, O'Fallon WM, et al. Lymphoid neogenesis in rheumatoid synovitis. *J Immunol* (2001) **167**:1072–80. doi:10.4049/jimmunol.167.2.1072
20. Salomonsson S, Jonsson MV, Skarstein K, Brokstad KA, Hjelmström P, Wahren-Herlenius M, et al. Cellular basis of ectopic germinal center formation and autoantibody production in the target organ of patients with Sjogren's syndrome. *Arthritis Rheum* (2003) **48**:3187–201. doi:10.1002/art.11311

18

Tertiary Lymphoid Organs in Central Nervous System Autoimmunity

Meike Mitsdoerffer[1,2] and Anneli Peters[3]**

[1] Klinikum Rechts der Isar, Department of Neurology, Technical University Munich, Munich, Germany, [2] Munich Cluster for Systems Neurology (SyNergy), Munich, Germany, [3] Department of Neuroimmunology, Max Planck Institute of Neurobiology, Martinsried, Germany

***Correspondence:**
Meike Mitsdoerffer
meike.mitsdoerffer@tum.de;
Anneli Peters
apeters@neuro.mpg.de

Multiple sclerosis (MS) is an autoimmune disease characterized by chronic inflammation in the central nervous system (CNS), which results in permanent neuronal damage and substantial disability in patients. Autoreactive T cells are important drivers of the disease; however, the efficacy of B cell depleting therapies uncovered an essential role for B cells in disease pathogenesis. They can contribute to inflammatory processes *via* presentation of autoantigen, secretion of pro-inflammatory cytokines, and production of pathogenic antibodies. Recently, B cell aggregates reminiscent of tertiary lymphoid organs (TLOs) were discovered in the meninges of MS patients, leading to the hypothesis that differentiation and maturation of autopathogenic B and T cells may partly occur inside the CNS. Since these structures were associated with a more severe disease course, it is extremely important to gain insight into the mechanism of induction, their precise function, and clinical significance. Mechanistic studies in patients are limited. However, a few studies in the MS animal model experimental autoimmune encephalomyelitis (EAE) recapitulate TLO formation in the CNS and provide new insight into CNS TLO features, formation, and function. This review summarizes what we know so far about CNS TLOs in MS and what we have learned about them from EAE models. It also highlights the areas that are in need of further experimental work, as we are just beginning to understand and evaluate the phenomenon of CNS TLOs.

Keywords: multiple sclerosis, EAE, TLO, ectopic lymphoid follicles, autoimmunity

INTRODUCTION

Multiple sclerosis (MS) is a chronic inflammatory disease of the central nervous system (CNS). Based on the disease course, three different subtypes of MS are distinguished. The vast majority of patients exhibit a relapsing-remitting disease course (RRMS) at first. However, after a variable period of time (usually 10–15 years), RRMS patients experience progressive disability independent of relapses. Hence, this subtype is called secondary progressive MS (SPMS). Few patients (about 10%) experience a progressive disease course from the beginning [primary progressive MS (PPMS)] (1).

Demyelination, axonal damage, and neuronal loss as a result of immune cell infiltration are hallmarks of the disease. A large body of evidence supports the concept of MS being a T cell-mediated autoimmune disease presumably directed against CNS antigens (2). However, it is not clear yet whether lesion formation requires additional immune mechanisms, such as antibody-mediated tissue destruction (3).

Intrathecal production of oligoclonal antibodies is a characteristic feature in MS patients (4). Moreover, plasma cells (PCs) accumulate in lesions and cerebrospinal fluid (CSF). Detection of immunoglobulin G (IgG) and activated complement fragments and complexes in close proximity to actively demyelinating lesions indicates the involvement of antibody-mediated effector mechanisms. Technical progress over the last decade has helped to further characterize the humoral immune response in MS patients. Detection of extensive somatic hypermutation and a high frequency of clonally expanded memory B cells in MS lesions and CSF suggest that the observed B cell response is antigen-specific and not a random bystander effect (5).

However, recent clinical trials with a B cell depleting agent (anti-CD20 antibody) indicate that B cells are significant in the pathogenesis of MS beyond the production of antibodies (6). Anti-CD20 therapy rapidly reduces recurrence of relapses in MS patients, while antibody levels in the CSF remain essentially unaffected (7). B cells may also act as efficient antigen-presenting cells (APCs), especially in the context of cognate B cell:T cell interactions (8). Furthermore, the release of pro- (IL-6, LTα, TNFα, GM-CSF) and anti-inflammatory (IL-10, IL-35) cytokines by B cells may affect the immune response. Interestingly, analysis of B cells in MS patients suggests a preponderance of pro-inflammatory cytokines (9).

In this context, it was a significant finding that a relevant fraction of SPMS patients show B cell-rich meningeal immune cell collections. These structures recapitulate lymphoid follicle-like features to some extent and, therefore, may provide an excellent microenvironment for the interaction of B and T cells (10, 11).

Initiation of adaptive immune responses as well as maintenance of immune homeostasis requires tightly regulated processes in our immune system. Secondary lymphoid organs (SLO) constitute an important platform of this sophisticated system (12). The architecture of SLOs allows intense interactions between the different cellular components and, therefore, facilitates antigen presentation to T and B cells. Encapsulated SLOs develop under the control of precise genetic programs at predefined key locations in the body during embryonic development and include the spleen and the lymph nodes. Those structures allow monitoring of self and foreign antigens displayed by APCs that survey tissues and traffic to SLOs. Lymphoid organs exhibit several typical features that allow the generation of a fast and efficacious anti-pathogen response. Germinal centers constitute one of them. These highly organized structures bring together antibody-secreting and proliferating B cells and follicular dendritic cells (FDCs) (13). Further characteristics are a T-cell zone populated by naïve T cells and central memory T cells recruited from the blood; high endothelial venules (HEV); and a network of stromal cells that provide chemokines and extracellular matrix (ECM) for cellular migration and structural integrity (14).

Inappropriate control of the immune system, for example, during autoimmunity, results in chronic inflammation. Under these circumstances, immune cells that infiltrate into peripheral tissues can shape highly organized follicle-like structures that share various features of SLOs. Accordingly, these ectopic lymphoid follicles are called tertiary lymphoid organs (TLOs) (12). Similarities include the presence of T and B compartmentalization, presence of APCs such as dendritic cells (DCs) and FDCs, stromal cells, HEV, and lymphatic vessels. However, in contrast to SLOs most TLOs lack a capsule. Moreover, TLOs are transient structures that often disintegrate upon clearance of the antigen.

Tertiary lymphoid organs have been observed in various forms of chronic inflammation, such as autoimmunity, chronic graft rejections, persistent infection, artherosclerosis, and cancer (12, 15–17).

Various factors of the local tissue microenvironment are involved in this process. Certain inflammatory mediators, such as members of the lymphotoxin (LT) family as well as different cytokines induce TLOs (18). Moreover, certain subsets of immune cells have been implicated in the development of TLOs (18). Even though their precise role is still elusive, it is assumed that they act as local sites of antigen presentation and lymphocyte activation, including somatic hypermutation and class switch recombination in B cells. Therefore, it stands to reason that they provide the ideal environment for antimicrobial responses, epitope spreading, as well as autoimmune exacerbation.

This review will discuss the occurrence and significance of TLOs in MS and its animal model experimental autoimmune encephalomyelitis (EAE).

OCCURRENCE AND SIGNIFICANCE IN MS

Features/Characteristics of TLOs in MS

A morphological study in the late 1970s described accumulations of immune cells in chronic MS lesions (19). The authors found lymphocytes, macrophages, and PCs interacting with reticular cells in the perivascular space of parenchymal blood vessels (19). In addition, recent studies discovered distinct inflammatory infiltrates around blood vessels of the leptomeninges of MS patients, in particular in SPMS patients at a late stage of the disease (10, 11). Interestingly, a subsequent study on biopsy specimens found similar conglomerates of lymphocytes in the meninges of MS patients at a very early stage of the disease (20).

The degree of meningeal inflammation varied between analyzed samples. However, it was shown that an increased level of general perivascular and meningeal inflammation was accompanied by meningeal aggregates of $CD20^+$ B cells, $CD138^+$ and Ig^+ PCs, and T cells buried in the sulci of the frontal, temporal, and parietal lobes, and in particular associated with the cingulate and precentral gyrus (10). Meningeal infiltrates exhibited various stages of organization, from elementary clusters of cells to highly organized follicle-like structures (10) (**Figure 1**). In line with this observation, some B cell aggregates featured a complex reticular network formed by $CD35^+$ FDCs (10).

Interestingly, the degree of meningeal inflammation in the forebrain correlated with the degree of cerebellar meningeal inflammation (21). Yet, cerebellar meninges did not exhibit lymphoid-like aggregates as detected in the forebrain. One could argue that specific properties of the cerebellar subarachnoid space restrain the formation of such structures. Furthermore, analysis of cerebellar meninges revealed a high density of $CD68^+$ macrophages, and the number of macrophages correlated with parenchymal microglial activation, fitting well with earlier reports that described an association between meningeal cellular infiltrates and parenchymal microglial/macrophage activation (21, 22).

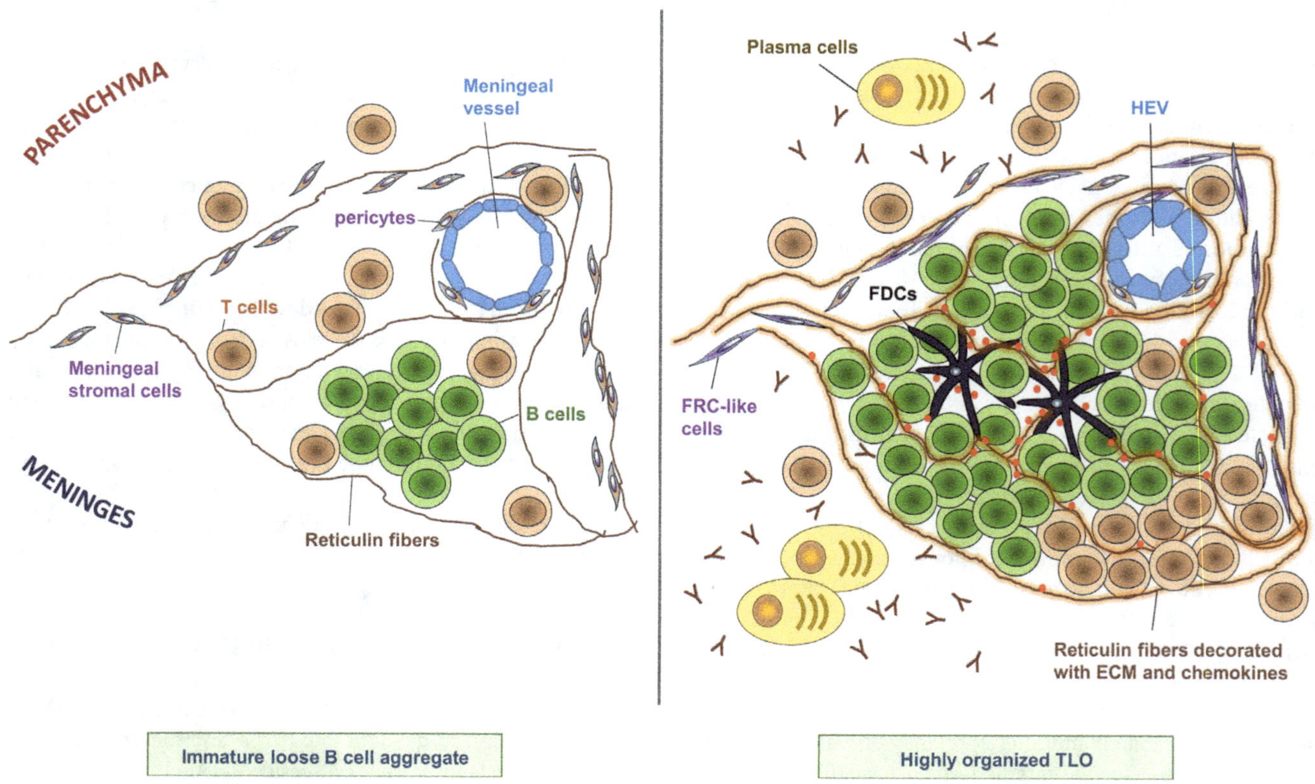

FIGURE 1 | Composition of CNS TLOs. TLOs in the CNS show different degrees of organization ranging from immature loose B cell aggregates (left) to highly organized lymphoid structures (right). Notably, at any time, only a minor fraction of cellular aggregates shows the highest degree of organization, however, the frequency of highly organized TLOs increases over time after onset of disease. Immature loose B cell aggregates show clustering of B cells in the meninges often in proximity to a meningeal blood vessel, scattered T cells, and a few reticulin fibers (left panel). In contrast, highly organized TLOs (right panel) are characterized by large B cell clusters next to a more or less defined T cell zone, and a dense network of reticulin fibers decorated with extracellular matrix (ECM) and chemokines. Reticulin fibers are produced by meningeal stromal cells that have differentiated into FRC-like cells. Sometimes FDCs can be detected at the center of the B cell follicle, which may have differentiated from pericytes. Plasma cells and antibodies are found in proximity to highly organized TLOs. In addition, HEVs can be detected in some highly organized TLOs, which may regulate infiltration of lymphocytes into the TLO.

Many B cells within follicles stained positive for the proliferation marker Ki67 (10). B cell aggregates with well-developed FDC networks showed clusters of Ki67$^+$ nuclei suggesting formation of germinal centers. However, these follicles lack an interfollicular T cell zone with HEV as it was observed in ectopic lymphoid tissue in other organs.

In conflict to these data, a recent report studying a different cohort of patients did not detect any follicle-like structures in the meninges of MS patients (23).

In summary, these observations suggest that some MS patients exhibit strong meningeal inflammation with formation of well-organized follicles. These intrameningeal structures feature some characteristics reminiscent of TLOs as they have been described in other persistently inflamed organs. Discrepancies in regard to the detection of these aggregates may be based on biological heterogeneity across patients. Furthermore, it is not clear whether these immune cell infiltrates persist for longer periods or whether they are only transiently present during periods of more active CNS inflammation. Technical difficulties may also contribute to this inconsistency as these structures tend to be very small (<100 μm in thickness), and meninges easily detach at autopsy. Therefore, these follicle-like structures may get lost during tissue processing. One challenge might be to provide guidelines on how to handle the tissue and to define criteria that allow the reproducible identification of these structures.

Induction/Formation of TLOs in MS

As only a fraction of MS patients shows B cell follicles in the meninges, ectopic lymphoid neogenesis must be controlled by a specific set of inflammatory signals. Likewise, it is known that some tissues and tumors are more prone to the development of TLOs than others indicating an important role of the microenvironment. The CNS holds a special status as several barriers, including the blood–brain barrier (BBB), the blood–meningeal barrier and the blood–CSF barrier control passage of macromolecules and immune cell infiltration (24). However, the CNS is rather an immune-specialized than an immune-privileged site, as it is controlled by extensive immune surveillance under physiologic conditions (24). Moreover, recent reports have described a functional lymphatic system in the CNS draining macromolecules and cells to deep cervical lymph nodes (cLN) (25, 26).

The question is what factors induce the formation of ectopic lymphoid follicles in this special environment. It is assumed that the formation of TLOs mimics significant steps of the organogenesis of SLOs. Initiation of SLOs is characterized by a close and reciprocal interaction of hematopoietic $CD4^{+}CD45^{+}CD3^{-}$ lymphoid tissue inducer (LTi) cells and lymphoid tissue organizer (LTo) cells of mesenchymal origin. The lymphoid chemokine CXCL13 released by LTo cells plays a crucial role as it attracts CXCR5-expressing LTi cells (12). CXCL13 is elevated in CSF and active lesions of MS patients and intrathecal Ig and occurrence of B cells and plasmablasts correlates with CXCL13 levels in the CSF (27–30). Furthermore, about 20% of CSF $CD4^{+}$ T cells and almost all B cells express CXCR5 suggesting that CXCL13 serves as an important chemoattractant to the CNS compartment (27). Moreover, FDCs in meningeal lymphoid aggregates express CXCL13 further indicating an important role for this chemokine in TLO formation (10).

Interestingly, untreated MS patients show elevated numbers of innate lymphoid cells in the peripheral blood and CSF (31, 32), and a recent study detected retinoic acid receptor-related orphan receptor γt (RORγt)-positive and CD3-negative cells in submeningeal B cell follicles (33). These cells may represent group 3 innate lymphoid cells, which comprise the LTi cell subset, and thus could potentially be involved in TLO formation.

In addition, there is evidence that, besides LTis, certain immune cell subsets in inflammatory lesions can trigger the development of TLOs. In particular, IL-17-secreting CD4 T helper (Th17) cells have been implicated in the pathogenesis of TLOs, and MS patients show an increased frequency of Th17 cells in peripheral blood and CSF compared with controls (34–36). Th17 cells secrete a variety of cytokines, among others IL-17, IL-21, and IL-22 (37). Interestingly, all of them have been linked to the formation of lymphoid follicles (18). As IL-17 was shown to induce CXCL13 (38), this might be an additional, indirect mechanism how Th17 cells contribute to the formation of TLOs.

In this context, it is interesting that there might be an ancestral link between adult LTi cells and Th17 cells (39, 40). Indeed, LTi cells and Th17 cells share several features as both cells express the transcriptional regulator RORγt; can respond to IL-23 and aryl hydrocarbon receptor ligands; and can produce IL-17, IL-22, and GM-CSF (41).

These factors and probably others like BAFF (B lymphocyte stimulator) and LT might contribute to create a permissive microenvironment for accumulation of B cells during chronic inflammatory conditions.

Function of TLOs in MS

Upon antigen encounter, naïve B lymphocytes develop into plasmablasts and undergo further maturation, e.g., hypermutation in germinal centers. TLOs, besides SLOs, are known to provide excellent niches where specific plasmablasts can further differentiate into PCs (12).

Detection of intrathecal Ig synthesis and oligoclonal bands (OCB) are typical features in MS patients. Ig synthesis occurs early in the course of the disease, and once acquired, persists unchanged throughout the disease in the majority of cases. Therefore, it serves as an important supportive diagnostic criterion (42).

Multiple sclerosis lesions often show deposition of antibodies and activated complement bound to disintegrating myelin (43, 44). Interestingly, the antibody repertoire in the CSF reflects Ig transcripts of B cells populating both CSF and brain lesions (45). Clonally related, antigen-experienced B cells are found in the CSF and peripheral blood as well as in the meninges and the parenchyma of MS patients suggesting an active immune axis between these different compartments (45–47). However, it remains unclear where these B cells encounter antigen and mature further. A recent study analyzed paired tissues comprising cLN and CNS by deep sequencing. Founding members of clonal families were primarily detected in cLNs while more mature members of these founders were found both in the cLNs and the CNS (48). These data provide further evidence that B cells can overcome tissue barriers between the periphery and the CNS. However, they also suggest that while the first antigen contact occurs in the periphery further maturation can happen both in the periphery and the CNS.

Meningeal immune cell aggregates recapitulate lymphoid follicle-like features to some extent and, therefore, may provide an excellent microenvironment for the interaction of B cells with T cells and FDC. Accordingly, they might support local B and T cell activation and further maturation. Therefore, one could speculate that antigen-experienced and clonally expanded B cells arise from these structures.

Overall, the above-mentioned studies suggest a role of meningeal TLOs in humoral- and cell-mediated immunity in MS patients.

Clinical Relevance of TLOs in MS

It is still not clear whether meningeal TLOs have a pathophysiological significance in MS or just represent an epiphenomenon. A recent postmortem study of chronic MS patients revealed extensive cortical demyelination affecting about 25% of the cerebral cortex in contrast to 5% of the subcortical/periventricular white matter (WM) (49). Similar observations were made in the cerebellum where demyelination of gray matter (GM) was far more pronounced than WM pathology (WM 3% versus GM 14%, representing % area of lesion in relation to total area) (21). Recently, MRI studies further broadened our knowledge about the prevalence of cortical lesions in various subtypes of MS and at different stages of the disease (50). Cortical lesions are clearly linked to cognitive impairment and disability progression (51). In this context, it is interesting that several studies suggested a correlation between the occurrence of meningeal inflammation and cortical demyelination (11, 20–22, 52, 53). Notably, formation of follicle-like structures in a fraction of SPMS cases was accompanied by increased meningeal inflammation and was associated with pronounced subpial cortical pathology. Concurrently, follicle positive cases showed a more severe disease course with younger age at disease onset, younger age at irreversible disability, and earlier death (11, 22). In addition, a study analyzing cortical biopsy specimens of early-stage MS patients also revealed a strong topographic association of moderate-to-marked meningeal inflammation with cortical demyelination (20). However, these findings are still a matter of debate and need validation in larger cohorts, especially since another study did not find evidence for an association of meningeal inflammation and cortical lesions in chronic MS (23).

Further histological analysis of follicle positive SPMS cases revealed a significant reduction in the thickness of the cortical GM layers in the precentral, frontal, and temporal gyrus (52). In line with this observation, these cases exhibited a substantial loss of neurons, which also included neurons with a pyramidal morphology. Interestingly, these pathologic changes exhibited a clear pial to WM gradient in the precentral gyrus, both in GM lesions and normal appearing GM (52). Overall, these observations strengthen the hypothesis that the meningeal inflammatory milieu is involved in the pathogenesis of cortical damage in a substantial number of SPMS cases. $CD8^+$ T cell-mediated immunopathology could be a potential cause as follicles harbor a considerable number of $CD8^+$ T cells (54). Both direct mechanisms *via* cytotoxic tissue damage and indirect mechanisms, e.g., by inducing activation of microglia might play a role. Other possible triggers are soluble factors released by inflammatory cells in the meninges. Finally, it could also be an antibody-mediated process, as an association between intrathecal immunoglobulin levels and cortical lesion load in patients with clinically isolated syndrome has been reported (55).

A striking difference between WM and GM damage is the lack of inflammatory cell infiltrates and rare deposition of immunoglobulin in cortical lesion (56–58). However, experimental models have shown that the GM does not support the persistence of inflammatory cells over extended periods of time (58). Thus, lack of inflammatory cells in GM with axonal damage or neuronal loss does not necessarily mean that these pathologic changes are not due to prior inflammatory events. However, an alternative hypothesis is that neurodegenerative processes unfold independently of inflammation and contribute to the attrition of GM structures in longstanding MS cases (59). Yet, axonal damage and neuronal loss in GM structures may also be a consequence of distant underlying WM lesions, e.g., *via* Wallerian degeneration. However, there was no correlation between the number of subpial GM lesions and WM lesions suggesting that inflammatory meningeal lesions actually determine GM damage (52).

Eventually, beyond further analysis of tissue samples from MS patients or autopsy tissue, advanced imaging technologies will contribute to solving these questions. In particular, development of MRI techniques that resolve meningeal inflammatory lesions and enable the unequivocal visualization of cortical lesions are sorely needed to analyze these issues in living patients.

Overall, the clinical relevance of meningeal TLOs in MS patients remains elusive. Validity of studies in human samples is limited as most of the tissues available are collected at a late stage of the disease. Poor quality of tissue, i.e., due to a long postmortem interval, might be another handicap. Thus, in order to further our understanding of CNS TLO formation, function, and impact, we can make use of the animal model for MS, EAE.

OCCURRENCE AND SIGNIFICANCE IN EAE

Experimental autoimmune encephalomyelitis has been employed for decades to study cellular and molecular pathogenic mechanisms that may also be relevant for MS pathogenesis and, in fact, many important mechanistic insights as well as successful therapeutic approaches have emerged from EAE studies. Thus, the EAE model was instrumental in demonstrating the importance of myelin-reactive CD4 T helper cells as disease drivers, as disease can be induced in healthy animals solely by transfer of these cells (60). Furthermore, the encephalitogenic properties of different T helper cell subsets were defined in numerous EAE studies, starting in the 1990s when IFN-γ-producing Th1 clones were described to be pathogenic while Th2 cells were characterized as non-pathogenic in the context of autoimmune CNS inflammation (61–64). When Tregs and Th17 cells entered the stage these studies were revisited and extended to show that both Th1 and Th17 cells can induce EAE, whereas Tregs aim to control the inflammatory processes (65). Since the majority of research efforts in the EAE field focused on T helper cells, the efficacy of B cell depleting therapies in MS came as quite a surprise for EAE researchers and raised the question why the obviously pathogenic role of B cells in the disease process was not recognized earlier in the EAE model. Rather than neglect and ignorance of the investigators, the most important reason lies in the experimental details of the model itself: the majority of EAE studies use immunization with myelin peptides together with adjuvant to induce disease. Since the self-peptide is already provided and, in this form, will most efficiently be taken up and presented by DCs, a potential role of B cells in processing/presentation of self-antigen and thereby activation of self-reactive T cells is largely bypassed in peptide immunization models. As a prominent example, it was shown that development of disease in C57Bl/6 mice immunized with MOG_{35-55} in CFA – the most widely used EAE model – is B cell independent and features very limited humoral responses (66, 67), whereas immunization of C57Bl/6 mice with recombinant human MOG protein relies on B cells to process and present the antigen and initiate the pathogenic cascade (66, 68, 69). Hence, moving away from the EAE blockbuster model, one can find several different EAE models in the literature that involve strong pathogenic (and also regulatory) B cell responses. Besides studying the role of B cells as antibody sources, APCs, and cytokine producers, a few studies have also described B cells to participate in TLOs in the CNS of EAE mice:

- After description of TLOs in MS brain, TLOs in EAE were first searched for and identified with relatively low frequency in SJL mice immunized with proteolipid protein $(PLP)_{139-151}$ – the only model, where TLOs develop after immunization with peptide (70, 71). In contrast, there is no robust evidence for TLO formation in the classical C57Bl/6-MOG_{35-55} immunization model. One reason for this difference may lie in the genetic background, since in the RRMS of the SJL background TLOs have more time to develop than in the relatively short acute–chronic disease course following immunization of C57Bl/6 mice with MOG_{35-55}.

- TLOs have also been described in C57Bl/6 mice immunized with a MBP–PLP fusion protein (MP4). In this model, mice develop a B cell-dependent chronic EAE that can be observed for up to 60 days post immunization (72).
- In the opticospinal EAE (OSE)-mouse, which features both a transgenic MOG-specific TCR as well as a MOG-specific BCR and spontaneously develops EAE, TLO-like structures were found in the CNS (73, 74).
- Following adoptive transfer of either MOG-specific Th17 cells in the C57Bl/6 background or PLP-specific Th17 cells in the SJL background, TLOs were identified with relatively high frequency in the CNS of sick mice (75, 76).

The fact that TLOs have been detected in several models that differ in regard to genetic background, identity and form of antigen, and method of disease induction implies that TLO formation is not just an exotic epiphenomenon, but will occur under varying conditions. However, characterization of EAE TLOs yielded very heterogeneous results not only between different models but also within the same model, suggesting that TLO development and regulation is very complex. Below, we are summarizing the results from different models regarding location, structural and cellular composition, induction, function, and clinical relevance of EAE TLOs to evaluate whether general principles important for CNS TLO formation can be identified, which could then also be applicable for MS TLOs.

TLO Location and Composition in EAE

Across the different EAE models and in agreement with the data from MS studies (see Features/Characteristics of TLOs in MS), TLOs are consistently found in association with meninges (**Figure 2**). Thus, both in the SJL immunization model as well as after transfer of Th17 cells on the SJL background, TLOs form primarily in the brain meninges, particularly those lining brainstem and ventricles (70, 71, 76). Similarly, in the MP4 immunization model TLOs form in the cerebral periventricular space, but also in the cerebellum and in association with spinal meninges (72). Upon transfer of Th17 cells in the C57Bl/6 background the majority of TLOs are located in the spinal meninges (75), and in the spontaneous OSE model TLOs are exclusively found in the spinal meninges (74). Whether TLOs form in the brain or spinal cord is most likely a consequence of the main route of infiltration, which differs between models. Thus, it has been shown that in the OSE model inflammation is restricted to optic nerve and spinal cord (73, 77). In addition, it is known that Th17 cells promote brain inflammation (78). However, whether in the brain or in the spinal cord, it is clear that TLOs preferentially form in association with meninges. This may be partly due to the high density of vessels in the meninges compared with the parenchyma, which have been shown to be an important point of entry for infiltrating leukocytes (79, 80). HEV, which express adhesion molecules like PNAd or MAdCAM to specifically attract naïve lymphocytes into SLOs and which have also been described in TLOs in other organs, were detected within TLOs in the MP4-immunization model (72). However, no evidence for HEVs was found in the spontaneous OSE model nor in the Th17 transfer model (C57Bl/6 background) (74, 75), while presence of HEVs was not determined in the SJL immunization and SJL Th17 transfer models. Since HEVs develop in response to cytokines like LT, their formation may require some time and occur only in the most mature TLOs. In addition, it is also possible that due to the abundance of meningeal vessels, which become permeable during CNS inflammation due to break-down of the BBB, the development of HEVs is not absolutely required for the recruitment of lymphocytes into CNS TLOs. In contrast, for example, tumor TLOs may be much more dependent on proper development of HEVs since the tumor environment is comparatively poorly vascularized.

Another important reason for the preferred formation of TLOs in association with meninges is the structural support that can be provided by the meningeal stromal cells. SLOs are structurally organized by fibroblastic reticular cells (FRCs), which line the

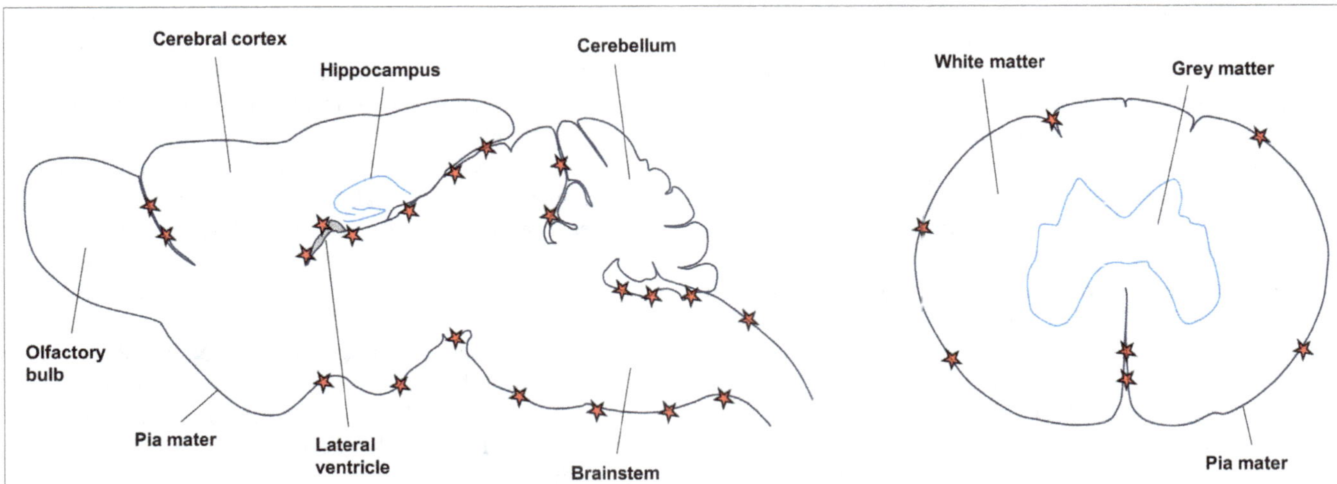

FIGURE 2 | Location of CNS TLOs. Sagittal view of the mouse brain (left) and horizontal view of the spinal cord (right) show preferential location of CNS TLOs (red stars) in association with the meninges.

subcapsular sinus and the conduits for antigen transport into the T cell zone, and secrete ECM components to form a dense network of reticulin fibers along which T cells, APCs, and B cells can migrate to their designated areas. FRCs are also an important source of the chemokines that retain T cells (CCL19 and CCL21) and B cells (CXCL13) in the SLO and organize it into separate B cell and T cell zones. In EAE TLOs, reticulin fibers suggestive of stromal FRC-like cells were described in several models, including the MP4-immunization model, the spontaneous OSE model, and the Th17 transfer model (C57Bl/6) (72, 73, 75). In a more detailed analysis, Pikor and colleagues could show that the fraction of FRC-like meningeal fibroblasts, which express Pdpn, PDGFRα, PDGFRβ, and Cadherin11 on their surface and secrete ECM components including fibronectin and ERTR7, increases during CNS inflammation (76). Therefore, the relative abundance of fibroblasts in the meninges, which can be stimulated to adopt FRC-like phenotype and function, may partly explain why TLOs are predominantly located in the meninges.

The other structurally essential stromal cell in the SLO is the FDC, which is positioned in the B cell follicles, where it presents opsonized antigen to induce affinity maturation of B cells and produces a network of reticulin fibers organizing migration into and structure of the follicle. In addition, FDCs are the main source of the B cell attracting chemokine CXCL13 in SLOs. Data from the different EAE models are heterogeneous in regard to the presence of FDCs in CNS TLOs. FDCs could not be identified in the spontaneous OSE model, nor in the Th17-transfer models (both C57Bl/6 and SJL), whereas FDCs were detected *via* the complement receptor CD35 or the marker FDC-M1 in the SJL- and the MP4-immunization model (71, 72). Like FRCs, FDCs are of stromal origin, and it has been suggested that they appear in TLOs as a consequence of differentiation/maturation of ubiquitous local precursors, namely PDGFRβ$^+$ pericytes (81), rather than migrating from SLOs. This maturation process requires the proper cytokine signals (primarily LT, TNF and potentially also others) and it may also take some time. Consistent with this idea, FDC-positive TLOs were observed late in the disease course, either upon relapses in the SJL-immunization model or in the chronic phase of EAE 30–57 days post onset in the MP4-immunization model (71, 72). Thus, absence of FDCs in the spontaneous OSE model and Th17 transfer models might be caused by lack of appropriate FDC maturation signals or by lack of time leading to an incomplete differentiation process. The latter may be especially true for the Th17 transfer models, where mice were analyzed comparatively early (5–20 days post onset) to prevent extended suffering due to severity of disease (75, 76). On the other hand, it is also unclear whether FDCs are required for antigen presentation in germinal center reactions in TLOs. Though presence of FDCs has been demonstrated in TLOs in other organs, it remains to be formally shown that they are required for antigen presentation. Thus, it is possible that other APCs can substitute for FDCs in CNS TLOs. Considering that meningeal macrophages have been shown to present antigen and reactivate infiltrating T cells during EAE (79, 80, 82, 83) and that they can be easily detected scattered in and around CNS TLOs they are certainly a good candidate.

Aside from structural components, segregated T and B cell zones are of course a hallmark characteristic for SLOs and TLOs. Across all EAE models, aggregation of B cells was considered a defining criterion for CNS TLOs. In contrast, T cells seemed to be scattered rather than clustered and were detected around and sporadically within the B cell zones (**Figure 1**). Their presence on the border or within the B cell zone may be a consequence of T cells acting as follicular T helper cells (TFH) to support the B cell maturation process (see TLO Function in EAE). Furthermore, the chemokines responsible for formation of a separate T cell zone (mainly CCL19 and CCL21) may not be so strongly expressed in the CNS, in contrast to the B cell zone-organizing chemokine CXCL13, which has been detected in several of the EAE models (see Induction/Formation of TLOs in EAE). Given that reactivation of T cells in the CNS and especially in the meninges has been clearly demonstrated also in the absence of TLOs (79, 80, 82, 83), T cells may also be less dependent on structure and clustering for their reactivation than B cells.

Induction/Formation of TLOs in EAE

For the formation of SLOs both LTo and LTi are required. During normal lymph node development, LTis (CD4$^+$CD3$^-$RORγt$^+$ IL7Rα^+) stimulate stromal cells to differentiate into LTos, which in turn start producing fibers and conduits and expressing adhesion molecules and chemokines that organize the SLO and guide lymphocytes to their designated areas. This stimulation of LTos by LTis is mediated primarily *via* cytokines of the TNF superfamily, especially LT. The heterotrimer LT$\alpha_1\beta_2$ expressed on the LTi cell surface engages with LTβ receptors on stromal cells to initiate the differentiation process. Additionally, LTis also secrete cytokines, including LTα_3, and TNFα which further activate LTos. In TLO formation, other cell types including type 3 innate lymphoid cells and T cells can perform the tasks of LTi, as long as they can provide the proper cytokine signals (84). Which cell type initiates the TLO formation process in the CNS was not investigated in detail in the immunization models nor in the spontaneous OSE model. However, increased expression of LT was detected in the SJL-immunization model at onset and upon relapses, and neutralization of LT prevented relapses and decreased expression of the B cell attracting chemokine CXCL13 in the CNS (71). These data suggested that LT-signaling is involved in activating LTos in the CNS, but did not identify the cellular source of LT. The Th17 adoptive transfer model (C57Bl/6) demonstrated that Th17 cells themselves are the cellular initiators for CNS TLO formation, since TLO formation was not observed after transfer of other T cell subsets, including Th1 cells, despite development of clinical disease (75, 85). Interestingly, Th17 cells and classical LTi share expression of several markers, including RORγt, IL-17, IL-22, CCR6, and IL-7Rα, and thus Th17 cells may also be able to function as LTi in stimulating CNS fibroblasts to act as LTo. This hypothesis was investigated in detail in the SJL Th17 adoptive transfer model (76): Pikor and colleagues could show that IL-17 and IL-22 together act on meningeal FRCs to induce remodeling of actin and collagen and production of ECM components, which ultimately leads to formation of fibrous networks providing proper structure for the TLO. Interestingly, IL-17 and IL-22 also induced expression of IL-6 and IL-23 in FRCs, which in turn supported *de novo* Th17 differentiation in the CNS, and may be a mechanism to ensure stable supply of Th17 cytokines for the FRCs to maintain their differentiation status. While FRC remodeling was independent of LT-signaling, production of CXCL13 by meningeal FRCs and therefore accumulation of B cells and deposition of complement in the lesion required intact LT-signaling. Together, these data suggest that the combination of LT and the Th17 cytokines IL-17 and IL-22 efficiently stimulates the meningeal fibroblasts to differentiate into FRCs (and potentially FDCs) and act as LTo in CNS TLOs. This also explains why there is almost no TLO formation in recipients of pure Th1 cells (75): although Th1 cells produce LT and TNFα and thus may even activate the meningeal fibroblast and stimulate them to produce CXCL13, complete maturation into FRCs (and potentially FDCs) additionally requires the presence of the Th17 cytokines IL-17 and IL-22. Importantly, both IL-17 and IL-22 have also been implicated in TLO formation in other organs/disease models including during iBALT formation in the lung (38), lymphoid follicle formation in the intestine during *Citrobacter* infection (86), and virus-induced TLO formation in salivary glands (87).

Data regarding the impact and requirement of chemokines for CNS TLO formation in EAE are limited. As already mentioned, CXCL13 is produced primarily by FDCs in SLOs to attract CXCR5-expressing B cells and TFH cells into the follicles and form a separate B cell zone. In all EAE models except the OSE model elevated CXCL13 mRNA levels were reported, and in some cases CXCL13 protein was also detected by immunohistochemistry at least in the more mature TLOs. CXCL13 was detected even in the absence of FDCs suggesting that in the CNS other cells can be a significant source of this chemokine. In fact, Pikor and colleagues showed that meningeal FRCs can produce CXCL13 in response to LT (76), and a recent study demonstrates that FRCs can also produce CXCL13 in response to IL-22 (87). While the evidence for presence of CXCL13 in CNS TLOs is comparatively robust, evidence that CXCL13 actually causes the attraction and aggregation of B cells into CNS TLOs is still missing. Another chemokine that may play a role in CNS TLO formation is CXCL12, which interacts with CXCR4$^+$ B cells. Intriguingly, Fleige and colleagues have shown that IL-17 can induce CXCL12 expression in stromal cells leading to FDC-independent TLO formation in the lung during *P. aeruginosa* infection (88), and another study showed that IL-22 can upregulate CXCL12 expression in epithelial cells (87). Given the importance of Th17 cells for CNS TLO formation in EAE, it is plausible that CXCL12 may contribute to B cell attraction and aggregation. While CXCL12 has been detected in standard EAE models, where it was suggested to retain infiltrating cells in the perivascular compartment (89), presence/relevance of CXCL12 was not tested in any of the TLO EAE models. The role of T cell chemokines for formation of CNS TLOs in EAE is even less understood. In SLOs, FRCs produce CCL19 and CCL21 to guide CCR7-positive T cells into the T cell zone. Constitutive expression of CCL19 has been detected in healthy CNS and increased levels of CCL19 and CCL21 were detected in the CNS in regular EAE and MS (90–92). The SJL Th17 adoptive transfer model showed a slight LT-independent upregulation of CCL21 in meningeal FRCs (76), but it remains to be determined whether this is relevant for CNS TLO formation. Taken together, the data suggest that CCL19/CCL21 produced by meningeal FRCs may recruit T cells into CNS TLOs in EAE. However, as mentioned already above, the fact that T cells seem to be much more scattered than B cells in CNS TLOs questions the presence and also the need for strong T cell chemokine signals that establish formation of a separate T cell zone. In summary, much more functional experimental work is needed to clearly define the role of chemokines in CNS TLO formation.

TLO Function in EAE

As for SLOs, the functions of a fully developed TLO comprise priming of naïve lymphocytes to new locally derived antigen resulting in differentiated antigen-specific T effector cells and B cells that underwent germinal center reactions yielding affinity-matured B memory cells and antibody-producing PCs. Studies in the MP4-immunization model, the spontaneous OSE model, and the SJL Th17 adoptive transfer model revealed T cell proliferation in TLOs (72, 74, 76). However, since T cells can also proliferate in the CNS in the absence of TLOs these data alone do not prove functionality of CNS TLOs. Additional evidence is provided in the MP4-immunization model, since T cells isolated from the CNS showed specificity not only for the immunizing antigen MP4 but also for the CNS-specific antigen MOG (72), suggesting that those MOG-specific T cells may have been primed directly in CNS TLOs. Although one cannot completely exclude the possibility that these MOG-specific T cells were primed in the periphery, the fact that MOG-specific T cells could not easily be detected in SLOs points toward T cell priming in the CNS. Similarly, in the SJL Th17 adoptive transfer model it was shown that in order to detect endogenous T cells differentiated into Th17 effector cells in the CNS, transferred T cells needed to express LT, which in turn stimulated meningeal FRC remodeling and expression of Th17 differentiation cytokines (76). These data – though not definite evidence – still support the idea that priming and differentiation of naïve T cells in response to CNS antigen may happen in CNS TLOs; however, more experimental evidence is needed to confirm this hypothesis. In regard to germinal center reactions, it was demonstrated in the C57Bl/6 Th17 adoptive transfer model that transferred Th17 cells in the CNS expressed markers associated with TFH cells including CXCR5 and Bcl6, as well as GC markers like GL7 and PNA (75). Thus, Th17 cells may function as TFH cells in CNS TLOs and provide help to B cells in GC reactions. In line with this, Th17 cells were shown previously to be excellent B cell helpers (93), and thus, the plasticity of Th17 cells to adopt TFH functions may be another reason why Th17 cells are superior to other T cell subsets in supporting TLO formation. Accordingly, some but not all CNS B cells also expressed GC markers including GL7, PNA, and Bcl6, some had undergone class switch recombination to IgG, and a few PCs were detectable in the CNS of Th17 recipients (75). Proliferating B cells were also found in the SJL and MP4-immunization model (70–72), and some B cells in the MP4-immunization model also expressed GC markers and AICD, the enzyme required for CSR and somatic hypermutation (72, 94). Consistent with this finding a germline transcript analysis indicated that B cells switched to IgG2b and IgG3 in the CNS, and sequencing of Ig transcripts revealed some CNS B cell clones that could not be detected in the spleen (94). Although these data support the hypothesis that GC reactions may happen in CNS TLOs, one has to keep in mind that it is extremely difficult to exclude that lymphocytes acquired the observed phenotype in the periphery and then migrated to the CNS. In contrast to these data, CNS B cells in the spontaneous OSE model showed no GC phenotype nor isotype switch, but appeared to be rather activated naïve B cells (74), confirming the notion that across the different models CNS TLOs are quite heterogeneous in their stage of development (**Figure 1**). Together the data from the different models suggest that definitely not all, but maybe the most organized and mature TLOs are also functional in supporting generation of differentiated T effector cells and affinity-matured B cells specific to CNS antigens.

Clinical Relevance of TLOs in EAE

Although CNS TLOs have been detected in several EAE models, their impact on the clinical disease course is completely unclear. Based on data from MS patients, where occurrence of TLOs was associated with a more aggressive disease course (10, 11), it has been postulated that TLOs in the CNS support differentiation and maturation of CNS antigen-specific effector lymphocytes, which continuously fuel the inflammatory process and thereby drive disease progression and chronicity. Except for the spontaneous OSE model, where TLO frequency and size was associated with a chronic and more severe disease course (74), presence of TLOs did not clearly correlate with disease severity in any of the other TLO EAE models. This may be explained by TLO frequency and kinetics of TLO development: In the SJL and MP4-immunization models TLO frequency increases in the late phases of disease, i.e., upon relapses or in the chronic phase of EAE 30–57 days post onset (71, 72). Although these late time points allow the TLOs to become comparatively mature and organized, the overall TLO frequency may still be too low (around 10 TLOs per mouse) to have a clinically visible effect. On the other hand, TLO frequency is significantly higher in the Th17 adoptive transfer models (around 60 TLOs per mouse) than in immunization models; however, mice were analyzed relatively early (2–15 days post onset) and thus TLOs may not yet be developed enough (reflected by lack of FDCs and HEVs) to affect the disease course (75, 76). In addition, the disease severity in Th17 adoptive transfer EAE is generally very pronounced and mice often show no recovery possibly due to irreversible tissue damage, making it very difficult to detect an exacerbation of clinical signs, especially using the rough scoring system common in the EAE field. Although it is likely, that CNS TLOs worsen clinical disease, especially considering that in the SJL Th17 adoptive transfer model TLOs promoted differentiation of endogenous Th17 effector cells (76), there is also the possibility that CNS TLOs counteract inflammation by generating regulatory T and B cells. This phenomenon has been observed in TLOs in the tumor microenvironment, but has never been investigated in CNS TLOs in EAE. A correlation of TLOs with cortical pathology, as described in MS brain (see Clinical relevance of TLOs in MS), has so far not been detected in TLO EAE models. Considering that cortical pathology may be caused by soluble and/or cellular factors emerging from meningeal TLOs over time, lack of cortical pathology in EAE may be a consequence of the short disease course when compared to human MS. On the other hand, it is also possible that this pathologic aspect of MS is simply not well recapitulated in EAE, since important cues (for example, presence and action of CD8 T cells) may be different in EAE and MS.

In order to define the clinical relevance of TLOs, an EAE model with reasonable frequency of TLOs and relatively mild disease course, which can be observed for long time periods, would be ideal. In addition, experimental methods need to be developed, which inhibit TLO formation in the CNS without disturbing the regular immune responses happening in the CNS and in the periphery during EAE. Thereby, one could gain detailed insight into the clinical relevance of TLOs in EAE.

CONCLUDING REMARKS

In summary, data from the last decade have revealed the existence of TLOs in the CNS of MS patients, and TLO formation can also be recapitulated in the MS animal model EAE, which will enable us to study the mechanisms of TLO formation as well as their precise functions and impact on disease development in more detail in the future. In general, the existence of TLOs further support an important role of B cells in MS pathogenesis, but the data also show a wide spectrum of TLO developmental stages ranging from simple B cell aggregates to highly organized structures (**Figure 1**), suggesting that a complex network of cellular players and cytokine signals is required to build these structures. Although some contributing factors and mechanisms like involvement of Th17 cells have now been exposed, considerable experimental work is needed to understand the phenomenon of CNS TLOs. The hypothesis that CNS TLOs support differentiation and maturation of CNS antigen-specific T and B effector cells, and thereby propagate continuous inflammation directly in the CNS – although attractive – remains to be first tested experimentally, and only then one can start thinking about CNS TLOs as therapeutic targets.

AUTHOR CONTRIBUTIONS

AP and MM contributed equally to the writing of this review article.

FUNDING

MM was supported by the Deutsche Forschungsgemeinschaft (SyNergy).

REFERENCES

1. Confavreux C, Vukusic S. The clinical course of multiple sclerosis. *Handb Clin Neurol* (2014) 122:343–69. doi:10.1016/B978-0-444-52001-2.00014-5
2. Hemmer B, Kerschensteiner M, Korn T. Role of the innate and adaptive immune responses in the course of multiple sclerosis. *Lancet Neurol* (2015) 14(4):406–19. doi:10.1016/S1474-4422(14)70305-9
3. Dendrou CA, Fugger L, Friese MA. Immunopathology of multiple sclerosis. *Nat Rev Immunol* (2015) 15(9):545–58. doi:10.1038/nri3871
4. Fitzner B, Hecker M, Zettl UK. Molecular biomarkers in cerebrospinal fluid of multiple sclerosis patients. *Autoimmun Rev* (2015) 14(10):903–13. doi:10.1016/j.autrev.2015.06.001
5. Blauth K, Owens GP, Bennett JL. The ins and outs of B cells in multiple sclerosis. *Front Immunol* (2015) 6:565. doi:10.3389/fimmu.2015.00565
6. Hauser SL, Waubant E, Arnold DL, Vollmer T, Antel J, Fox RJ, et al. B-cell depletion with rituximab in relapsing-remitting multiple sclerosis. *N Engl J Med* (2008) 358(7):676–88. doi:10.1056/NEJMoa0706383
7. Piccio L, Naismith RT, Trinkaus K, Klein RS, Parks BJ, Lyons JA, et al. Changes in B- and T-lymphocyte and chemokine levels with rituximab treatment in multiple sclerosis. *Arch Neurol* (2010) 67(6):707–14. doi:10.1001/archneurol.2010.99
8. Lanzavecchia A. Receptor-mediated antigen uptake and its effect on antigen presentation to class II-restricted T lymphocytes. *Annu Rev Immunol* (1990) 8:773–93. doi:10.1146/annurev.iy.08.040190.004013
9. Li R, Rezk A, Healy LM, Muirhead G, Prat A, Gommerman JL, et al. Cytokine-defined B cell responses as therapeutic targets in multiple sclerosis. *Front Immunol* (2015) 6:626. doi:10.3389/fimmu.2015.00626
10. Serafini B, Rosicarelli B, Magliozzi R, Stigliano E, Aloisi F. Detection of ectopic B-cell follicles with germinal centers in the meninges of patients with secondary progressive multiple sclerosis. *Brain Pathol* (2004) 14(2):164–74. doi:10.1111/j.1750-3639.2004.tb00049.x
11. Magliozzi R, Howell O, Vora A, Serafini B, Nicholas R, Puopolo M, et al. Meningeal B-cell follicles in secondary progressive multiple sclerosis associate with early onset of disease and severe cortical pathology. *Brain* (2007) 130(Pt 4):1089–104. doi:10.1093/brain/awm038
12. Drayton DL, Liao S, Mounzer RH, Ruddle NH. Lymphoid organ development: from ontogeny to neogenesis. *Nat Immunol* (2006) 7(4):344–53. doi:10.1038/ni1330
13. Allen CD, Okada T, Cyster JG. Germinal-center organization and cellular dynamics. *Immunity* (2007) 27(2):190–202. doi:10.1016/j.immuni.2007.07.009
14. Roozendaal R, Mebius RE. Stromal cell-immune cell interactions. *Annu Rev Immunol* (2011) 29:23–43. doi:10.1146/annurev-immunol-031210-101357
15. Grabner R, Lotzer K, Dopping S, Hildner M, Radke D, Beer M, et al. Lymphotoxin beta receptor signaling promotes tertiary lymphoid organogenesis in the aorta adventitia of aged ApoE-/- mice. *J Exp Med* (2009) 206(1):233–48. doi:10.1084/jem.20080752
16. Pitzalis C, Jones GW, Bombardieri M, Jones SA. Ectopic lymphoid-like structures in infection, cancer and autoimmunity. *Nat Rev Immunol* (2014) 14(7):447–62. doi:10.1038/nri3700
17. Hu D, Mohanta SK, Yin C, Peng L, Ma Z, Srikakulapu P, et al. Artery tertiary lymphoid organs control aorta immunity and protect against atherosclerosis via vascular smooth muscle cell lymphotoxin beta receptors. *Immunity* (2015) 42(6):1100–15. doi:10.1016/j.immuni.2015.05.015
18. Jones GW, Jones SA. Ectopic lymphoid follicles: inducible centres for generating antigen-specific immune responses within tissues. *Immunology* (2016) 147(2):141–51. doi:10.1111/imm.12554
19. Prineas JW. Multiple sclerosis: presence of lymphatic capillaries and lymphoid tissue in the brain and spinal cord. *Science* (1979) 203(4385):1123–5. doi:10.1126/science.424741
20. Lucchinetti CF, Popescu BF, Bunyan RF, Moll NM, Roemer SF, Lassmann H, et al. Inflammatory cortical demyelination in early multiple sclerosis. *N Engl J Med* (2011) 365(23):2188–97. doi:10.1056/NEJMoa1100648
21. Howell OW, Schulz-Trieglaff EK, Carassiti D, Gentleman SM, Nicholas R, Roncaroli F, et al. Extensive grey matter pathology in the cerebellum in multiple sclerosis is linked to inflammation in the subarachnoid space. *Neuropathol Appl Neurobiol* (2015) 41(6):798–813. doi:10.1111/nan.12199
22. Howell OW, Reeves CA, Nicholas R, Carassiti D, Radotra B, Gentleman SM, et al. Meningeal inflammation is widespread and linked to cortical pathology in multiple sclerosis. *Brain* (2011) 134(Pt 9):2755–71. doi:10.1093/brain/awr182
23. Kooi EJ, Geurts JJ, van Horssen J, Bo L, van der Valk P. Meningeal inflammation is not associated with cortical demyelination in chronic multiple sclerosis. *J Neuropathol Exp Neurol* (2009) 68(9):1021–8. doi:10.1097/NEN.0b013e3181b4bf8f
24. Louveau A, Harris TH, Kipnis J. Revisiting the mechanisms of CNS immune privilege. *Trends Immunol* (2015) 36(10):569–77. doi:10.1016/j.it.2015.08.006
25. Aspelund A, Antila S, Proulx ST, Karlsen TV, Karaman S, Detmar M, et al. A dural lymphatic vascular system that drains brain interstitial fluid and macromolecules. *J Exp Med* (2015) 212(7):991–9. doi:10.1084/jem.20142290
26. Louveau A, Smirnov I, Keyes TJ, Eccles JD, Rouhani SJ, Peske JD, et al. Structural and functional features of central nervous system lymphatic vessels. *Nature* (2015) 523(7560):337–41. doi:10.1038/nature14432
27. Krumbholz M, Theil D, Cepok S, Hemmer B, Kivisakk P, Ransohoff RM, et al. Chemokines in multiple sclerosis: CXCL12 and CXCL13 up-egulation is differentially linked to CNS immune cell recruitment. *Brain* (2006) 129(Pt 1):200–11. doi:10.1093/brain/awh680
28. Ragheb S, Li Y, Simon K, VanHaerents S, Galimberti D, De Riz M, et al. Multiple sclerosis: BAFF and CXCL13 in cerebrospinal fluid. *Mult Scler* (2011) 17(7):819–29. doi:10.1177/1352458511398887
29. Kowarik MC, Cepok S, Sellner J, Grummel V, Weber MS, Korn T, et al. CXCL13 is the major determinant for B cell recruitment to the CSF during neuroinflammation. *J Neuroinflammation* (2012) 9:93. doi:10.1186/1742-2094-9-93
30. Alvarez E, Piccio L, Mikesell RJ, Klawiter EC, Parks BJ, Naismith RT, et al. CXCL13 is a biomarker of inflammation in multiple sclerosis, neuromyelitis optica, and other neurological conditions. *Mult Scler* (2013) 19(9):1204–8. doi:10.1177/1352458512473362
31. Perry JS, Han S, Xu Q, Herman ML, Kennedy LB, Csako G, et al. Inhibition of LTi cell development by CD25 blockade is associated with decreased intrathecal inflammation in multiple sclerosis. *Sci Transl Med* (2012) 4(145):145ra106. doi:10.1126/scitranslmed.3004140
32. Degn M, Modvig S, Dyring-Andersen B, Bonefeld CM, Frederiksen JL, Geisler C, et al. Increased prevalence of lymphoid tissue inducer cells in the cerebrospinal fluid of patients with early multiple sclerosis. *Mult Scler* (2016) 22(8):1013–20. doi:10.1177/1352458515609795
33. Serafini B, Rosicarelli B, Veroni C, Zhou L, Reali C, Aloisi F. RORgammat expression and lymphoid neogenesis in the brain of patients with secondary progressive multiple sclerosis. *J Neuropathol Exp Neurol* (2016) 75(9):877–88. doi:10.1093/jnen/nlw063
34. Matusevicius D, Kivisakk P, He B, Kostulas N, Ozenci V, Fredrikson S, et al. Interleukin-17 mRNA expression in blood and CSF mononuclear cells is augmented in multiple sclerosis. *Mult Scler* (1999) 5(2):101–4. doi:10.1177/135245859900500206
35. Vaknin-Dembinsky A, Balashov K, Weiner HL. IL-23 is increased in dendritic cells in multiple sclerosis and down-regulation of IL-23 by antisense oligos increases dendritic cell IL-10 production. *J Immunol* (2006) 176(12):7768–74. doi:10.4049/jimmunol.176.12.7768
36. Brucklacher-Waldert V, Stuerner K, Kolster M, Wolthausen J, Tolosa E. Phenotypical and functional characterization of T helper 17 cells in multiple sclerosis. *Brain* (2009) 132(Pt 12):3329–41. doi:10.1093/brain/awp289
37. Sie C, Korn T, Mitsdoerffer M. Th17 cells in central nervous system autoimmunity. *Exp Neurol* (2014) 262(Pt A):18–27. doi:10.1016/j.expneurol.2014.03.009
38. Rangel-Moreno J, Carragher DM, de la Luz Garcia-Hernandez M, Hwang JY, Kusser K, Hartson L, et al. The development of inducible bronchus-associated lymphoid tissue depends on IL-17. *Nat Immunol* (2011) 12(7):639–46. doi:10.1038/ni.2053
39. Takatori H, Kanno Y, Watford WT, Tato CM, Weiss G, Ivanov II, et al. Lymphoid tissue inducer-like cells are an innate source of IL-17 and IL-22. *J Exp Med* (2009) 206(1):35–41. doi:10.1084/jem.20072713
40. Sawa S, Cherrier M, Lochner M, Satoh-Takayama N, Fehling HJ, Langa F, et al. Lineage relationship analysis of RORgammat+ innate lymphoid cells. *Science* (2010) 330(6004):665–9. doi:10.1126/science.1194597
41. Artis D, Spits H. The biology of innate lymphoid cells. *Nature* (2015) 517(7534):293–301. doi:10.1038/nature14189
42. Milo R, Miller A. Revised diagnostic criteria of multiple sclerosis. *Autoimmun Rev* (2014) 13(4–5):518–24. doi:10.1016/j.autrev.2014.01.012

43. Storch MK, Piddlesden S, Haltia M, Iivanainen M, Morgan P, Lassmann H. Multiple sclerosis: in situ evidence for antibody- and complement-mediated demyelination. *Ann Neurol* (1998) 43(4):465–71. doi:10.1002/ana.410430409
44. Genain CP, Cannella B, Hauser SL, Raine CS. Identification of autoantibodies associated with myelin damage in multiple sclerosis. *Nat Med* (1999) 5(2):170–5. doi:10.1038/5532
45. Obermeier B, Lovato L, Mentele R, Bruck W, Forne I, Imhof A, et al. Related B cell clones that populate the CSF and CNS of patients with multiple sclerosis produce CSF immunoglobulin. *J Neuroimmunol* (2011) 233(1–2):245–8. doi:10.1016/j.jneuroim.2011.01.010
46. Lovato L, Willis SN, Rodig SJ, Caron T, Almendinger SE, Howell OW, et al. Related B cell clones populate the meninges and parenchyma of patients with multiple sclerosis. *Brain* (2011) 134(Pt 2):534–41. doi:10.1093/brain/awq350
47. Palanichamy A, Apeltsin L, Kuo TC, Sirota M, Wang S, Pitts SJ, et al. Immunoglobulin class-switched B cells form an active immune axis between CNS and periphery in multiple sclerosis. *Sci Transl Med* (2014) 6(248):248ra106. doi:10.1126/scitranslmed.3008930
48. Stern JN, Yaari G, Vander Heiden JA, Church G, Donahue WF, Hintzen RQ, et al. B cells populating the multiple sclerosis brain mature in the draining cervical lymph nodes. *Sci Transl Med* (2014) 6(248):248ra107. doi:10.1126/scitranslmed.3008879
49. Bo L, Geurts JJ, van der Valk P, Polman C, Barkhof F. Lack of correlation between cortical demyelination and white matter pathologic changes in multiple sclerosis. *Arch Neurol* (2007) 64(1):76–80. doi:10.1001/archneur.64.1.76
50. Calabrese M, Filippi M, Gallo P. Cortical lesions in multiple sclerosis. *Nat Rev Neurol* (2010) 6(8):438–44. doi:10.1038/nrneurol.2010.93
51. van Munster CE, Jonkman LE, Weinstein HC, Uitdehaag BM, Geurts JJ. Gray matter damage in multiple sclerosis: impact on clinical symptoms. *Neuroscience* (2015) 303:446–61. doi:10.1016/j.neuroscience.2015.07.006
52. Magliozzi R, Howell OW, Reeves C, Roncaroli F, Nicholas R, Serafini B, et al. A gradient of neuronal loss and meningeal inflammation in multiple sclerosis. *Ann Neurol* (2010) 68(4):477–93. doi:10.1002/ana.22230
53. Choi SR, Howell OW, Carassiti D, Magliozzi R, Gveric D, Muraro PA, et al. Meningeal inflammation plays a role in the pathology of primary progressive multiple sclerosis. *Brain* (2012) 135(Pt 10):2925–37. doi:10.1093/brain/aws189
54. Serafini B, Rosicarelli B, Franciotta D, Magliozzi R, Reynolds R, Cinque P, et al. Dysregulated Epstein-Barr virus infection in the multiple sclerosis brain. *J Exp Med* (2007) 204(12):2899–912. doi:10.1084/jem.20071030
55. Calabrese M, Federle L, Bernardi V, Rinaldi F, Favaretto A, Varagnolo MC, et al. The association of intrathecal immunoglobulin synthesis and cortical lesions predicts disease activity in clinically isolated syndrome and early relapsing-remitting multiple sclerosis. *Mult Scler* (2012) 18(2):174–80. doi:10.1177/1352458511418550
56. Bo L, Vedeler CA, Nyland H, Trapp BD, Mork SJ. Intracortical multiple sclerosis lesions are not associated with increased lymphocyte infiltration. *Mult Scler* (2003) 9(4):323–31. doi:10.1191/1352458503ms917oa
57. Brink BP, Veerhuis R, Breij EC, van der Valk P, Dijkstra CD, Bo L. The pathology of multiple sclerosis is location-dependent: no significant complement activation is detected in purely cortical lesions. *J Neuropathol Exp Neurol* (2005) 64(2):147–55. doi:10.1093/jnen/64.2.147
58. Merkler D, Ernsting T, Kerschensteiner M, Bruck W, Stadelmann C. A new focal EAE model of cortical demyelination: multiple sclerosis-like lesions with rapid resolution of inflammation and extensive remyelination. *Brain* (2006) 129(Pt 8):1972–83. doi:10.1093/brain/awl135
59. Friese MA, Schattling B, Fugger L. Mechanisms of neurodegeneration and axonal dysfunction in multiple sclerosis. *Nat Rev Neurol* (2014) 10(4):225–38. doi:10.1038/nrneurol.2014.37
60. Ben-Nun A, Wekerle H, Cohen IR. The rapid isolation of clonable antigen-specific T lymphocyte lines capable of mediating autoimmune encephalomyelitis. *Eur J Immunol* (1981) 11(3):195–9. doi:10.1002/eji.1830110307
61. Baron JL, Madri JA, Ruddle NH, Hashim G, Janeway CA Jr. Surface expression of alpha 4 integrin by CD4 T cells is required for their entry into brain parenchyma. *J Exp Med* (1993) 177(1):57–68. doi:10.1084/jem.177.1.57
62. Kuchroo VK, Martin CA, Greer JM, Ju ST, Sobel RA, Dorf ME. Cytokines and adhesion molecules contribute to the ability of myelin proteolipid protein-specific T cell clones to mediate experimental allergic encephalomyelitis. *J Immunol* (1993) 151(8):4371–82.
63. Das MP, Nicholson LB, Greer JM, Kuchroo VK. Autopathogenic T helper cell type 1 (Th1) and protective Th2 clones differ in their recognition of the autoantigenic peptide of myelin proteolipid protein. *J Exp Med* (1997) 186(6):867–76. doi:10.1084/jem.186.6.867
64. Lafaille JJ, Keere FV, Hsu AL, Baron JL, Haas W, Raine CS, et al. Myelin basic protein-specific T helper 2 (Th2) cells cause experimental autoimmune encephalomyelitis in immunodeficient hosts rather than protect them from the disease. *J Exp Med* (1997) 186(2):307–12. doi:10.1084/jem.186.2.307
65. Jäger A, Kuchroo VK. Effector and regulatory T-cell subsets in autoimmunity and tissue inflammation. *Scand J Immunol* (2010) 72(3):173–84. doi:10.1111/j.1365-3083.2010.02432.x
66. Lyons JA, San M, Happ MP, Cross AH. B cells are critical to induction of experimental allergic encephalomyelitis by protein but not by a short encephalitogenic peptide. *Eur J Immunol* (1999) 29(11):3432–9. doi:10.1002/(SICI)1521-4141(199911)29:11<3432::AID-IMMU3432>3.0.CO;2-2
67. Fillatreau S, Sweenie CH, McGeachy MJ, Gray D, Anderton SM. B cells regulate autoimmunity by provision of IL-10. *Nat Immunol* (2002) 3(10):944–50. doi:10.1038/ni833
68. Lyons JA, Ramsbottom MJ, Cross AH. Critical role of antigen-specific antibody in experimental autoimmune encephalomyelitis induced by recombinant myelin oligodendrocyte glycoprotein. *Eur J Immunol* (2002) 32(7):1905–13. doi:10.1002/1521-4141(200207)32:7<1905:AID-IMMU1905>3.0.CO;2-L
69. Oliver AR, Lyon GM, Ruddle NH. Rat and human myelin oligodendrocyte glycoproteins induce experimental autoimmune encephalomyelitis by different mechanisms in C57BL/6 mice. *J Immunol* (2003) 171(1):462–8. doi:10.4049/jimmunol.171.9.4934
70. Magliozzi R, Columba-Cabezas S, Serafini B, Aloisi F. Intracerebral expression of CXCL13 and BAFF is accompanied by formation of lymphoid follicle-like structures in the meninges of mice with relapsing experimental autoimmune encephalomyelitis. *J Neuroimmunol* (2004) 148(1–2):11–23. doi:10.1016/j.jneuroim.2003.10.056
71. Columba-Cabezas S, Griguoli M, Rosicarelli B, Magliozzi R, Ria F, Serafini B, et al. Suppression of established experimental autoimmune encephalomyelitis and formation of meningeal lymphoid follicles by lymphotoxin beta receptor-Ig fusion protein. *J Neuroimmunol* (2006) 179(1–2):76–86. doi:10.1016/j.jneuroim.2006.06.015
72. Kuerten S, Schickel A, Kerkloh C, Recks MS, Addicks K, Ruddle NH, et al. Tertiary lymphoid organ development coincides with determinant spreading of the myelin-specific T cell response. *Acta Neuropathol* (2012) 124(6):861–73. doi:10.1007/s00401-012-1023-3
73. Bettelli E, Baeten D, Jäger A, Sobel RA, Kuchroo VK. Myelin oligodendrocyte glycoprotein-specific T and B cells cooperate to induce a Devic-like disease in mice. *J Clin Invest* (2006) 116(9):2393–402. doi:10.1172/JCI28334
74. Dang AK, Tesfagiorgis Y, Jain RW, Craig HC, Kerfoot SM. Meningeal infiltration of the spinal cord by non-classically activated B cells is associated with chronic disease course in a spontaneous B cell-dependent model of CNS autoimmune disease. *Front Immunol* (2015) 6:470. doi:10.3389/fimmu.2015.00470
75. Peters A, Pitcher LA, Sullivan JM, Mitsdoerffer M, Acton SE, Franz B, et al. Th17 cells induce ectopic lymphoid follicles in central nervous system tissue inflammation. *Immunity* (2011) 35(6):986–96. doi:10.1016/j.immuni.2011.10.015
76. Pikor NB, Astarita JL, Summers-Deluca L, Galicia G, Qu J, Ward LA, et al. Integration of Th17- and lymphotoxin-derived signals initiates meningeal-resident stromal cell remodeling to propagate neuroinflammation. *Immunity* (2015) 43(6):1160–73. doi:10.1016/j.immuni.2015.11.010
77. Krishnamoorthy G, Lassmann H, Wekerle H, Holz A. Spontaneous opticospinal encephalomyelitis in a double-transgenic mouse model of autoimmune T cell/B cell cooperation. *J Clin Invest* (2006) 116(9):2385–92. doi:10.1172/JCI28330
78. Pierson E, Simmons SB, Castelli L, Goverman JM. Mechanisms regulating regional localization of inflammation during CNS autoimmunity. *Immunol Rev* (2012) 248(1):205–15. doi:10.1111/j.1600-065X.2012.01126.x
79. Bartholomaus I, Kawakami N, Odoardi F, Schlager C, Miljkovic D, Ellwart JW, et al. Effector T cell interactions with meningeal vascular structures in nascent autoimmune CNS lesions. *Nature* (2009) 462(7269):94–8. doi:10.1038/nature08478

80. Pesic M, Bartholomaus I, Kyratsous NI, Heissmeyer V, Wekerle H, Kawakami N. 2-photon imaging of phagocyte-mediated T cell activation in the CNS. *J Clin Invest* (2013) 123(3):1192–201. doi:10.1172/JCI67233
81. Krautler NJ, Kana V, Kranich J, Tian Y, Perera D, Lemm D, et al. Follicular dendritic cells emerge from ubiquitous perivascular precursors. *Cell* (2012) 150(1):194–206. doi:10.1016/j.cell.2012.05.032
82. Kivisakk P, Imitola J, Rasmussen S, Elyaman W, Zhu B, Ransohoff RM, et al. Localizing central nervous system immune surveillance: meningeal antigen-presenting cells activate T cells during experimental autoimmune encephalomyelitis. *Ann Neurol* (2009) 65(4):457–69. doi:10.1002/ana.21379
83. Mues M, Bartholomaus I, Thestrup T, Griesbeck O, Wekerle H, Kawakami N, et al. Real-time in vivo analysis of T cell activation in the central nervous system using a genetically encoded calcium indicator. *Nat Med* (2013) 19(6):778–83. doi:10.1038/nm.3180
84. Grogan JL, Ouyang W. A role for Th17 cells in the regulation of tertiary lymphoid follicles. *Eur J Immunol* (2012) 42(9):2255–62. doi:10.1002/eji.201242656
85. Jäger A, Dardalhon V, Sobel RA, Bettelli E, Kuchroo VK. Th1, Th17, and Th9 effector cells induce experimental autoimmune encephalomyelitis with different pathological phenotypes. *J Immunol* (2009) 183(11):7169–77. doi:10.4049/jimmunol.0901906
86. Ota N, Wong K, Valdez PA, Zheng Y, Crellin NK, Diehl L, et al. IL-22 bridges the lymphotoxin pathway with the maintenance of colonic lymphoid structures during infection with *Citrobacter rodentium*. *Nat Immunol* (2011) 12(10):941–8. doi:10.1038/ni.2089
87. Barone F, Nayar S, Campos J, Cloake T, Withers DR, Toellner KM, et al. IL-22 regulates lymphoid chemokine production and assembly of tertiary lymphoid organs. *Proc Natl Acad Sci U S A* (2015) 112(35):11024–9. doi:10.1073/pnas.1503315112
88. Fleige H, Ravens S, Moschovakis GL, Bolter J, Willenzon S, Sutter G, et al. IL-17-induced CXCL12 recruits B cells and induces follicle formation in BALT in the absence of differentiated FDCs. *J Exp Med* (2014) 211(4):643–51. doi:10.1084/jem.20131737
89. McCandless EE, Wang Q, Woerner BM, Harper JM, Klein RS. CXCL12 limits inflammation by localizing mononuclear infiltrates to the perivascular space during experimental autoimmune encephalomyelitis. *J Immunol* (2006) 177(11):8053–64. doi:10.4049/jimmunol.177.11.8053
90. Alt C, Laschinger M, Engelhardt B. Functional expression of the lymphoid chemokines CCL19 (ELC) and CCL 21 (SLC) at the blood-brain barrier suggests their involvement in G-protein-dependent lymphocyte recruitment into the central nervous system during experimental autoimmune encephalomyelitis. *Eur J Immunol* (2002) 32(8):2133–44. doi:10.1002/1521-4141(200208)32:8<2133::AID-IMMU2133>3.0.CO;2-W
91. Krumbholz M, Theil D, Steinmeyer F, Cepok S, Hemmer B, Hofbauer M, et al. CCL19 is constitutively expressed in the CNS, up-regulated in neuroinflammation, active and also inactive multiple sclerosis lesions. *J Neuroimmunol* (2007) 190(1–2):72–9. doi:10.1016/j.jneuroim.2007.07.024
92. Bielecki B, Jatczak-Pawlik I, Wolinski P, Bednarek A, Glabinski A. Central nervous system and peripheral expression of CCL19, CCL21 and their receptor CCR7 in experimental model of multiple sclerosis. *Arch Immunol Ther Exp (Warsz)* (2015) 63(5):367–76. doi:10.1007/s00005-015-0339-9
93. Mitsdoerffer M, Lee Y, Jäger A, Kim HJ, Korn T, Kolls JK, et al. Proinflammatory T helper type 17 cells are effective B-cell helpers. *Proc Natl Acad Sci U S A* (2010) 107(32):14292–7. doi:10.1073/pnas.1009234107
94. Batoulis H, Wunsch M, Birkenheier J, Rottlaender A, Gorboulev V, Kuerten S. Central nervous system infiltrates are characterized by features of ongoing B cell-related immune activity in MP4-induced experimental autoimmune encephalomyelitis. *Clin Immunol* (2015) 158(1):47–58. doi:10.1016/j.clim.2015.03.009

19

Artery Tertiary Lymphoid Organs: Powerhouses of Atherosclerosis Immunity

Changjun Yin[1,2†], Sarajo Kumar Mohanta[1†], Prasad Srikakulapu[3], Christian Weber[1,2] and Andreas J. R. Habenicht[1]*

[1] Institute for Cardiovascular Prevention, Ludwig-Maximilians-University, Munich, Germany, [2] German Centre for Cardiovascular Research (DZHK), Partner Site Munich Heart Alliance, Munich, Germany, [3] Cardiovascular Research Center (CVRC), University of Virginia, Charlottesville, VA, USA

***Correspondence:**
Changjun Yin
changjun.yin@med.uni-muenchen.de

†Changjun Yin and Sarajo Kumar Mohanta contributed equally to this work.

Artery tertiary lymphoid organs (ATLOs) are atherosclerosis-associated lymphoid aggregates with varying degrees of complexity ranging from small T/B-cell clusters to well-structured lymph node-like though unencapsulated lymphoid tissues. ATLOs arise in the connective tissue that surrounds diseased arteries, i.e., the adventitia. ATLOs have been identified in aged atherosclerosis-prone hyperlipidemic apolipoprotein E-deficient (ApoE$^{-/-}$) mice: they are organized into distinct immune cell compartments, including separate T-cell areas, activated B-cell follicles, and plasma cell niches. Analyses of ATLO immune cell subsets indicate antigen-specific T- and B-cell immune reactions within the atherosclerotic arterial wall adventitia. Moreover, ATLOs harbor innate immune cells, including a large component of inflammatory macrophages, B-1 cells, and an aberrant set of antigen-presenting cells. There is marked neoangiogenesis, irregular lymphangiogenesis, neoformation of high endothelial venules, and *de novo* synthesis of lymph node-like conduits. Molecular mechanisms of ATLO formation remain to be identified though media vascular smooth muscle cells may adopt features of lymphoid tissue organizer-like cells by expressing lymphorganogenic chemokines, i.e., CXCL13 and CCL21. Although these data are consistent with the view that ATLOs participate in primary T- and B-cell responses against elusive atherosclerosis-specific autoantigens, their specific protective or disease-promoting roles remain to be identified. In this review, we discuss what is currently known about ATLOs and their potential impact on atherosclerosis and make attempts to define challenges ahead.

Keywords: atherosclerosis, aging, adventitia, autoimmune responses, artery tertiary lymphoid organs

ATHEROSCLEROSIS

Atherosclerosis leading to cardiovascular diseases is the major cause of death worldwide (1–8). The pathological hallmark of atherosclerosis is the atherosclerotic plaque in the intima layer of the arterial wall. Plaques ultimately clog the artery with life-threatening consequences, resulting in tissue infarcts such as myocardial infarcts (heart attacks) and stroke (9). Little is known about molecular mechanisms of atherosclerosis. Health organizations have proposed recommendations regarding risk factor reduction (smoking, diabetes mellitus, obesity, hypertension, hyperlipidemia, and sedentary lifestyle). The most important, but least understood, risk factor is aging. However, there is currently no clue as to the mechanisms of its impact on atherosclerosis progression.

A generally accepted hypothesis is that the immune system is critically involved in the pathogenesis of atherosclerosis, but major issues of atherosclerosis immunity remain to be addressed: it is not clear where and when atherosclerosis-specific immune responses are organized; what are the relative contributions of the innate *vis-à-vis* the adaptive immune systems during the various stages of the disease; and, most importantly, is atherosclerosis a *bona fide* antigen-dependent autoimmune disease or a chronic autoinflammatory condition? Answers to these questions are needed to develop therapeutic strategies to directly target the atherosclerotic plaque in the intima of arteries.

IMMUNE HYPOTHESIS OF ATHEROSCLEROSIS

Each innate and adaptive immune cell lineage and their subtypes has been implicated in the pathogenesis of atherosclerosis including platelets, neutrophils, monocytes/macrophages, mast cells, various dendritic cell (DC) subsets, numerous T- and B-cell subtypes, and innate lymphoid cells (3, 4, 7, 10–22). However, there is no generally accepted concept which immune cells trigger the disease, at which step distinct subsets promote or attenuate the disease, and how plaque growth unfolds at the molecular level. Indeed, widely different hypotheses have been proposed [reviewed in Ref. (23)].

Concepts regarding atherogenesis have been deduced from observations in mouse models including low-density lipoprotein receptor-deficient (LDLR$^{-/-}$) or apolipoprotein E-deficient (ApoE$^{-/-}$) mice (24) and human tissue specimens. Mouse models on hyperlipidemic backgrounds have been generated to disrupt one or more molecules that control the systemic immune system. The worrying fact of the matter, however, is that – given the complex nature of the disease involving multiple genetic and life-style- and aging-driven risk factors – atherosclerosis research is in a dismal state.

Fundamental questions remain: the specific roles of each immune cell subset and their interplay, the timing and sites of their actions, the relative shares of the innate and adaptive immune systems in the organization of atherosclerosis immune responses over time, and the impacts and location of disease-causing and disease-suppressing leukocyte subsets, all remain to be determined. The major challenge, however, concerns the principal nature of the underlying disease-causing immune responses: Is plaque formation a chronic autoinflammatory tissue reaction (without generation of autoimmune B- or T-cells) or are elusive disease-causing autoantigens driving generation and action of autoimmune lymphocyte subsets?

Thus, atherosclerosis research shares major unanswered questions with other clinically important chronic inflammatory diseases such as rheumatoid arthritis, multiple sclerosis, and inflammatory bowel diseases (25–28). Based on circumstantial evidence, some of these diseases are considered *bona fide* autoimmune diseases although – similar to atherosclerosis – their *disease-triggering autoantigens* have not been identified [see review in Ref. (23, 29, 30)]. Moreover, atherosclerosis-specific immune responses have long been assumed to be organized in atherosclerotic plaques in the intima layer of arteries or systemically in secondary lymphoid organs (SLOs), but the evidence for these views is scarce if not non-existing. Thus, it is safe to say that neither the existence, their nature (T- versus B-cell responses), nor the location of autoimmune reactions in atherosclerosis have been identified.

ATHEROSCLEROTIC PLAQUES

The normal intima layer consists of an endothelial cell monolayer attached to the internal basement membrane (7). Vascular DCs have been described in the intima layer of normal mouse arteries, but their role in the maintenance of artery homeostasis or their impact on disease has not been determined (31, 32). The disease ultimately affects all layers of the arterial wall including the media layer [largely consisting of vascular smooth muscle cells (VSMCs)] and the adventitial layer (the outer connective tissue coat; see below): advanced atherosclerosis can therefore be viewed as a chronic *transmural inflammatory arterial wall disease*. Early plaques undergo major alterations of cellular composition over time: during the early stages of the disease, subsequent or concomitantly with the influx of monocytes into the arterial wall, T-cells home into the intima. VSMCs may migrate into the intima and increase in number by self-renewal. Monocytes/macrophages, T-cells, and VSMCs undergo activation and proliferation during the various stages of the disease. It should be pointed out that other views on the early stages of atherosclerosis emphasize the role of platelets and/or neutrophils (12, 21).

STAGING OF ATHEROSCLEROSIS AND DISTINCT IMMUNE CELL SUBSETS IN ARTERIAL WALL LAYERS

Human atherosclerotic plaques have been staged into types I–VI according to the histological and clinical criteria (9). However, only the late V and VI stages become clinically significant when artery lumen narrowing compromises oxygen supply to the downstream tissue and the plaque becomes unstable. Atherosclerotic plaques in ApoE$^{-/-}$ mice recapitulate some – but not all – features of the different stages of human plaques. Of note, plaques lack B-cells and consequently B-cell follicles including follicular dendritic cells (FDCs). Plaques are also devoid of nerve axons, lymph vessels, high endothelial venules (HEVs), and lymph node-like conduits, which are all critically involved in efficient recruitment of lymphocytes and the subsequent organization of adaptive immune responses (see below) (**Figures 1** and **2**). It is therefore difficult to envision that immune cells in atherosclerotic plaques participate in adaptive cellular and humoral immune responses though they may be involved in antigen presentation to T-cells through vascular DCs or monocyte-derived DCs (mDCs) that emigrate from plaques to home to SLOs [see contribution of antigen presentation by Hughes et al. (under review)[1]; this Research Topic].

[1]Hughes C, Bedaj M, Benson RA, Maffia P. Antigen presenting cells and antigen presentation in tertiary lymphoid organs. (under review in this Research topic).

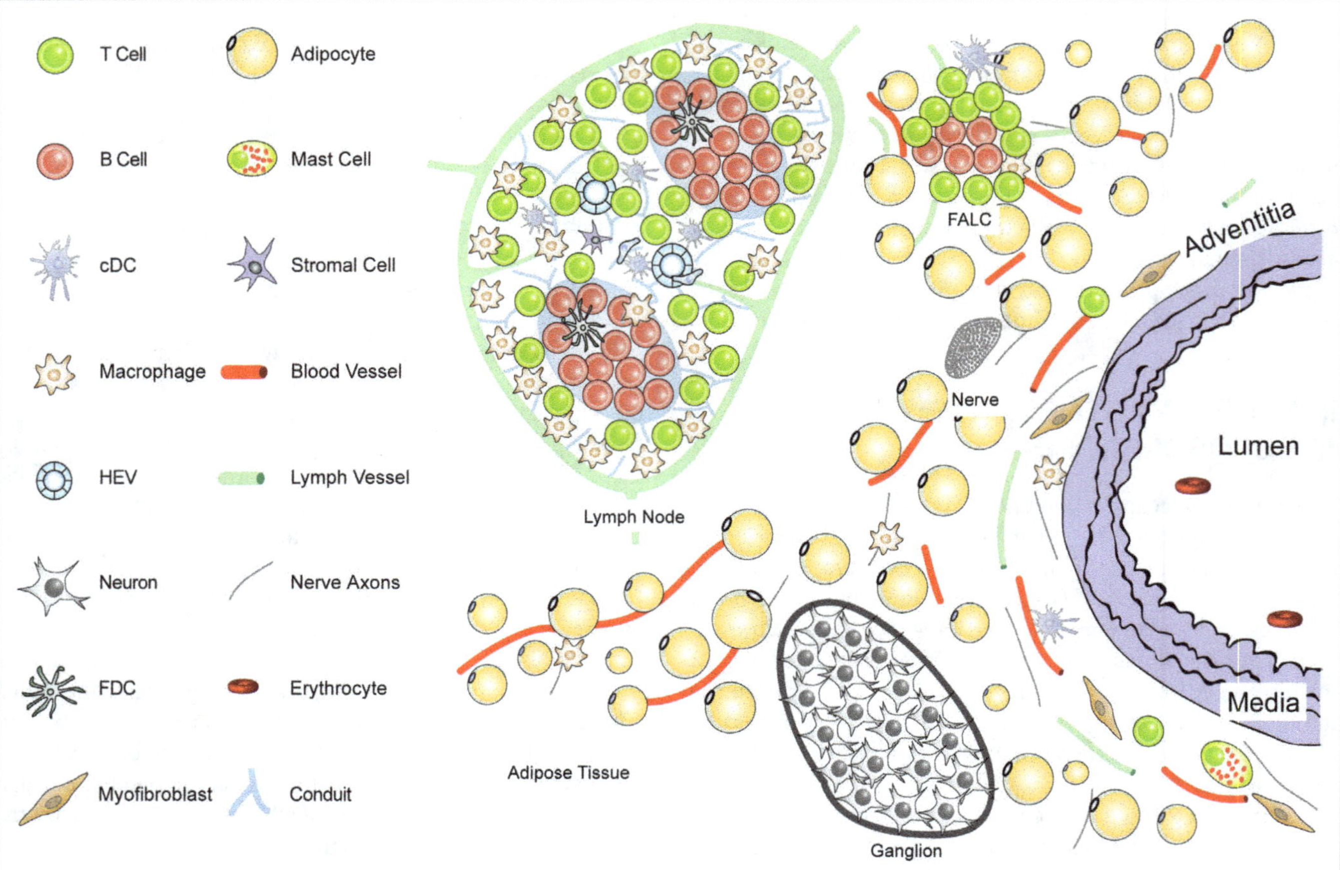

FIGURE 1 | Anatomy of the normal aorta adventitia and adjacent tissues. The normal adventitial layer of the mouse aorta constitutively contains T-cells (but no B-cells), tissue macrophages, cDCs, stromal cells or myofibroblasts, and mast cells. The adjacent tissues including the periaortic adipose tissue harbors fat-associated lymphoid clusters (FALCs) in wild-type mice. FALCs represent T/B-cell aggregates of various sizes that are exclusively observed in adipose tissue. In the adventitia, axons of both the sensory and the sympathetic nervous systems have been identified as well as vasa vasorum and lymph vessels. Ganglia of the peripheral nervous system are embedded in the adipose tissue, and their axons reach the external lamina that separates the adventitia from the media layer.

THE ADVENTITIA: AN ELUSIVE CONNECTIVE TISSUE COAT OF ARTERIES

A commonly accepted notion states that the adventitia (33–37) forms the *outer connective tissue coat that surrounds blood vessels or arteries*. Given the complexity of the connective tissue surrounding arteries and the lack of size definition together with recent progress in understanding the potential impact of the adventitia in arterial wall remodeling and atherosclerosis, the shortcomings of this definition are apparent (35). However, as we discuss below, the adventitia is a highly active and complex tissue whose roles in the maintenance and homeostasis of the artery is only beginning to be unraveled (38–50).

To delineate the impact the adventitia may have on arterial wall remodeling and atherosclerosis in future studies, a more sophisticated definition should be attempted. The normal connective tissue coat surrounding arteries (in the mouse within 100 μm extending from the aorta external lamina separating the media from the adventitia) includes blood vessels (vasa vasorum), small lymph vessels, and an axon network of both the sympathetic and the sensory peripheral nervous systems (**Figure 1**).

Unlike the resistance arteries (muscular arterioles) involved in blood pressure regulation, axons of both of these peripheral autonomous nervous systems, but not of the parasympathetic nervous system, reach out to the external lamina; however, they do not cross into the media of medium- and large-sized arteries in mice. Major cellular constituents in the normal adventitia are mast cells, T-cells, and tissue macrophages, a meshwork of fibroblasts or myofibroblasts, classical DCs (cDCs), and most likely pericytes [see contribution of Kranich and Krautler (51); this Research Topic]. Furthermore, the adjacent adipose tissue (containing FALCs) needs to be considered as a tissue in the immediate vicinity of the adventitia (**Figure 1**). Thus, in mice, the immediate connective tissue coat within a diameter of 100 μm contains myofibroblasts, a loose network of extracellular matrix components, small blood and lymph vessels, and nerve axons. In addition, few tissue macrophages, T-cells, cDCs, and mast cells are important cellular constituents of the normal adventitia (33, 52) (**Figure 1**).

Each of these immune cell subsets may participate in immune surveillance of arteries (35, 53). Adventitia progenitor cells maintain the endothelial and VSMC pools (52). The vasa vasorum is a network of small blood vessels that reach the external lamina

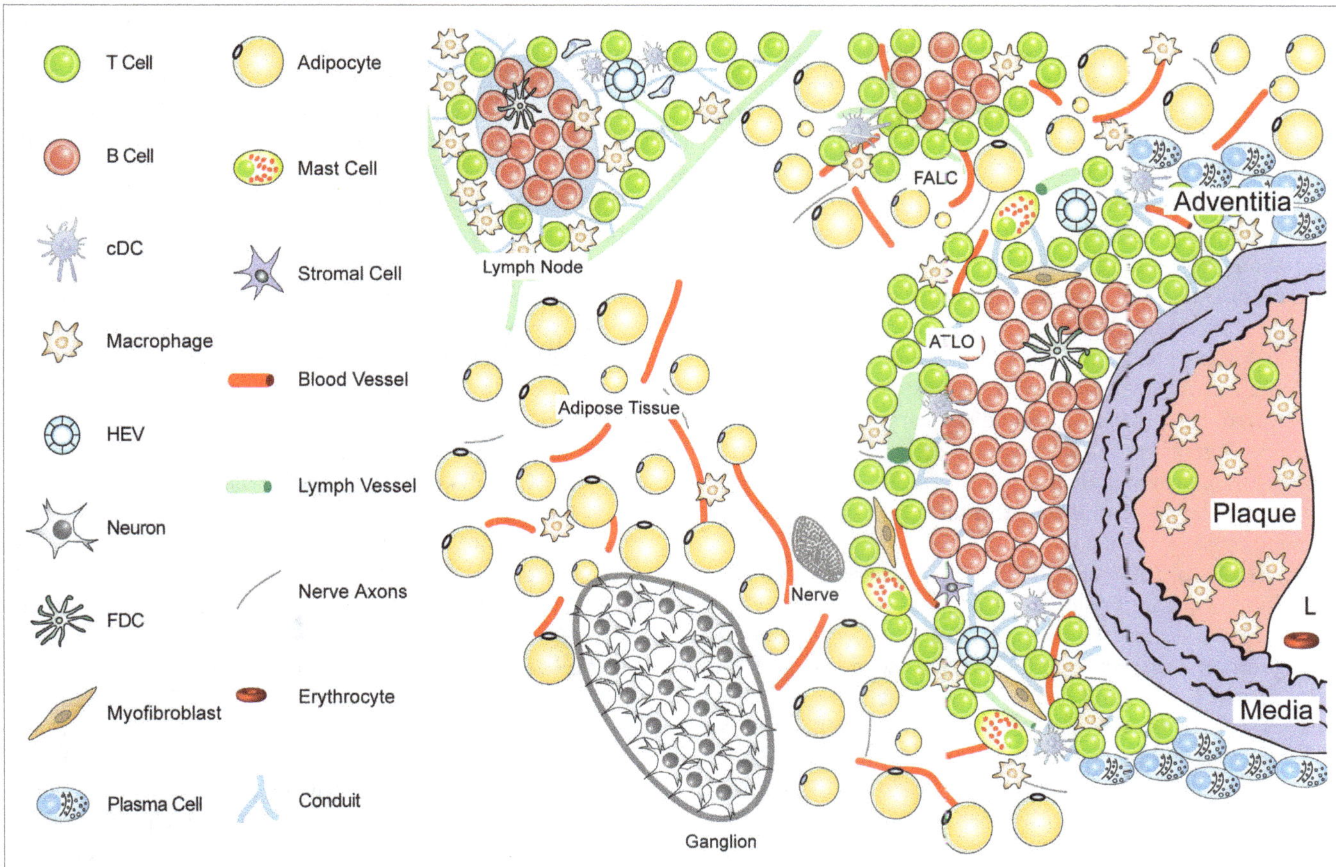

FIGURE 2 | Anatomy of the diseased aorta adventitia in aged hyperlipidemic mice. Aged hyperlipidemic mice develop ATLOs in the adventitia layer of the aorta selectively adjacent to atherosclerotic plaques with a preference for the abdominal aorta segment. ATLOs range from small T/B-cell aggregates to well-structured TLOs with separate T- and B-cell areas. The most advanced forms of ATLOs contain B-cell follicles including FDCs, newly formed conduits, HEVs, and aberrant lymph vessels (see **Figure 4**).

providing nutrients and oxygen to large- and medium-sized arteries (36, 38, 54, 55). Though little is known about their functional impact, conceivably, each of these adventitia constituents could affect arterial wall homeostasis. We have begun to systematically delineate the aorta adventitia of wild-type (WT) mice and hyperlipidemic ApoE$^{-/-}$ mice (**Figures 1** and **2**). The normal adventitia is neighboring the para-aortic adipose tissue, which contains FALCs recently described in the omentum of the peritoneum of mice [(56); observations; contribution of Caamano et al. (under review)[2]; this Research Topic]. Although little is known about them in atherosclerosis, it is conceivable that FALCs may participate in atherosclerosis immune responses. It is important to distinguish each of the adventitia and adjacent tissues as it is recognized that cells in the adventitia and the adjacent tissues are capable of sensing and responding to a wide range of stimuli (37).

DISCOVERY AND STAGING OF ATLOs

Tissues that are invaded by antigen are targeted by leukocytes which form – within hours – an acute form of inflammatory infiltrate. This rapid and vigorous action of the innate immune system is carried out with the aim to eliminate the antigen before it can spread and/or inflict harm. However, if the immune system fails to eliminate the invaders, the immune system doubles down on its efforts: the nature of the inflammatory infiltrate will change over time including a reduction of neutrophils, further recruitment of blood monocytes, *de novo* recruitment of T-cells and DCs and form – within days – a predominantly monocyte/macrophage/T-cell/DC-driven inflammatory tissue response (57–59).

Can this type of immune cell infiltrate qualify as a TLO? It probably does or should not qualify for the following reasons: lymphorganogenesis during ontogeny and in adult organisms requires action of lymphorganogenic chemokines, i.e., CCL21 and CXCL13 (60, 61), which are essential for the attraction of B-cells and the formation of T/B-cell aggregates (various contributions in this Research Topic). Without lymphorganogenic chemokines, the immune system is severely impaired (60, 62). There may be exceptions to this paradigm as recent studies on colitis models in mice suggest that the nervous system is not only triggering the earliest forms of lymph node anlagen (63) but also TLO neogenesis in the gastrointestinal tract (64). In addition, early and chronic inflammatory infiltrates without major structural

[2] Caamano J et al. (manuscript in preparation for this Research topic).

components of SLOs including HEVs, lymph vessels, and conduits, and T-cell areas and B-cell follicles may be less efficient in recruiting and activating naïve lymphocytes to generate T- and B-memory cells in response to antigen [(65); see Ruddle (under review)[3]; this Research Topic].

In 2004, we reported that the number of inflammatory leukocytes, in particular monocyte/macrophages and T-cells, when determined by morphometry of the innominate artery and throughout the arterial tree, increase progressively in the adventitia during aging (66). We systematically studied the relation between plaque and adventitial leukocytes in $ApoE^{-/-}$ mice that were adolescent/young (16 weeks; small atherosclerotic plaques), adult (32 weeks; significant atherosclerosis in the aortic arch; little atherosclerosis in the abdominal aorta); advanced adult (52 weeks; significant aortic arch atherosclerosis; beginning atherosclerosis of the abdominal aorta), and aged (78 weeks; significant atherosclerosis throughout the aorta including abdominal segments) (46).

The results of these studies can be summarized as follows: the inflammatory infiltrate of atherosclerotic plaques decreased in cellularity over time; by contrast, adventitial T-cells and macrophages increased over time in adventitia segments areas that were afflicted with atherosclerosis throughout all major arteries; the size of the adventitial infiltrates correlated with atherosclerotic plaque burden in a highly territorialized way; the ratio between adventitia T-cell density over plaque T-cell density reached a dramatic approximately 80-fold in aged $ApoE^{-/-}$ mice in some segments (46); T-cells were both $CD4^+$ and $CD8^+$ T helper cells and also included a large T regulatory cell component (see below); the cellularity of the ubiquitous adventitial infiltrate in areas such as the innominate artery and the thoracic aorta could be distinguished from that in the upper abdominal portion of the aorta, however, which was being infiltrated by B-cells at around 52 weeks of age. We therefore suggested that the lymphocyte aggregate of the earliest TLO stage (Stage I) should be characterized by a combined T-/B-cell aggregate. Stage I TLOs have not yet been fully separated T-cell and B-cell compartments, but they are precursors of the well-developed later artery tertiary lymphoid organ (ATLO) stages as indicated by kinetic experiments (41, 46). We suggested three stages of ATLOs.

ATLO Stage I: B-cells begin to infiltrate the adventitia as loosely arranged leukocytes without forming distinct T- and B-cell areas; ATLO Stage I emerges parallel to the formation of atherosclerotic plaques in the intima during aging and has not been observed in young mice; this first ATLO stage strongly indicates the action of lymphorganogenic chemokines, i.e., CCL21 and CXCL13, which may be important chemoattractants for T- and B-cells, respectively, and thus ATLO neogenesis. It is noteworthy that not all adventitial leukocyte infiltrates adjacent to atherosclerotic plaques develop into ATLOs. In hyperlipidemic mice, ATLO Stage I, as all subsequent stages, has a strong preference for the upper abdominal aorta adventitia. However, we have little cues as to the molecular mechanisms for this predilection site. *ATLO Stage II*: separate T- and B-cell areas emerge; lymph vessel neogenesis becomes prominent together with a dense network of lymph node-like conduits connecting the arterial wall with newly formed HEVs. *ATLO Stage III*: a well-structured ATLO contains separate T-cell and B-cell follicles with activated germinal centers (GCs) including FDCs, plasma cell (PC) niches, prominent lymph vessel, and blood vessel neogenesis of vasa vasorum.

It should be noted, however, that ATLO stages and the onset of lymph vessel, blood vessel, and HEV neogenesis have not yet been defined. Following this reasoning, TLO Stage II can be distinguished from Stage I by the development of separate T- and B-cell areas. Although TLO Stage II lacking FDCs does not appear to be able to mount affinity maturation of B-cell receptors (BCRs) in a GC reaction [see Kranich and Krautler (51); this Research Topic], it is likely that activation of T-cells and B-cells and somatic hypermutation of BCRs can be organized in ATLOs stages I and II (67, 68). Finally, TLO Stage III shows activated GCs containing FDCs in B-cell follicles as their defining hallmark (see also **Figures 3** and **4**).

Although not directly demonstrated for any TLO, it is conceivable to assume that there is – at least for some TLOs – an antigen-driven T-cell activation and memory T-cell generation pathway (69, 70). In addition, in Stage III TLOs, an affinity maturation pathway leading to memory B-cells and/or PC generation is likely to occur (see below). Our proposal of TLO staging in general and that of ATLO staging in particular is debatable from a number of perspectives and should be regarded as an exercise to begin a discussion on the pros and cons of these definitions.

Our rationale to define the TLO stage is as follows: ATLOs Stage I already harbors proliferating T- and B-cells, which appear to be vigorously activated (note that both T-cell and B-cell activation occurs or can occur outside of GCs and in the absence of FDCs to mount a protective and/or proinflammatory adaptive immune response); the emergence of CCL21 and CXCL13 signals as strong drivers of lymphorganogenesis (71–74); CCL21 and CXCL13 expression indicate – in adult organisms – the activation of the lymphotoxin receptor and the tumor necrosis factor receptor on lymphoid tissue organizer (LTo) cells, which appear to be required for differentiation of stromal cells to become LTo cells (41, 67, 75–77).

It is of interest to note that major underlying mechanisms of ATLO neogenesis are distinct when compared with similar structures in the lung. Inducible bronchus-associated lymphoid tissues (iBALTs) preferentially form in young mice, whereas well-developed ATLOs are not observed before the age of 52 weeks (41, 78) [see article by Hwang et al. (79); this Research Topic]. However, there are also similarities, i.e., some iBALTs develop in the perivascular space of pulmonary blood vessels in addition to the connective tissue underneath the bronchial epithelium.

ATLO IMMUNE CELLS AND STRUCTURES

To understand atherosclerosis-related adaptive immune responses in the diseased arterial wall better, we determined

[3]Ruddle N. High endothelial venules and lymphatic vessels in tertiary lymphoid organs: characteristics, functions, and regulation. (under review in this Research topic).

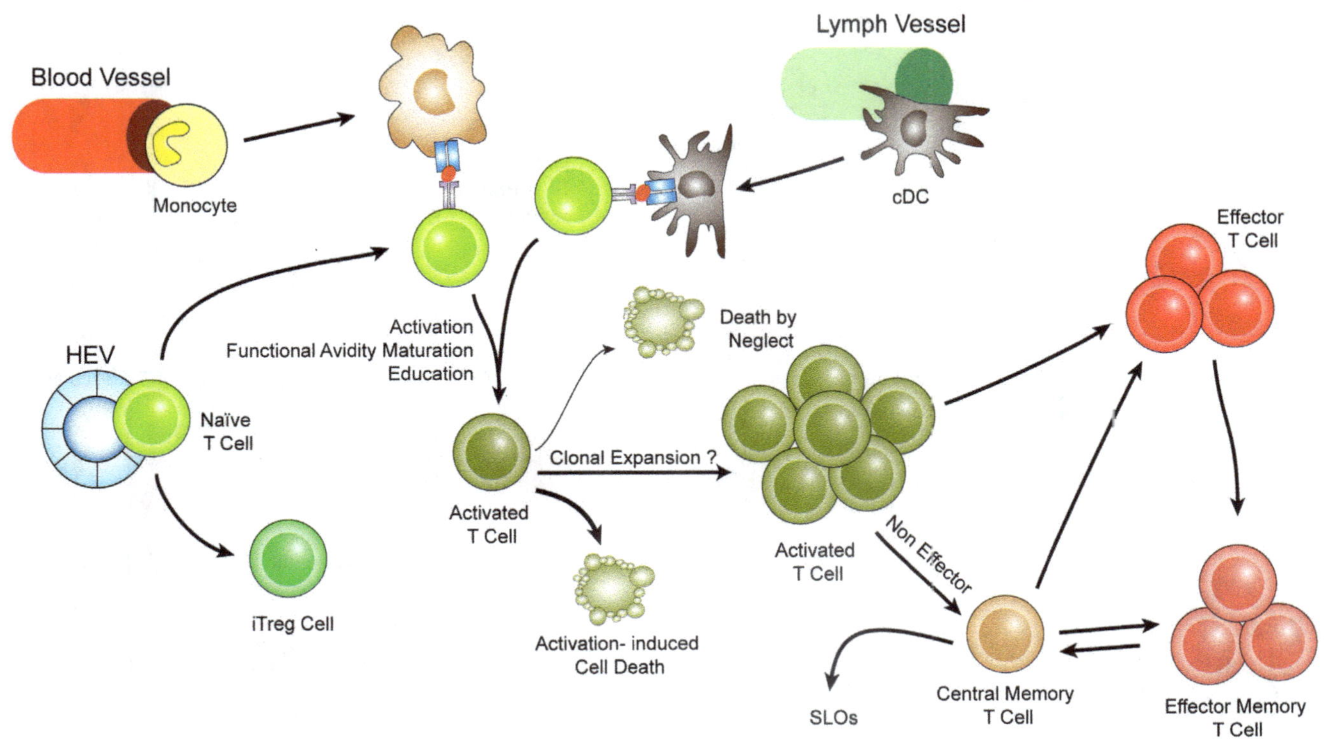

FIGURE 3 | Hypothetical choreography for antigen-dependent ATLO T-cell response pathways. ATLOs are powerhouses of T-cell immunity. They promote T-cell recruitment and suppress T-cell egress allowing for extended T/DC interactions, activation, proliferation, and education of T-cells. ATLOs also mediate conversion of naïve CD4+ T-cells into iT_{reg} cells. This schematic representation has been modified from Hu et al. reported earlier [see Ref. (67) for detailed data].

leukocyte subtypes in the abdominal aorta during aging in $ApoE^{-/-}$ mice, which we had tentatively termed *tertiary lymphoid follicles* (46, 66). As the high leukocyte density in these developing follicles prevented morphometric analyses, we established single cell suspension protocols of aorta segments to perform FACS analyses (67): T-cell subtypes include $CD4^+$, $CD8^+$, $FoxP3^+$ $CD4^+$, and few $FoxP3^+$ $CD8^+$ cells; a significant number of B-cells accumulate in the follicles though B-cells are rarely seen in other parts of the arterial tree; no lymphoid follicles develop in plaque-free aorta segments; leukocyte follicles are absent in young mice before 52 weeks of age; there is marked neogenesis of HEVs, lymph node-like conduits, and lymph vessels; the lymph vessels are aberrant in that they show dilated lumina with large numbers of luminal leukocytes; semi-quantitative analyses revealed that the follicles promote recruitment of T-cells after adoptive transfer through HEVs, whereas little recruitment occurs in atherosclerotic plaques; the conduits resemble lymph node conduits as they exclude fluorescent dextran particles of 500 kDa (which were seen in the HEV lumen only) though they transport 10-kDa dextran particles; VSMCs in segments afflicted with atherosclerosis and lymphocyte follicles in the adventitia express lymphorganogenic chemokines CCL21 and CXCL13; *in vivo* blockade using an antagonistic decoy lymphotoxin β receptor antiserum eliminated FDCs from the aggregates and significantly reduced the number of HEVs (41). These data indicated that atherosclerosis is associated with TLO formation.

CONDUITS, ANGIOGENESIS, LYMPHANGIOGENESIS, AND NEOFORMATION OF HEVs

There is considerable information on the structure and function of conduits in SLOs (41, 63, 80–83). In SLOs, stromal cells in the subcapsular sinus of lymph nodes play a major role in the traffic of molecules and of distinct immune cells (65, 84). Although little is known about conduits in TLOs, we identified conduit-like structures in ATLOs using immunohistochemistry and fluorescent dextran labeling *in vivo* [(41); **Figure 2**]. We observed that ATLO conduits share a series of structural and cellular similarities of LN conduits. Moreover, using fluorescently labeled microbeads, we observed that ATLO conduits sieve low molecular weight molecules from the circulation into the conduit network (41). However, the normal lymph node conduits are structures that connect afferent lymph and HEVs.

This anatomy of lymph node conduits is probably different from that of ATLOs: in lymph nodes, conduits form a reticular network connecting the subcapsular sinus and HEVs [see Ager (under review)[4]; this Research Topic]. Instead, we found that ATLO conduits connect the outer media of the arterial wall with newly formed HEVs within the T-cell areas of ATLOs. This distinctive

[4]Ager A. High endothelial venules. (manuscript in preparation for this Research topic).

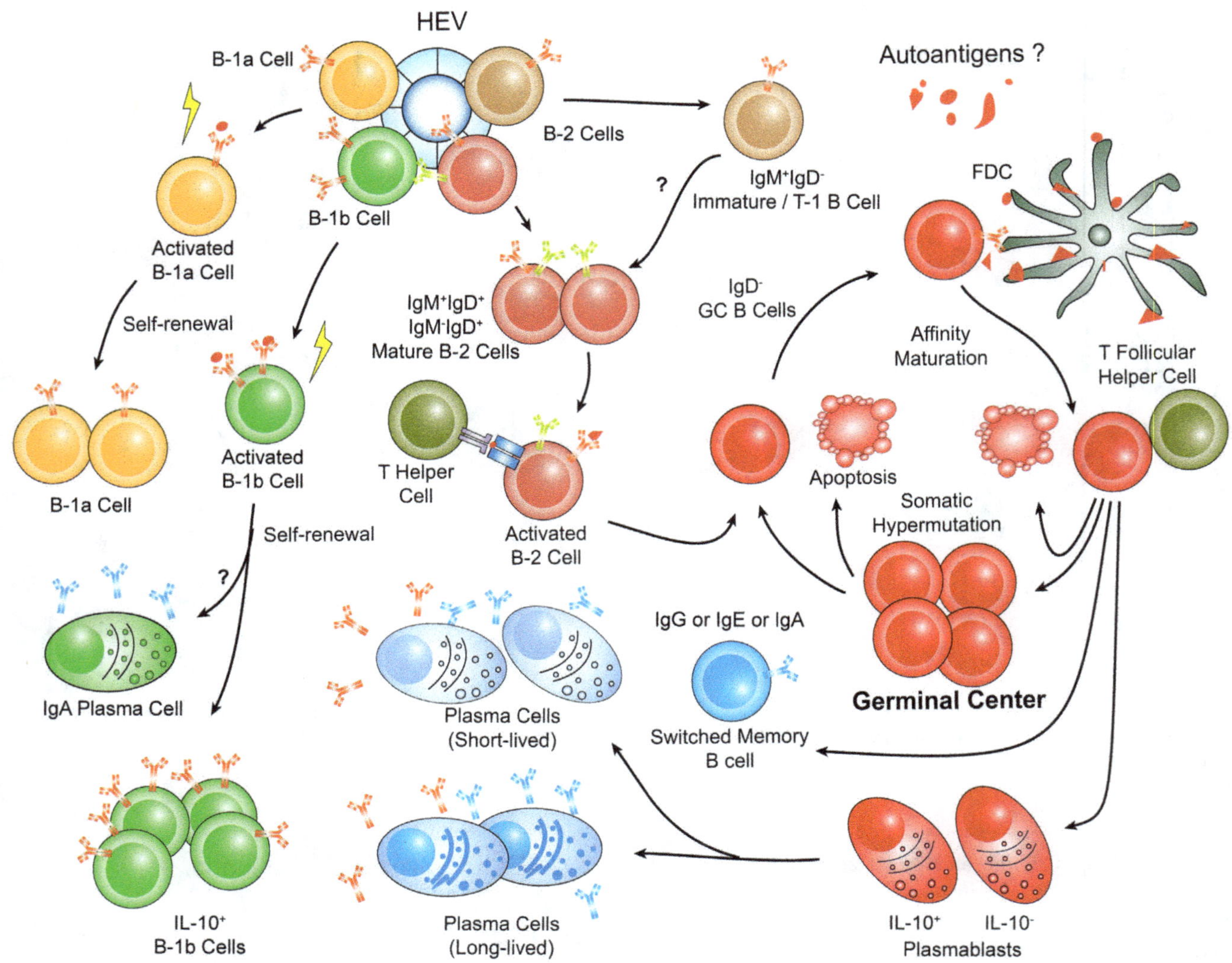

FIGURE 4 | Hypothetical choreography of antigen-dependent ATLO B-cell response pathways. Advanced ATLOs are powerhouses of B-cell immunity. ATLO B-cell responses are two-pronged in nature containing a comprehensive B-1 and a multi-faceted B-2 maturation pathway. Although similarities of B-cell immunity in ATLOs and SLOs are apparent, differences include a large PC component and a distinct B-1 B cell compartment which differs from that in the peritoneal cavity. This schematic figure has been modified from Srikakulapu et al. (68) [see Ref. (68) for detailed data].

anatomy of conduits in SLOs versus TLOs is interesting in view of the hypothesis that chemokine gradients may exist within ATLOs with possible CXCL13 derived from activated media segments adjacent to atherosclerotic plaques. Furthermore, small molecular weight soluble antigens could be transported from the media to T-cell areas or B-cell follicles. It is possible that the lymph vessels of ATLOs also connect with conduits, but this has not yet been studied. We therefore speculate that molecules in the range of the size of chemokines (which can enter conduits) and possibly soluble antigen may be transported from the media compartment to HEVs, i.e., the entry sites of lymphocytes into ATLOs. Given the capacity of several ATLO antigen-presenting cells (APCs) to present exogenous antigen to T-cells [see contribution of Maffia et al. (33); this Research Topic], ATLO conduits may therefore have functional roles in the maintenance of atherosclerosis immunity.

However, ATLOs lack capsules and therefore no apparent subcapsular sinus, i.e., the anatomical structure that allows afferent lymph vessels to drain cells and antigen *via* conduits into the parenchyma of the lymph node. Although there are clearly differences in conduit architecture between lymph nodes and ATLOs, the function of the latter may be to facilitate draining of the inflamed artery to allow antigen access the T-cell areas of ATLOs. However, the precise function of ATLO conduits remains to be determined. It will be of interest to test the possibility whether the atherosclerosis immune response within the arterial wall may be altered by crossing ApoE$^{-/-}$ with PLVAP$^{-/-}$ mice that have a pathological conduit system (82).

ATHEROSCLEROSIS, AGING, AND ATLO T-CELL IMMUNITY

Our data on ATLOs raise several questions: Is aging of the immune system (also referred to as immune senescence) (85–87) affected by hyperlipidemia? What is the relationship between local and systemic, i.e., SLO-dependent, atherosclerosis immunity during aging? Are there principal differences in T-cell immunity-related gene expression and inflammation-related gene expression in atherosclerotic plaques versus ATLOs? What is the territoriality of atherosclerosis T-cell responses in diseased arterial walls? (**Figure 3**) How are the ATLO T-cell responses organized as opposed to those in SLOs? Are VSMC lymphotoxin β receptors important in shaping the anatomy and function of ATLOs? Answers to these questions may be of general interest to understand TLO immunity in a wide range of disease conditions.

At the level of renal lymph nodes (RLNs) which drain the aorta, we characterized major T-cell subtypes during aging by FACS and genome-wide transcript expression arrays. Although the results of these studies identified major age-related gene expression changes, transcriptomes of WT versus ApoE$^{-/-}$ RLNs were principally identical (67), indicating that hyperlipidemia does not affect T-cells and their activation systemically in major ways including aorta-draining LNs. However, transcriptome analyses of RLNs, spleen, and blood during aging showed marked aging/senescence-dependent changes. In sharp contrast, immune response-related and inflammation-related changes in aorta territories, i.e., plaques versus ATLOs, were dramatic, indicating that T-cell immunity in atherosclerosis appears to be regulated locally rather than systemically (67).

We used laser capture microdissection-based mRNA expression analyses to construct transcript atlases and to delineate the territoriality of T-cell immunity in the arterial wall in comparison with SLOs. Gene ontology (GO) terms *immune response, inflammation, T-cell activation, positive regulation of T-cell regulation,* and *T-cell proliferation* were examined. Again, these analyses failed to identify significant differential gene expression in WT versus ApoE$^{-/-}$ RLNs (2 genes), but major changes between RLNs and ATLOs (1251 genes), between atherosclerotic plaques and ATLOs (1102 genes), and major changes between adventitia segments afflicted with versus those without atherosclerotic plaques in the intima (1274 genes). The transcript atlases of ATLOs and other affected diseased tissues in atherosclerosis (88, 89) will be important to address a variety of questions regarding atherosclerosis immunity and other issues including remodeling of extracellular matrix components during disease progression. The data were published in the NCBI Gene Expression Omnibus (GSE 40156) to be used to address a series of questions such as B-cell immunity in the arterial wall [see Ref. (68); below].

T-CELL PHENOTYPES IN ATLOs ARE DISTINCT FROM THOSE IN SLOs

FACS analyses yielded additional information on the activation status of ATLO T-cell subtypes: naïve T-cells were rare in ATLOs yielding a 27-fold ratio of ATLO CD4$^+$ T effector memory cells (T_{EM}) and also considerable numbers of T central memory (T_{CM}) T-cells over their naïve counterparts; similar data were obtained for T regulatory cells (T_{reg} cells) yielding an 87-fold ratio of T_{reg} cells with an EM or CM phenotype over their naïve counterparts, and in a similar, though less pronounced, way, the data were similar for CD8$^+$ T-cells. Functional impacts of TLOs in general and of ATLOs in particular are only beginning to be understood. In peripheral tissues, immunosurveillance is carried out by tissue-specific homing and education of T_{EM} and T_{CM} T-cells as exemplified in skin and intestine (90–97). Thus, T-cells home into inflamed tissues, but they are also retained in these tissues to account for preferential action of T-cells in the diseased versus healthy tissues.

To study T-cell tropism in atherosclerosis, a series of adoptive transfer experiments were conducted to test the ability of ATLOs as *homing hubs* and *education centers* of T-cell immunity. Sizable numbers of ATLO CD4$^+$, CD8$^+$, and T_{reg} cells expressed CD103, PD-1, CD69, and other activation and homing molecules contrasting to their SLO counterparts. Moreover, there were little changes in these T-cell education signatures in WT versus ApoE$^{-/-}$ SLOs. As T-cell recirculation is rapid, we used adoptive transfers using highly FACS-purified naïve T-cells in splenectomized and FTY720-treated mice: splenectomy was necessary to prevent recirculation of T-cells through the spleen, while FTY720 was required to prevent T-cell egress from lymph nodes. These data showed that ATLOs are effective in both recruitment and preventing egress of T-cells. FTY720 acts through sphingosine 1-phosphate receptors type 1 expressed by efferent lymph vessel endothelial cells in SLOs (98, 99). Our data also indicated that ATLO lymph vessels are functional and therefore may be involved in T-cell recruitment and recirculation into and out of the arterial wall bearing strong similarities to the function of lymph vessels in lymph nodes (67) (See text footnote 3).

Leukocyte movement in ATLOs versus WT adventitia was also assessed using multiphoton microscopy. These data showed striking similarities of T-cell movement that had been observed when naïve T-cells undergo a primary immune response in SLOs during activation and priming including length of migration per time interval, track velocity, and displacement (67, 100–102). In contrast, movement parameters of naïve T-cells in the WT adventitia showed nearly motionless cells. Detailed studies of movement parameters of T-cells in WT versus ApoE$^{-/-}$ lymph nodes including the popliteal lymph node which does not drain the aorta showed identical characteristics. Furthermore, we identified a series of APCs in ATLOs using two independent assays of *in vivo* antigen presentation [see article of Maffia et al. (33); this Research Topic]. The composition of ATLO APCs, however, was aberrant in that the majority was mDCs followed by B-cells, cDCs, macrophages, and a minor population of lymphoid DCs (lyDCs).

ATLOs CONTAIN LARGE NUMBERS OF T REGULATORY CELLS AND CONVERT NAÏVE T-CELLS INTO INDUCED T REGULATORY CELLS

T-cell-specific ATLO immunity is dichotomic in nature in that both proinflammatory and anti-inflammatory lymphocyte subsets including a large number of T_{reg} cells have been observed using immunohistochemistry and FACS analyses (41, 103). It is well established that T_{reg} cells accumulate in inflamed tissues (104–106). There are two major T_{reg} subtypes, i.e., one that is generated in the thymus (nT_{reg} cells) and another that is generated in the periphery from naïve CD4$^+$ precursors (105) termed induced T_{reg} (iT_{reg}) cells. The functional significance of these two T_{reg} subtypes for the regulation of T-cell immunity in various diseases remains to be fully understood, but it is possible that the TCR repertoire of naïve CD4$^+$ T-cells gives rise to memory T_{reg} cells that have potent immunosuppressive properties under chronic inflammatory disease conditions as judged from other model systems in mice (105, 107). Moreover, regulatory T memory cells have been identified and may contribute to antigen-specific immunosuppression (108).

In view of our observation that ATLOs contain large numbers of T_{reg} cells (41), we attempted to characterize ATLO T_{reg} cells in more detail using subtype-specific markers and to delineate the activation status of ATLO T_{reg} cells. Naïve GFP-T_{reg} cells purified from spleens and lymph nodes of transgenic FoxP3-DTR-GFP mice (106) were adoptively transferred into aged ApoE$^{-/-}$ mice and their phenotype was examined in ATLOs. The adoptively transferred T_{reg} cells did not show the activated endogenous phenotype even 3 weeks after transfer. These data were surprising and indicated that the endogenous ATLO T_{reg} cell population may be generated locally through an extended period of time during aging and that there may be clonal selection of endogenous T_{reg} cells in an antigen-specific way (67). We then examined the ability of ATLOs to convert CD4$^+$ T-cells into iT_{reg} cells. FACS-purified naïve CD4$^+$ T cells were transferred into aged ApoE$^{-/-}$ mice. Although at 24 h, ATLOs did not show significant iT_{reg} cells, after 3 weeks, a considerable number of T_{reg} cells in ATLOs became Helios$^-$/FoxP3$^+$ iT_{reg} cells consistent with the ability of ATLOs to generate T_{reg} cells from CD4$^+$/FoxP3$^-$ precursors in the periphery (67).

ATLO B-CELL SUBSETS INDICATE ANTIGEN-SPECIFIC HYPERMUTATION, AFFINITY MATURATION, AND ISOTYPE SWITCHING IN ATLO GCs

We explored aorta B-cell immunity in aged ApoE$^{-/-}$ mice (**Figure 4**). Inspection of B-cell-related aorta transcriptomes (see above) revealed large numbers of differentially expressed transcripts in the GO terms *B-cell-mediated immunity*, *B-cell activation*, *positive regulation of B-cell-mediated immunity*, *positive regulation of B-cell activation*, *B-cell proliferation*, and *B-cell differentiation* during aging (68). At the systemic immune system level, aging was associated with large numbers of age-dependent differentially expressed B-cell-related transcripts, but no major changes were observed in B-cell-related transcripts when WT and ApoE$^{-/-}$ SLOs or blood were compared. These data demonstrated that the systemic B-cell transcriptome underwent strong aging/senescence-specific changes but that hyperlipidemia did not affect these changes.

B-cell-related transcripts of whole aortas specifically emerged during the time window of 52–78 weeks correlating with the appearance of ATLOs. *Bona fide* B-cell genes, such as IgM transcripts, were induced by a factor of up to 135. In sharp contrast, young WT or young ApoE$^{-/-}$ aortas did not express B-cell genes as confirmed by immunohistochemistry. Furthermore, we never observed B-cells in atherosclerotic plaques either in the thoracic or abdominal aortas at any age using a variety of marker antibodies. However, as small lymph nodes lining the adventitia contained large numbers of B-cells, the FACS analyses – but not the immunohistochemical analyses – showed few B-cells indicating that the preparations of single cell suspensions from aortas were contaminated by lymph node-derived B-cells (109).

Laser capture microdissection-derived transcriptome atlases were constructed from distinct aorta tissues. Genes associated with B-cell survival, proliferation, differentiation, and activation were expressed in ATLOs including immunoglobulin genes, TACI (*tnfrsf13b*), B-cell activating factor receptor (*tnfrsf13c*), CD40 antigen (*cd40*), complement components (*c1qb*), and *myD88* (68). The degree of territoriality of adventitial B-cell transcripts was high as adventitial tissues adjacent to adventitia segments that were not afflicted with atherosclerotic lesions in the intima and did not or to a much lesser extent expressed these genes. Moreover, the *igj* chain gene involved in somatic hypermutation of the BCR, and B-cell memory cell generation (110) was expressed at a significant level in ATLOs. Expression of B-cell-related genes in the atherosclerotic plaque versus ATLOs showed marked differences: *bona fide* B-cell genes showed strong expression in the adventitia versus low expression in plaques [*ighm*; *cd19*; *ms4a1* (CD20), *igj*, and *cd79a/b*], whereas atherosclerotic plaques expressed inflammation-related B-cell-related genes that are expressed in B-cell target cells including macrophages. As expected from the global comparisons between WT and ApoE$^{-/-}$ RLNs, no differential expression of B-cell-related genes were observed though – as pointed out above – aging/senescence was significant. We determined B-cell subtypes using an improved protocol to prepare single cell suspensions for FACS analyses (109).

HETEROGENEOUS B-CELL SUBTYPES IN ATLOs VERSUS LYMPH NODES AND SPLEEN

B-cell subtype data indicated three distinct major B-cell subtypes: B-2 cells, B-1 cells, and PCs. B-2 B-cell subtypes contained IgM$^+$/IgD$^-$ (immature or transitional B-cells are either immature B-cells that have left the bone marrow or they represent B-1 cells), IgM$^+$/IgD$^+$, and IgM$^-$/IgD$^+$ B-cells (mature B-cell maturation stages). Among mature IgD$^+$ B-cells, IgM$^-$/IgD$^+$ B-cells represent follicular B-2 cells. IgM$^-$/IgD$^-$ cells represent either switched Ig$^+$ B-cells, GC B-cells that have transiently lost Ig expression during somatic hypermutation of their Ig genes or they are GC memory B cells. Of special interest regarding impacts of ATLOs to control B-cell immunity was the identification of GC B-cells, i.e., IgD$^-$/PNA$^+$/GL-7$^+$ B-2 cells, indicating GC reactions (somatic hypermutation and affinity maturation). These data indicated that ATLOs conduct the entire B-cell maturation pathway including antigen-specific B-cell GC reactions. Furthermore, we sought evidence for isotype switching within ATLOs, which follows the GC reaction in SLOs. We observed CD19$^+$/IgD$^-$/IgG1$^+$, CD19$^+$/

IgD⁻/IgA⁺, and CD19⁺/IgD⁻/IgE⁺ B-2 cells in ATLOs. Although class switching is not restricted to GCs, the totality of our morphological, transcript atlas transcriptome, and FACS analyses are consistent with the possibility that class switching follows ATLO GC reactions (68).

PCs FORM A LARGE ATLO B-CELL SUBSET

We had observed earlier that ATLOs contain PCs in the periphery adjacent to T-cell zones (41). PCs constitute a major part of B-cell memory (29, 111, 112): two major PC subtypes had been identified in SLOs, i.e., the short-lived and long-lived PCs (113, 114), whereby short-lived PCs – after their generation – home to SLOs, whereas long-lived PCs largely home to the bone marrow. Both PC subtypes were identified in ATLOs using a BrdU labeling protocol (68). As it is known that PCs use inflammatory tissues as survival niches, our data fall short of demonstrating the generation of short-lived or long-lived PCs within ATLOs. Further work needs to address the important question where the ATLO PCs are generated and whether they provide B-cell memory that is atherosclerosis antigen-specific or whether they merely reflect the influx of atherosclerosis-unrelated PCs into the inflammatory arterial wall adventitia. In attempts to determine the potential functions of the arterial wall PCs, we determined their marker profile: a fraction of them express IL-10 indicating that at least some of them exert immunosuppressive activities. The second major B-cell subtype was B-1 cells. Two major observations deserve attention: (i) The B-1 cell subtypes, unlike their peritoneal cavity counterparts, were skewed toward B-1b cells versus B-1a cells. (ii) As the two B-1 subtypes have different functions to contribute to T-cell-independent B-cell immunity, further studies are needed to determine the functional impact of each of these subtypes to contribute to atherosclerosis immunity. As many of the ATLO B-1 cells express markers of immunosuppressive B regulatory cells (115–121) (TGFβ1, IL-10, PD-L1, and FasL), it is conceivable that the majority of B-1 cells have anti-atherosclerosis impacts on the disease.

EXPLORATION OF TLOs: TRICKS AND DELUSIONS AROUND EVERY CORNER

As potential roles of TLOs in an expanding number of clinically important diseases are being recognized, robust methods for their exploration need to be established. ATLOs are among the best characterized TLOs in any disease: however, they are located in a complex tissue environment (see above) which asks for a combination of analytical techniques to avoid methodological flaws. Analyses of ATLOs – let alone other TLOs – pose considerable challenges: their formation occurs at inconsistent rates and variable sizes; ATLOs' structures and cellular compositions range from small T/B lymphocyte aggregates to large lymphoid clusters containing distinct T-cell areas, B-cell follicles including activated GCs, and PC niches; similar to the dichotomic nature of SLOs, ATLOs generate both effector and immunosuppressive T and B lymphocytes; boundaries between ATLOs and other periaortic or perivascular tissues are difficult to define: they are located close to numerous small paraaortic lymph nodes, periaortic adipose tissue compartments, and ganglia of the sympathetic nervous system (**Figure 1**).

It is important to note: very little is known about these previously overlooked lymphoid aggregates (122). Consequently, major questions arose soon after they had been discovered: how to define a TLO? Should small T/B aggregates qualify as an early stage of a TLO or is the presence of FDCs in GCs essential to qualify a lymphocyte aggregate as TLO? How to distinguish between *bona fide* TLO cells and cells of neighboring tissues if tissue borders of the unencapsulated TLOs are ill-defined? Other challenges relate to determination of the size of TLOs, define the molecular cues of their interaction with the adjacent diseased tissue, determine their specific cellular constituents, quantify and determine the activation status of their immune cell subsets, characterize the properties and gene expression signatures of their connective tissue mesenchymal cells, and most importantly examine their functional impact on disease progression.

Analyses so far applied to ATLOs include laser capture microdissection-based large-scale microarray analyses. This method has been shown valuable to understand the territoriality of atherosclerosis-specific immune cells (41, 46, 67, 68, 88, 89, 109). If combined with immunohistochemical analyses and FACS analyses, it provides guidelines and specific information on many aspects of ATLO immunity. We have applied this technique to identify specific features of atherosclerosis immunity including lymphocyte activation and proliferation and the relation between artery immune responses and those in the draining RLNs. When carefully applied, laser capture microdissection-based mRNA expression analyses have helped to construct transcript atlases of both B-cell and T-cell immunity from which a series of conclusion can be drawn. These include lack of differential transcript expression in WT versus ApoE$^{-/-}$ RLNs, a large inflammation-related transcriptome in ATLOs when compared to the RLN, lack of *bona fide* B-cell genes in plaques, and differences in gene expression in adventitia with atherosclerotic plaque versus adventitia without plaque. Another important technique applied to ATLOs has been FACS analyses together with morphometric assays to quantify distinct lymphocyte subsets and their activation status. However, when we performed comparative analyses of aorta single cell suspensions and immunofluorescent microscopy analyses, we became aware of distinct shortcomings of FACS analyses: since the adventitia or by the same token ATLOs are not visible with the naked eye, there was a tendency to detect immune cell subsets including B-cells in WT adventitia that were undetectable by immunohistochemistry indicating contamination of TLO preparations by neighboring tissues including FALCs.

ARE ATLOs ATHEROSCLEROSIS PROTECTIVE? NOT SO FAST!

In the past, TLOs have often been viewed as *disease-promoting* aggregates of immune cells largely because TLOs were exclusively *disease-associated* and because their size correlated with disease severity (123–126). However, as the immune cell composition of TLOs is being evaluated, concepts regarding their impact on disease have changed: it has been shown that immunosuppressive immune cells including T_{reg} cells, B-1 cells, and innate immune cells are major TLO constituents (**Figures 1–4**).

As mentioned above, we observed that VSMCs that are sandwiched between aorta atherosclerotic plaques and ATLOs express the lymphorganogenic chemokines, i.e., CCL21 and CXCL13. As these chemokines are both indispensable and sufficient to organize lymph nodes and TLOs [see contribution by Watanabe (127); this Research Topic], we hypothesized that VSMCs may adopt features of LTo cells. In cultured aorta VSMCs, we observed that a combination of TNF and agonistic antibodies directed against the lymphotoxin β receptor, but not each cytokine alone, led to a strong induction of CXCL13 mRNA and protein (77). To test the hypothesis that CXCL13 expression in VSMCs affects ATLO homeostasis, we generated $ApoE^{-/-}Ltbr^{fl/fl}$Tagln-cre mice using the late VSMC differentiation marker, i.e., Tagln/SM22α (67, 128). Unlike their $Ltbr^{-/-}$ counterparts, $ApoE^{-/-}Ltbr^{fl/fl}$Tagln-cre mice showed no major alteration of the systemic immune system, indicating that the deletion of the Ltbr was specific for VSMCs. At the level of the arterial wall, however, $ApoE^{-/-}Ltbr^{fl/fl}$Tagln-cre mice showed two distinct phenotypes when compared to their $ApoE^{-/-}$ controls: their ATLO structure was disrupted as evidenced by smaller ATLOs, less HEVs, loose mixed T-/B-cell aggregates rather than separate T- and B-cell areas; and the mice showed marked exacerbation of atherosclerosis. We interpreted these combined results as evidence that the VSMC lymphotoxin β receptor may be involved in atherosclerosis protection *via* ATLOs (67).

There are several caveats, however, regarding the veracity of this conclusion: VSMCs are also constituents of atherosclerotic plaques and the VSMC lymphotoxin β receptor may have affected atherosclerosis directly rather than *via* ATLOs; the mechanisms of an apparent atherosclerosis protection by ATLOs is complex as immunosuppressive leukocyte subsets have been described including T_{reg} cells (67) and a series of $IL\text{-}10^{+}$ B regulatory cells (68). It is therefore possible that the promotion of atherosclerosis in $ApoE^{-/-}Ltbr^{fl/fl}$Tagln-cre mice is due to mechanisms other than *via* ATLO's impact on the disease and that – under different conditions – ATLOs may even promote the disease. What these conditions may be will be a subject of future studies, but it could either include activation of the various effector lymphocyte subsets that have already been described to be major cellular constituents of ATLOs or the generation of autoimmune lymphocytes. Yet, we have shown – as a proof of principal experiment – that interference with the lymphotoxin β receptor in presumptive tissue-specific LTo cells is an experimentally feasible approach and that this interference has an effect on the outcome of the associated disease. Similar approaches could lead to interference with the lymphotoxin β receptor in lymphoid tissue-organizer-like cells in other disease models if the receptor can be targeted specifically as shown for the Tagln/SM22α gene.

CHALLENGES AHEAD

We still do not know much about the specific impacts of any TLO on disease progression. Data from the characterization of the dichotomic nature of TLO immunity suggest that there is not a black or white picture: like SLOs, TLOs generate opposing immune responses that promote generation of antigen-specific lymphocyte subsets. Following this reasoning, it is probably naïve to give or ask for only one answer to this important question. However, we assume that the initial purpose of TLO neogenesis is to eliminate antigen and/or fight inflammation but whether and when the TLO turns into autoimmune responses and/or disease is – at present – difficult or impossible to assess. Analyses of the inflammatory cytokine/chemokine environment of TLOs and its chronicity versus the transient nature of antigen presentation in SLOs may yield additional distinguishing features of TLOs to examine their specific disease impacts.

Other distinguishing features of TLOs relate to the characterization of PC niches, the analysis of innate lymphoid cells, the composition and impact of the macrophage phenotypes in TLOs, and last but not least the T-cell receptor and BCR repertoire of TLOs versus those of SLOs. One approach to identify the specific impact of TLOs in disease may be to delete the lymphotoxin β receptor in presumptive LTo cells as exemplified for ATLOs in atherosclerosis.

Although it seems clear from TLO research during recent years that disease-associated lymphoid clusters are powerhouses of disease immunity, new experimental approaches are needed. These include next-generation sequencing, specific tissue-targeted disruption of the lymphotoxin β receptor or of lymphorganogenic chemokines, improved methods to identify potential antigen-specific lymphocytes, a better understanding and characterization of iT_{reg} cells, isolation of B memory cells and PCs, and cloning of their immunoglobulin genes. It will be of utmost interest to study tolerance mechanisms in TLOs. If TLOs fail to maintain tolerance, autoimmune lymphocytes are likely to be generated in them, which may have major implications for disease immunity. Understanding TLO immunity better may lead the way to exploit the amazing ability of the immune system to target disease mechanisms by developing immunotherapeutics for both chronic autoinflammatory and autoimmune diseases.

CONCLUSION

Artery tertiary lymphoid organs are complex atherosclerosis-associated lymphoid aggregates that generate dichotomically acting immunosuppressive and immune response-promoting immune cells. Their structural organization and cellular composition suggest three major pillars of disease immunity: a large inflammatory component, a considerable antigen-independent element, and a possible antigen-specific domain. ATLO structures promote immune responses by recruitment of naïve lymphocytes, impaired egress, and extended DC/lymphocyte cluster formation. Until today, although many TLOs occur in autoimmune diseases, TLOs have not been demonstrated to generate autoreactive lymphocytes.

AUTHOR CONTRIBUTIONS

All authors contributed to the design, writing, and editing of the submitted manuscript.

FUNDING

This work was funded by the German Research Council: YI 133/2-1 to CY; MO 3054/1-1 to SM; and HA 1083/15-4 to AH; and the German Centre for Cardiovascular Research (MHA VD1.2), SFB 1123/A1 and Z3, the European Research Council (AdG 249929) to CW.

REFERENCES

1. Ait-Oufella H, Sage AP, Mallat Z, Tedgui A. Adaptive (T and B cells) immunity and control by dendritic cells in atherosclerosis. *Circ Res* (2014) 114:1640–60. doi:10.1161/CIRCRESAHA.114.302761
2. Glass CK, Witztum JL. Atherosclerosis. the road ahead. *Cell* (2001) 104:503–16. doi:10.1016/S0092-8674(01)00238-0
3. Hansson GK, Hermansson A. The immune system in atherosclerosis. *Nat Immunol* (2011) 12:204–12. doi:10.1038/ni.2001
4. Libby P. Mechanisms of acute coronary syndromes and their implications for therapy. *N Engl J Med* (2013) 368:2004–13. doi:10.1056/NEJMra1216063
5. Swirski FK, Nahrendorf M. Leukocyte behavior in atherosclerosis, myocardial infarction, and heart failure. *Science* (2013) 339:161–6. doi:10.1126/science.1230719
6. Tabas I, Glass CK. Anti-inflammatory therapy in chronic disease: challenges and opportunities. *Science* (2013) 339:166–72. doi:10.1126/science.1230720
7. Weber C, Noels H. Atherosclerosis: current pathogenesis and therapeutic options. *Nat Med* (2011) 17:1410–22. doi:10.1038/nm.2538
8. Witztum JL, Lichtman AH. The influence of innate and adaptive immune responses on atherosclerosis. In: Abbas AK, Galli SJ, Howley PM, editors. *Annual Review of Pathology: Mechanisms of Disease* (Vol. 9), Palo Alto: Annual Reviews (2014). p. 73–102.
9. Stary HC, Chandler AB, Dinsmore RE, Fuster V, Glagov S, Insull W Jr, et al. A definition of advanced types of atherosclerotic lesions and a histological classification of atherosclerosis. A report from the Committee on Vascular Lesions of the Council on Arteriosclerosis, American Heart Association. *Circulation* (1995) 92:1355–74. doi:10.1161/01.CIR.92.5.1355
10. Binder CJ, Shaw PX, Chang MK, Boullier A, Hartvigsen K, Horkko S, et al. The role of natural antibodies in atherogenesis. *J Lipid Res* (2005) 46:1353–63. doi:10.1194/jlr.R500005-JLR200
11. Daugherty A, Rateri DL. T lymphocytes in atherosclerosis: the Yin-Yang of Th1 and Th2 influence on lesion formation. *Circ Res* (2002) 90:1039–40. doi:10.1161/01.RES.0000021397.28936.F9
12. Gawaz M, Langer H, May AE. Platelets in inflammation and atherogenesis. *J Clin Invest* (2005) 115:3378–84. doi:10.1172/JCI27196
13. Le Borgne M, Caligiuri G, Nicoletti A. Once upon a time: the adaptive immune response in atherosclerosis – a fairy tale no more. *Mol Med* (2015) 21:S13–8. doi:10.2119/molmed.2015.00027
14. Ley K, Miller YI, Hedrick CC. Monocyte and macrophage dynamics during atherogenesis. *Arterioscler Thromb Vasc Biol* (2011) 31:1506–16. doi:10.1161/ATVBAHA.110.221127
15. Libby P, Lichtman AH, Hansson GK. Immune effector mechanisms implicated in atherosclerosis: from mice to humans. *Immunity* (2013) 38:1092–104. doi:10.1016/j.immuni.2013.06.009
16. Lichtman AH, Binder CJ, Tsimikas S, Witztum JL. Adaptive immunity in atherogenesis: new insights and therapeutic approaches. *J Clin Invest* (2013) 123:27–36. doi:10.1172/JCI63108
17. Moore KJ, Sheedy FJ, Fisher EA. Macrophages in atherosclerosis: a dynamic balance. *Nat Rev Immunol* (2013) 13:709–21. doi:10.1038/nri3520
18. Nording HM, Seizer P, Langer HF. Platelets in inflammation and atherogenesis. *Front Immunol* (2015) 6:98. doi:10.3389/fimmu.2015.00098
19. Randolph GJ. Mechanisms that regulate macrophage burden in atherosclerosis. *Circ Res* (2014) 114:1757–71. doi:10.1161/CIRCRESAHA.114.301174
20. Silvestre-Roig C, de Winther MP, Weber C, Daemen MJ, Lutgens E, Soehnlein O. Atherosclerotic plaque destabilization: mechanisms, models, and therapeutic strategies. *Circ Res* (2014) 114:214–26. doi:10.1161/CIRCRESAHA.114.302355
21. Soehnlein O. Multiple roles for neutrophils in atherosclerosis. *Circ Res* (2012) 110:875–88. doi:10.1161/CIRCRESAHA.111.257535
22. Woollard KJ, Geissmann F. Monocytes in atherosclerosis: subsets and functions. *Nat Rev Cardiol* (2010) 7:77–86. doi:10.1038/nrcardio.2009.228
23. Mohanta SK, Yin C, Peng L, Srikakulapu P, Bontha V, Hu D, et al. Artery tertiary lymphoid organs contribute to innate and adaptive immune responses in advanced mouse atherosclerosis. *Circ Res* (2014) 114:1772–87. doi:10.1161/CIRCRESAHA.114.301137
24. Potteaux S, Ait-Oufella H, Mallat Z. Mouse models of atherosclerosis. *Drug Discov Today* (2007) 4(4):165–70. doi:10.1016/j.ddmod.2007.11.005
25. Goodnow CC. Multistep pathogenesis of autoimmune disease. *Cell* (2007) 130:25–35. doi:10.1016/j.cell.2007.06.033
26. Grundtman C, Wick G. The autoimmune concept of atherosclerosis. *Curr Opin Lipidol* (2011) 22:327–34. doi:10 1097/MOL.0b013e32834aa0c2
27. Kuchroo VK, Ohashi PS, Sartor RB, Vinuesa CG. Dysregulation of immune homeostasis in autoimmune diseases. *Nat Med* (2012) 18:42–7. doi:10.1038/nm.2621
28. Lang KS, Recher M, Junt T, Navarini AA, Harris NL, Freigang S, et al. Toll-like receptor engagement converts T-cell autoreactivity into overt autoimmune disease. *Nat Med* (2005) 11:138–45. doi:10.1038/nm1176
29. Hiepe F, Radbruch A. Plasma cells as an innovative target in autoimmune disease with renal manifestations. *Nat Rev Nephrol* (2016) 12:232–40. doi:10.1038/nrneph.2016.20
30. van Kempen TS, Wenink MH, Leijten EF, Radstake TR, Boes M. Perception of self: distinguishing autoimmunity from autoinflammation. *Nat Rev Rheumatol* (2015) 11:483–92. doi:10.1038/nrrheum.2015.60
31. Choi JH, Cheong C, Dandamudi DB, Park CG, Rodriguez A, Mehandru S, et al. Flt3 signaling-dependent dendritic cells protect against atherosclerosis. *Immunity* (2011) 35:819–31. doi:10.1016/j.immuni.2011.09.014
32. Steinman RM. Decisions about dendritic cells: past, present, and future. *Annu Rev Immunol* (2012) 30:1–22. doi:10.1146/annurev-immunol-100311-102839
33. Hu Y, Xu Q. Adventitial biology: differentiation and function. *Arterioscler Thromb Vasc Biol* (2011) 31:1523–9. doi:10.1161/ATVBAHA.110.221176
34. Majesky MW. Adventitia and perivascular cells. *Arterioscler Thromb Vasc Biol* (2015) 35:e31–5. doi:10.1161/ATVBAHA.115.306088
35. Majesky MW, Dong XR, Hoglund V, Mahoney WM Jr, Daum G. The adventitia: a dynamic interface containing resident progenitor cells. *Arterioscler Thromb Vasc Biol* (2011) 31:1530–9. doi:10.1161/ATVBAHA.110.221549
36. Sartore S, Chiavegato A, Faggin E, Franch R, Puato M, Ausoni S, et al. Contribution of adventitial fibroblasts to neointima formation and vascular remodeling: from innocent bystander to active participant. *Circ Res* (2001) 89:1111–21. doi:10.1161/hh2401.100844
37. Stenmark KR, Yeager ME, El Kasmi KC, Nozik-Grayck E, Gerasimovskaya EV, Li M, et al. The adventitia: essential regulator of vascular wall structure and function. *Annu Rev Physiol* (2013) 75:23–47. doi:10.1146/annurev-physiol-030212-183802
38. Campbell KA, Lipinski MJ, Doran AC, Skaflen MD, Fuster V, McNamara CA. Lymphocytes and the adventitial immune response in atherosclerosis. *Circ Res* (2012) 110:889–900. doi:10.1161/CIRCRESAHA.111.263186
39. Galkina E, Kadl A, Sanders J, Varughese D, Sarembock IJ, Ley K. Lymphocyte recruitment into the aortic wall before and during development of atherosclerosis is partially L-selectin dependent. *J Exp Med* (2006) 203:1273–82. doi:10.1084/jem.20052205
40. Gerlis LM. The significance of adventitial infiltrations in coronary atherosclerosis. *Br Heart J* (1956) 18:166–72. doi:10.1136/hrt.18.2.166
41. Grabner R, Lotzer K, Dopping S, Hildner M, Radke D, Beer M, et al. Lymphotoxin beta receptor signaling promotes tertiary lymphoid

organogenesis in the aorta adventitia of aged ApoE-/- mice. *J Exp Med* (2009) 206:233–48. doi:10.1084/jem.20080752
42. Houtkamp MA, de Boer OJ, van der Loos CM, van der Wal AC, Becker AE. Adventitial infiltrates associated with advanced atherosclerotic plaques: structural organization suggests generation of local humoral immune responses. *J Pathol* (2001) 193:263–9. doi:10.1002/1096-9896(2000)9999:9999<::AID-PATH774>3.0.CO;2-N
43. Hu Y, Zhang Z, Torsney E, Afzal AR, Davison F, Metzler B, et al. Abundant progenitor cells in the adventitia contribute to atherosclerosis of vein grafts in ApoE-deficient mice. *J Clin Invest* (2004) 113:1258–65. doi:10.1172/JCI19628
44. Kortelainen M-L, Porvari K. Adventitial macrophage and lymphocyte accumulation accompanying early stages of human coronary atherogenesis. *Cardiovasc Pathol* (2014) 23:193–7. doi:10.1016/j.carpath.2014.03.001
45. Michel JB, Thaunat O, Houard X, Meilhac O, Caligiuri G, Nicoletti A. Topological determinants and consequences of adventitial responses to arterial wall injury. *Arterioscler Thromb Vasc Biol* (2007) 27:1259–68. doi:10.1161/ATVBAHA.106.137851
46. Moos MP, John N, Grabner R, Nossmann S, Gunther B, Vollandt R, et al. The lamina adventitia is the major site of immune cell accumulation in standard chow-fed apolipoprotein E-deficient mice. *Arterioscler Thromb Vasc Biol* (2005) 25:2386–91. doi:10.1161/01.ATV.0000187470.31662.fe
47. Okamoto E-I, Couse T, De Leon H, Vinten-Johansen J, Goodman RB, Scott NA, et al. Perivascular inflammation after balloon angioplasty of porcine coronary arteries. *Circulation* (2001) 104:2228–35. doi:10.1161/hc4301.097195
48. Sakamoto S, Tsuruda T, Hatakeyama K, Imamura T, Asada Y, Kitamura K. Impact of age-dependent adventitia inflammation on structural alteration of abdominal aorta in hyperlipidemic mice. *PLoS One* (2014) 9:e105739. doi:10.1371/journal.pone.0105739
49. Wilcox JN, Scott NA. Potential role of the adventitia in arteritis and atherosclerosis. *Int J Cardiol* (1996) 54:S21–35. doi:10.1016/S0167-5273(96)02811-2
50. Xu F, Liu Y, Hu W. Adventitial fibroblasts from apoE(−/−) mice exhibit the characteristics of transdifferentiation into myofibroblasts. *Cell Biol Int* (2013) 37:160–6. doi:10.1002/cbin.10027
51. Kranich F, Krautler NJ. How follicular dendritic cells shape the B-cell antigenome. *Front Immunol* (2016) 7:225. doi:10.3389/fimmu.2016.00225
52. Passman JN, Dong XR, Wu SP, Maguire CT, Hogan KA, Bautch VL, et al. A sonic hedgehog signaling domain in the arterial adventitia supports resident Sca1+ smooth muscle progenitor cells. *Proc Natl Acad Sci U S A* (2008) 105:9349–54. doi:10.1073/pnas.0711382105
53. Ensan S, Li A, Besla R, Degousee N, Cosme J, Roufaiel M, et al. Self-renewing resident arterial macrophages arise from embryonic CX3CR1(+) precursors and circulating monocytes immediately after birth. *Nat Immunol* (2016) 17:159–68. doi:10.1038/ni.3343
54. Cheema AN, Hong T, Nili N, Segev A, Moffat JG, Lipson KE, et al. Adventitial microvessel formation after coronary stenting and the effects of SU11218, a tyrosine kinase inhibitor. *J Am Coll Cardiol* (2006) 47:1067–75. doi:10.1016/j.jacc.2005.08.076
55. Kwon HM, Sangiorgi G, Ritman EL, Lerman A, McKenna C, Virmani R, et al. Adventitial vasa vasorum in balloon-injured coronary arteries: visualization and quantitation by a microscopic three-dimensional computed tomography technique. *J Am Coll Cardiol* (1998) 32:2072–9. doi:10.1016/S0735-1097(98)00482-3
56. Benezech C, Luu N-T, Walker JA, Kruglov AA, Loo Y, Nakamura K, et al. Inflammation-induced formation of fat-associated lymphoid clusters. *Nat Immunol* (2015) 16:819–28. doi:10.1038/ni.3215
57. Fullerton JN, Gilroy DW. Resolution of inflammation: a new therapeutic frontier. *Nat Rev Drug Discov* (2016) 15(8):551–67. doi:10.1038/nrd.2016.39
58. Medzhitov R. Origin and physiological roles of inflammation. *Nature* (2008) 454:428–35. doi:10.1038/nature07201
59. Nathan C, Ding A. Nonresolving inflammation. *Cell* (2010) 140:871–82. doi:10.1016/j.cell.2010.02.029
60. Luther SA, Ansel KM, Cyster JG. Overlapping roles of CXCL13, interleukin 7 receptor α, and CCR7 ligands in lymph node development. *J Exp Med* (2003) 197:1191–8. doi:10.1084/jem.20021294
61. Luther SA, Bidgol A, Hargreaves DC, Schmidt A, Xu Y, Paniyadi J, et al. Differing activities of homeostatic chemokines CCL19, CCL21, and CXCL12 in lymphocyte and dendritic cell recruitment and lymphoid neogenesis. *J Immunol* (2002) 169:424–33. doi:10.4049/jimmunol.169.1.424
62. van de Pavert SA, Olivier BJ, Goverse G, Vondenhoff MF, Greuter M, Beke P, et al. CXCL13 is essential for lymph node initiation and is induced by retinoic acid and neuronal stimulation. *Nat Immunol* (2009) 10:1193–9. doi:10.1038/ni.1789
63. Mebius RE. Organogenesis of lymphoid tissues. *Nat Rev Immunol* (2003) 3:292–303. doi:10.1038/nri1054
64. Olivier BJ, Cailotto C, van der Vliet J, Knippenberg M, Greuter MJ, Hilbers F, et al. Vagal innervation is required for the formation of tertiary lymphoid tissue in colitis. *Eur J Immunol* (2016) 1–14. doi:10.1002/eji.201646370
65. Bajenoff M, Egen JG, Koo LY, Laugier JP, Brau F, Glaichenhaus N, et al. Stromal cell networks regulate lymphocyte entry, migration, and territoriality in lymph nodes. *Immunity* (2006) 25:989–1001. doi:10.1016/j.immuni.2006.10.011
66. Zhao L, Moos MP, Grabner R, Pedrono F, Fan J, Kaiser B, et al. The 5-lipoxygenase pathway promotes pathogenesis of hyperlipidemia-dependent aortic aneurysm. *Nat Med* (2004) 10:966–73. doi:10.1038/nm1099
67. Hu D, Mohanta, Sarajo K, Yin C, Peng L, Ma Z, et al. Artery tertiary lymphoid organs control aorta immunity and protect against atherosclerosis via vascular smooth muscle cell lymphotoxin β receptors. *Immunity* (2015) 42:1100–15. doi:10.1016/j.immuni.2015.05.015
68. Srikakulapu P, Hu D, Yin C, Mohanta SK, Bontha SV, Peng L, et al. Artery tertiary lymphoid organs control multilayered territorialized atherosclerosis B-cell responses in aged ApoE-/- mice. *Arterioscler Thromb Vasc Biol* (2016) 36:1174–85. doi:10.1161/ATVBAHA.115.306983
69. Geginat J, Sallusto F, Lanzavecchia A. Cytokine-driven proliferation and differentiation of human naive, central memory, and effector memory CD4(+) T cells. *J Exp Med* (2001) 194:1711–9. doi:10.1084/jem.194.12.1711
70. Woodland DL, Kohlmeier JE. Migration, maintenance and recall of memory T cells in peripheral tissues. *Nat Rev Immunol* (2009) 9:153–61. doi:10.1038/nri2496
71. Drayton DL, Liao S, Mounzer RH, Ruddle NH. Lymphoid organ development: from ontogeny to neogenesis. *Nat Immunol* (2006) 7:344–53. doi:10.1038/ni1330
72. Drayton DL, Ying X, Lee J, Lesslauer W, Ruddle NH. Ectopic LT alpha beta directs lymphoid organ neogenesis with concomitant expression of peripheral node addressin and a HEV-restricted sulfotransferase. *J Exp Med* (2003) 197:1153–63. doi:10.1084/jem.20021761
73. Futterer A, Mink K, Luz A, Kosco-Vilbois MH, Pfeffer K. The lymphotoxin beta receptor controls organogenesis and affinity maturation in peripheral lymphoid tissues. *Immunity* (1998) 9:59–70. doi:10.1016/S1074-7613(00)80588-9
74. Kratz A, Campos-Neto A, Hanson MS, Ruddle NH. Chronic inflammation caused by lymphotoxin is lymphoid neogenesis. *J Exp Med* (1996) 183:1461–72. doi:10.1084/jem.183.4.1461
75. Bobik A, Kyaw TS, Tipping P, Toh B-H. M1 macrophages, key contributors to lymphoid neogenesis in atherosclerotic aorta. *Cardiovasc Res* (2014) 101:339–41. doi:10.1093/cvr/cvu019
76. Clement M, Guedj K, Andreata F, Morvan M, Bey L, Khallou-Laschet J, et al. Control of the T follicular helper–germinal center B-cell axis by CD8+ regulatory T cells limits atherosclerosis and tertiary lymphoid organ development. *Circulation* (2015) 131:560–70. doi:10.1161/CIRCULATIONAHA.114.010988
77. Lotzer K, Dopping S, Connert S, Grabner R, Spanbroek R, Lemser B, et al. Mouse aorta smooth muscle cells differentiate into lymphoid tissue organizer-like cells on combined tumor necrosis factor receptor-1/lymphotoxin beta-receptor NF-kappaB signaling. *Arterioscler Thromb Vasc Biol* (2010) 30:395–402. doi:10.1161/ATVBAHA.109.191395
78. Moyron-Quiroz JE, Rangel-Moreno J, Kusser K, Hartson L, Sprague F, Goodrich S, et al. Role of inducible bronchus associated lymphoid tissue

(iBALT) in respiratory immunity. *Nat Med* (2004) 10:927–34. doi:10.1038/nm1091
79. Hwang JY, Randall TD, Silva-Sanchez A. Inducible bronchus-associated lymphoid tissue: taming inflammation in the lung. *Front Immunol* (2016) 7:258. doi:10.3389/fimmu.2016.00258
80. Hons M, Sixt M. The lymph node filter revealed. *Nat Immunol* (2015) 16:338–40. doi:10.1038/ni.3126
81. Nolte MA, Belien JA, Schadee-Eestermans I, Jansen W, Unger WW, van Rooijen N, et al. A conduit system distributes chemokines and small blood-borne molecules through the splenic white pulp. *J Exp Med* (2003) 198:505–12. doi:10.1084/jem.20021801
82. Rantakari P, Auvinen K, Jappinen N, Kapraali M, Valtonen J, Karikoski M, et al. The endothelial protein PLVAP in lymphatics controls the entry of lymphocytes and antigens into lymph nodes. *Nat Immunol* (2015) 16:386–96. doi:10.1038/ni.3101
83. Sixt M, Kanazawa N, Selg M, Samson T, Roos G, Reinhardt DP, et al. The conduit system transports soluble antigens from the afferent lymph to resident dendritic cells in the T cell area of the lymph node. *Immunity* (2005) 22:19–29. doi:10.1016/j.immuni.2004.11.013
84. Roozendaal R, Mebius RE. Stromal cell-immune cell interactions. *Annu Rev Immunol* (2011) 29:23–43. doi:10.1146/annurev-immunol-031210-101357
85. Goronzy JJ, Weyand CM. Aging, autoimmunity and arthritis: T-cell senescence and contraction of T-cell repertoire diversity – catalysts of autoimmunity and chronic inflammation. *Arthritis Res Ther* (2003) 5:225–34. doi:10.1186/ar751
86. Lindstrom TM, Robinson WH. Rheumatoid arthritis: a role for immunosenescence? *J Am Geriatr Soc* (2010) 58:1565–75. doi:10.1111/j.1532-5415.2010.02965.x
87. Linton PJ, Dorshkind K. Age-related changes in lymphocyte development and function. *Nat Immunol* (2004) 5:133–9. doi:10.1038/ni1033
88. Beer M, Doepping S, Hildner M, Weber G, Grabner R, Hu D, et al. Laser-capture microdissection of hyperlipidemic/ApoE-/- mouse aorta atherosclerosis.*MethodsMolBiol*(2011)755:417–28.doi:10.1007/978-1-61779-163-5_35
89. Yin C, Mohanta S, Ma Z, Weber C, Hu D, Weih F, et al. Generation of aorta transcript atlases of wild-type and apolipoprotein E-null mice by laser capture microdissection-based mRNA expression microarrays. *Methods Mol Biol* (2015) 1339:297–308. doi:10.1007/978-1-4939-2929-0_20
90. Gebhardt T, Whitney PG, Zaid A, Mackay LK, Brooks AG, Heath WR, et al. Different patterns of peripheral migration by memory CD4+ and CD8+ T cells. *Nature* (2011) 477:216–9. doi:10.1038/nature10339
91. Lathrop SK, Bloom SM, Rao SM, Nutsch K, Lio CW, Santacruz N, et al. Peripheral education of the immune system by colonic commensal microbiota. *Nature* (2011) 478:250–4. doi:10.1038/nature10434
92. Lathrop SK, Santacruz NA, Pham D, Luo J, Hsieh CS. Antigen-specific peripheral shaping of the natural regulatory T cell population. *J Exp Med* (2008) 205:3105–17. doi:10.1084/jem.20081359
93. Mackay CR. Dual personality of memory T cells. *Nature* (1999) 401:659–60. doi:10.1038/44309
94. Mackay CR, von Andrian UH. Immunology. memory T cells – local heroes in the struggle for immunity. *Science* (2001) 291:2323–4. doi:10.1126/science.1059984
95. Mikhak Z, Strassner JP, Luster AD. Lung dendritic cells imprint T cell lung homing and promote lung immunity through the chemokine receptor CCR4. *J Exp Med* (2013) 210:1855–69. doi:10.1084/jem.20130091
96. Sallusto F, Geginat J, Lanzavecchia A. Central memory and effector memory T cell subsets: function, generation, and maintenance. *Annu Rev Immunol* (2004) 22:745–63. doi:10.1146/annurev.immunol.22.012703.104702
97. Sheridan BS, Lefrancois L. Regional and mucosal memory T cells. *Nat Immunol* (2011) 12:485–91. doi:10.1038/ni.2029
98. Matloubian M, Lo CG, Cinamon G, Lesneski MJ, Xu Y, Brinkmann V, et al. Lymphocyte egress from thymus and peripheral lymphoid organs is dependent on S1P receptor 1. *Nature* (2004) 427:355–60. doi:10.1038/nature02284
99. Schwab SR, Cyster JG. Finding a way out: lymphocyte egress from lymphoid organs. *Nat Immunol* (2007) 8:1295–301. doi:10.1038/ni1545
100. Mempel TR, Scimone ML, Mora JR, von Andrian UH. In vivo imaging of leukocyte trafficking in blood vessels and tissues. *Curr Opin Immunol* (2004) 16:406–17. doi:10.1016/j.coi.2004.05.018
101. Miller MJ, Safrina O, Parker I, Cahalan MD. Imaging the single cell dynamics of CD4+ T cell activation by dendritic cells in lymph nodes. *J Exp Med* (2004) 200:847–56. doi:10.1084/jem.20041236
102. Schneider H, Downey J, Smith A, Zinselmeyer BH, Rush C, Brewer JM, et al. Reversal of the TCR stop signal by CTLA-4. *Science* (2006) 313:1972–5. doi:10.1126/science.1131078
103. Weih F, Grabner R, Hu D, Beer M, Habenicht AJ. Control of dichotomic innate and adaptive immune responses by artery tertiary lymphoid organs in atherosclerosis. *Front Physiol* (2012) 3:226. doi:10.3389/fphys.2012.00226
104. Ait-Oufella H, Salomon BL, Potteaux S, Robertson AK, Gourdy P, Zoll J, et al. Natural regulatory T cells control the development of atherosclerosis in mice. *Nat Med* (2006) 12:178–80. doi:10.1038/nm1343
105. Bilate AM, Lafaille JJ. Induced CD4+Foxp3+ regulatory T cells in immune tolerance. *Annu Rev Immunol* (2012) 30:733–58. doi:10.1146/annurev-immunol-020711-075043
106. Kim JM, Rasmussen JP, Rudensky AY. Regulatory T cells prevent catastrophic autoimmunity throughout the lifespan of mice. *Nat Immunol* (2007) 8:191–7. doi:10.1038/ni1428
107. Curotto de Lafaille MA, Lafaille JJ. Natural and adaptive foxp3+ regulatory T cells: more of the same or a division of labor? *Immunity* (2009) 30:626–35. doi:10.1016/j.immuni.2009.05.002
108. Rosenblum MD, Way SS, Abbas AK. Regulatory T cell memory. *Nat Rev Immunol* (2016) 16:90–101. doi:10.1038/nri.2015.1
109. Hu D, Yin C, Mohanta S, Weber C, Habenicht AJ. Preparation of single cell suspensions from mouse aorta. *Bio Protoc* (2016) 6(11):e1832.
110. Källberg E, Leanderson T. Joining-chain (J-chain) negative mice are B cell memory deficient. *Eur J Immunol* (2006) 36:1398–403. doi:10.1002/eji.200635981
111. Radbruch A, Muehlinghaus G, Luger EO, Inamine A, Smith KG, Dorner T, et al. Competence and competition: the challenge of becoming a long-lived plasma cell. *Nat Rev Immunol* (2006) 6:741–50. doi:10.1038/nri1886
112. Schroder AE, Greiner A, Seyfert C, Berek C. Differentiation of B cells in the nonlymphoid tissue of the synovial membrane of patients with rheumatoid arthritis. *Proc Natl Acad Sci U S A* (1996) 93:221–5. doi:10.1073/pnas.93.1.221
113. Hoyer BF, Moser K, Hauser AE, Peddinghaus A, Voigt C, Eilat D, et al. Short-lived plasmablasts and long-lived plasma cells contribute to chronic humoral autoimmunity in NZB/W mice. *J Exp Med* (2004) 199:1577–84. doi:10.1084/jem.20040168
114. Manz RA, Thiel A, Radbruch A. Lifetime of plasma cells in the bone marrow. *Nature* (1997) 388:133–4. doi:10.1038/40540
115. Chousterman BG, Swirski FK. Innate response activator B cells: origins and functions. *Int Immunol* (2015) 27:537–41. doi:10.1093/intimm/dxv028
116. Lykken JM, Candando KM, Tedder TF. Regulatory B10 cell development and function. *Int Immunol* (2015) 27:471–7. doi:10.1093/intimm/dxv046
117. Mauri C, Menon M. The expanding family of regulatory B cells. *Int Immunol* (2015) 27:479–86. doi:10.1093/intimm/dxv038
118. Miyagaki T, Fujimoto M, Sato S. Regulatory B cells in human inflammatory and autoimmune diseases: from mouse models to clinical research. *Int Immunol* (2015) 27(10):495–504. doi:10.1093/intimm/dxv026
119. Ray A, Basu S, Williams CB, Salzman NH, Dittel BN. A novel IL-10–independent regulatory role for B cells in suppressing autoimmunity by maintenance of regulatory T cells via GITR ligand. *J Immunol* (2012) 188:3188–98. doi:10.4049/jimmunol.1103354
120. Shen P, Fillatreau S. Antibody-independent functions of B cells: a focus on cytokines. *Nat Rev Immunol* (2015) 15:441–51. doi:10.1038/nri3857
121. Tedder TF. B10 cells: a functionally defined regulatory B cell subset. *J Immunol* (2015) 194:1395–401. doi:10.4049/jimmunol.1401329
122. Leslie M. Immunity goes local. *Science* (2016) 352:21–3. doi:10.1126/science.352.6281.21
123. Aloisi F, Pujol-Borrell R. Lymphoid neogenesis in chronic inflammatory diseases. *Nat Rev Immunol* (2006) 6:205–17. doi:10.1038/nri1786
124. Cupedo T, Jansen W, Kraal G, Mebius RE. Induction of secondary and tertiary lymphoid structures in the skin. *Immunity* (2004) 21:655–67. doi:10.1016/j.immuni.2004.09.006
125. Pitzalis C, Jones GW, Bombardieri M, Jones SA. Ectopic lymphoid-like structures in infection, cancer and autoimmunity. *Nat Rev Immunol* (2014) 14:447–62. doi:10.1038/nri3700

126. Weyand CM, Kurtin PJ, Goronzy JJ. Ectopic lymphoid organogenesis: a fast track for autoimmunity. *Am J Pathol* (2001) 159:787–93. doi:10.1016/S0002-9440(10)61751-8
127. Kobayashi Y, Watanabe T. Gel-trapped lymphorganogenic chemokines trigger artificial tertiary lymphoid organs and mount adaptive immune responses in vivo. *Front. Immunol* (2016) 7:316. doi:10.3389/fimmu.2016.00316
128. Owens GK, Kumar MS, Wamhoff BR. Molecular regulation of vascular smooth muscle cell differentiation in development and disease. *Physiol Rev* (2004) 84:767–801. doi:10.1152/physrev.00041.2003

20

Gel-Trapped Lymphorganogenic Chemokines Trigger Artificial Tertiary Lymphoid Organs and Mount Adaptive Immune Responses *In Vivo*

Yuka Kobayashi and Takeshi Watanabe*

The Tazuke-Kofukai Medical Research Institute, Kitano Hospital, Kita-ku, Osaka, Japan

Correspondence:
Takeshi Watanabe
takeshi-watanabe@kitano-hp.or.jp

We previously generated artificial lymph node-like tertiary lymphoid organs (artTLOs) in mice using lymphotoxin α-expressing stromal cells. Here, we show the construction of transplantable and functional artTLOs by applying soluble factors trapped in slow-releasing gels in the absence of lymphoid tissue organizer stromal cells. The resultant artTLOs were easily removable, transplantable, and were capable of attracting memory B and T cells. Importantly, artTLOs induced a powerful antigen-specific secondary immune response, which was particularly pronounced in immune-compromised hosts. Synthesis of functionally stable immune tissues/organs like those described here may be a first step to eventually develop immune system-based therapeutics. Although much needs to be learned from the precise mechanisms of action, they may offer ways in the future to reestablish immune functions to overcome hitherto untreatable diseases, including severe infection, cancer, autoimmune diseases, and various forms of immune deficiencies, including immune-senescence during aging.

Keywords: artificial tertiary lymphoid organs, immune therapeutics, primary immune deficiencies

INTRODUCTION

It is well established that the function of the immune system may be compromised in a variety of diseases resulting in clinically significant immune deficiencies. Secondary immune deficiencies may be caused by overwhelming microbial infections, surgical removal of secondary lymphoid organs (SLOs), or destruction by tumor invasion leaving the host immune system incapable to mount effective immune responses with often lethal clinical outcomes. The function of the immune system is also severely compromised during aging due to immune senescence. Until today, no effective treatment regimens are available for such conditions. In order to restore the exhausted function of lymphoid tissues, a trial has recently been reported using therapeutic formation of TLOs in tumor-bearing hosts by delivering molecules known to be involved in immune system homeostasis, such as lymphotoxin-α1β2 or LIGHT, which stimulate lymphotoxin-β receptors on tissue-resident stromal cells (1–7). Newly synthesized TLOs appear to be effective to suppress tumor growth under distinct experimental conditions (2, 3, 8). Although TLO formation has been thought to be associated with autoimmune disease progression rather than suppression, TLOs may play beneficial roles by enhancing protective immunity in a variety of disease conditions (8, 9).

Structures of both SLOs and TLOs resemble each other in many ways, including segregated T and B cell compartments, the presence of CD11c^{+} dendritic cells (DCs), networks of fibroblastic reticular cells (FRCs) and follicular DCs (FDCs), and the formation of high endothelial venules (HEV)

(10–15). It is well known that TLO neogenesis recapitulates many features of SLO formation involving molecules secreted from lymphoid inducer (LTi) cells, such as lymphotoxin α1β2 and LIGHT (4–7). Rat insulin promoter (RIP)-LTα transgenic mice, which express Lta (lymphotoxin-α) gene driven by the RIP, develop TLOs in pancreatic islets, skin, and kidney (16). Transgenic mice expressing both LTα and LTβ (LTα1β2) under the control of RIP had larger lymphoid tissues with distinct T and B cell areas, well-developed FDC networks, and higher expression of CCL19, CCL21, and CXCL13 chemokines (also referred to as lymphorganogenic chemokines) in the pancreatic islets when compared to transgenic mice expressing only LTα (4).

Overexpression of CCL21 under control of either the thyroglobulin or RIP promoters developed TLOs in the thyroid or in the pancreatic islets, respectively (17, 18). The TLOs also showed PNAd positive HEVs and lymphatic vessels (19–21). Mice expressing CXCL13 under the control of RIP also developed TLOs with distinct B cell follicles and T cell areas in the pancreas (4, 22). Moreover, mice overexpressing CXCL12 in the pancreas showed lymphoid aggregates with accumulation of DCs, B cells, and plasma cells but few T cells (22). Transgenic mice with CCL19 gene expression under control of RIP showed small cell infiltrates composed of lymphocytes and DCs (22). CXCL13 stimulated LTαβ expression in B cells, while CCL19 and CCL21 trigger LTαβ expression in CD4 T cells (22). LTαβ expression was also induced by the stimulation of naive T cells by IL-4 and IL-7 (19).

In tertiary lymphoid organs located in inflammatory tissues in humans, CCL19 and CCL21 are apparently secreted from the smooth muscle actin-positive stromal cells, in close proximity to HEVs (23). Mature DCs and lymph vessels also promote CCL21 expression. The ligand for CXCR4, i.e., CXCL12, contributes to T cell trafficking in lymph nodes and Peyer's patches together with CCR7 ligands, i.e., CCL19 and CCL21 (24). Another important chemokine for lymphocyte trafficking is CXCL13, which is expressed by stromal cells, including FDCs in germinal centers of SLOs. CXCL13 initiates migration of CXCR5-expressing B cells into follicles and thereby contributes to lymphoid organ formation (25). Importantly, CXCL13 also recruits follicular helper T (T-FH) cell into B cell follicles (26, 27). LTα1β2 is not only expressed by B cells but also by LTi cells thereby further promoting generation of an FDC network, including CXCL13 expression in FDCs (28). These cell/cell interactions driven by lymphorganogenic chemokines stimulate recruitment of B cells and establish a positive feedback loop for B cell follicle homeostasis (29). A crosstalk between lymphotoxin-expressing B cells and FRCs plays a role in promoting B cell follicle formation through activation of B cells expressing type 2 inflammatory cytokines (30). FRC networks containing lymph node-like conduits that promote lymph flow also provide tracks for T cell migration, which is promoted by CCR7 ligands, CCL19 and CCL21. FRCs produce various survival factors for lymphocytes besides CCL19 and CCL21, such as IL-6, IL-7, and B cell survival factor BAFF (31), VEGF (32), and retinoic acid (RA) (33, 34). The conduit system is not only en-sheathed by FRCs and connected to the FRC network but FRCs generate conduits (35). Conduits also link to lymph vessels in draining lymph nodes (see contribution by Nancy Ruddle, this Research Topic). CCL21 secreted from FRCs promotes fluid flow in conduits, which enhances the organization of FRC networks (36). Blocking lymph flow in peripheral lymph nodes downregulates CCL21 and CCL19 gene expression in FRCs. All these data together suggest that the increased lymph flow in inflammatory tissues promotes FRC networks resulting in enhancement of immune cell trafficking, sampling of lymph, and enhancing antigen-specific immune responses. CD4 depletion results in FRC loss because of lack of lymphotoxin-β produced by CD4 T cells. Thus, CD4 T cells appear to play a central role in maintaining lymphoid tissue structure and homeostasis through secretion of lymphotoxin-β (37). Thus, mutual interactions between FRC and CD4 T cells may play a role for formation of TLOs. RA may participate in homing of activated T cells through activation of DCs (38). The interaction of signal regulatory protein α (SIRPα), Ig superfamily protein, expressed on the DCs, and T cells with its counterpart CD47, expressed on non-hematopoietic cells such as lymphoid stromal cells, play crucial roles in T cell homeostasis and formation of T cell area in the spleen white pulp (20), suggesting that interaction between SIRPα and its binding partner CD47 may be required for formation of SLOs as well as TLOs. These data indicate mutual interactions between lymphoid tissue organizer (LTo)-like stromal cells and immune cells, such as T cells, B cells, and DCs and these principles known for SLOs may also apply to TLOs. At inflammatory sites, such as aortic smooth muscle cells adjacent to atherosclerotic plaques (37, 39, 40) and local resident fibroblasts (41) give rise to LTo-like stromal cells, which express chemokines, such as CXCL13, CCL19, and CCL21 upon stimulation with lymphotoxin-αβ through lymphotoxin-β receptor (LTβR).

Appearance of TLOs has been reported during allograft rejection (42–45), indicating that TLOs may play a role in induction of an effective immune response upon alloantigen stimulation and serve as a site for local adaptive immune responses. Transplantation of skin grafts prepared from RIP-LTα transgenic mice into allogeneic splenectomized aly/aly mice, which lack SLOs, resulted in the rejection of skin grafts containing TLOs. Mice, which lack both spleen and peripheral lymph nodes, were resistant against viral infection but they mounted a strong immune defense by generating TLOs (9, 43). These reports indicated that antigen-specific activation of host-derived naive T cells as well as the establishment of memory T cells had taken place in the TLO. Thus, TLOs also play a role as an activation site of naive T cells to effector and memory T cells similarly to SLOs. It has been recently reported that TLO in the artery such as aorta could control aorta immunity and protect against atherosclerosis (39, 40). Taken together, TLOs may organize highly localized immune responses against microbial-derived antigens, tumor-derived antigens, and auto- or alloantigens. It, therefore, appears a promising concept to construct artificial lymph node-like tertiary lymphoid organs (artTLOs) for the treatment of various clinically important diseases (46).

Lymph node FRCs ectopically expressed peripheral tissue antigen (PTA) and directly presented it to naive T cells under steady state as well as inflammatory conditions (47). Moreover, lymph node-resident lymphatic endothelial cells directly present PTA to T cells and mediate peripheral tolerance independently of autoimmune regulator (Aire) (48). These findings suggest that lymph node stromal cells (LTo) appear to be involved in not only the TLO formation but also the maintenance of tolerance to self-antigens in the periphery at adult stage. As discussed above, artery TLO, which emerge in the aorta adventitia adjacent to atherosclerotic plaques, regulate immunity in aorta, and protect against atherosclerosis through LTβR expressed on vascular smooth muscle cells (40). These diverse function displayed by stromal cells suggests that the artTLO may acquire the immunological function when the stromal cells adopt or differentiate into LTo cells. These diverse functions may include not only promotion of antigen-specific protective immune response to treat autoimmune diseases. Therefore, our principal tenet has been to create artTLOs with various and even opposite functions to foster maintenance of immune homeostasis depending on the disease conditions.

We had previously reported synthesis of artTLOs with the ability to induce immune responsiveness *in vivo* by applying lymphoid stromal cells and bone marrow-derived DCs (49–52). The stromal cell line TEL-2 (53), which had been established from neonatal mouse thymus, was transfected with LTα cDNA. The LTα-expressing stromal cells or TEL-2 cells stimulated with LTα-coated beads expressed VCAM-1 and ICAM-1, and secreted lymphorganogenic chemokines, including CCL19, CCL21, and CXCL13. LTα-expressing stromal cells were then mixed with bone marrow-derived DCs (49, 50). The cell suspension was first incorporated into collagen sponges, which were subsequently transplanted into the renal subcapsular space of mice. After 2–3 weeks, lymphocyte-rich cell-aggregates had emerged in the collagen sponges. The resulting structures consisted of clearly segregated clusters of T and B cells, FDCs in B cell follicles, and FRC networks in T cell areas. HEVs, lymph vessels, and germinal center formation upon antigen stimulation were also evident (49). Thus, the grafts were termed as artificial lymph node tissues (aLN) but are more appropriately called *artTLOs*. When the artTLOs were generated in mice that had been preimmunized with antigen, they were capable of inducing a strong secondary immune response *in vivo* upon antigen re-stimulation, as evidenced by the accumulation of effector memory and T-FH cells, as well as antigen-specific memory B cells (50). In addition, the artTLOs were capable of inducing a strong secondary immune response when re-transplanted into naive mice upon immunization with the antigen. Also, re-transplantation of the artTLOs into SCID mice, followed by immunization, let to a robust secondary immune response. The artTLOs as well as spleen cells in SCID mice produced large amounts of antigen-specific high affinity IgG class antibodies consistent with the possibility that somatic hypermutation, germinal center reaction, affinity maturation, and Ig class switching were conducted in the artTLOs (50). Furthermore, the artTLOs appeared to suppress tumor growth when they were transplanted into tumor-bearing mice (51, 52). This was the first proof of principle that artificial lymphoid tissues are transplantable and immunologically active.

Taken together, these previous data led us to develop new strategies to artificially synthesize transplantable and immunologically functional lymphoid tissues/organs in the absence of stromal cells, i.e., LTo cells. We hypothesized that *in vivo* transplantation of a combination of lymphorganogenic chemokines and cytokines as a substitute for LTo cells would be feasible. Here, we report that functionally highly active artTLOs can indeed be generated by applying slow-releasing gels containing lymphotoxin-α1β2 and additional chemokines on a collagen matrix.

RESULTS

Preparation of Gels and Formation of artTLOs

Although application of stromal cell lines is an effective strategy for the construction of artificial lymphoid tissues (47, 48), the approach has major limitations in clinical practice. Consequently, we sought to establish a cell-free method. For this purpose, we transplanted collagen sponge scaffolds containing the slow-releasing Medgel beads in which lymphotoxin-α1β2, CCL19, CCL21, CXCL12, CXCL13, and soluble RANK ligand (sRANKL) were trapped (experimental strategy is outlined in Section "Materials and Methods" and legend for **Figure 1A**). Gel-beads gradually release each protein over extended period of time and are concomitantly resolved by the endogenous collagenase. The collagen sponge containing randomly arranged gel-beads was transplanted into the renal subcapsular space of mice. After 3 weeks, grafts were removed and the resulting cell aggregates were examined by immunofluorescence microscopy. Medgel alone without any chemokine did not give rise to any tissue graft. Although Medgels containing lymphotoxin-α1β2 or any of each recombinant CCL19, CCl21, CXCL12, or CXCL13 chemokine formed more or less of a tertiary lymphoid tissue-like cell mass, referred to as artTLO, as suggested by the previous reports mentioned in the Section "Introduction," mixtures of gels containing lymphotoxin-α1β2 and four different types of chemokines, CCL19, CCL21, CXCL12, and CXCL13, together with sRANKL gave constantly the most advanced lymphoid structures. They consist of segregated B cell and T cell areas (**Figure 1B**), DCs in T cell areas (**Figure 1C**), FDC and FRC networks (**Figure 1D**), and appearance of HEVs-like structure (**Figure 1B**, right side). Besides, angiogenesis was prominent in the lymphoid tissues and lymph capillary vessels appeared in the periphery (**Figure 1B**, middle).

Memory B and T Cells Are Major Cellular Constituents in artTLO

artTLOs were formed in renal subcapsuler space of Balb/c mice that had been preimmunized with NP hapten-coupled chicken egg albumin (NP-OVA) in alum more than 1 month before artTLO formation was initiated. ArtTLOs and spleens of recipient Balb/c mice were then excised. The artTLOs and spleens were minced and single-cell suspension was prepared from each artTLO or spleen, followed by fluorescence flow cytometer analysis (**Figure 2**). A large number of anti-NP antibody-secreting cells were detected in artTLO but few in the recipient spleen (the second column from left). Furthermore, $B220^+CD38^+IgG^+$ memory B cells (third column from left) and $CD3^+CD4^+CD44^+$ $CD62L^-$ effector memory T cells (fourth column from left) were

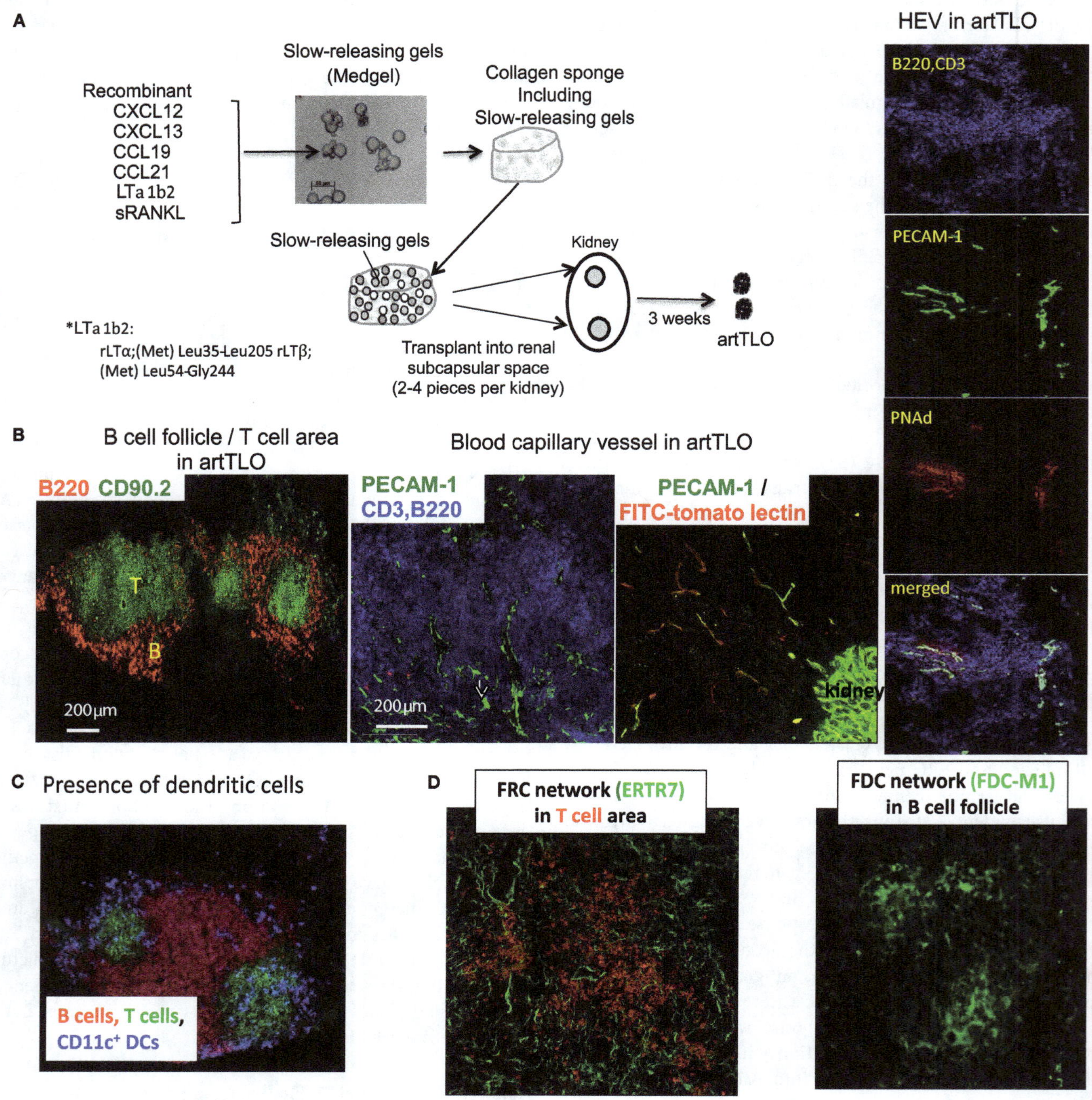

FIGURE 1 | **Strategy to construct functional artTLOs. (A)** The slow-releasing gel-beads (Medgel) containing each recombinant chemokine and cytokine protein indicated in the Figure were prepared. Briefly, solution (100 μg/ml) of each soluble recombinant protein (CXCL12, CXCL13, CCL19, CCL21, LTα1β2, and sRANKL) was added to the dry powder of the Medgel in 1.5 ml micro tube, respectively, and was incubated for 2 h at 37°C. Then, Medgels containing each chemokine and LTα1β2 were combined and mixed. The combined gels were incorporated into the collagen sponges as described in the Section "Materials and Methods." The collagen sponges were then transplanted into the renal subcapsular space of NP-OVA preimmunized Balb/c mouse. After 3 weeks, artTLO had formed. **(B)** Lymphoid cell assembly consisted of segregation of T cell area and B cell follicles. Functional capillaries and lymph vessels were detected. Functional arteries and high endothelial venules (HEV) were well developed. **(C)** Distribution of dendritic cells in T cell area. **(D)** FDC network in B cell follicle and FRC network in T cell area.

highly enriched in artTLOs when compared to recipient spleens. IgG class anti-NP antibody-forming cells (AFCs) were also enriched (second column). These results indicated that artTLOs possess a remarkable property to efficiently accumulate memory T and memory B cells as well as antigen-specific AFCs that had been recruited from the recipient Balb/c mouse lymphoid tissues during lymphocyte cell trafficking between recipient mouse and artTLO tissue through blood vessel. The artTLOs, which were

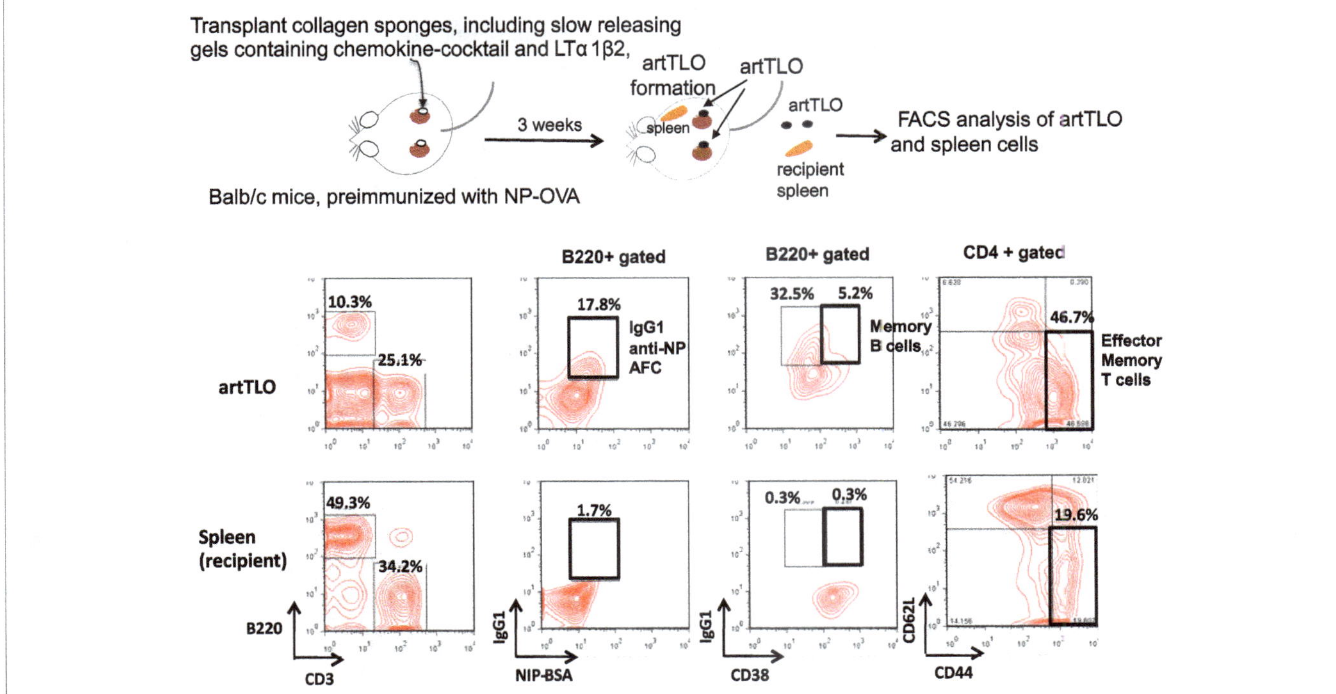

FIGURE 2 | Accumulation of antigen-specific memory B cells and CD4 positive T cells in artTLOs. artTLOs were constructed in Balb/c mice, which had been preimmunized with 100 μg NP-hapten conjugated ovalbumin (NP-OVA) in alum as described in the Section "Materials and Methods." After 3 weeks, artTLO were formed in the subcapsular space of kidney. artTLO and spleen were removed from recipients for flow cytometer analysis. Flow cytometer profiles of artTLO and spleen cells of recipient mice are shown. Note that IgG1 class anti-NP antibody-forming cells as well as memory B cells and effector memory T cells are remarkably enriched in artTLOs, compared to the recipient spleen cells. Representative data are shown from FACS analysis of 10 individual artTLO. Data were highly reproducible.

constructed in antigen-primed recipients by applying the gel-trapped chemokines, work as an efficient reservoir for memory T and B cells and also for antigen-specific AFCs.

artTLOs Function as Highly Active Immune Tissues Following Transplantation into Immuno-Compromised Recipients

artTLOs, which had been formed in antigen (NP-OVA)-preimmunized mice and then excised, were re-transplanted into renal subcapsular spaces of immune-deficient SCID mice having no mature T and B lymphocyte (**Figure 3**). Two weeks after transplantation, half of the SCID mice carrying artTLO were intravenously immunized with the same antigen. The other half of the SCID mice carrying artTLO remained un-immunized. One week later, artTLOs and spleen of recipient SCID mice were removed. Cell suspension was prepared from each individual artTLO and spleen. IgG1 class anti-NP-specific AFCs in artTLOs as well as recipient SCID spleens were counted as shown in **Figure 3**. Total (NP30) and high affinity (NP3) of NP-specific AFCs were measured. Low but significant numbers of anti-NP AFCs were detected in re-transplanted artTLO in non-immunized SCID mice. They were remnant of the AFCs that had been migrated from the first NP-OVA preimmunized Babl/c mouse. On the other hand, numbers of antigen (NP)-specific high affinity as well as total IgG class antibody-producing cells were remarkably increased in re-transplanted artTLOs upon immunization (**Figure 3**, left side), indicating that secondary immune response was efficiently induced by memory B and T cells that had been accumulated in the re-transplanted artTLO as shown in **Figure 2**. Anti-NP AFCs were hardly detected in spleen of artTLO-re-transplanted SCID mice without immunization of SCID mice with NP-OVA (**Figure 3**, right side), indicating that no migration of AFCs occurred in the artTLO-carrying SCID mice even though the presence of empty space in SCID mouse spleen for lymphoid cells and even though that lymphocyte could freely communicate between artTLO and SCID mouse immune tissues through blood vessels. Surprisingly, extraordinarily large numbers of anti-NP AFCs appeared in spleens of the artTLO-carrying SCID mice as shown in **Figure 3** (right side), suggesting that NP-specific memory B cells and T cells are migrating from artTLO into empty SCID spleen and they quickly maturate and explosively expand into NP-specific AFCs in the empty space in SCID mouse spleen upon antigen stimulation. Thus, artTLOs constructed by the present gel-trapped lymphoorganogenic chemokines are effective immune tissues, especially in immune-compromised hosts, in which the artTLO could induce a strong specific immune response upon antigen stimulation.

DISCUSSION

The major conclusion of the data detailed above is that immunologically highly active and transplantable artTLOs can be generated in the absence of LTo cells in mice by providing suitable

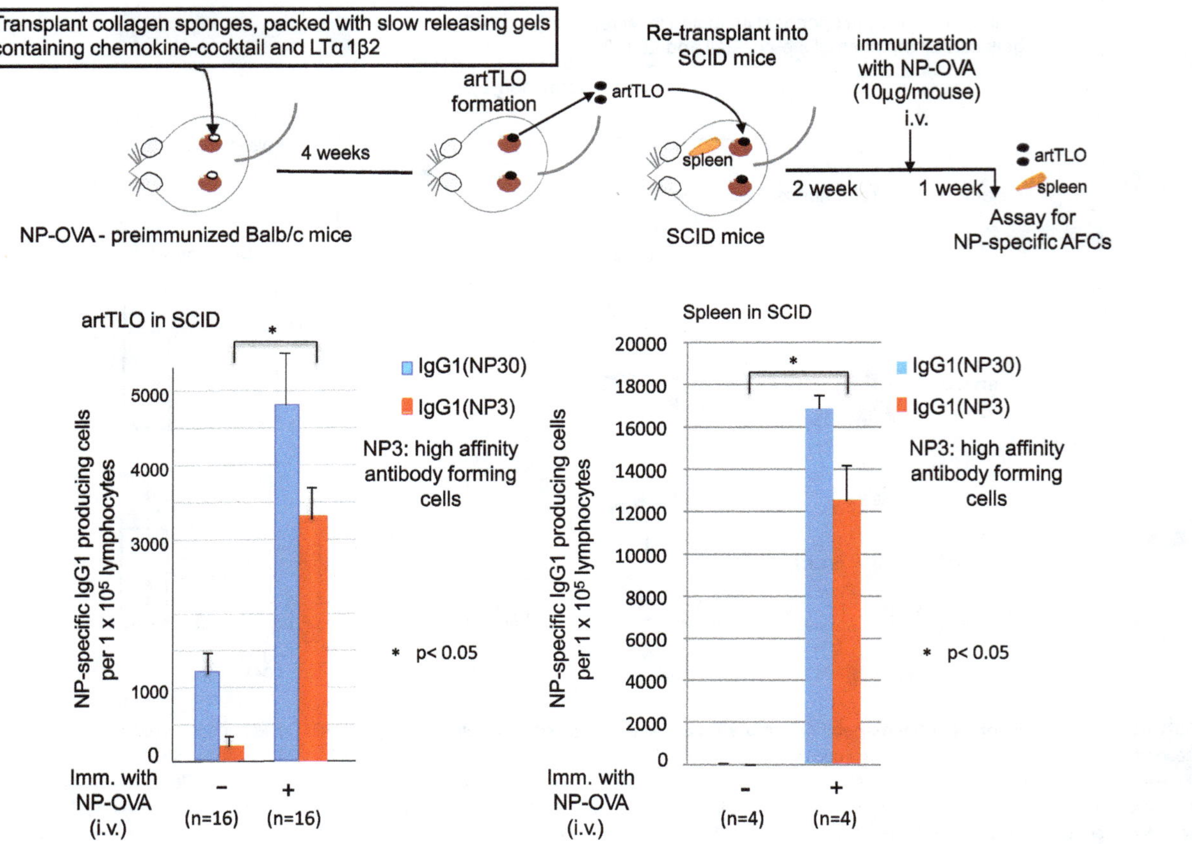

FIGURE 3 | Enrichment of antigen-specific high-affinity antibody-producing cells in artTLO upon transplantation into immunodeficient SCID mice. ArtTLO were first formed in eight NP-OVA preimmunized Balb/c mice as described in **Figure 2**. Four artTLO (two artTLO in each kidney) in one mouse were constructed. Then, artTLO were individually extirpated and collected from Balb/c mice and re-transplanted into renal subcapsular space of eight SCID mice. Four artTLO were re-transplanted into each SCID mouse. Two weeks after re-transplantation, four of artTLO-carrying SCID mice were intravenously immunized with 10 μg NP-OVA. The other four SCID mice were not immunized. One week after, artTLO and recipient spleen were extirpated individually from SCID mice and single cell suspensions were prepared. Numbers of high affinity as well as total IgG class anti-NP antibody-forming cells (AFCs) in individual artTLO and in spleens of recipient SCID mice were counted by an immunospot analyzer. Numbers of AFCs were calculated from 16 individual artTLO for each group.

factors that are usually secreted from LTo upon stimulation by lymphoid tissue inducer cells (LTi). We successfully constructed immunologically functional artTLO by applying slow-releasing gels containing combination of four chemokines (CXCL12, CXCL13, CCL19, and CCL21) and sRANKL together with lymphotoxin α1β2 protein. We propose that the strategy applied here may lead the way to the generation of artTLOs not only in mouse but also in human to ameliorate untreatable diseases as varied as severe infection (sepsis), primary and secondary immune deficiency syndromes, autoimmunity, and a large number of clinically important chronic inflammatory diseases, including atherosclerosis, rheumatoid arthritis, and inflammatory bowel and brain diseases (37, 39, 40, 54–62). It is well known that T cell immune responses are actively induced in tumors (63). However, tumors have evolved to acquire immunosuppressive mechanisms or they apply other immune evasion mechanisms. Recent advances in checkpoint therapy for cancers will be an effective strategy to overcome some of these hurdles (64, 65). The artTLO may provide the machinery to assist checkpoint therapy for cancers. Also, atrophy of primary and SLOs, which occur during aging associated with immuno-senescence (66, 67), gives rise to fatal infectious diseases in the elderly. The artTLO may play a role in reinforcement of immune function in the elderly. Moreover, artTLOs should be examined for their ability to counteract the compromised immune system in patients who receive radiation therapy or chemotherapy. We further envisage application of artTLO in patients that undergo hematopoitic stem cell transplantation during conditioning regimens, including non-myeloablative conditioning to overcome a window in time of severely compromised immune function, since the immune cells in the artTLO rapidly may expand and maturate in the patients much as they would in a SCID mouse as shown in **Figure 3**.

Since artTLOs in the present study are formed on the scaffold of a collagen sponge, it is easily removable and transplantable. As the characteristics of biomaterials are important in tissue engineering strategies, a collagen sponge was applied. In order to efficiently generate artTLOs, the scaffold should be carefully prepared to mimic the natural environment of TLO neo-genesis.

Scaffolds for the synthesis of immune tissues are required to allow the LTo cells and respective immune cell populations to organize themselves to create microenvironments that allow artTLO neo-genesis. Such scaffolds should also maintain the three-dimensional structure that allows immune cells to move effectively for both optimal recruitment and egression (through the newly formed HEVs, blood vessels, and lymphatics), and maintain a reservoir of soluble factors, such as chemokines and cytokines expressed by stromal cells. A number of synthetic biomaterials have been developed, which are all able to duplicate the three-dimensional microenvironments that are provided by natural extracellular matrices, such as fibril or non-fibril collagen, proteoglycans, matrix cellular proteins (68), and their hydrogels (69). It has been demonstrated that structurally engineered macro-porous scaffolds, which combine polyethylene glycol hydrogels with collagen, support T cell, and DC migration (70). The first *in vivo* synthesis of artificial lymphoid tissues was achieved by using a porous biocompatible collagen matrix, prepared from the bovine Achilles tendon (referred to as a collagen sponge) (49). It has a non-homogeneous pore size ranging from 50 to 300 μm. A key in lymphoid tissue engineering is to properly modulate and mimic dynamics of lymphocyte trafficking. In addition, it is important to recruit the appropriate immune cells to the lymphoid tissues. Finally, the gradients of the soluble factors secreted from stromal cells need to be adjusted. Biomaterials that release soluble factors simultaneously not only uniformly but also gradually with temporal differences have been described (71). In the present study, Medgels, which consist of collagen gels, were applied. Medgels maintain and slowly release soluble protein molecules. The 3D scaffold in which cell-specific chemokines/cytokines are geometrically positioned and fixed based on the histological patterns are expected to be advantageous for the formation of more sophisticated and functional artTLOs. In order to do so, a manufacturing approach using 3D bioprinters should be attempted.

There has been much progress in the establishment and analysis of humanized mice (72–77). As a result, humanized mice will be utilized as human disease models. They can be experimentally manipulated and used to directly study infectious diseases, immunological disorders, and cancers (78–80). These model systems could be suitable candidates for generating human artTLOs in future by applying the present slow-releasing gels containing chemokine cocktail and lymphotoxin-α1β2.

CONCLUSION

Tertiary lymphoid organs are unique lymphoid tissues in which interaction of antigen-presenting cells with effector T- and B-lymphocytes is organized and followed by induction of protective adaptive as well as innate immune responses. The synthesis of artificially constructed TLO tissues (artTLOs) that function as the effective substitutes for SLOs may be a promising novel strategy to treat both local and systemic infections, autoimmune diseases, and cancer. Development of functionally active human artTLOs or similar devices is expected in the near future. In this report, we have attempted to construct artificially made functional TLOs by applying gel-trapped lymphorganogenic soluble factors, instead of using lymphoid tissue stromal cells. They showed a remarkable immune function especially as a reservoir of antigen-specific memory B and T cells.

MATERIALS AND METHODS

Antibodies and Reagents

Fluorescein-, phycoerythrin-, or biotin- labeled anti-B220 (clone:RA3-6B2), anti-CD3 (Clone:145-2c11), anti-Thy1.2 (clone: 30-H12), anti-CD11c (clone:N418), anti-CD21/35 (clone:7G6), anti-FDC-M1 (clone:FDC-M2) were obtained from BD Pharmingen. Anti-ER-TR7 was from Abcam plc., anti-PCAM-1 (clone:390), and anti-PNAd (clone:MECA-79) were from Biolegend. Anti-IgG1 and goat anti-hamster IgG and fluorescein- or phycoerythrin-labeled streptavidin were all purchased from BD Bioscience. NP-OVA and NIP-BSA were purchased from Bioresearch Technology. Lymphotoxin α1β2 was purchased from R&D System. CXCL13 (cat no.:300-47), CCL19 (cat. No:300-29B), CCL21 (cat. No:300-35), CXCL12 (cat no:300-28A), and sRANKL (cat. No:310-01) were purchased from Peprotech. Medgel was obtained from MeDGEL Co., LTD (Japan).

Mice

Balb/cAnNcrj mice and SCID mice (C.B.-17/IcrCrj-scid/scid) were purchased from Japan SLC, Inc. All mice were housed under specific pathogen-free condition in the animal facility of Medical Research Institute, Kitano Hospital. All experiments described herein were approved by the Kitano Hospital animal use committee and were performed in accordance with the applicable guidelines and regulation.

Immunization

For pre-immunization, 100 μg NP15-OVA precipitated in alum was injected i.p. into 7- to 10-week-old Balb/c mice. Four or more weeks after immunization, mice were used as donors for the generation of artTLO.

Synthesis of artTLOs

Since Medgel releases the protein (chemokines, lymphotoxin) very slowly *in vivo* and it is difficult to determine the optimal dose of each protein for *in vivo* formation of lymphoid tissues, large excess amounts of chemokine or lymphotoxin were added to Medgel. Twenty-microliter solution of each kind of soluble factor (CXCL12, CXCL13, CCL19, CCL21, LTα1β2, and sRANKL; 100 μg/ml each) was added to dry powder of Medgel (400 μg) in 1.5 ml microtubes followed by an incubation for 2 h at 37°C. Then, all soluble factor-containing Medgels were once mixed in a microtube. About 50 μg of the mixtures of Medgels was absorbed into a collagen sponge piece (2 × mm × 2 × mm square, CS-35; KOKEN). Approximately 30–40 Medgel-adsorbed collagen sponges were prepared at once and transplanted into renal subcapsular space of 8–10 adult (7- to 10-week-old) Balb/c mice (4 pieces in one mouse). The artTLOs were constantly formed 3 weeks after transplantation.

Immunohistochemical Staining

artTLOs and lymphoid tissues from recipient mice were embedded in Tissue-Tek OCT compound (SAKURA FINETEK), and snap frozen in liquid nitrogen. Five-micrometer-thick cryostat sections were prepared and placed on APS-coated glass slides (Matsunami Glass Ind. Ltd.). Sections were fixed with cold acetone for 5 min, dried, and kept at −80°C until use. After blocking with 5% normal rat serum and 1% BSA in TBS-T (Tris-buffered saline with 0.005% Tween20) for 1 h at 20°C, sections were incubated for 1 h at 20°C with appropriate antibodies or streptavidin-fluorochrome reagents diluted in blocking buffer and washed with PBS three times every 5 min.

ELISPOT for Measurement of NP-Specific IgG1 and IgM Antibody-Forming Cells

The frequency of high- and low-affinity NP-specific AFCs among cells collected from artTLOs or spleen cells from donor mice was measured by ELISPOT using NP3-BSA- and NP30-BSA-coated filter paper for low-affinity AFC, respectively, as shown previously (50). Hydrophobic PVDF filters on MultiScreenIP Filter Plates (MAIPS4510, Millipore) were coated with 50 µg/ml NP3-BSA, NP30-BSA, or BSA in PBS at 4°C overnight, and then blocked with 1% BSA in PBS. Cells (0.2–1 $\times$ 10^5 cells/well) were incubated for 2 h at 37°C and washed once with PBS containing 50 mM EDTA, twice with TBS-T, and once with PBS. After washing, filters were visualized with BCIP/NBT (Chemical International) and AEC (BD Biosciences-Pharmingen). Numbers of AFCs were counted by ImmunoSpot Analyzer (C.T.L.).

Statistics

All the statistical analysis were performed by using an unpaired two-tailed Student's test. A *P*-value of less than 0.05 was considered significant.

STUDIES INVOLVING ANIMAL RESEARCH

Animal research in this review were approved by the ethics committee of The Tazuke-Kofukai Medical Research Institute and Kitano Hospital, Osaka, Japan, and carried out in accordance with the recommendation of animal research guidelines issued from the ethics committee.

AUTHOR CONTRIBUTIONS

YK performed all experiments. TW planned experiments and wrote the manuscript.

ACKNOWLEDGMENTS

This work was supported by a Grant-in-Aid for Scientific Research on Priority Areas from MEXT, Japan (Grant No. 24111009). We especially thank Peter Burrows for helpful discussions and assistance with translation of the manuscript.

FUNDING

Grant-in-Aid for Scientific Research on Priority Areas from MEXT, Japan (Grant No. 24111009).

REFERENCES

1. Dieu-Nosjean MC, Goc J, Giraldo NA, Friedman CS, Friedman WH. Tertiary lymphoid structures in cancer and beyond. *Trends Immunol* (2014) 35:571–80. doi:10.1016/j.it.2014.09.006
2. Chen L, Fabian KL, Taylor JL, Storkus WL. Therapeutic use of dendritic cells to promote the extranodal priming of anti-tumor immunity. *Front Immunol* (2013) 4:388. doi:10.3389/fimm.2013.00388
3. Tang H, Wang Y, Chlewicki LK, Zhang Y, Guo J, Liang W, et al. Facilitating T cell infiltration in tumor microenvironement overcomes resistance to PD-L1 blockade. *Cancer Cell* (2016) 29:285–96. doi:10.1016/j.ccell.2016.02.004
4. Drayton DL, Ying X, Lee J, Lesslauer W, Ruddle NH. Ectopic LT alpha beta directs lymphoid organ neogenesis with concomitant expression of peripheral node addressin and a HEV-restricted sulfotransferase. *J Exp Med* (2003) 197(9):1153–63. doi:10.1084/jem.20021761
5. Wang J, Foster A, Chin R, Yu P, Sun Y, Wang Y, et al. The complementation of lymphotoxin deficiency with LIGHT, a newly discovered TNF family member, for the restoration of secondary lymphoid structure and function. *Eur J Immunol* (2002) 32:1969–79. doi:10.1002/1521-4141(200207)32:7<1969::AID-IMMU1969>3.0.CO;2-M
6. Gommerman JL, Browning JL. Lymphotoxin/LIGHT, lymphoid microenvironments and disease. *Nat Rev Immunol* (2003) 3:642–55. doi:10.1038/nri1151
7. Scheu S, Alferink J, Potzel T, Barchet W, Kalinke U, Pfeffer K. Targeted disruption of LIGHT causes defects in costimulatory T cell activation and reveals cooperation with lymphotoxinbeta in mesenteric lymph node genesis. *J Exp Med* (2002) 195:1613–24. doi:10.1084/jem.20020215
8. Leslie M. Features: immunity goes local. *Science* (2016) 352:21–3. doi:10.1126/science.352.6281.21
9. Carragher DM, Rangel-Moreno J, Randall TD. Ectopic lymphoid tissues and local immunity. *Semin Immunol* (2008) 20:26–42. doi:10.1016/j.smin.2007.12.004
10. Roozendaal R, Mebius RE. Stromal cell-immune cell interactions. *Annu Rev Immunol* (2011) 29:23–43. doi:10.1146/annurev-immunol-031210-101357
11. Drayton DL, Liao S, Mounzer RH, Ruddle NH. Lymphoid organ development: from ontogeny to neogenesis. *Nat Immunol* (2006) 7(4):344–53. doi:10.1038/ni1330
12. Thaunat O, Field AC, Dai J, Louedec L, Patey N, Bloch MF, et al. Lymphoid neogenesis in chronic rejection: evidence for a local humoral alloimmune response. *Proc Natl Acad Sci U S A* (2005) 102(41):14723–8. doi:10.1073/pnas.0507223102
13. Krautler NJ, Kana V, Kranich J, Tian Y, Perera D, Lemm D, et al. Follicular dendritic cells emerge from ubiquitous perivascular precursors. *Cell* (2012) 150(1):194–206. doi:10.1016/j.cell.2012.05.032
14. Fletcher AL, Malhotra D, Acton SE, Lukacs-Kornek V, Bellemare-Pelletier A, Curry M, et al. Reproducible isolation of lymph node stromal cells reveals site-dependent differences in fibroblastic reticular cells. *Front Immunol* (2011) 2:35. doi:10.3389/fimmu.2011.00035
15. Chai Q, Onder L, Scandella E, Gil-Cruz C, Perez-Shibayama C, Cupovic J, et al. Maturation of lymph node fibroblastic reticular cells from myofibroblastic precursors is critical for antiviral immunity. *Immunity* (2013) 38(5):1013–24. doi:10.1016/j.immuni.2013.03.012
16. Kraz A, Campos-Neto A, Hanson MS, Ruddle NH. Chronic inflammation caused by lymphotoxin is lymphoid neogenesis. *J Exp Med* (1996) 183:1461–72. doi:10.1084/jem.183.4.1461
17. Martin AP, Coronal EC, Sano G, Chen SC, Vassiliva G, Canasto-Chibuque C, et al. A novel model for lymphocytic infiltration of the thyroid gland generated by transgenic expression of the CC Chemokine CCL21. *J Immunol* (2004) 173:4791–8. doi:10.4049/jimmunol.173.8.4791
18. Furtado GC, Marinkovic T, Martin AP, Garin A, Hoch B, Hubner W, et al. Lymphotoxin beta receptor signaling is required for inflammatory lymphangiogenesis in the thyroid. *Proc Natl Acad Sci USA* (2007) 104:5026–31. doi:10.1073/pnas.0606697104

19. Zeng M, Paiardini M, Engram JC, Beilman GJ, Chipman JG, Schacker TW, et al. Critical role of CD4 T cells in maintaining lymphoid tissue structure for immune cell homeostasis and reconstitution. *Blood* (2012) 120(9):1856–67. doi:10.1182/blood-2012-03-418624
20. Sato-Hashimoto M, Saito Y, Ohnishi H, Iwamura H, Kanazawa Y, Kaneko T, et al. Signal regulator protein alpha regulates the homeostasis of T lymphocytes in the spleen. *J Immunol* (2011) 187:291–7. doi:10.4049/jimmunol.1100528
21. Pikor NB, Astarita JL, Summers-Deluca L, Galicia G, Qu J, Ward LA, et al. Integration of Th17- and lymphotoxin-derived signals initiates meningeal-resident stromal cell remodeling to propagate neuroinflammation. *Immunity* (2015) 43(6):1160–73. doi:10.1016/j.immuni.2015.11.010
22. Luther SA, Bidgol A, Hargreaves DC, Schmidt A, Xu Y, Paniyadi J, et al. Differing activities of homeostatic chemokines CCL19, CCL21, and CXCL12 in lymphocyte and dendritic cell recruitment and lymphoid neogenesis. *J Immunol* (2002) 169(1):424–33. doi:10.4049/jimmunol.169.1.424
23. Manzo A, Bugatti S, Caporali R, Prevo R, Jackson DG, Uguccioni M, et al. CCL21 expression pattern of human secondary lymphoid organ stroma is conserved in inflammatory lesions with lymphoid neogenesis. *Am J Pathol* (2007) 171(5):1549–62. doi:10.2353/ajpath.2007.061275
24. Shields JD, Kourtis IC, Tomei AA, Roberts JM, Swartz MA. Induction of lymphoidlike stroma and immune escape by tumors that express the chemokine CCL21. *Science* (2010) 328(5979):749–52. doi:10.1126/science.1185837
25. van de Pavert SA, Olivier BJ, Goverse G, Vondenhoff MF, Greuter M, Beke P, et al. Chemokine CXCL13 is essential for lymph node initiation and is induced by retinoic acid and neuronal stimulation. *Nat Immunol* (2009) 10(11):1193–9. doi:10.1038/ni.1789
26. Schaerli P, Willimann K, Lang AB, Lipp M, Loetscher P, Moser B. CXC chemokine receptor 5 expression defines follicular homing T cells with B cell helper function. *J Exp Med* (2000) 192(11):1553–62. doi:10.1084/jem.192.11.1553
27. Schmitt N, Bentebibel SE, Ueno H. Phenotype and functions of memory Tfh cells in human blood. *Trends Immunol* (2014) 35(9):436–42. doi:10.1016/j.it.2014.06.002
28. Aguzzi A, Kranich J, Krautier NJ. Follicular dendritic cells: origin, phenotype, and function in health ans disease. *Trends Immunol* (2014) 35:105–13. doi:10.1016/j.it.2013.11.001
29. Ansel KM, Ngo VN, Hyman PL, Luther SA, Forster R, Sedgwick JD, et al. A chemokine-driven positive feedback loop organizes lymphoid follicles. *Nature* (2000) 406(6793):309–14. doi:10.1038/35018581
30. Dubey LK, Lebbon L, Mosconi I, Yang CY, Scandella E, Ludewig B, et al. Lymphotoxin-dependent B cell-FRC crosstalk promotes de novo follicle formation and antibody production following intestinal helminth infection. *Cell Rep* (2016) 15:1–15. doi:10.1016/j.celrep.2016.04.020
31. Cremasco V, Woodruff MC, Onder L, Cupovic J, Nieves-Bonilla JM, Schildberg FA, et al. B cell homeostasis and follicle confines are governed by fibroblastic reticular cells. *Nat Immunol* (2014) 15(10):973–81. doi:10.1038/ni.2965
32. Chyou S, Ekland EH, Carpenter AC, Tzeng TC, Tian S, Michaud M, et al. Fibroblast-type reticular stromal cells regulate the lymph node vasculature. *J Immunol* (2008) 181(6):3887–96. doi:10.4049/jimmunol.181.6.3887
33. Hammerschmidt SI, Ahrendt M, Bode U, Wahl B, Kremmer E, Forster R, et al. Stromal mesenteric lymph node cells are essential for the generation of gut-homing T cells in vivo. *J Exp Med* (2008) 205(11):2483–90. doi:10.1084/jem.20080039
34. Molenaar R, Greuter M, van der Marel AP, Roozendaal R, Martin SF, Edele F, et al. Lymph node stromal cells support dendritic cell-induced gut-homing of T cells. *J Immunol* (2009) 183(10):6395–402. doi:10.4049/jimmunol.0900311
35. Katakai T, Hara T, Sugai M, Gonda H, Shimizu A. Lymph node fibroblastic reticular cells construct the stromal reticulum via contact with lymphocytes. *J Exp Med* (2004) 200(6):783–95. doi:10.1084/jem.20040254
36. Tomei AA, Siegert S, Britschgi MR, Luther SA, Swartz MA. Fluid flow regulates stromal cell organization and CCL21 expression in a tissue-engineered lymph node microenvironment. *J Immunol* (2009) 183(7):4273–83. doi:10.4049/jimmunol.0900835
37. Grabner R, Lotzer K, Dopping S, Hildner M, Radke D, Beer M, et al. Lymphotoxin beta receptor signaling promotes tertiary lymphoid organogenesis in the aorta adventitia of aged ApoE-/- mice. *J Exp Med* (2009) 206(1):233–48. doi:10.1084/jem.20080752
38. Iwata M, Hirakiyama A, Eshima Y, Kagechika H, Kato C, Song SY. Retinoic acid imprints gut-homing specificity on T cells. *Immunity* (2004) 21(4):527–38. doi:10.1016/j.immuni.2004.08.011
39. Lotzer K, Dopping S, Connert S, Grabner R, Spanbroek R, Lemser B, et al. Mouse aorta smooth muscle cells differentiate into lymphoid tissue organizer-like cells on combined tumor necrosis factor receptor-1/lymphotoxin beta-receptor NF-kappaB signaling. *Arterioscler Thromb Vasc Biol* (2010) 30(3):395–402. doi:10.1161/atvbaha.109.191395
40. Hu D, Mohanta SK, Yin C, Peng L, Ma Z Srikakulapu P, et al. Artery tertiary lymphoid organs control aorta immunity and protect against atherosclerosis via vascular smooth muscle cell lymphotoxin beta receptors. *Immunity* (2015) 42(6):1100–15. doi:10.1016/j.immuni.2015.05.015
41. Peduto L, Dulauroy S, Lochner M, Spath GF, Morales MA, Cumano A, et al. Inflammation recapitulates the ontogeny of lymphoid stromal cells. *J Immunol* (2009) 182(9):5789–99. doi:10.4049/jimmunol.0803974
42. Nasr IW, Reel M, Oberbarnscheidt MH, Mounzer RH, Baddoura FK, Ruddle NH, et al. Tertiary lymphoid tissues generate effector and memory T cells that lead to allograft rejection. *Am J Transplant* (2007) 7(5):1071–9. doi:10.1111/j.1600-6143.2007.01756.x
43. Randall TD, Carragher DM, Rangel-Moreno J. Development of secondary lymphoid organs. *Annu Rev Immunol* (2008) 26:627–50. doi:10.1146/annurev.immunol.26.021607.090257
44. Thaunat O, Graff-Dubois S, Brouard S, Gautreau C, Varthaman A, Fabien N, et al. Immune responses elicited in tertiary lymphoid tissues display distinctive features. *PLoS One* (2010) 30:e11398 doi:10.1371/journal.pone.0011398
45. Sicard A, Chen CC, Morelon E, Thaunat O. Alloimmune-induced intragraft lymphoid neogenesis promotes B-cell tolerance breakdown that accelerates chronic rejection. *Curr Opin Organ Transplant* (2016) 21:368–73. doi:10.1097/MOT.0000000000000329
46. Cupedo T, Stroock A, Coles M. Application of tissue engineering to the immune system: development of artificial lymph nodes. *Front Immunol* (2012) 3:343. doi:10.3389/fimmu.2012.00343
47. Fletcher AL, Lukacs-Kornek V, Reynoso ED, Pinner SE, Bellemare-Pelletier A, Curry MS, et al. Lymph node fibroblastic reticular cells directly present peripheral tissue antigen under steady-state and inflammatory conditions. *J Exp Med* (2010) 207(4):689–97. doi:10.1084/jem.20092642
48. Cohen JN, Guidi CJ, Tewalt EF, Qiao H, Rouhani SJ, Ruddell A, et al. Lymph node-resident lymphatic endothelial cells mediate peripheral tolerance via aire-independent direct antigen presentation. *J Exp Med* (2010) 207(4):681–8. doi:10.1084/jem.20092465
49. Suematsu S, Watanabe T. Generation of a synthetic lymphoid tissue-like organoid in mice. *Nat Biotechnol* (2004) 22(12):1539–45. doi:10.1038/nbt1039
50. Okamoto N, Chihara R, Shimizu C, Nishimoto S, Watanabe T. Artificial lymph nodes induce potent secondary immune responses in naive and immunodeficient mice. *J Clin Invest* (2007) 117(4):997–1007. doi:10.1172/jci30379
51. Kobayashi Y, Kato K, Watanabe T. Synthesis of functional artificial lymphoid tissues. *Discov Med* (2011) 12(65):351–62.
52. Kobayashi Y, Watanabe T. Synthesis of artificial lymphoid tissue with immunological function. *Trends Immunol* (2010) 31(11):422–8. doi:10.1016/j.it.2010.09.002
53. Nakashima M, Mori K, Maeda K, Kishi H, Hirata K, Kawabuchi M, et al. Selective elimination of double-positive immature thymocytes by a thymic epithelial cell line. *Eur J Immunol* (1990) 20(1):47–53. doi:10.1002/eji.1830200108
54. Young CL, Adamson TC III, Vaughan JH, Fox RI. Immunohistologic characterization of synovial membrane lymphocytes in rheumatoid arthritis. *Arthritis Rheum* (1984) 27(1):32–9. doi:10.1002/art.1780270106
55. Kobayashi S, Murata K, Shibuya H, Morita M, Ishikawa M, Furu M, et al. A distinct human CD4+ T cell subset that secretes CXCL13 in rheumatoid synovium. *Arthritis Rheum* (2013) 65(12):3063–72. doi:10.1002/art.38173
56. Salomonsson S, Jonsson MV, Skarstein K, Brokstad KA, Hjelmstrom P, Wahren-Herlenius M, et al. Cellular basis of ectopic germinal center formation and autoantibody production in the target organ of patients with Sjogren's syndrome. *Arthritis Rheum* (2003) 48(11):3187–201. doi:10.1002/art.11311
57. Stott DI, Hiepe F, Hummel M, Steinhauser G, Berek C. Antigen-driven clonal proliferation of B cells within the target tissue of an autoimmune disease.

The salivary glands of patients with Sjogren's syndrome. *J Clin Invest* (1998) 102(5):938–46. doi:10.1172/jci3234

58. Kielczewski JL, Horai R, Jittayasothorn Y, Chan CC, Caspi RR. Tertiary lymphoid tissue forms in retinas of mice with spontaneous autoimmune uveitis and has consequences on visual function. *J Immunol* (2016) 196(3):1013–25. doi:10.4049/jimmunol.1501570
59. Sura R, Colombel JF, Kruiningen HJ. Lymphatics, tertiary lymphoid organs and the granuloma of Crohn's disease: an immunohistochemical study. *Aliment Pharmacol Ther* (2011) 33:930–9. doi:10.1111/j.1365-2036.2011.04605x
60. McNamee EN, Masterson C, Jedlicka P, Collins CB, William IR, Rivera-Nieves J. Ectopic lymphoid tissue alters the chemokine gradient, inctreases lymphoid lymphocyte retention and exacerbates murine ileitis. *Gut* (2016) 62:53–62. doi:10.1136/gutjnl-2011-301272
61. Aloisi F, Columba-Cabezas S, Franciotta D, Rosicarelli B, Magliozzi R, Reynolds R, et al. Lymphoid chemokines in chronic neuroinflammation. *J Neuroimmunol* (2008) 198:106–12. doi:10.1016/j.jneuroim.2008.04.025
62. Kuerten S, Schickel A, Kerkloh C, Recks MS, Addicks K, Ruddie NH, et al. Tertiary lymphoid organ development coincides with determinant spreading of the myelin-specific T cell response. *Acta Neuropathol* (2012) 124:861–73. doi:10.1007/s00401-012-1023-3
63. Thompson ED, Enriquez HL, Fu YX, Engelhard VH. Tumor masses support naive T cell infiltration, activation, and differentiation into effectors. *J Exp Med* (2010) 207(8):1791–804. doi:10.1084/jem.20092454
64. Littman DR. Releasing the brakes on cancer immunotherapy. *Cell* (2015) 162(6):1186–90. doi:10.1016/j.cell.2015.08.038
65. Sharma P, Allison JP. The future of immune checkpoint therapy. *Science* (2015) 348(6230):56–61. doi:10.1126/science.aaa8172
66. Pan WR, Suami H, Taylor GI. Senile changes in human lymph nodes. *Lymphat Res Biol* (2008) 6(2):77–83. doi:10.1089/lrb.2007.1023
67. Hadamitzky C, Spohr H, Debertin AS, Guddat S, Tsokos M, Pabst R. Age-dependent histoarchitectural changes in human lymph nodes: an underestimated process with clinical relevance? *J Anat* (2010) 216(5):556–62. doi:10.1111/j.1469-7580.2010.01213.x
68. Lutolf MP, Hubbell JA. Synthetic biomaterials as instructive extracellular microenvironments for morphogenesis in tissue engineering. *Nat Biotechnol* (2005) 23(1):47–55. doi:10.1038/nbt1055
69. Aberle T, Franke K, Rist E, Benz K, Schlosshauer B. Cell-type specific four-component hydrogel. *PLoS One* (2014) 9(1):e86740. doi:10.1371/journal.pone.0086740
70. Stachowiak AN, Irvine DJ. Inverse opal hydrogel-collagen composite scaffolds as a supportive microenvironment for immune cell migration. *J Biomed Mater Res A* (2008) 85(3):815–28. doi:10.1002/jbm.a.31661
71. Richardson TP, Peters MC, Ennett AB, Mooney DJ. Polymeric system for dual growth factor delivery. *Nat Biotechnol* (2001) 19(11):1029–34. doi:10.1038/nbt1101-1029
72. Ishikawa F, Yasukawa M, Lyons B, Yoshida S, Miyamoto T, Yoshimoto G, et al. Development of functional human blood and immune systems in NOD/SCID/IL2 receptor γ chain(null) mice. *Blood* (2005) 106(5):1565–73. doi:10.1182/blood-2005-02-0516
73. Ito M, Hiramatsu H, Kobayashi K, Suzue K, Kawahata M, Hioki K, et al. NOD/SCID/gamma(c)(null) mouse: an excellent recipient mouse model for engraftment of human cells. *Blood* (2002) 100(9):3175–82. doi:10.1182/blood-2001-12-0207
74. Shultz LD, Saito Y, Najima Y, Tanaka S, Ochi T, Tomizawa M, et al. Generation of functional human T-cell subsets with HLA-restricted immune responses in HLA class I expressing NOD/SCID/IL2rγ(null) humanized mice. *Proc Natl Acad Sci U S A* (2010) 107(29):13022–7. doi:10.1073/pnas.1000475107
75. Shultz LD, Brehm MA, Garcia-Martinez JV, Greiner DL. Humanized mice for immune system investigation: progress, promise and challenges. *Nat Rev Immunol* (2012) 12(11):786–98. doi:10.1038/nri3311
76. Traggiai E, Chicha L, Mazzucchelli L, Bronz L, Piffaretti JC, Lanzavecchia A, et al. Development of a human adaptive immune system in cord blood cell-transplanted mice. *Science* (2004) 304(5667):104–7. doi:10.1126/science.1093933
77. Danner R, Chaudhari SN, Rosenberger J, Surls J, Richie TL, Brumeanu TD, et al. Expression of HLA class II molecules in humanized NOD.Rag1KO.IL2RgcKO mice is critical for development and function of human T and B cells. *PLoS One* (2011) 6(5):e19826. doi:10.1371/journal.pone.0019826
78. Jaiswal S, Smith K, Ramirez A, Woda M, Pazoles P, Shultz LD, et al. Dengue virus infection induces broadly cross-reactive human IgM antibodies that recognize intact virions in humanized BLT-NSG mice. *Exp Biol Med (Maywood)* (2015) 240(1):67–78. doi:10.1177/1535370214546273
79. Saito Y, Uchida N, Tanaka S, Suzuki N, Tomizawa-Murasawa M, Sone A, et al. Induction of cell cycle entry eliminates human leukemia stem cells in a mouse model of AML. *Nat Biotechnol* (2010) 28(3):275–80. doi:10.1038/nbt.1607
80. Zhang L, Kovalev GI, Su L. HIV-1 infection and pathogenesis in a novel humanized mouse model. *Blood* (2007) 109(7):2978–81. doi:10.1182/blood-2006-07-033159

21

Antigen-Presenting Cells and Antigen Presentation in Tertiary Lymphoid Organs

*Catherine E. Hughes[1], Robert A. Benson[1], Marija Bedaj[1,2] and Pasquale Maffia[1,3,4]**

[1] Centre for Immunobiology, Institute of Infection, Immunity and Inflammation, College of Medical, Veterinary and Life Sciences, University of Glasgow, Glasgow, UK, [2] Rheumatology Research Group, Centre for Translational Inflammation Research, School of Immunity and Infection, College of Medical and Dental Sciences, University of Birmingham, Birmingham, UK, [3] BHF Centre of Excellence in Vascular Science and Medicine, College of Medical, Veterinary and Life Sciences, University of Glasgow, Glasgow, UK, [4] Department of Pharmacy, University of Naples Federico II, Naples, Italy

***Correspondence:**
Pasquale Maffia
pasquale.maffia@glasgow.ac.uk

Tertiary lymphoid organs (TLOs) form in territorialized niches of peripheral tissues characterized by the presence of antigens; however, little is known about mechanism(s) of antigen handling by ectopic lymphoid structures. In this mini review, we will discuss the role of antigen-presenting cells and mechanisms of antigen presentation in TLOs, summarizing what is currently known about this facet of the formation and function of these tissues as well as identifying questions yet to be addressed.

Keywords: antigen presentation, antigen-presenting cells, B cells, dendritic cells, follicular dendritic cells, macrophages, tertiary lymphoid organs

INTRODUCTION

The ability to respond rapidly and effectively to damage or infection is mediated by the immune system. Secondary lymphoid organs (SLOs) such as lymph nodes (LNs) and spleen provide critical meeting points for immune cells and antigens, promoting interactions that result in a prompt, targeted immune response. A key process in initiating and sustaining such an adaptive response is in the delivery of antigen for interrogation by lymphocyte populations. Networks of lymphatic vessels channel free and cell-borne antigen to the lymph node where it is then further directed to appropriate lymphocyte compartments through additional structural and cellular filters. However, during chronic inflammation, ectopic lymphoid tissue can form in the periphery, outside the normal sites of secondary lymphoid organogenesis. This tissue shares common features with SLOs, including segregated T and B cell areas, germinal centers (GCs), development of structural stromal components, and vascularization, with high endothelial venules (HEVs) often observed (1). These so-called tertiary lymphoid organs (TLOs) are thought to function as a local site for perpetuation of adaptive immune responses providing a local source of antibody, generated as the result of local antigen presentation, and lymphocyte activation and maturation in the newly formed structure. In some settings, development of these lymphoid structures may be advantageous, as in bacterial and viral infections (2–4), atherosclerosis (5, 6), and cancer (7, 8), while in a number of diseases, particularly autoimmune disorders, the development of TLOs may be associated with non-resolving inflammation, with a vigorous and sustained response to self-antigen amplifying severe and chronic pathology [reviewed in Ref. (9); see also Ref. (10–12)]. In this review, we will outline the role of antigen-presenting cells (APCs) and mechanisms of antigen presentation in the TLO, summarizing what is currently known about this facet of the formation and function of these tissues as well as identifying questions yet to be addressed.

A spectrum of TLO development has been documented in the literature, with ectopic lymphoid tissue ranging from relatively loose aggregates of B and T cells to highly compartmentalized, complex structures that include stromal scaffolding supporting distinct T cell zones and secondary B cell follicles containing GCs, i.e., *bona fide* lymphoid organs with clear parallels to secondary lymphoid tissue (9, 13). The initial steps leading to development of TLOs are unclear, as a number of distinct but inter-related signals can prompt development of organized lymphoid structures in non-lymphoid tissue. Determining the "tipping point" beyond which development of functional, relatively stable ectopic lymphoid tissue is inevitable is inherently difficult. However, a number of features are known to affect formation and stability of the structure. Several studies, described in more detail elsewhere in this research topic issue, variously indicate increased expression of cytokines such as lymphotoxin (LT) and other TNF family members (14), IL-22 (15), and chemokines such as CXCL13 and CCL21 (16–18) as being capable of inducing TLO formation. In a patho-physiological setting, specific cell types (19), including T cells (16), and APCs, such as macrophages (20), dendritic cells (DCs) (2, 3), and activated B cells (21), are all described as possible key players in early expression of cytokines and chemokines that promote increased tissue infiltration by leukocytes, development of lymphoid stromal cells such as follicular dendritic cells (FDCs), and construction and maintenance of the functional TLO. Fluid accumulation at the site of infection has also been suggested to influence TLO development (22).

ANTIGEN-PRESENTING CELL POPULATIONS WITHIN TLOs

Dendritic Cells

Although an ever-increasing number of cell types have been shown to be capable of presenting antigen to immune cells, the classical professional antigen-presenting cell is the conventional dendritic cell (23).

Their involvement in various types of TLO has been demonstrated by a number of studies. In a model of viral lung infection, Halle et al. (2) showed that early infiltration of $CD11c^+$ cells into the perivascular and peribronchiolar space (4 days post infection) precipitated recruitment of lymphocytes to the infected tissue, with subsequent development of organized inducible bronchus-associated lymphoid tissue (iBALT) structures. Within these highly developed structures, DCs resided primarily within the T cell area, as in SLOs. When $CD11c^+$ cells were selectively depleted at various time points using a diphtheria toxin receptor (DTR) transgenic model, the size, but not frequency, of iBALT was reduced, suggesting an important role for DCs, and possibly alveolar macrophages, in maintaining TLO integrity (2). A concurrent study, investigating induction of iBALT in a model of influenza infection, also demonstrated a key role for $CD11c^+$ cells in maintenance of these lymphoid structures. Again, using a DTR-transgenic model, this study showed that selective depletion of $CD11c^+$ cells from lungs with mature iBALT led to disintegration of the TLO and gradual dispersal of lymphocytes from the lung (3). Notably, influenza-specific plasma cells were found to be undetectable soon after DT-induced depletion of $CD11c^+$ cells, while total B cells and peanut agglutinin $(PNA)^+$ GC B cells were also substantially reduced. The level of class-switched immunoglobulin, specifically IgA, was also significantly reduced in bronchoalveolar lavage fluid. These results indicate a prominent role for DCs in the function and maintenance of iBALT following influenza infection, as well as suggesting an important role for the TLO in local production of class-switched antibodies. Somewhat surprisingly, depletion of $CD11c^+$ cells also led to a significant reduction in the level of systemic hemagglutinin-specific antibody present, indicating a potential role for TLO GCs in generation of long-lived plasma cells that home to the bone marrow (BM). To investigate the role of antigen presentation by DCs in this tissue, lung DCs were isolated from animals challenged with influenza virus expressing the MHC-II $OVA_{323-339}$ epitope, at days 4 and 17 post infection. While these DCs were able to activate OVA-specific $CD4^+$ T cells (OT-II) at day 4, this was no longer the case at the later time point. However, they retained antigen-presenting ability, as demonstrated by DC-mediated activation of OT-II cells after addition of pre-processed OVA peptide. The authors suggest that the primary role of the DC population in maintenance of the iBALT is production of LTβ, which in turn induces high levels of CXCL13, an important chemokine in B cell migration and retention. Finally, the study also demonstrated that adoptive transfer of granulocyte-macrophage colony-stimulating factor (GM-CSF)-cultured BM-derived cells (a mix of conventional DCs and monocyte-derived macrophages) intratracheally into the lungs of naïve mice leads to iBALT development (3).

In a model of thyroid TLO development, where high levels of CCL21 were artificially induced in the thyroid, $CD3^+CD4^+$ T cells from an adoptively transferred mixed splenocyte population were found to be the initiating cell type in development of ectopic lymphoid tissue. Subsequent recruitment of host DCs and DC/T cell interactions were found to be important for the formation of peripheral-node addressin-positive $(PNAd^+)$ HEVs in the developing TLO, in a LTα-/LTβR-dependent manner (16). A subsequent paper by the same group confirmed that depletion of $CD11c^+$ DCs led to reduced lymphangiogenesis in the thyroid (24).

LTβR is known to have an important role in the maintenance of HEVs within LNs (25), again indicating that these structures are *bona fide* lymphoid organs. Interestingly, in a model of insulin-dependent diabetes mellitus induced by adoptive transfer of specific antigen-expressing DCs, only mice that showed early infiltration of leukocytes and formation of islet-associated organized lymphoid structures in the pancreatic parenchyma went on to develop diabetes, suggesting a link between antigen presentation by DCs to T cells, TLO formation, and development of autoimmunity (26). More recently, the presence of mature DCs in tumor TLOs was highly associated with a favorable clinical outcome in patients with lung cancers (27, 28); however, to date, there is no direct demonstration that APCs in TLOs permit efficient local T-cell priming against tumor-associated antigens.

Macrophages

Macrophages are some of the earliest immune cells to encounter antigen at sites of infection or injury. The response to antigenic stimulus is context-dependent but production of inflammatory cytokines is a key function of these cells in the early stages of inflammation. In the case of atherosclerosis, macrophages that infiltrate the early plaque take up oxidized low-density lipoprotein (ox-LDL) particles and are activated, including upregulation of antigen-presentation genes and increased production of inflammatory cytokines (29). Recently, work from Guedj et al. has proposed a role for pro-inflammatory macrophages as a kind of lymphoid tissue inducer (LTi) cell in the development of artery tertiary lymphoid organs (ATLOs) during atherosclerosis. In this study, BM-derived macrophages were incubated with both LPS and IFNγ to yield a "pro-inflammatory" phenotype or with IL-4 to generate "alternatively activated" macrophages. Vascular smooth muscle cells (VSMCs) incubated with LPS/IFNγ-stimulated macrophages, which produced TNFα and LTα, developed a lymphoid tissue organizer (LTo) phenotype, while those incubated with IL-4-stimulated macrophages did not (20). This activity did not require LTβR signaling but was dependent on TNF receptor involvement. In addition, Jupelli et al. (4) have reported that iNOS-expressing macrophage involvement in early stages of bacterial lung infection precedes development of iBALT in the lungs of infected mice in their model. Intratracheal transfer of "pro-inflammatory" macrophages (generated from BM-derived macrophages cultured with IFNγ) into infected lungs leads to increased lung inflammation and iBALT formation. It should be also noted that, although the recruitment of CD11c$^+$ DCs is clearly a crucial step in the development of iBALT in the viral infection model from Halle et al. (2), the earliest infiltrate recorded was that of alveolar macrophages, within 5–7 h of infection, with DC accumulation described from 4 days post infection. As TLOs, by their nature, form during inflammatory events, and particularly during sustained inflammation, it is logical to assume that macrophage production of inflammatory cytokines following antigen encounter is a necessary, but probably not sufficient, primary event in TLO formation. As described for ATLO formation, a possible role for macrophages as a type of inducible LTi remains to be demonstrated for other types of ectopic lymphoid tissues.

B Cells

The main role of B cells in an immune response is production of antibodies. B cell presentation of antigen to T cells is an integral aspect of this function. These interactions allow B cells to receive survival signals and direct them appropriately to generate high affinity antibody specific to the antigen encountered (30). Well-established, highly organized TLOs contain secondary B cell follicles, which form following antigen encounter and activation of B cells (31–33). The GCs of these follicles are structurally and functionally similar to those within SLOs, with FDC development described within a number of ectopic lymphoid tissues. This lends credence to the hypothesis that TLOs provide a venue for local production of antibody proximal to the site of inflammation, with either beneficial (e.g., during infection, cancer, or atherosclerosis) or deleterious (e.g., autoimmunity) effects depending on the context in which the TLO forms.

B cells are involved in FDC development (34) in a LT- and TNF-dependent manner, with B cell aggregates shown to induce FDC through LTα1β2 production in SLOs (35, 36). LTα1β2 expression by naïve B cells is induced by CXCL13 (also known as B-lymphocyte chemoattractant), which is itself induced by LTα1β2 in a positive feedback loop (37), with FDCs likely the major source of CXCL13 in the follicle (36). In mice with B cells lacking LTβ, FDC structures in the spleen were disrupted, though not wholly absent (13). Similarly, LTα is not fully required for formation of iBALT, as lymphocytic aggregates form in influenza-infected *Lta*$^{-/-}$ mice and lymphoid chemokines CXCL13 and CCL21 are detectable. However, these structures lack the level of development and organization of the TLO observed in mice expressing LTα (17). A similar role in promoting FDC formation has been suggested for B cells in TLOs that arise in the salivary glands of Sjögrens syndrome patients (38).

Follicular Dendritic Cells

Follicular dendritic cells are cells of the immune system found in B cell follicles. FDCs are integral to the function of the follicle, presenting antigen in the form of immune complexes bound to their surface (39, 40). FDCs are believed to provide a uniquely long-lasting "depot" of antigen that can be accessed by B cells well beyond clearance of the initial infection or injury from which the antigen was acquired. They are thought to be important in the affinity maturation of the B-cell receptor (BCR). Only B cells expressing a receptor of high enough affinity will be successful in acquiring sufficient antigen from the FDC to in turn present the antigen to their cognate T cell and receive survival signals (36). A recent study has shown that disruption of the FDC network in a model of arthritis led to reduced GC formation in lymphoid follicles, impaired recruitment of follicular helper T (Tfh) cells into B cell areas, diminished autoantibody production, and attenuation of disease (41).

Although there is some debate over how B cells within a TLO might perceive antigen due to the likelihood of increased availability of local antigen compared to SLOs, a number of studies have identified FDCs within ectopic lymphoid structures (5, 42–45). The source of these cells within TLOs is unclear, but, as discussed above, various studies indicate that B cell production of LTα1β2 is important for differentiation of FDCs within ectopic lymphoid organs (1, 35, 38), even though follicle formation in BALT has been reported also in the absence of differentiated FDCs (46). In addition to providing a platform for antigen presentation, FDCs are also known to produce a variety of cytokines and chemokines involved in B cell migration survival and proliferation, as well as recruitment of Tfh cells into B cell areas, such as CXCL13, BAFF, IL-15, and IL-6 (45, 47). Therefore, a similarly multi-faceted role for these cells in mature TLOs is anticipated.

Other Antigen-Presenting Cells

As reviewed by Kambayashi and Laufer recently, a number of cells not traditionally considered "professional" APC may nonetheless under specific circumstances be induced to express MHC-II on their surface and have been shown to interact with T cells in an antigen-specific manner (23, 48). In Sjögrens syndrome, salivary gland epithelial cells (SGECs) may play an important role in the presentation of self-antigen. Numerous lines of evidence point to this ability, including expression of co-stimulatory molecules, such as CD80, CD86, and CD40 (49, 50), the ability to express adhesion molecules and human leukocyte antigen (HLA)-DR (51), and the ability to activate antigen-specific T cells (48). Ishimaru et al. also suggest expression of IFNγ by SGECs may be involved in increased expression of MHC-II by these cells (48). Self-antigen presentation by thyroid epithelial cells – indicated by MHC-II expression and an ability to induce T cell activation – was described more than 30 years ago, with the authors suggesting that the cells might preferentially present self-antigen (52). Other non-hematopoietic cells have also been implicated in presentation of self-antigen. In 2010, Cohen and colleagues described a role for lymphatic endothelial cells (LECs) in the induction of peripheral tolerance through autoimmune regulator (AIRE)-independent presentation of self-antigen (53). Additionally, extrathymic AIRE-expressing cells (eTACs) have been identified in pancreatic TLO of non-obese diabetic (NOD) mice (54). The ability of eTACs to induce peripheral tolerance in TLOs is yet to be demonstrated, but expression of AIRE in these cells has been linked to non-canonical NF-κB activation, which contributes to peripheral tolerance induction (55). Finally, fibroblastic reticular cells (FRCs) express and present peripheral tissue-restricted antigen to T cells as part of the peripheral tolerance mechanism, and their ability to stimulate T cells is altered depending on the inflammatory state of the tissue (56). These cell types have also been detected in TLOs, again pointing to roles in directing the immune response that unfolds within (5, 45, 57).

While the presence in TLOs of each of the APCs described thus far has been robustly reported in the literature and across a variety of TLOs, in the vast majority of cases there has been limited or no direct investigation of actual antigen presentation in these tissues. What mechanisms exist to allow TLO-associated APCs access to antigen? Who are the main APCs presenting antigen, what are the nature of the antigens, and what are the ultimate immunological consequences of antigen presentation in TLOs?

ACQUIRING ANTIGEN FOR PRESENTATION

In the case of LNs, DCs carrying antigen acquired directly in a peripheral tissue migrate *via* the lymphatic vessels and enter the subcapsular sinus (SCS). Here, the DCs must traverse from the SCS ceiling to the floor, cross the dense parenchyma, and enter the paracortex. Small antigens can also drain freely through the lymphatic bed to the SCS. These antigens can be accessed by DCs already residing within the LN as they pass through conduits linking the SCS and HEVs (58, 59). A comparable conduit system is present in the follicular regions, allowing similar access to antigen by B cells (60, 61). The follicles themselves are positioned directly adjacent to the SCS and may facilitate B cell acquisition of soluble antigen, potentially draining through SCS pores (62, 63) or presented by SCS macrophages (64–66). Another possibility is that B cells could acquire unprocessed antigen from DCs (67). In this instance, uptake by the DC would likely involve the FcγRIIB receptor, allowing the antigen to remain unprocessed and recycled to the cell surface (68). Larger antigens acquired by non-cognate B cells can be further transported to FDCs in a complement-dependent way.

But what happens in a TLO? To date, direct data pertaining to antigen handling within TLOs is scarce. One might speculate as to the relevance of lymphatics and conduits to antigen transport to/within TLOs since, in general, the majority of TLOs do not demonstrate a distinct capsule or SCS, and form locally at the peripheral site of antigenic challenge. Yet lymphatic vessels do appear to be present in TLOs, such as those seen in ATLOs, iBALT, and pancreatic and thyroid infiltrate (5, 18, 24, 69). But their direct contribution in antigen transport is open for debate [as reviewed in Ref. (22)]. Splenic white pulp lacks afferent lymphatics but demonstrates series of organized cellular transport mechanisms [involving marginal zone macrophages, B cells and DCs (70)] along with a conduit network directly linked to the blood stream (71). As in the LN conduit system, transport of antigen/molecules is similarly size restricted, but does represent one way in which small molecules can be transported to particular compartments within the TLO. ATLOs demonstrate ER-TR7$^+$ reticular networks consistent with the presence of conduits. Indeed, conduit structures were seen to extend through the T cell areas terminating adjacent to HEVs of the ATLO. In addition, these conduits were able to channel only small particles (10 kDa) and not larger particles from the adventitia following i.v. administration (5). Evidence of conduit-like structures have been reported in both human and murine studies and in a variety of tertiary lymphoid tissues found in pancreas, kidney, salivary glands, and liver (57). So, it seems likely that an additional contribution of conduits and lymphatics in the instance of TLOs may relate to antigen transport, allowing small molecule percolation throughout the ectopic lymphoid organ, while, as in other lymphoid organs, their major role likely relates to cellular trafficking (transport of chemokines to HEVs in the case of conduits, and perhaps efferent lymphatic functions for removal of inflammatory cells and mediators from the affected tissue). Mechanisms of antigen handling and presentation in LNs vs. TLOs are illustrated in **Figure 1**.

ANTIGEN PRESENTATION IN TLOs

We have recently extensively studied antigen presentation in ATLOs (72), by using the Eα-GFP/Y-Ae system to visualize antigen uptake through a GFP tag and tracking of Eα peptide/MHC-II presentation using a commercially available (Y-Ae) Ab (73–75). In the case of ATLO APCs, acquisition and presentation of soluble antigen upon MHC class II occurs within a matter of hours (72). However, unlike in the LN, presentation in the ATLO occurs equally across the major APC populations, perhaps more consistent with free diffusion of the antigen rather than transport to defined niches and compartments (72). Around 80% of the CD11c^{hi}MHC-II$^+$ APCs were monocyte-derived CD11b$^+$DC-SIGN$^+$ cells, 15% were CD11b$^+$DC-SIGN$^-$ conventional DCs, and 5% CD11b$^-$DC-SIGN$^-$ lymphoid DCs. The majority (80%) of MHC-II$^+$CD11c$^{lo/-}$ APCs were CD19$^+$CD11b$^-$ B cells and 10%

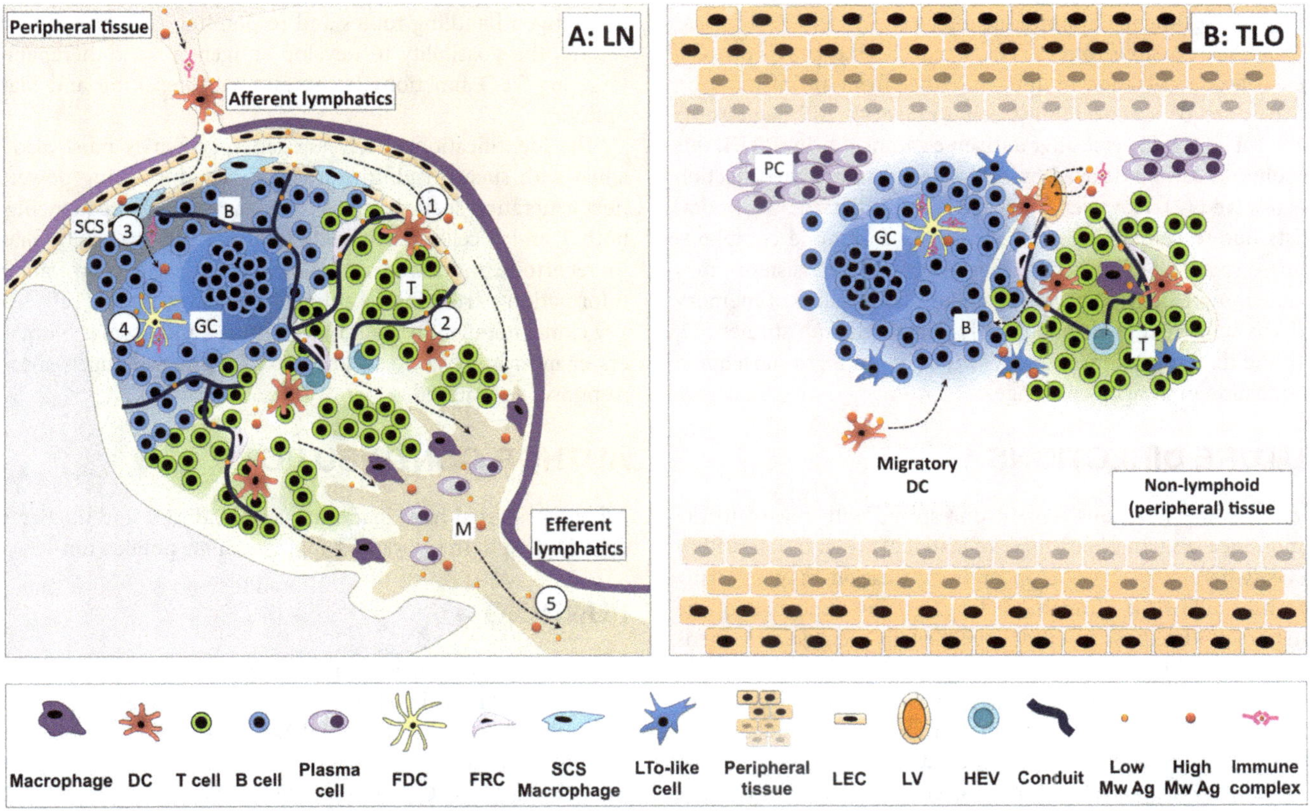

FIGURE 1 | Antigen handling and presentation in lymph nodes vs. TLOs. (A) Antigen reaches lymph nodes (LNs) *via* the afferent lymphatics, transported by dendritic cells (DCs) or freely draining from the peripheral tissues. Migratory DCs cross the subcapsular sinus (SCS) and enter the paracortex (T cell area), migrating in response to appropriate chemotactic cues (1). Here, they encounter T cells searching for cognate peptide–MHC complexes. DCs residing within T cell areas can also sample small soluble molecules from a network of conduits traversing the paracortex (2). Additionally, small soluble antigens may be accessed by B cells *via* pores in the endothelial layer or transported by SCS macrophages, as is the case for larger antigens and immune complexes (3). Such antigen can be further transferred to FDCs for presentation to B cells (4). Freely draining antigen may also exit the LN efferent lymphatic and reach the next lymph node in the chain (5). **(B)** In general, tertiary lymphoid organs (TLOs) lack a defined capsule, which may allow more free diffusion of antigen through the structure. Lymphatic and conduit-like structures have been identified in TLOs, and may function in an analogous fashion to those in SLOs, although this has yet to be formally demonstrated. Similar cellular compartmentalization is observed between TLOs and SLOs, and they share many common antigen-presenting cell populations. Indeed, the migration of DCs from surrounding tissues to the TLOs has been observed in several models of TLO formation. Thus, TLOs likely share common pathways for handling cell-associated and free antigen with SLOs to optimize the functioning of adaptive immune responses. *Key:* B, B cell follicle; T, T cell area; SCS, subcapsular sinus; GC, germinal center; M, medulla; PC, plasma cell niche; DC, dendritic cell; FDC, follicular DC; FRC, fibroblastic reticular cells; LTo, lymphoid tissue organizer; LEC, lymphatic endothelial cell; LV, lymphatic vessel; HEV, high endothelial venule; low/high Mw Ag, low/high molecular weight antigen.

were CD19$^-$CD11b$^+$ macrophages. 1–2% of CD11c^{lo}SiglecH$^+$ plasmacytoid dendritic cells (pDCs) were also detectable within the ATLO. Following Eα i.v. administration, around 55% of MHC-II^{hi}Y-Ae$^+$ APCs were CD11c$^+$CD11b$^+$DC-SIGN$^+$, followed by B cells, conventional DCs, CD11c$^{lo/-}$ macrophages, and lymphoid DCs. None of the pDCs were Y-Ae$^+$, in contrast with what was previously observed by us in the aorta of early atherosclerotic mice (73, 74). In summary, DCs, macrophages and B cells were the major ATLO APCs.

Altering the kinetics of antigen presentation is known to influence the outcome of T cell responses (76–81). How, or even if, differences in antigen handling between TLOs and LNs impact on the ensuing immune response is unknown. While TLOs form at sites of active antigen presentation and functional lymphocyte responses, they also support entry and priming of naïve T cells within the tissue. Intranasal delivered mature BM-derived DCs pulsed with OVApeptide (SIINFEKL) were readily detected in iBALT and able to induce proliferative responses in naïve OT-I CD8$^+$ T cells (2). Similarly, OT-I T cells proliferated in tumor-associated tertiary lymphoid structures following interaction with DCs (82). Notably, multiphoton imaging revealed that the dynamics of naïve T cell migration and interaction with antigen-bearing DCs in iBALT (2) was consistent with the three phases of T cell priming reported by Mempel et al. (83). A similar observation relating to CD4$^+$ T cell behavior showed OT-II T cells clustering around ATLO resident CD11c$^+$ cells following antigen challenge (72), reminiscent of that seen in LN priming of CD4$^+$ T cells (84). Priming of naïve T cells within ectopic structures may have beneficial or detrimental effects depending upon context of the ongoing immune response, being beneficial in infectious disease where secondary infection is a risk or contributing to epitope spreading in autoimmune disease.

Another possible role of TLOs may be the provision of a localized concentration of antigen, either from an infection or, in the case of autoimmunity, self-antigen(s). Although some transient TLOs disperse after antigen clearance, as in iBALT, this dissolution can be delayed by up to 3 weeks after the infection has resolved (2). However, it may be possible that this lag period exists due to some antigen in the form of immune complexes being displayed by FDCs. In either respect, this persistence may enable more efficient development and maintenance of memory cells, as suggested by data from ATLO and allograft studies (72, 85), and therefore a more effective *in situ* response to subsequent re-infection or antigen challenge.

FUTURE DIRECTIONS

Clearly, many questions remain unresolved with regard to the importance and mechanism(s) of antigen presentation within TLOs, where lack of isolation or encapsulation may, in many instances, allow for a much greater degree of exposure to free antigen for all cells within the tissue. Details such as *in situ* neo-antigen availability, the timing of antigen arrival and presentation, the context in which antigen is encountered by specific cells, and the ability of those cells to receive appropriate co-stimulatory or tolerogenic signals remain to be elucidated.

With advances in cellular imaging techniques, in combination with trackable antigens and cell populations, the answers to such questions are becoming increasingly tangible. The elegant application of such approaches has successfully furthered our understanding of soluble antigen and immune complex trafficking and related immune cell interactions in SLOs (86–88). By identifying key antigen handling routes and responding cells in a dynamic setting, the possibility to develop antigen-specific therapeutics targeting TLO functions becomes a more exciting and viable option.

The identification of key antigen specificities must also be allied with such imaging approaches. The increasing power of next generation sequencing techniques makes the sequencing of both T and B cell repertoires (89, 90) in TLOs a reality. Biases in repertoire indicating clonal responses could yield valuable information pertaining to antigen specificity. At the very least, key clonal populations could be identified and used as biomarkers or even be targeted to prevent or augment antigen-specific responses as required.

AUTHOR CONTRIBUTIONS

All authors listed have made substantial, direct, and intellectual contribution to the work and approved it for publication.

FUNDING

This work was supported by the British Heart Foundation grants PG/06/083/21198, PG/12/81/29897 and RE/13/5/30177; the Medical Research Scotland grant 276 FRG-L-0806; the European Commission Marie Skłodowska-Curie Individual Fellowships 661369; and an Oliver Bird Studentship by the Nuffield Foundation. MB and RB are members of the Arthritis Research UK - Rheumatoid Arthritis Pathogenesis Centre of Excellence (RACE) - part-funded by Arthritis Research UK through grant number 20298.

REFERENCES

1. Aloisi F, Pujol-Borrell R. Lymphoid neogenesis in chronic inflammatory diseases. *Nat Rev Immunol* (2006) 6(3):205–17. doi:10.1038/nri1786
2. Halle S, Dujardin HC, Bakocevic N, Fleige H, Danzer H, Willenzon S, et al. Induced bronchus-associated lymphoid tissue serves as a general priming site for T cells and is maintained by dendritic cells. *J Exp Med* (2009) 206(12):2593–601. doi:10.1084/jem.20091472
3. GeurtsvanKessel CH, Willart MA, Bergen IM, van Rijt LS, Muskens F, Elewaut D, et al. Dendritic cells are crucial for maintenance of tertiary lymphoid structures in the lung of influenza virus-infected mice. *J Exp Med* (2009) 206(11):2339–49. doi:10.1084/jem.20090410
4. Jupelli M, Shimada K, Chiba N, Slepenkin A, Alsabeh R, Jones HD, et al. *Chlamydia pneumoniae* infection in mice induces chronic lung inflammation, iBALT formation, and fibrosis. *PLoS One* (2013) 8(10):e77447. doi:10.1371/journal.pone.0077447
5. Grabner R, Lotzer K, Dopping S, Hildner M, Radke D, Beer M, et al. Lymphotoxin beta receptor signaling promotes tertiary lymphoid organogenesis in the aorta adventitia of aged ApoE-/- mice. *J Exp Med* (2009) 206(1):233–48. doi:10.1084/jem.20080752
6. Yin C, Mohanta SK, Srikakulapu P, Weber C, Habenicht AJR. Artery tertiary lymphoid organs: powerhouses of atherosclerosis immunity. *Front Immunol* (2016) 7:387. doi:10.3389/fimmu.2016.00387
7. Hiraoka N, Ino Y, Yamazaki-Itoh R. Tertiary lymphoid organs in cancer tissues. *Front Immunol* (2016) 7:244. doi:10.3389/fimmu.2016.00244
8. Sautès-Fridman C, Lawand M, Giraldo NA, Kaplon H, Germain C, Fridman WH, et al. Tertiary lymphoid structures in cancers: prognostic value, regulation, and manipulation for therapeutic intervention. *Front Immunol* (2016) 7:407. doi:10.3389/fimmu.2016.00407
9. Pitzalis C, Jones GW, Bombardieri M, Jones SA. Ectopic lymphoid-like structures in infection, cancer and autoimmunity. *Nat Rev Immunol* (2014) 14(7):447–62. doi:10.1038/nri3700
10. Weyand CM, Goronzy JJ. Ectopic germinal center formation in rheumatoid synovitis. *Ann N Y Acad Sci* (2003) 987:140–9. doi:10.1111/j.1749-6632.2003.tb06042.x
11. Bombardieri M, Pitzalis C. Ectopic lymphoid neogenesis and lymphoid chemokines in Sjogren's syndrome: at the interplay between chronic inflammation, autoimmunity and lymphomagenesis. *Curr Pharm Biotechnol* (2012) 13(10):1989–96. doi:10.2174/138920112802273209
12. Serafini B, Rosicarelli B, Magliozzi R, Stigliano E, Aloisi F. Detection of ectopic B-cell follicles with germinal centers in the meninges of patients with secondary progressive multiple sclerosis. *Brain Pathol* (2004) 14(2):164–74. doi:10.1111/j.1750-3639.2004.tb00049.x
13. Tumanov A, Kuprash D, Lagarkova M, Grivennikov S, Abe K, Shakhov A, et al. Distinct role of surface lymphotoxin expressed by B cells in the organization of secondary lymphoid tissues. *Immunity* (2002) 17(3):239–50. doi:10.1016/S1074-7613(02)00397-7
14. Kratz A, Campos-Neto A, Hanson MS, Ruddle NH. Chronic inflammation caused by lymphotoxin is lymphoid neogenesis. *J Exp Med* (1996) 183(4):1461–72. doi:10.1084/jem.183.4.1461
15. Barone F, Nayar S, Campos J, Cloake T, Withers DR, Toellner KM, et al. IL-22 regulates lymphoid chemokine production and assembly of tertiary lymphoid organs. *Proc Natl Acad Sci U S A* (2015) 112(35):11024–9. doi:10.1073/pnas.1503315112
16. Marinkovic T, Garin A, Yokota Y, Fu YX, Ruddle NH, Furtado GC, et al. Interaction of mature CD3+CD4+ T cells with dendritic cells triggers the development of tertiary lymphoid structures in the thyroid. *J Clin Invest* (2006) 116(10):2622–32. doi:10.1172/jci28993

17. Moyron-Quiroz JE, Rangel-Moreno J, Kusser K, Hartson L, Sprague F, Goodrich S, et al. Role of inducible bronchus associated lymphoid tissue (iBALT) in respiratory immunity. *Nat Med* (2004) 10(9):927–34. doi:10.1038/nm1091
18. Rangel-Moreno J, Hartson L, Navarro C, Gaxiola M, Selman M, Randall TD. Inducible bronchus-associated lymphoid tissue (iBALT) in patients with pulmonary complications of rheumatoid arthritis. *J Clin Invest* (2006) 116(12):3183–94. doi:10.1172/jci28756
19. Jones GW, Hill DG, Jones SA. Understanding immune cells in tertiary lymphoid organ development: it is all starting to come together. *Front Immunol* (2016) 7:401. doi:10.3389/fimmu.2016.00401
20. Guedj K, Khallou-Laschet J, Clement M, Morvan M, Gaston AT, Fornasa G, et al. M1 macrophages act as LTβR-independent lymphoid tissue inducer cells during atherosclerosis-related lymphoid neogenesis. *Cardiovasc Res* (2014) 101(3):434–43. doi:10.1093/cvr/cvt263
21. McDonald KG, McDonough JS, Newberry RD. Adaptive immune responses are dispensable for isolated lymphoid follicle formation: antigen-naive, lymphotoxin-sufficient B lymphocytes drive the formation of mature isolated lymphoid follicles. *J Immunol* (2005) 174(9):5720–8. doi:10.4049/jimmunol.174.9.5720
22. Ruddle NH. Lymphatic vessels and tertiary lymphoid organs. *J Clin Invest* (2014) 124(3):953–9. doi:10.1172/jci71611
23. Kambayashi T, Laufer TM. Atypical MHC class II-expressing antigen-presenting cells: can anything replace a dendritic cell? *Nat Rev Immunol* (2014) 14(11):719–30. doi:10.1038/nri3754
24. Muniz LR, Pacer ME, Lira SA, Furtado GC. A critical role for dendritic cells in the formation of lymphatic vessels within tertiary lymphoid structures. *J Immunol* (2011) 187(2):828–34. doi:10.4049/jimmunol.1004233
25. Browning JL, Allaire N, Ngam-Ek A, Notidis E, Hunt J, Perrin S, et al. Lymphotoxin-beta receptor signaling is required for the homeostatic control of HEV differentiation and function. *Immunity* (2005) 23(5):539–50. doi:10.1016/j.immuni.2005.10.002
26. Ludewig B, Odermatt B, Landmann S, Hengartner H, Zinkernagel RM. Dendritic cells induce autoimmune diabetes and maintain disease *via* de novo formation of local lymphoid tissue. *J Exp Med* (1998) 188(8):1493–501. doi:10.1084/jem.188.8.1493
27. Dieu-Nosjean MC, Antoine M, Danel C, Heudes D, Wislez M, Poulot V, et al. Long-term survival for patients with non-small-cell lung cancer with intratumoral lymphoid structures. *J Clin Oncol* (2008) 26(27):4410–7. doi:10.1200/JCO.2007.15.0284
28. Germain C, Gnjatic S, Tamzalit F, Knockaert S, Remark R, Goc J, et al. Presence of B cells in tertiary lymphoid structures is associated with a protective immunity in patients with lung cancer. *Am J Respir Crit Care Med* (2014) 189(7):832–44. doi:10.1164/rccm.201309-1611OC
29. Cho HJ, Shashkin P, Gleissner CA, Dunson D, Jain N, Lee JK, et al. Induction of dendritic cell-like phenotype in macrophages during foam cell formation. *Physiol Genomics* (2007) 29(2):149–60. doi:10.1152/physiolgenomics.00051.2006
30. Chen X, Jensen PE. The role of B lymphocytes as antigen-presenting cells. *Arch Immunol Ther Exp* (2008) 56(2):77–83. doi:10.1007/s00005-008-0014-5
31. Srikakulapu P, Hu D, Yin C, Mohanta SK, Bontha SV, Peng L, et al. Artery tertiary lymphoid organs control multilayered territorialized atherosclerosis B-cell responses in aged ApoE-/- mice. *Arterioscler Thromb Vasc Biol* (2016) 36(6):1174–85. doi:10.1161/ATVBAHA.115.306983
32. Germain C, Gnjatic S, Dieu-Nosjean MC. Tertiary lymphoid structure-associated B cells are key players in anti-tumor immunity. *Front Immunol* (2015) 6:67. doi:10.3389/fimmu.2015.00067
33. Jones GW, Jones SA. Ectopic lymphoid follicles: inducible centres for generating antigen-specific immune responses within tissues. *Immunology* (2016) 147(2):141–51. doi:10.1111/imm.12554
34. MacLennan IC. Germinal centers. *Annu Rev Immunol* (1994) 12:117–39. doi:10.1146/annurev.iy.12.040194.001001
35. Fu YX, Huang G, Wang Y, Chaplin DD. B lymphocytes induce the formation of follicular dendritic cell clusters in a lymphotoxin alpha-dependent fashion. *J Exp Med* (1998) 187(7):1009–18. doi:10.1084/jem.187.7.1009
36. Allen CD, Cyster JG. Follicular dendritic cell networks of primary follicles and germinal centers: phenotype and function. *Semin Immunol* (2008) 20(1):14–25. doi:10.1016/j.smim.2007.12.001
37. Ansel KM, Ngo VN, Hyman PL, Luther SA, Forster R, Sedgwick JD, et al. A chemokine-driven positive feedback loop organizes lymphoid follicles. *Nature* (2000) 406(6793):309–14. doi:10.1038/35018581
38. Le Pottier L, Devauchelle V, Fautrel A, Daridon C, Saraux A, Youinou P, et al. Ectopic germinal centers are rare in Sjogren's syndrome salivary glands and do not exclude autoreactive B cells. *J Immunol* (2009) 182(6):3540–7. doi:10.4049/jimmunol.0803588
39. Heesters BA, Myers RC, Carroll MC. Follicular dendritic cells: dynamic antigen libraries. *Nat Rev Immunol* (2014) 14(7):495–504. doi:10.1038/nri3689
40. Kranich J, Krautler NJ. How follicular dendritic cells shape the B-cell antigenome. *Front Immunol* (2016) 7:225. doi:10.3389/fimmu.2016.00225
41. Victoratos P, Kollias G. Induction of autoantibody-mediated spontaneous arthritis critically depends on follicular dendritic cells. *Immunity* (2009) 30(1):130–42. doi:10.1016/j.immuni.2008.10.019
42. Drayton DL, Ying X, Lee J, Lesslauer W, Ruddle NH. Ectopic LT alpha beta directs lymphoid organ neogenesis with concomitant expression of peripheral node addressin and a HEV-restricted sulfotransferase. *J Exp Med* (2003) 197(9):1153–63. doi:10.1084/jem.20021761
43. Moser B, Schaerli P, Loetscher P. CXCR5(+) T cells: follicular homing takes center stage in T-helper-cell responses. *Trends Immunol* (2002) 23(5):250–4. doi:10.1016/S1471-4906(02)02218-4
44. Barone F, Bombardieri M, Manzo A, Blades MC, Morgan PR, Challacombe SJ, et al. Association of CXCL13 and CCL21 expression with the progressive organization of lymphoid-like structures in Sjogren's syndrome. *Arthritis Rheum* (2005) 52(6):1773–84. doi:10.1002/art.21062
45. Stranford S, Ruddle NH. Follicular dendritic cells, conduits, lymphatic vessels, and high endothelial venules in tertiary lymphoid organs: parallels with lymph node stroma. *Front Immunol* (2012) 3:350. doi:10.3389/fimmu.2012.00350
46. Fleige H, Ravens S, Moschovakis GL, Bölter J, Willenzon S, Sutter G, et al. IL-17-induced CXCL12 recruits B cells and induces follicle formation in BALT in the absence of differentiated FDCs. *J Exp Med* (2014) 211(4):643–51. doi:10.1084/jem.20131737
47. El Shikh ME, Pitzalis C. Follicular dendritic cells in health and disease. *Front Immunol* (2012) 3:292. doi:10.3389/fimmu.2012.00292
48. Ishimaru N, Arakaki R, Yoshida S, Yamada A, Noji S, Hayashi Y. Expression of the retinoblastoma protein RbAp48 in exocrine glands leads to Sjogren's syndrome-like autoimmune exocrinopathy. *J Exp Med* (2008) 205(12):2915–27. doi:10.1084/jem.20080174
49. Kapsogeorgou EK, Moutsopoulos HM, Manoussakis MN. Functional expression of a costimulatory B7.2 (CD86) protein on human salivary gland epithelial cells that interacts with the CD28 receptor, but has reduced binding to CTLA4. *J Immunol* (2001) 166(5):3107–13. doi:10.4049/jimmunol.166.5.3107
50. Dimitriou ID, Kapsogeorgou EK, Moutsopoulos HM, Manoussakis MN. CD40 on salivary gland epithelial cells: high constitutive expression by cultured cells from Sjogren's syndrome patients indicating their intrinsic activation. *Clin Exp Immunol* (2002) 127(2):386–92. doi:10.1046/j.1365-2249.2002.01752.x
51. Tsunawaki S, Nakamura S, Ohyama Y, Sasaki M, Ikebe-Hiroki A, Hiraki A, et al. Possible function of salivary gland epithelial cells as nonprofessional antigen-presenting cells in the development of Sjogren's syndrome. *J Rheumatol* (2002) 29(9):1884–96.
52. Londei M, Lamb JR, Bottazzo GF, Feldmann M. Epithelial cells expressing aberrant MHC class II determinants can present antigen to cloned human T cells. *Nature* (1984) 312(5995):639–41. doi:10.1038/312639a0
53. Cohen JN, Guidi CJ, Tewalt EF, Qiao H, Rouhani SJ, Ruddell A, et al. Lymph node-resident lymphatic endothelial cells mediate peripheral tolerance *via* Aire-independent direct antigen presentation. *J Exp Med* (2010) 207(4):681–8. doi:10.1084/jem.20092465
54. Gardner JM, Devoss JJ, Friedman RS, Wong DJ, Tan YX, Zhou X, et al. Deletional tolerance mediated by extrathymic Aire-expressing cells. *Science* (2008) 321(5890):843–7. doi:10.1126/science.1159407
55. van Delft MA, Huitema LF, Tas SW. The contribution of NF-κB signalling to immune regulation and tolerance. *Eur J Clin Invest* (2015) 45(5):529–39. doi:10.1111/eci.12430
56. Fletcher AL, Lukacs-Kornek V, Reynoso ED, Pinner SE, Bellemare-Pelletier A, Curry MS, et al. Lymph node fibroblastic reticular cells directly present

peripheral tissue antigen under steady-state and inflammatory conditions. *J Exp Med* (2010) 207(4):689–97. doi:10.1084/jem.20092642
57. Link A, Hardie DL, Favre S, Britschgi MR, Adams DH, Sixt M, et al. Association of T-zone reticular networks and conduits with ectopic lymphoid tissues in mice and humans. *Am J Pathol* (2011) 178(4):1662–75. doi:10.1016/j.ajpath.2010.12.039
58. Bajenoff M, Granjeaud S, Guerder S. The strategy of T cell antigen-presenting cell encounter in antigen-draining lymph nodes revealed by imaging of initial T cell activation. *J Exp Med* (2003) 198(5):715–24. doi:10.1084/jem.20030167
59. Sixt M, Kanazawa N, Selg M, Samson T, Roos G, Reinhardt DP, et al. The conduit system transports soluble antigens from the afferent lymph to resident dendritic cells in the T cell area of the lymph node. *Immunity* (2005) 22(1):19–29. doi:10.1016/j.immuni.2004.11.013
60. Roozendaal R, Mempel TR, Pitcher LA, Gonzalez SF, Verschoor A, Mebius RE, et al. Conduits mediate transport of low-molecular-weight antigen to lymph node follicles. *Immunity* (2009) 30(2):264–76. doi:10.1016/j.immuni.2008.12.014
61. Bajenoff M, Germain RN. B-cell follicle development remodels the conduit system and allows soluble antigen delivery to follicular dendritic cells. *Blood* (2009) 114(24):4989–97. doi:10.1182/blood-2009-06-229567
62. Clark SL Jr. The reticulum of lymph nodes in mice studied with the electron microscope. *Am J Anat* (1962) 110:217–57. doi:10.1002/aja.1001100303
63. Pape KA, Catron DM, Itano AA, Jenkins MK. The humoral immune response is initiated in lymph nodes by B cells that acquire soluble antigen directly in the follicles. *Immunity* (2007) 26(4):491–502. doi:10.1016/j.immuni.2007.02.011
64. Carrasco YR, Batista FD. B cells acquire particulate antigen in a macrophage-rich area at the boundary between the follicle and the subcapsular sinus of the lymph node. *Immunity* (2007) 27(1):160–71. doi:10.1016/j.immuni.2007.06.007
65. Junt T, Moseman EA, Iannacone M, Massberg S, Lang PA, Boes M, et al. Subcapsular sinus macrophages in lymph nodes clear lymph-borne viruses and present them to antiviral B cells. *Nature* (2007) 450(7166):110–4. doi:10.1038/nature06287
66. Phan TG, Grigorova I, Okada T, Cyster JG. Subcapsular encounter and complement-dependent transport of immune complexes by lymph node B cells. *Nat Immunol* (2007) 8(9):992–1000. doi:10.1038/ni1494
67. Qi H, Egen JG, Huang AY, Germain RN. Extrafollicular activation of lymph node B cells by antigen-bearing dendritic cells. *Science* (2006) 312(5780):1672–6. doi:10.1126/science.1125703
68. Delamarre L, Pack M, Chang H, Mellman I, Trombetta ES. Differential lysosomal proteolysis in antigen-presenting cells determines antigen fate. *Science* (2005) 307(5715):1630–4. doi:10.1126/science.1108003
69. Penaranda C, Tang Q, Ruddle NH, Bluestone JA. Prevention of diabetes by FTY720-mediated stabilization of peri-islet tertiary lymphoid organs. *Diabetes* (2010) 59(6):1461–8. doi:10.2337/db09-1129
70. Kraal G. Cells in the marginal zone of the spleen. *Int Rev Cytol* (1992) 132:31–74. doi:10.1016/S0074-7696(08)62453-5
71. Nolte MA, Belien JA, Schadee-Eestermans I, Jansen W, Unger WW, van Rooijen N, et al. A conduit system distributes chemokines and small blood-borne molecules through the splenic white pulp. *J Exp Med* (2003) 198(3):505–12. doi:10.1084/jem.20021801
72. Hu D, Mohanta SK, Yin C, Peng L, Ma Z, Srikakulapu P, et al. Artery tertiary lymphoid organs control aorta immunity and protect against atherosclerosis *via* vascular smooth muscle cell lymphotoxin beta receptors. *Immunity* (2015) 42(6):1100–15. doi:10.1016/j.immuni.2015.05.015
73. Macritchie N, Grassia G, Sabir SR, Maddaluno M, Welsh P, Sattar N, et al. Plasmacytoid dendritic cells play a key role in promoting atherosclerosis in apolipoprotein E-deficient mice. *Arterioscler Thromb Vasc Biol* (2012) 32(11):2569–79. doi:10.1161/ATVBAHA.112.251314
74. Sage AP, Murphy D, Maffia P, Masters LM, Sabir SR, Baker LL, et al. MHC Class II-restricted antigen presentation by plasmacytoid dendritic cells drives proatherogenic T cell immunity. *Circulation* (2014) 130(16):1363–73. doi:10.1161/CIRCULATIONAHA.114.011090
75. Maddaluno M, MacRitchie N, Grassia G, Ialenti A, Butcher JP, Garside P, et al. Murine aortic smooth muscle cells acquire, though fail to present exogenous protein antigens on major histocompatibility complex class II molecules. *Biomed Res Int* (2014) 2014:949845. doi:10.1155/2014/949845
76. Obst R, van Santen HM, Melamed R, Kamphorst AO, Benoist C, Mathis D. Sustained antigen presentation can promote an immunogenic T cell response, like dendritic cell activation. *Proc Natl Acad Sci U S A* (2007) 104(39):15460–5. doi:10.1073/pnas.0707331104
77. Celli S, Lemaitre F, Bousso P. Real-time manipulation of T cell-dendritic cell interactions in vivo reveals the importance of prolonged contacts for CD4+ T cell activation. *Immunity* (2007) 27(4):625–34. doi:10.1016/j.immuni.2007.08.018
78. Baumjohann D, Preite S, Reboldi A, Ronchi F, Ansel KM, Lanzavecchia A, et al. Persistent antigen and germinal center B cells sustain T follicular helper cell responses and phenotype. *Immunity* (2013) 38(3):596–605. doi:10.1016/j.immuni.2012.11.020
79. Henrickson SE, Perro M, Loughhead SM, Senman B, Stutte S, Quigley M, et al. Antigen availability determines CD8(+) T cell-dendritic cell interaction kinetics and memory fate decisions. *Immunity* (2013) 39(3):496–507. doi:10.1016/j.immuni.2013.08.034
80. Rabenstein H, Behrendt AC, Ellwart JW, Naumann R, Horsch M, Beckers J, et al. Differential kinetics of antigen dependency of CD4+ and CD8+ T cells. *J Immunol* (2014) 192(8):3507–17. doi:10.4049/jimmunol.1302725
81. Benson RA, MacLeod MK, Hale BG, Patakas A, Garside P, Brewer JM. Antigen presentation kinetics control T cell/dendritic cell interactions and follicular helper T cell generation in vivo. *Elife* (2015) 4. doi:10.7554/eLife.06994
82. Joshi NS, Akama-Garren EH, Lu Y, Lee DY, Chang GP, Li A, et al. Regulatory T cells in tumor-associated tertiary lymphoid structures suppress anti-tumor T cell responses. *Immunity* (2015) 43(3):579–90. doi:10.1016/j.immuni.2015.08.006
83. Mempel TR, Henrickson SE, Von Andrian UH. T-cell priming by dendritic cells in lymph nodes occurs in three distinct phases. *Nature* (2004) 427(6970):154–9. doi:10.1038/nature02238
84. Zinselmeyer BH, Dempster J, Gurney AM, Wokosin D, Miller M, Ho H, et al. In situ characterization of CD4+ T cell behavior in mucosal and systemic lymphoid tissues during the induction of oral priming and tolerance. *J Exp Med* (2005) 201(11):1815–23. doi:10.1084/jem.20050203
85. Nasr IW, Reel M, Oberbarnscheidt MH, Mounzer RH, Baddoura FK, Ruddle NH, et al. Tertiary lymphoid tissues generate effector and memory T cells that lead to allograft rejection. *Am J Transplant* (2007) 7(5):1071–9. doi:10.1111/j.1600-6143.2007.01756.x
86. Itano AA, Jenkins MK. Antigen presentation to naive CD4 T cells in the lymph node. *Nat Immunol* (2003) 4(8):733–9. doi:10.1038/ni957
87. Cyster JG. B cell follicles and antigen encounters of the third kind. *Nat Immunol* (2010) 11(11):989–96. doi:10.1038/ni.1946
88. Germain RN, Robey EA, Cahalan MD. A decade of imaging cellular motility and interaction dynamics in the immune system. *Science* (2012) 336(6089):1676–81. doi:10.1126/science.1221063
89. Robins H. Immunosequencing: applications of immune repertoire deep sequencing. *Curr Opin Immunol* (2013) 25(5):646–52. doi:10.1016/j.coi.2013.09.017
90. Calis JJ, Rosenberg BR. Characterizing immune repertoires by high throughput sequencing: strategies and applications. *Trends Immunol* (2014) 35(12):581–90. doi:10.1016/j.it.2014.09.004

Permissions

All chapters in this book were first published by Frontiers; hereby published with permission under the Creative Commons Attribution License or equivalent. Every chapter published in this book has been scrutinized by our experts. Their significance has been extensively debated. The topics covered herein carry significant findings which will fuel the growth of the discipline. They may even be implemented as practical applications or may be referred to as a beginning point for another development.

The contributors of this book come from diverse backgrounds, making this book a truly international effort. This book will bring forth new frontiers with its revolutionizing research information and detailed analysis of the nascent developments around the world.

We would like to thank all the contributing authors for lending their expertise to make the book truly unique. They have played a crucial role in the development of this book. Without their invaluable contributions this book wouldn't have been possible. They have made vital efforts to compile up to date information on the varied aspects of this subject to make this book a valuable addition to the collection of many professionals and students.

This book was conceptualized with the vision of imparting up-to-date information and advanced data in this field. To ensure the same, a matchless editorial board was set up. Every individual on the board went through rigorous rounds of assessment to prove their worth. After which they invested a large part of their time researching and compiling the most relevant data for our readers.

The editorial board has been involved in producing this book since its inception. They have spent rigorous hours researching and exploring the diverse topics which have resulted in the successful publishing of this book. They have passed on their knowledge of decades through this book. To expedite this challenging task, the publisher supported the team at every step. A small team of assistant editors was also appointed to further simplify the editing procedure and attain best results for the readers.

Apart from the editorial board, the designing team has also invested a significant amount of their time in understanding the subject and creating the most relevant covers. They scrutinized every image to scout for the most suitable representation of the subject and create an appropriate cover for the book.

The publishing team has been an ardent support to the editorial, designing and production team. Their endless efforts to recruit the best for this project, has resulted in the accomplishment of this book. They are a veteran in the field of academics and their pool of knowledge is as vast as their experience in printing. Their expertise and guidance has proved useful at every step. Their uncompromising quality standards have made this book an exceptional effort. Their encouragement from time to time has been an inspiration for everyone.

The publisher and the editorial board hope that this book will prove to be a valuable piece of knowledge for researchers, students, practitioners and scholars across the globe.

List of Contributors

Alice Koenig and Olivier Thaunat
Service de Transplantation, Néphrologie et Immunologie Clinique, Hôpital Edouard Herriot, Hospices Civils de Lyon, Lyon, France
INSERM UMR1111, Lyon, France
Université de Lyon, Lyon, France

Ann Ager
Division of Infection and Immunity, School of Medicine and Systems Immunity Research Institute, Cardiff University, Cardiff, UK

Jan Kranich
Institute for Immunology, Ludwig Maximilian University Munich, Munich, Germany

Nike Julia Krautler
Institute of Microbiology, ETH Zurich, Zurich, Switzerland

James A. Butler and Jason Cosgrove
Centre for Immunology and Infection, Department of Biology, Hull York Medical School, York, UK
Department of Electronics, University of York, York, UK
York Computational Immunology Laboratory, University of York, York, UK

Kieran Alden and Jon Timmis
Department of Electronics, University of York, York, UK,
York Computational Immunology Laboratory, University of York, York, UK

Mark Christopher Coles
Centre for Immunology and Infection, Department of Biology, Hull York Medical School, York, UK
York Computational Immunology Laboratory, University of York, York, UK

Nancy H. Ruddle
Department of Epidemiology of Microbial Diseases, School of Public Health, Yale University School of Medicine, New Haven, CT, USA

Katrijn Neyt, Kim Deswarte and Hamida Hammad
Laboratory of Immunoregulation, VIB Inflammation Research Center, Ghent, Belgium
Department of Respiratory Medicine, Ghent University, Ghent, Belgium,

Corine H. GeurtsvanKessel
Department of Viroscience, Erasmus MC, Rotterdam, Netherlands

Bart N. Lambrecht
Laboratory of Immunoregulation, VIB Inflammation Research Center, Ghent, Belgium
Department of Respiratory Medicine, Ghent University, Ghent, Belgium
Department of Pulmonary Medicine, Erasmus MC, Rotterdam, Netherlands

Francesca Barone, David H. Gardner, Saba Nayar, Nathalie Steinthal and Christopher D. Buckley
Rheumatology Research Group, Institute of Inflammation and Ageing, University of Birmingham, Birmingham, UK

Sanjiv A. Luther
Department of Biochemistry, Center for Immunity and Infection, University of Lausanne, Lausanne, Switzerland

Gareth W. Jones, David G. Hill and Simon A. Jones
Division of Infection and Immunity, Systems Immunity URI, The School of Medicine, Cardiff University, Cardiff, UK

Elisa Corsiero, Alessandra Nerviani, Michele Bombardieri and Costantino Pitzalis
Centre for Experimental Medicine and Rheumatology, William Harvey Research Institute, Barts and The London School of Medicine and Dentistry, Queen Mary University of London, London, UK

Aliyah M. Weinstein
Department of Immunology, University of Pittsburgh School of Medicine, Pittsburgh, PA, USA

Walter J. Storkus
Department of Immunology, University of Pittsburgh School of Medicine, Pittsburgh, PA, USA
Department of Dermatology, University of Pittsburgh School of Medicine, Pittsburgh, PA, USA
University of Pittsburgh Cancer Institute, Pittsburgh, PA, USA

Catherine Sautès-Fridman, Myriam Lawand, Nicolas A. Giraldo, Hélène Kaplon, Claire Germain, Wolf Herman Fridman and Marie-Caroline Dieu-Nosjean
INSERM, UMR_S 1138, Team "Cancer, Immune Control and Escape", Cordeliers Research Center, Paris, France
UMR_S 1138, Centre de Recherche des Cordeliers, University Paris Descartes, Paris, France
UMR_S 1138, Centre de Recherche des Cordeliers, Sorbonne University, UPMC University Paris 06, Paris, France

Sara Cruz-Migoni and Jorge Caamaño
College of Medical and Dental Sciences, Institute of Immunology and Immunotherapy, University of Birmingham, Birmingham, UK

Eóin N. McNamee
Mucosal Inflammation Program, Department of Anesthesiology, School of Medicine, University of Colorado - Anschutz Medical Campus, Aurora, CO, USA

Ji Young Hwang, Troy D. Randall and Aaron Silva-Sanchez
Division of Clinical Immunology and Rheumatology, Department of Medicine, University of Alabama at Birmingham, Birmingham, AL, USA

Manuela Buettner
Central Animal Facility, Institute of Laboratory Animal Science, Hannover Medical School, Hannover, Germany

Matthias Lochner
Institute of Infection Immunology, TWINCORE, Centre for Experimental and Clinical Infection Research, a joint venture between the Medical School Hannover (MHH) and the Helmholtz Centre for Infection Research (HZI), Hannover, Germany

Nobuyoshi Hiraoka
Division of Pathology and Clinical Laboratories, National Cancer Center Hospital, Tokyo, Japan
Division of Molecular Pathology, National Cancer Center Research Institute, Tokyo, Japan
Division of Analytical Pathology, National Cancer Center Research Institute, Tokyo, Japan

Rie Yamazaki-Itoh
Division of Molecular Pathology, National Cancer Center Research Institute, Tokyo, Japan

Yoshinori Ino
Division of Molecular Pathology, National Cancer Center Research Institute, Tokyo, Japan
Division of Analytical Pathology, National Cancer Center Research Institute, Tokyo, Japan

Marc Clement and Marion Morvan
INSERM U1148, Université Paris Diderot, PRES Sorbonne Paris Cité, Paris, France

Anneli Peters
Department of Neuroimmunology, Max Planck Institute of Neurobiology, Martinsried, Germany

Prasad Srikakulapu
Cardiovascular Research Center (CVRC), University of Virginia, Charlottesville, VA, USA

Adrien Galy
Département de Médecine Interne, Hôpital Bichat, Assistance Publique Hôpitaux de Paris, Université Paris Diderot, PRES Sorbonne Paris Cité, Paris, France

Jesús Rivera-Nieves
Division of Gastroenterology, Inflammatory Bowel Disease Center, San Diego VAMC, University of California San Diego, La Jolla, CA, USA

Patrick Bruneval
Département de Pathologie, Hôpital Européen Georges Pompidou, Assistance Publique Hôpitaux de Paris, Université Paris Descartes, PRES Sorbonne Paris Cité, Paris, France

Fabien Hyafil
INSERM U1148, Université Paris Diderot, PRES Sorbonne Paris Cité, Paris, France
Département de Médecine Nucléaire, Hôpital Bichat, Assistance Publique Hôpitaux de Paris, Université Paris Diderot, PRES Sorbonne Paris Cité, Paris, France

Khadija Benali
Département de Médecine Nucléaire, Hôpital Bichat, Assistance Publique Hôpitaux de Paris, Université Paris Diderot, PRES Sorbonne Paris Cité, Paris, France

Nicoletta Pasi
Département de Radiologie, Hôpital Bichat, Assistance Publique Hôpitaux de Paris, Université Paris Diderot, PRES Sorbonne Paris Cité, Paris, France

Lydia Deschamps
Département de Pathologie, Hôpital Bichat, Assistance Publique Hôpitaux de Paris, Université Paris Diderot, PRES Sorbonne Paris Cité, Paris, France

Quentin Pellenc
Département de Chirurgie Vasculaire, Hôpital Bichat, Assistance Publique Hôpitaux de Paris, Université Paris Diderot, PRES Sorbonne Paris Cité, Paris, France

Thomas Papo and Karim Sacre
Département de Médecine Interne, Hôpital Bichat, Assistance Publique Hôpitaux de Paris, Université Paris Diderot, PRES Sorbonne Paris Cité, Paris, France
INSERM U1149, Laboratoire d'excellence INFLAMEX, Université Paris Diderot, PRES Sorbonne Paris Cité, Paris, France
Département Hospitalo-Universitaire FIRE (Fibrosis, Inflammation and Remodelling in Renal and Respiratory Diseases), Université Paris Diderot, PRES Sorbonne Paris Cité, Paris, France

Antonino Nicoletti
INSERM U1148, Université Paris Diderot, PRES Sorbonne Paris Cité, Paris, France
Département Hospitalo-Universitaire FIRE (Fibrosis, Inflammation and Remodelling in Renal and Respiratory Diseases), Université Paris Diderot, PRES Sorbonne Paris Cité, Paris, France

Meike Mitsdoerffer
Klinikum Rechts der Isar, Department of Neurology, Technical University Munich, Munich, Germany
Munich Cluster for Systems Neurology (SyNergy), Munich, Germany

Changjun Yin and Christian Weber
Institute for Cardiovascular Prevention, Ludwig-Maximilians-University, Munich, Germany
German Centre for Cardiovascular Research (DZHK), Partner Site Munich Heart Alliance, Munich, Germany

Sarajo Kumar Mohanta and Andreas J. R. Habenicht
Institute for Cardiovascular Prevention, Ludwig-Maximilians-University, Munich, Germany

Yuka Kobayashi and Takeshi Watanabe
The Tazuke-Kofukai Medical Research Institute, Kitano Hospital, Kita-ku, Osaka, Japan

Catherine E. Hughes and Robert A. Benson
Centre for Immunobiology, Institute of Infection, Immunity and Inflammation, College of Medical, Veterinary and Life Sciences, University of Glasgow, Glasgow, UK

Pasquale Maffia
Centre for Immunobiology, Institute of Infection, Immunity and Inflammation, College of Medical, Veterinary and Life Sciences, University of Glasgow, Glasgow, UK
BHF Centre of Excellence in Vascular Science and Medicine, College of Medical, Veterinary and Life Sciences, University of Glasgow, Glasgow, UK
Department of Pharmacy, University of Naples Federico II, Naples, Italy

Marija Bedaj
Centre for Immunobiology, Institute of Infection, Immunity and Inflammation, College of Medical, Veterinary and Life Sciences, University of Glasgow, Glasgow, UK
Rheumatology Research Group, Centre for Translational Inflammation Research, School of Immunity and Infection, College of Medical and Dental Sciences, University of Birmingham, Birmingham, UK

Index

M

P

R

S

T

V

Printed in the USA
CPSIA information can be obtained
at www.ICGtesting.com
LVHW080734221023
761596LV00011B/2118

9 781646 466047